ISBN 978-0-282-13649-9
PIBN 10843202

EDINBURGH MEDICAL AND SURGICAL JOURNAL:

EXHIBITING

A CONCISE VIEW

OF THE LATEST AND MOST IMPORTANT

DISCOVERIES IN MEDICINE, SURGERY, AND PHARMACY.

1806.

VOLUME SECOND.

EDINBURGH:

PRINTED FOR ARCHIBALD CONSTABLE & COMPANY, EDINBURGH; AND JOHN MURRAY, LONDON; AND GILBERT & HODGES, DUBLIN.

1806.

D. RAMSAY & SON, PRINTERS.

CONTENTS.

ORIGINAL COMMUNICATIONS.

NO. V.

Page

Art. I. Observations on the Formation and Structure of the Human Ovum. By Mr John Burns, Lecturer on Midwifery, Glasgow - - - - - - 1
II. On the degree to which Exercise should be carried in some varieties of Dyspepsia. By Dr Faulkner, London - - - - - - - - - - 5
III. On the use of Sulphurated Hydrogen in Stomachic Complaints. By Mr Forbes, Peterhead - - - - - - - - - - - - - - - - 9
IV. Account of Dr Rousseau's Experiments on Cutaneous Absorption. By Dr Stock, Bristol - 10
V. Analysis of a Stearoid Tumour. By Dr Bostock, Liverpool - - - - - - - - - - - - 14
VI. History of a Case of Diabetes Mellitus successfully treated. By Dr Fraser, London - - - 16
VII. Account of a Fœtus found in the Abdomen of a Woman 83 years of age. By M. Grivel, Dresden. Communicated by Dr George Pearson, London - - - - - - - - - - 19
VIII. Case of an Ossified Fœtus and Uterus in a Woman 60 years of age. By Dr Caldwell, Preland, Londonderry - - - - - - - - - - - 22
IX. Essay on Erythema Mercuriale. By Dr M'Mullin 25
X. Second Essay on the Analysis of Animal Fluids. By Dr Bostock, Liverpool - - - - - - - 37
XI. Medical Biography, No. I. Dr Currie - - - 46
XII. Inquirer, No. IV. On the Diagnosis between Hydrocephalus and Worms - - - - - - - 52

NO. VI.

Art. I. Case of Abscess in the Abdominal Muscles, which terminated fatally - - - - - - - 129
Case of Syphilitic Ulceration of the Skin, accompanied with Caries of the Tibia. By Caleb Crowther, M.D. Wakefield - - - - - 133

Art.

Page

ART. II. Remarks on the Internal Use of Tincture of Cantharides in Gleet or Leucorrhoea. By Mr John Roberton - - - - - - - - - - - 134
III. Remarks on the Dracunculus or Guinea Worm, as it appears in the Peninsula of India. By Mr Ninian Bruce - - - - - - - - - - - 145
IV. Cases of Guinea Worm, with Observations. By Mr Paton - - - - - - - - - - - - - - 151
V. Case of Encysted Ascites, with Hydatids. By Dr Macleay Oban - - - - - - - - 170
VI. Description of the Koutam-poulli, shewing, contrary to the commonly received opinion, that it does not afford Gum-Gamboge. By Dr White, Cananore - - - - - - - - - - - 171
VII. The Inquirer, No. V. Observations on Secondary Hemorrhage, and on the Ligature of Arteries, after Amputation and other Operations 176
VIII. Case of Teeth and Hairs found in the right Ovarium. By Mr James Anderson - - - - 180
IX. The Efficacy of Inoculated Small Pox in promoting the Population of Great Britain. By Dr Gillum - - - - - - - - - - - - - - - 182
X. Essay on the External use of Oil. By Mr Hunter 185
XI. Case of Crural Hernia, in which the Obturator Artery surrounded the Mouth of the Sac. By Mr James Wardrop - - - - - - - - 203

NO. VII.

ART. I. Observations on the Structure of the parts concerned in Crural Hernia. By Mr Allan Burns, Glasgow - - - - - - - - - - - 265
II. Observations on the State of the Venereal Disease in the South Sea Islands. By Mr John Wilson, R. N. - - - - - - - - - - 274
III. Remarks on the Depopulation of Otaheite and Eimeo, with an Account of some of the most common Diseases. By Mr John Wilson, R. N. 281
IV. Report of the Physical and Mathematical Class of the French National Institute, upon the question, "Are those Manufactories which emit a disagreeable Smell prejudicial to Health." By M. M. Guyton-Morveau and Chaptal - - - - - - - - - - - 290
Observations by the Editors on the Laws relating to Nuisances - - - - - - - - - 297

Page

Art. V. History of the Guinea Worm, and the Method of Cure employed by the Hindoos. By Mr Dubois, and Dr Anderson, Madras - - 300
VI. Case of Sphacelated Hernia, with Observations. By Dr Kellie - - - - - - - - 307
VII. Case of Sphacelated Hernia. By a Physician in Edinburgh - - - - - - - - - 313
VIII. Case of a Tumour of the Tongue, cured by Calomel and Cicuta. By G. Atkinson, Surgeon to the Sunderland Dispensary - - - 318
IX. Case of Tic Douloureux. By Mr Kitson, Bath 319
X. Account of Dr Gall's Anatomical Discoveries regarding the Structure of the Brain. By Prof. Rosenmuller, Leipsic - - - - 320
XI. The Inquirer, No. VI. On Herpes - - 325

NO. VIII.

Art. I. An Account of the Illness and Death of H. B. de Saussure. By Professor Odier - - 393
II. Remarks on the White Indurations of Organs. By Dr G. L. Bayle - - - - - 401
III. Observations on Tubercles found in the Brain of two Scrofulous Subjects. By Dr F. V. Merat - - - - - - - 405
IV. History of a Case of Diseased Spleen, with the appearances on Dissection. By Dr Drake 409
V. Case of Chorea Sancti Viti cured by Purgatives. By Dr Kellie - - - - - - 422
VI. On the Application of Galvanism in the Cure of Connate Deafness. By Professor Volta 424
VII. Explanation of a supposed Case of Small Pox after Vaccination. By Mr Johnston - 426
VIII. Case of Epilepsy Cured by Trepanning the Skull. By Mr H. Coates - - - - - - 428
IX. Cases of Idiopathic Tetanus, with Observations. By Professor Mursinna - - - - 430
X. On the Plan for Medical Reform By Senex - 437
XI. The Inquirer. No. VIII. On the Study of Mental Pathology - - - - - - 440

CRITICAL ANALYSIS.

NO. V.

	Page
ART. I. Description and Treatment of Cutaneous Diseases. By Robert Willan, M.D. &c. - - -	56
II. A Treatise on Febrile Diseases. By Alexander Philips Wilson, M.D. &c. - - - - -	72
III. The Modern Practice of Physic. By E. G. Clarke, M.D. &c. - - - - - - - -	81
IV. The Edinburgh Practice of Physic - - -	82
V. Osservazioni Mediche sulla Malattia Febrile di Livorno. Del D. G. Palloni - - - - -	83
VI. Parere Medico sulla stessa Malattia. Del D. G. Palloni - - - - - - - - - - -	83
VII. Dr Pulteney's View of the Writings of Linnæus. By Dr Maton - - - - - - -	91
VIII. Observations on the Utility and Administration of Purgative Medicines. By James Hamilton, M.D. - - - - - - - - - -	97

NO. VI.

ART. I. Coup d'Oeil sur les Revolutions et sur la Reforme de la Medicine. Par P. J. G. Cabanis	206
II. Relation Historique et Chirurgicale de l'Expedition de l'Armée d' Orient, en Egypt et en Syrie. Par D. J. Larrey, &c. - - -	213
III. A Treatise on the Process employed by Nature in suppressing the Hemorrhage from divided and punctured Arteries, &c. By J. F. D. Jones, M.D. &c. - - - - - - - -	224
IV. Chirurgical Observations relating to the Eye, &c. By James Ware, Surgeon, F.R.S. -	233
V. Letters to Dr Rowley on his Pamphlet entitled "Cow-Pock Inoculation no Security against Infection." By Aculeus. - - - - -	240
VI. The Anatomy and Surgical Treatment of Inguinal and Congenital Hernia. By Astley Cooper, F.R.S. &c. - - - - - - - - -	241

NO. VII.

ART. I. Ricerche sulla Quina. Di Giovanni Fabbroni	333
II. Medical Collections on the Effects of Cold. By J E. Stock, M.D. - - - - - -	340

Page

ART. III. Cases of Pulmonary Consumption treated with Uva Ursi. By Robert Bourne, M.D. &c. - 346
IV. On Epilepsy, and the Use of Viscus Quercinus, in the Cure of that Disease. By Henry Fraser, M.D. - - - - - - - - - - - 352
V. Darstelling der Gallschen Gehirn-und Schädel Lehre. Von Dr C. H. Bischoff - - - - 354
Bemerkungen über diese Lehre. Von Dr C. W. Hufeland - - - - - - - - - ib.
Etwas über Dr Gall's Hirnschädel Lehre. Von Prof. J. G. Walter - - - - - - - - ib.
VI. Observations on Abortion. By Mr John Burns 366
VII. On the Effects of Carbonate of Iron upon Cancer. By Mr R. Carmichael - - - - 372

NO. VIII.

ART. I. Manuel de Medicine pratique. Par Louis Odier, M.D.-& P. - - - - 446
II. Observations on the Utility and Administration of Purgative Medicines. By Dr Hamilton, 2d edit. - - - - - - - - 454
III. Practical Observations concerning Sea Bathing. By Dr Buchan - - - - - - 456
IV. Surgical Observations. Part II. By Mr Abernethy - - - - - - - - - - 463
V. Institutions for the Education of *Empirical Practioners*, necessary in the present state of Society. By Professor Reil - - - - 472
VI. On the Cure of Intermittent Fever by Gelatine. By Dr Gautieri and Professor Bischoff - 479
VII. Equinoctial Plants. By Humboldt and Bonpland - - - - - - - - - - 483

MEDICAL INTELLIGENCE.

NO. V.

Second Report of the Board of Health - - - - 111
Resolutions of the Vaccine Pock Institution, Broad-street 117
Honours to the Memory of Bichat and Dessault - - ib.
Intended Publications - - - - - - - - ib.
Repetition of Pacchioni's Experiments on the composition of Muriatic Acid. By Biot - - - - - 118

Page

Prize Questions from Wilna, on Diabetes - - - 118
————————, on Plica Polonica - - 121
————————, on Diseases of Vegetables - ib.
Carey-street Dispensary Report - - - - - 123
Letters on Vaccination, from Doctors Reeve and De Carro, Vienna - - - - - - - - 126

NO. VI.

Association for Medical Reform - - - - - 252
Report of the Royal Jennerian Society - - - 254
Report of the Vaccine Institution at Edinburgh - - 257
Quarterly Report of Carey-street Dispensary - - 258
Annual Report of the Liverpool Dispensary - - 261
Fourcroy on the Phosphate of Lime in Bones - - 262

NO. VII.

Medical Topography of Berlin - - - - - - - 376
Dr R. Pearson's Method of treating Hooping-cough - - 380
M. Wilkinson on the Decomposition of Water by Galvanism 381
Queries published by the Institution for investigating the Nature and Cure of Cancer - - - - - - 382
List of Graduations at Edinburgh, June 1806 - - 387
Quarterly Report of the Carey-street Dispensary - - 390
To Correspondents - - - - - - - - 392

NO. VIII.

Advertisement from the Royal College of Physicians in London - - - - - - - - - - - - 487
Proceedings of the Association for Medical Reform - 489
Account of the General Hospital and Medical School at Vienna - - - - - - - - - - - 491
Quarterly Report of the Carey-street Dispensary. By Dr Bateman - - - - - - - - - - - 496
Letter from Dr Joseph Frank, Professor at Wilna - 499
—— from a Gentleman connected with the University of Wilna - - - - - - - - - - - 500
—— from Mr Elder, Missionary, Otaheite - - 502
—— from a Surgeon at Madras - - - - - 503
Resolutions of Original Vaccine Pock Institution - 504
Medical Graduations at Edinburgh, September 1806 505
Medical Lectures at Edinburgh, Glasgow, and London 506
Letter from Paris - - - - - - - - - - 509
List of New Publications - - - - - - 510
Index - - - - - - - - - - - - 514

THE

EDINBURGH

MEDICAL AND SURGICAL JOURNAL.

JANUARY 1. 1806.

PART I.

ORIGINAL COMMUNICATIONS.

I.

Obſervations on the Formation and Structure of the Human Ovum.
By Mr John Burns, Lecturer on Midwifery in Glaſgow.

It has been the opinion of all the anatomiſts who have written on the ſubject of the gravid uterus, that the vaſcular part of the ovum, or the membrana decidua, is originally formed from lymph or extravaſated blood. But the formation of organized animal matter is accompliſhed by a proceſs very different from the inſpiſſation of lymph, or the production of new veſſels through the medium of coagulated blood.

This opinion I have already controverted in my account of the gravid uterus, which was publiſhed in 1799. Since that time, I have had an opportunity of examining an additional number of uteri and abortions, in all the ſtages of advancement. By theſe means, and with my brother's aſſiſtance, I am able now to elucidate ſtill more the formation of the human ovum.

Very ſoon after conception, the vaſcular action of the uterus is conſiderably increaſed: its ſubſtance becomes ſofter, its ſize rather greater. The fibres are more ſeparated from each other, and a larger quantity of interſtitial fluid is formed. The cavity alſo enlarges a little, particularly in point of length, and the membrane which lines it ſeems to be ſomewhat ſofter and redder. The lacunæ at the os uteri are more diſtinct.

Next we find that, confiderably within a month after impregnation, a number of veffels fhoot out from that part of the membrane which lines the fundus uteri. Thefe veffels have fomewhat the appearance of the down which proceeds from putrid flefh. They are, however, of a different colour, thickly planted, and pretty clofely united at their roots, but more feparated at their extremities; fo that, when the uterus is put in water, this part of it has a flocculent appearance. They never exceed the twelfth part of an inch in length. By degrees, ftill more of the uterine furface yields this vafcular production, but it never is formed by the glandular part at the os uteri. This part fecretes a jelly of a reddifh colour, which is decompofed, and efcapes very foon after death. The furface, however, immediately above the lacunæ yields a thin vafcular production, which ftretches acrofs the uterus, and is evident as foon as the fundus has produced its down, whilft the intervening body of the uterus has as yet formed none.

This vafcular production forms the outer layer of the decidua. It has at firft a ftriated appearance, from the direction of the veffels which go off at right angles to the uterine furface, which yields them. The ftriæ are alternately white and red, or black, owing to the empty arteries and diftended veins; but if the uterus has been injected, then they are altogether coloured. This ftriated ftructure of the outer layer of decidua feems, in the courfe of geftation, to be deftroyed chiefly by preffure; for, by the end of the fecond or the beginning of the third month, it has more of a laminated appearance.

I now go on to obferve, that, almoft immediately after this efflorefcence of veffels proceeds from the uterus, (forming the outer layer of decidua, or what may, at this period, be called the decidua ftriata), a fecond fet of veffels is produced from the extremities of the firft. Thefe veffels are very different from the former, which are fhort, ftraight, and parallel to each other. Thefe, on the contrary, are more extended, intermix and ramify together, fo as to form an irregular tiffue or fheet of vafcular fubftance, the fibres or veffels of which affume a direction at right angles to the fhag or primary veffels which formed them. This direction is very naturally given by the weight of the veffels themfelves, which makes them hang down, or point toward the os uteri. This production conftitutes the internal layer of the decidua,—the decidua interna. It is much more irregular than the outer layer; many ragged flocculent proceffes hang down in the cavity of the uterus, and extend toward the cervix; fo that this layer prefently appears to confift of a number of torn floating membranes, like portions of fpider's web, hanging pendulous in whose listlessness and enfeebled system were but ill calculated to support any very violent exertion. To speak in the phrase of the science, *to it* they went, and *at it* they kept for a good hour ever morning fasting, until master, as well as pupil, got a pretty well-warmed jacket. Nay, the pupil seemed to have odds in his favour here, as he was much *harder to sweat* than his instructor. In the course of a very few days, not less to his joy than surprise, the invalid found himself free from almost all his dyspeptic ailments, and his powers of digestion were now scarcely outdone by his abilities for consuming food. The great dislike which he bore at first against the fatigue of exertion was shortly overcome, and his depressed and occasionally fluctuating spirits were elevated once more to their ordinary level of hilarity and steadiness. Such a very speedy and happy revolution in the patient's health readily pointed out the source from which it was derived; and as no other change had been made in his diet or regimen, nor any new plan adopted in the treatment of his complaint, those good effects, which so speedily and unexpectedly showed themselves, were, upon very fair and just grounds of reasoning, ascribed to the active nature of the exercise which he had lately undertaken. He always found it exceedingly difficult to bring out a sweat; but, when this was effected, his aversion for the fatigue was changed into pleasure and entertainment, and he sat down to breakfast with an appetite as much diminished as his powers of digestion were refitted for their office. But he likewise found, that if sweating had not been previously induced, as sometimes happened when the rounds of fencing were shorter than usual, his digestive organs were not at all aided by the exercise he had taken. Thus we have a satisfactory explanation why the customary stated exercise, which my patient had been for so long a time in the habit of taking with unremitted regularity, was not attended with the happy consequences which it was designed to secure. He had altogether overlooked how essential and indispensable sweating was to ensure its effects, without which, exercise brings little else with it than fatigue, and aversion to its repetition. The very reverse of this takes place when it has been employed to the extent of inducing perspiration. Besides, there is very generally present in dyspeptics, along with listlessness and exhaustion, two powerful enemies to the proper employment of exercise, an unconquerable dryness of the skin, which renders it extremely difficult to elicit perspiration, when exercise is enjoined, as it is almost in every instance, to dyspeptic persons. I know it is generally directed in the unfortunate terms of regular moderate exercise; practitioners, in my opinion, attaching too great importance to the caution of not fatiguing their patients. Hence it invariably almost happens that it is never pushed to its proper extent, never exhibited in a proper dose; a circumstance of as much consequence here as in the exhibition of medicines. To unfold this error has been the purpose for which I have trespassed so much on the patience of my reader, whose indulgence I must necessarily solicit.

Since the above was written, some considerable time ago, I have been enabled, by experiments repeatedly and cautiously instituted, to ascertain that a few minutes only of exercise, conducted so as induce perspiration, have enabled a dyspeptic person to digest a quantity of food which a whole day of his accustomed sluggish exercise was insufficient for. It was necessary, however, to employ the exercise just before eating. I hold it, therefore, as a circumstance of indispensable consequence in the treatment of dyspepsia that exercise be employed to the extent of promoting a free and copious perspiration; and I conceive that the less violent the exertions are for this purpose, the effects will be the more happy and permanent. It should be an object of the first consequence, in the treatment of this disease, to derive to the skin in those cases where dryness of the cuticle opposes this derivation. In such cases, those means which have been termed indirect are the only ones upon which any perfect confidence can be placed. The exhibition of medicines, and the regulations of diet, in such cases, ought to be regarded only as auxiliary and co-operative.

It has long been observed, that there subsists a very remarkable sympathy between the stomach and surface of the body. There is scarcely an aphorism in medicine more hackneyed. It seems, therefore, extraordinary that it should not be more attended to in the treatment of the disease I have been considering. Since it is our great object to effect a change in the functions of depraved digestion, when the cure of dyspepsia is undertaken, one obvious method of effecting this, according to the principle I have alluded to, is to produce a change in the surface. But this does not seem to be accomplished by exercise, except by inducing its perspiring condition.

Finsbury Place, Sept. 1805.

III.

III.

Letter on the Use of Sulphurated Hydrogen in Stomachic Complaints. By Mr WILLIAM FORBES, Surgeon, Peterhead.

GENTLEMEN,

I WISH, through the medium of your valuable publication, to recommend to the attention of practitioners a medicine which I take to be much seldomer employed than it deserves to be; I mean the sulphuret of potash. It is a remedy which will be found particularly serviceable in disorders of the stomach, whether acute or chronic, and, of consequence, in other diseases proceeding from a disordered state of that organ. The dose is from a few grains to half a drachm, to be taken dissolved in milk, water, or beer. If this do not relieve in a short time, the medicine ought to be repeated; for a small quantity will often fail, when a larger dose will succeed. A little volatile alkali forms an excellent addition to it, and conceals the disagreeable smell of the sulphuret. When the stomach is in such a condition as not easily to bear the taking of cold liquids, the medicine may be advantageously dissolved in warm water.

Sulphurated hydrogen and the simple sulphuret are known to be the best remedies for the mineral poisons, and, when employed for this purpose, they are very usefully given along with opium and milk, &c.

If sulphurated hydrogen be preferred to the sulphuret, and it is, no doubt, in some respects preferable, it may easily be obtained, by adding to the sulphuret, dissolved in water, a quantity of sulphuric or muriatic acid sufficient to saturate it. If this be kept for some days in a vessel perfectly full and close, the precipitated sulphur subsides, and we obtain the gas combined with the water, along with some sulphate or muriate of potash. Thus an artificial water impregnated with sulphurated hydrogen, analogous to the natural sulphureous waters, is easily obtained. Care should be taken not to add the precipitating acid to excess, otherwise the water becomes disagreeably bitter. This, however, might be corrected by adding some alkaline carbonate, which would also disengage a portion of carbonic acid. A pound of sulphuret is sufficient for ten gallons of water.

Of all the alkalis, the volatile is the only one in common use; the sulphurets are scarcely ever used, and sulphurated hydrogen only when afforded by nature; yet I have no doubt that the more general and free use of it in remedies, especially of the

sulphureous

ſulphureous ones, would be found highly beneficial in fever, diarrhœa, and many other ordinary diſeaſes, acute as well as chronic.

Peterhead, 14*th September*, 1805.

IV.

Account of Dr Rouſſeau's Experiments on Cutaneous Abſorption. By J. G. Stock, M. D. Briſtol.

Gentlemen,

I have peruſed, with much intereſt, Dr Kellie's paper on the functions of the ſkin, in the ſecond Number of your Journal. If you think the following abſtract of ſome experiments on abſorption worthy a place in your next Number, it is much at your ſervice. They are contained in an inaugural eſſay on that ſubject, written by Dr Rouſſeau, a native of St Domingo, who graduated in the univerſity of Pennſylvania in the year 1800. They appear ſtrongly to militate againſt cutaneous abſorption, and to render it probable that even the moſt active ſubſtances do not affect the ſyſtem through that medium, unleſs the cuticle be previouſly in ſome degree deſtroyed or abraded. I do not pretend, however, to decide upon the queſtion myſelf, but offer the ſubſequent facts to you as a valuable appendix to Dr Kellie's paper. I remain, &c. J. C. Stock.

The Doctor begins his eſſay with a brief ſtatement of his objections to the commonly received doctrine of cutaneous abſorption. He attempts to account for the apparent abſorption of mercury, by friction upon the external ſurface, in the following manner: "Were the mercury abſorbed in friction, it would certainly, after a long uſe, be found in ſome parts of the body; but I have never been able to diſcover any marks of the preſence of mercury in the urine, milk, or other fluids of animals, upon whom it had not been ſpared."

From ſeveral experiments, which are not yet ſufficient to enable me to ſay any thing poſitive upon this ſubject, I am induced to believe, that mercury being a ſubſtance volatile enough to be capable of riſing and diffuſing emanations by a moderate degree of heat, (as has been proved by Mr Achard's experiments),

experiments *), it may, with the assistance of the heat of the body of those using the frictions, be raised in very minute particles, as musk, camphor, spirit of turpentine, garlic, and others, and absorbed in the same manner as these volatile substances are. May it not be supposed also, that, during the frictions, some of the mercury is, by the action of the air, assisted by the heat of the body, oxided, that it afterwards parts by degrees with its oxygen, which carries along with it to the lungs (which, I am to prove, are the organs performing absorption) some parts of the mercury, which is with difficulty separated from it? †

He goes on to observe, that, "From all the facts and observations that he has been able to collect from others, as well as from his own observations and inquiries, he had never been able to determine the absorption of any substance by the lymphatics; on the contrary, that every experiment which he had made, with the view to come at such discovery, had convinced him that the lungs are the only organs by which absorption is performed. He admits that various active substances may be introduced *under* the cuticle; but this, he says, "cannot certainly be called absorption. In such cases the virus is carried on by the circulating fluid with which it has been mixed. Anatomists dissect putrid bodies with perfect safety, and no noxious matter is absorbed by their hands, as long as the cuticle is not injured. Would not surgeons be exposed every day to the most dangerous consequences, if the matter of venereal and gangrenous ulcers could be absorbed by the entire skin? Even the venom of the viper may be laid upon the skin without any accident ensuing."

The above is a very superficial abstract of the Doctor's opinions. I hasten to the experimental part of his essay, which contains many striking facts in support of them. The substance made use of in them was the spirit of turpentine. The test of its

* This gentleman, having left a dish containing twenty pounds of mercury over a furnace which was daily heated, after some days experienced a salivation, as did two other persons who had not quitted the room. This heat he estimates to be about 72° of Fahrenheit.—*Journal de Physique, Octobre* 1762.

One of the professors of this university (Pennsylvania) experienced a similar effect in his own person, in consequence of being repeatedly in a close room with a patient under a profuse salivation from mercurial frictions. And two others have noticed a similar effect to have been produced upon persons who resided in a ward in the Pennsylvania hospital, where mercurial friction was administered to several patients.

† Oxygenous gas, obtained from the mercurial oxides, almost always holds a small quantity of mercury in solution. I have been a witness to its having produced a speedy salivation on two persons who used it for disorders of the lungs.

Chaptal's Chemistry.

its introduction into the ſyſtem was the violet ſmell imparted to the urine; and with a view to accelerate its ſecretion, in a majority of his experiments, he took a few grains of the nitrate of potaſh.

In the firſt experiment he took a few drops of ſpiritus terebinthinæ on ſugar with water. In the ſecond he expoſed himſelf to its exhalations only, by walking backwards and forwards in a cloſe room, after pouring ſome of it from a phial into an open bowl, during the ſpace of half an hour. The violet ſmell was perceptible in the urine in both theſe caſes, and to an equal degree.

In his third experiment, he provided a long tube communicating with the air of another apartment. Through this he breathed, while he remained expoſed to ſimilar exhalations, as in the ſecond experiment, for the ſpace of two hours. At the expiration of this period, he changed all his clothes, and withdrew to another apartment. No violet ſmell could be detected, although his urine was carefully examined for upwards of twenty-four hours.

In his fourth experiment, he introduced his right arm, about 10 A. M. into a large glaſs jar, with a phial of turpentine in his hand. The jar was then luted round his arm; he uncorked the phial, and immerſed his fingers and thumb into the fluid, while the whole arm was expoſed, without covering, to its exhalations. At the end of an hour, his urine began to be plentifully ſecreted in conſequence of his draughts of nitrate of potaſh; no violet ſmell was perceptible. He continued his arm and hand in this ſituation during the ſpace of three hours; at the expiration of which period, great pain and redneſs induced him to withdraw. While this was doing, he breathed through the tube, as in experiment third; his arm was waſhed, and he withdrew to another apartment. No violet ſmell was detected at any future period; though the urine was examined during the whole of the day and ſucceeding night. The inflammation of the finger laſted during the whole day, but went off in the night.

In a fifth experiment, he previouſly took his diuretic draught, and then breathing through his tube, as in the two preceding experiments, an aſſiſtant applied ſpirit of turpentine, by means of a ſpunge, to the whole of his naked body, during the ſpace of an hour. During this interval the urine was evacuated three times, but without any violet ſmell. This experiment the author deſcribes as a very painful one, or he ſhould have perſiſted in it for a longer time. He concludes his hiſtory of it with ſome cautions to any who may have the curioſity to repeat it, with reſpect to the careful excluſion of the exhalations of the turpentine,

pentine, by ſtopping the noſe, and adjuſting the mouth-piece of the tube with accuracy.

An interval of a few days took place between each of the experiments above related. The violet ſmell was perceptible in the firſt and ſecond within an hour.

After a ſhort interval, he began a ſecond ſeries of experiments with analogous reſults; the former ſet being, as he obſerves, deſigned to diſprove the idea of abſorption by the cuticle; the ſecond to eſtabliſh the performance of this function by the lungs.

About twelve o'clock on a windy day, he took a narrow-necked bottle, containing ſpirit of turpentine, and, applying his noſe to the opening, inſpired twelve times, and then put the bottle by, and left the room. He took a walk in the ſtreet, and, in an hour and a half afterwards, the ſmell of the turpentine was perceptible in his breath to his friends. On his firſt making water after this experiment, which was at the expiration of an hour, it imparted a ſtrong violet ſmell, and gave a ſimilar teſt every time it was evacuated, till he went to bed. The ſmell was retained for twenty-four hours.

He adds, that he has detected ſimilar effects, after being preſent at ſome chemical experiments, in which ſpirit of turpentine was inflamed.

In his ſecond experiment, being deſirous to aſcertain how little of the turpentine was neceſſary to produce a ſenſible effect upon the ſyſtem, he emptied his lungs by a long expiration, and inhaled once the emanation of ſpirit of turpentine. In the ſpace of half an hour, the urine was very ſenſibly impregnated with the ſmell of violets, and retained it for three or four hours. The author obſerves, that the reſult of this experiment ſhows how very cautious the experimenter ought to be in performing the experiments in which the organs of reſpiration are to have any ſhare; becauſe, if the ſmell of the turpentine have once reached the noſe, it is ſufficient to render the whole experiment fallacious.

In a third, he made uſe of the long tube already ſpoken of, and inhaled the emanation of the turpentine from a glaſs jar, ſet at ſuch a diſtance that none could reach him where he ſtood, except through the medium of the tube. The urine imparted a violet ſmell within half an hour, which might be diſcovered in every part of the room where he was, and continued as long as in his former experiments.

"I could adduce," ſays the author, "a number of other experiments made with muſk, garlic, and camphor, yielding all the ſame reſults, to reinforce all that I have ſaid upon the abſorption of the ſpirit of turpentine; but as the ſmall limits of a diſſerta-

dissertation will not permit so extensive an undertaking, I have preferred the spirit of turpentine for the subject of my experiments in the present dissertation; and I would recommend it to those who would faithfully repeat the same experiments, on account of its certain characteristic property of imparting a strong smell of violets to the urine, whenever and howsoever it is received in the body. Such a smell cannot leave any doubt of its presence in the system, as soon as it has been perceived; while, on the other hand, the proofs given by other volatile substances of their existence in the body are often fallacious, and may easily elude observation.

V.

Analysis of a Stearoid Tumour. By John Bostock, M. D. Liverpool.

I was requested by Mr Mather of this place to examine the contents of a tumour which he had removed from the forehead of a young man of about 18 years of age. It made its appearance soon after birth, and gradually increased until it arrived at the size of a walnut. Upon opening the sac, the contents seemed to have no attachment to it, but were expressed from it without difficulty. They were not intersected by any membranes, nor did they appear in any degree vascular or organized.

The substance itself was of the consistence and colour of butter, and appeared homogeneous, and uniform in its texture; by means, however, of a microscope, a slight tendency to granulation might be detected. It was liquified by the application of a moderate degree of heat, and, by increasing the temperature, it was consumed, the combustion being attended with a succession of explosions. A portion was exposed to the action of caustic potash, but no effect was produced at the temperature of the atmosphere: upon keeping it for some time at the boiling heat the substance was broken down, and diffused through the fluid, but, upon cooling, very nearly the whole of it subsided. There did not appear to be any of that saponaceous emulsion formed, such as is usually produced by the action of potash upon an adipose substance. Portions of this alkaline liquor were successively neutralized by the sulphuric, nitric, and acetous acids; but there was scarcely any precipitate thrown down, nor was there any change of colour in the fluid indicating that the potash contained

any

any of the fatty matter in solution. Exactly similar effects were produced by treating the substance with pure ammonia; it appeared that scarcely any portion of it was dissolved.

It was in some degree acted on by boiling alcohol; a precipitate was thrown down by the addition of water; a little was deposited as the alcohol cooled, and still more by its evaporation: the matter deposited did not exhibit any tendency to crystallization.

No effect was produced upon the substance by keeping it immersed for some time in boiling oil of turpentine, nor was it dissolved when suspended in the vapour of this fluid; it merely became softened, and assumed a reddish brown hue. It was dissolved by boiling ether, though sparingly; when the ethereal solution was added to water, the substance was instantly separated in the form of an oily film, which swam on the surface of the fluid, and the evaporation of the ether also left behind a layer of fatty matter.

When the substance was boiled for some time in sulphuric acid, the fluid was rendered of a dark brown colour, while the fatty matter swam at the top in the form of black globules. After the acid became cool, it was passed through a filter, and the globules were retained on the paper, exhibiting a black, shining appearance, and pitchy consistence, much resembling the bitumen occasionally mixed with pitcoal. Scarcely any precipitate was formed by the addition of an alkali to the sulphuric acid. The pitchy matter tinged boiling alcohol of a deep brown colour, but did not appear to be properly soluble in it.

When the fatty matter was boiled in nitric acid, the fluid was tinged of a golden hue, while the substance was converted into a mass of a deep yellow colour, and somewhat waxy consistence. The acid did not appear to hold any of it in solution. The yellow mass was boiled in alcohol; it tinged it of a light brown hue, and was sparingly dissolved, as was evident from the precipitation produced by the addition of water, and the deposit formed by evaporation.

The results of these experiments indicated that the substance, though forming what is usually called a fatty tumour, and certainly much resembling fat in external appearance, yet differed from it essentially in its chemical properties. As far as my information extends, it indeed differs from every other animal substance which has hitherto been submitted to chemical analysis. It neither resembles fat, cellular substance, the muscular fibre, medullary matter, jelly, nor adipo-cire. I was not possessed of a sufficient quantity of it to examine the products of its combustion, which would perhaps have thrown some light upon its chemical

chemical compoſition. I am induced to conjecture, that it is principally compoſed of carbonaceous matter, a circumſtance which I infer, both from its general intractability, and more particularly from the effect produced on it by the ſulphuric acid. It may be neceſſary to add, that the experiment with potaſh was repeated with different ſpecimens of this reagent, until I could no longer doubt of its accuracy; the reſult appeared to me ſo ſingular, that I ſuſpected ſome imperfection in the alkali which I employed in the firſt trial.

Though the inferences that can be deduced from theſe experiments are almoſt entirely negative, ſtill, I apprehend, you may think the facts worth recording in your Journal, as giving an account of the chemical properties of an animal ſubſtance hitherto unexamined, and particularly as they point out that the name by which tumours, ſimilar to the one under conſideration, have been deſignated, is altogether unappropriate *.

I am your obedient ſervant,

JOHN BOSTOCK.

Liverpool, Auguſt 20. 1805.

VI.

The Hiſtory of a Caſe of Diabetes Mellitus ſucceſsfully treated. By HENRY FRASER, M. D. London.

GENTLEMEN,

A FAVOURABLE termination of the diabetes mellitus being rather a rare occurrence, I am induced to offer the following caſe for inſertion in your valuable Journal; you will therefore have the goodneſs to publiſh it, if you think it worthy. It is not my intention to enter into any diſcuſſion of the theory of diabetes, but merely to give a brief narrative of this caſe, and the remedies effectually employed for its cure.

Mr M——e, a wine-merchant, between 60 and 70 years of age, reſident about 30 miles weſt of this metropolis, became the ſubject of diabetes in the autumn of 1804. Although he had been always in the habit of indulging without reſerve in the luxuries of life, yet there was no evident diſeaſe of the liver; he had, however, been occaſionally afflicted with the gout, the two laſt

* If it be thought neceſsary to invent a term for them, we may, according to the custom observed on similar occasions, call them *stearoid tumours*.

last regular paroxysms of which, in the latter end of the year 1803, were removed by the refrigerative plan of treatment so zealously recommended by the ingenious Dr Kinglake. Since that period, he has experienced no return of the gout, nor has he, to use his own words, enjoyed one day's perfect health.

Whether this circumstance could have any share in producing the disease in question, is not for me to determine; for I have no ambition to become a controvertist on a subject where illiberality and invective have long since usurped the place of logic and reason.

As soon as the nature of his complaint was ascertained, the well-known fatality of it alarmed both himself and his friends, and the advice of a skilful surgeon was immediately obtained. Under the management of this gentleman, the patient took most, if not all, of the remedies usually resorted to upon such occasions, but without being enabled to arrest the progress of the disease; for, in spite of the combined efforts of skill and attention, the complaint rapidly gained ground. He consulted me on the 15th of January 1805. Upon examination, I found him labouring under a confirmed diabetes. His urine was perfectly sweet to the taste, entirely clear, and generally colourless, sometimes, however, tinged with a yellowish green. As he was in the habit of frequently measuring the quantity of urine discharged in the course of the twenty-four hours, we were enabled to ascertain it with correctness, and, at this period of the disorder, it was found to average from twelve to fourteen pints. His thirst was insatiable; but he had no appetite for solid food, and the body was become greatly emaciated. His tongue was constantly coated with a thick brown-coloured fur, and very dry. He also complained of an obtuse pain in the lumbar region, and of great prostration of strength. His pulse was very irregular, having a remarkable intermission about every fifth stroke; the frequency of the pulsations but seldom exceeded eighty-four in a minute. He had also at this time nocturnal pains in his feet and knees, somewhat resembling gout, which he was advised by all means to encourage by the use of a topical warm bath, in which a considerable quantity of the flour of mustard had been previously dissolved. This pediluvium did not obtain the desired effect; nor were other means, employed with the same intent, more efficient.

When I considered the general fatality of this complaint, and revolved the opinion of my learned friend Dr Willan, whose soundness of judgment is equalled only by the sedulous attention he has uniformly paid to the phenomena of diseases, "That all confirmed cases of diabetes are attended with some considerable disorder of the constitution, or a defect of some organ essential to life," my hope of seeing this patient recover was very faint. As it was impossible to restrain him from the use of liquids, I recommended him to drink old bottled porter, and laid no restriction upon his diet, except forbearance from vegetables. I prescribed for him a draught, containing half an ounce of the acetite of ammonia, twenty drops of tartarized antimonial wine, and thirty drops of laudanum, in the camphorated mixture of the London Pharmacopoeia, which was ordered to be taken every third night, the astringent effect of the opium being carefully obviated by a gentle laxative. This draught was soon discontinued. He was also directed to use a chalybeate medicine, prepared according to the formula recommended by the late Dr Griffiths, beginning with a dose of two grains of the ferrum vitriolatum, and gradually increasing it to five grains. After he had steadily pursued this plan for more than a month, I was informed, by letter, of his gradual amendment, although he was still considered to be in a very precarious state; the taste of the urine was changed from sweetness to insipidity; the quantity discharged was diminished; the patient's appetite was improved, and he thought himself stronger. On the 25th of February, I again saw the patient, who was now frequently harassed by symptoms analogous to those which have been regarded by authors as pathognomic of the angina pectoris, or, according to Dr Parry, syncope anginosa. These distressing symptoms were, however, fortunately soon relieved by a combination of camphor, castor, and æther, given in considerable quantities, and did not return during the further progress of the disease.

It was now deemed prudent to substitute another tonic for the steel, lest, by too long continuance, it should become at last useless, if not noxious; a property I have more frequently observed to follow the use of this medicine, for an immoderate length of time, than any other article in the materia medica. At this time, the yellow bark, in union with the sulphuric acid, was prescribed, in the dose of one drachm of the powder, two drachms of the compound tincture, and twenty drops of the diluted acid. The disease now began to yield more speedily, and, at the expiration of two months from the commencement of the use of the bark, no trace of diabetes was to be found.

On the 12th of August, I was again consulted by this gentleman, on account of an aphthous sore throat, which, for several days, was so severe as to threaten his life; at this time, his former disease manifested no disposition to return; and having, since his recovery from the latter complaint, spent a month amidst the gaieties of Cheltenham, he now enjoys good health and spirits.

M. GRIVEL'S CASE.

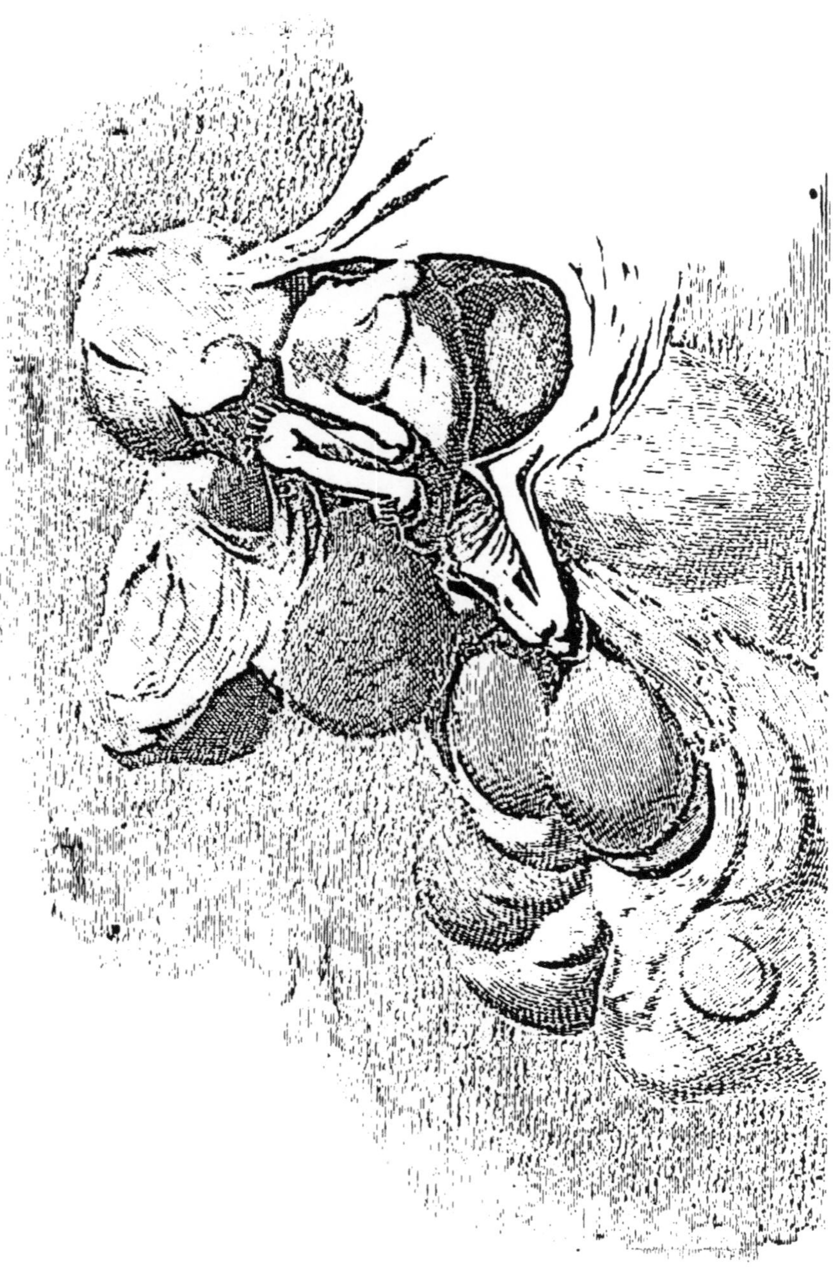

Published by A Constable & C° Edinburgh Jany 1806

I had frequent conversations on this case with my late much-lamented friend and tutor, Dr Woodville, who approved of this plan of treatment; his medical science was surpassed by none, equalled but by few of the many physicians of this metropolis; and his various merits, to use the elegant language of Mr Highmore, the trump of eulogy can never tarnish by exaggeration. It is a national loss, and a matter of universal regret, that his second volume of the History of Inoculation, which has been long ready for the press, was not published before his death; for although the vaccine inoculation, introduced by the ingenious Dr Jenner, and supported, and in a great measure established, by the zeal and ability of Dr Woodville, may eventually entirely supersede variolous inoculation (an occurrence which unfortunately it is more reasonable to wish for than to expect at present), still the importance of its contents would render it a valuable acquisition to the library of every natural philosopher.

VII.

An Account of a Fœtus found in the Abdomen of a Woman 83 years of age. By J. Grivel, Accoucheur in the Hospital of Villeneuve at Dresden, as communicated in the following Letter to Dr Pearson, Leicester-Square.

Sir,

I take the liberty of addressing to you a few lines, to desire you to accept the two drawings which I have sent, done as faithfully as my poor talent in the art enables me. You must know that we are in no want of bodies at Dresden, having, besides those of the hospital, all those of murderers and suicides. We lately received the body of Maria Walther, born at Meissen, widow of a Prussian hussar, who had attended in several campaigns in the capacity of a sutler to Frederic II. King of Prussia's army. She has been kept in the Lazarus hospital since 1794 through charity, on account of her great age only, being in perfect health, and having never complained of any pain in the belly. She talked of nothing but of the wars in her former days, and assisted as a nurse to the sick in the Lazarus hospital till within two hours of her death. On opening her body, the young surgeon who was employed was surprised to find a child in an indurated state, and blended, as it were, with the intestines. It appeared as repre-

sented

sented in the drawing, No. 1. A more distinct view appeared after washing the parts, and as represented in the drawing, No. 2. (See plate, No. 1.) We consider this as a most rare case, the woman being 83 *years of age*, as was proved by an extract of her baptism. I wished much to have purchased for you the original; but I was unable, it being reserved for the cabinet of the Elector. I have the honour of recommending myself to your protection, and of being your very humble servant,

J. Grivel.

P. S. We have a girl (*une fille nine* *) now in the hospital, who is much deformed, and far advanced in pregnancy. Her pelvis is not two inches, English, wide. We shall be obliged to perform the Cæsarean operation. This is the second of this description which we have had at the hospital within these 18 months.

Dresden, June 28. 1803.

REMARKS.

1. Although the above statement by no means contains a relation of many particulars, which a well-informed person would desire, and although, from the want of a more full account, it will be impossible to make many inferences, which otherwise could have been established, there is no just reason to question the fact that a fœtus † was found in the abdomen as described.

2. I have heard, within the last six months, of three similar cases, viz. one which fell under the observation of a very experienced physician of the first reputation in Gloucestershire. I have been favoured with a sight of the drawings of this case, and I know it is destined for publication: it will, there is no doubt, be given very correctly, and will contain a minute history of all the particulars belonging to so extraordinary an occurrence. A second instance of the same sort fell under the observation of a physician at Glasgow; and, as I was informed by a young physician, my pupil, in Edinburgh, it was so similar to the Gloucestershire case, that, while I was relating it in a lecture the last winter, he supposed it was the same as that with which he was acquainted at Glasgow. A third instance was communicated to me yesterday at Woolwich by Dr Rollo: it occurred in Ireland, of which an account had been seen a few days ago in a letter.

3. Even if I had leisure, I should not be disposed to make a number

* *Nine* is not a classical word in the French language, in which the letter was written, but we understand it to be a cant term used in some hospitals on the Continent for those cases of deformity in the female in which parturition must be difficult, if not impossible.—*Editors.*

† It is supposed to have been five months old before it escaped from the uterus.

number of remarks, and endeavour to explain the nature of these occurrences, there being so many professional men better qualified. However, one question I shall venture to propose, in order to obtain from others a satisfactory explanation. What are the powers or circumstances which prevent the fœtus from undergoing the compositions and decompositions usual in the process of putrefaction? Three different reasons may be assigned.

1. That the fœtus is in a dead state; but the exclusion of air containing oxygen gas is the circumstance which prevents putrefaction.

2. That the fœtus is in a dead state; but the agency of living surfaces in contact with it counteracts the putrefactive process.

3. That the vitality of the fœtus is not extinguished, although the mode of agency of the principle of life is different from what is usual.

The first supposition does not appear to me satisfactory, because air certainly does permeate through every part of the animal economy; and it is common for dead animal matter to become putrid in many cavities to which air has not a more free access than into the cavity of the abdomen. Also, out of the animal body, we know that animal fluids, kept in glass vessels quite full, and hermetically sealed, afford new compositions by the play of chemical attraction.

The second supposition may, perhaps, be thought not altogether improbable, being supported by analogy. So the fluid in dropsies, and in many other diseases, remains for months, and even years, in cavities, without alteration in its composition, seemingly owing to its being in contact with living matter. Generally, however, when lifeless animal matter is exposed to living surfaces, and confined so as to be much excluded from the air, it is either absorbed, or it excites the formation of pus, or it putrefies. The late Mr Pierce Smith, my most ingenious pupil, wrote a paper, which was read at the Royal Society about the year 1795, containing many experiments to show, that when flesh of various sorts was inserted into the cavities of wounds purposely inflicted, it was absorbed, if in a certain quantity, and if the animal was in vigorous health; but if the quantity was too great, then purulent matter was formed, and, in some cases, the flesh introduced became putrid.

The third supposition, viz. that vitality remains, appears most reasonable, because certain actions go on, which produce changes only known in living bodies; such as the ossification of a great part of the fœtus; the process of induration; the thickening of parts, and perhaps adhesion, from the communication of new vessels between the confined extraneous body, and the cavity in which it is contained.

VIII.

Remarkable Case of an Ossified Fœtus and Uterus in a Woman 60 years of age. By JOHN CALDWELL, M. D. Preland, Londonderry.

MRS MARY DELAP, aged 60, a woman of good character, on the 17th day of June 1805, four months after the death of her husband, to whom she had been married 26 years, complained, without any known cause, of great pain and uneasiness in her abdomen and pelvis, with obstinate costiveness, and difficulty of passing her urine, for which she took a gentle purgative without any effect. Her husband had been twice married, but had no children by either of his wives.

The 18th. She swallowed castor oil freely, and submitted to purging injections, with some little effect, by stool and urine. The injections could not be forced high enough, as there was a very hard, large lump in the vagina, obstructing the passage, like a child's head advancing by labour. The pain continued, was increasing, and more resembling labour. She said that she never had a child, but imagined herself pregnant soon after her marriage, and *then* had a large discharge, supposed to be a miscarriage. But, after that supposed miscarriage, she had menstruated regularly to her 49th or 50th year of age; and since that time, for ten years at least, she had not any change of constitution. She said that her health had been generally good, and she had frequently walked six miles a-day; but occasionally she had complaints like colic or gravel, accompanied with costiveness, and strange irregularity and difficulty in passing her urine. *She had not considered herself pregnant.*

The 19th. Labour continued, and was very troublesome; but there was no change on the cervix uteri, which was very long in form, and not in the least dilated, though very far down, like prolapsus. The cervix, at its top, was not bulbous in structure; and the orifice could only admit a catheter or goose-quill, and was too much turned to the ossa pubis. The vagina seemed to be not more than an inch and a quarter long; bones could be distinctly felt through the substance of the uterus, behind its long neck; and there was not any appearance of water before the bones.

During these three days, her skin was cool, her respiration easy, and her pulse from 65 to 90, natural in strength. But her

IX.

Essay on Erythema Mercuriale, or that Eruption which sometimes occurs from the Use of Mercury. By JOHN M'MULLIN, M. D.

WHEN, from the use of any remedy, unusual effects are produced, it cannot fail to embarrass the practitioner; and if these effects be of such a nature that they are liable to be confounded with the original disease for which the remedy was exhibited, the patient must be subjected to much inconvenience, and even danger. The truth of this remark is strongly exemplified in that species of eruption which sometimes arises from the use of mercury.

Eruptions of various kinds are very common symptoms of syphilis, but a very unusual effect of mercury; therefore, until the real nature of this erythema was lately discovered, whenever it occurred in patients undergoing a mercurial course for syphilitic complaints, it was naturally enough considered as an anomalous form of lues venerea. The mercury was consequently pushed to a greater extent, in proportion to the violence of the symptoms, and, from the cause of the disease being thus unconsciously applied for its removal, it could not fail to be aggravated, and hurried on to a fatal termination. The observation of this fact, conjoined with another of less frequent occurrence, namely, that a similar eruption did sometimes appear in patients using mercury for other complaints, and in whom no suspicion of syphilis could be entertained, at last led some judicious practitioners in Dublin to the important discovery, that the eruption was entirely an effect of the mercury, and not at all connected with the original disease. This discovery was not published until the year 1804 *; and much still remains to be done, in order to render the history of this troublesome disease perfect, and to enable us to recognise it at its first appearance, on which our success in treating it in a great measure depends. Having had several opportunities of accurately observing its progress, and having carefully studied the observations of those who have at all mentioned it, I shall endeavour, in the following essay,

* An Essay on a peculiar Eruptive Disease, arising from the Exhibition of Mercury. By GEORGE ALLEY. Dublin. 1804.
A Description of the Mercurial Lepra. By Dr MORIARTY. Dublin. 1804.
History of three Cases of Erythema Mercuriale, with Observations. By THOMAS SPENS, M. D. &c. Edinburgh.—See this Journal, vol. i. p. 7.

eſſay, to condenſe all that I have been able to learn concerning it, either from others, or from perſonal obſervation.

The different appearances which this diſeaſe aſſumes, according to its ſeverity and duration, will be beſt underſtood by deſcribing it as conſiſting of three diſtinct ſtages.

The firſt ſtage commences with languor, laſſitude, and cold ſhiverings; theſe ſymptoms are ſucceeded by increaſed temperature of the body, quick pulſe, nauſea, headach, and thirſt. The patient is troubled with a dry cough, and complains of difficult reſpiration, anxiety, and ſenſe of ſtricture about the præcordia. The tongue is uſually moiſt, and covered with a white glutinous ſlime; it ſometimes appears clean and bright red in the centre, whilſt the margins remain foul. The ſkin feels unuſually hot and itchy, with a ſenſe of prickling, not unlike the ſenſation experienced from the application of nettles. The belly is generally coſtive, but a diarrhœa is often produced by very ſlight cauſes.

On the firſt or ſecond day an eruption moſt commonly ſhows itſelf, the colour of which is either dark or bright red: the papulæ * are at firſt diſtinct and elevated, reſembling very much thoſe in rubeola. Sometimes, but rarely, the eruption appears like urticaria, and in ſuch inſtances the diſeaſe is obſerved to be very mild. The papulæ very ſpeedily run together in ſuch a manner as to form a ſuffuſed redneſs, which diſappears on preſſure. In moſt caſes it begins firſt on the ſcrotum, inſide of the thighs, fore arm, or where mercurial friction had been applied, and the integuments of the parts affected become much ſwoln. There have alſo been obſerved inſtances where an eruption of a purpliſh colour, and unaccompanied by papulæ, has diffuſed itſelf ſuddenly over the entire body †. This, however, may be conſidered as uncommon. In every inſtance which came under my obſervation, it was confined at firſt to a few places, and from thence gradually extended, until the different portions of the eruption had united, and the papulæ were alſo rough to the feel. But in thoſe caſes which reſemble urticaria, a number of minute veſicles, which contain a ſerous fluid, appear, from the commencement, interſperſed among the papulæ. Contrary to what happens in moſt diſeaſes accompanied with cutaneous affections, the febrile ſymptoms are much aggravated, and continue to

* *Papula*; a very ſmall and acuminated elevation of the cuticle, with an inflamed baſe, not containing a fluid, not tending to ſuppuration.
The duration of papulæ is uncertain; but they terminate for the moſt part in ſcurf.—*Willan on Cutaneous Diseases*, p. 13.

† Dr Moriarty on Lepra Mercurialis.

to increase after the eruption has been completed. The pulse in general beats from 120 to 130 in a minute, the thirst continues urgent, and the patient, extremely restless, seldom enjoys quiet sleep. When the eruption has continued in this manner for a certain period, the cuticle begins to peel off in thin, whitish, scurfy * exfoliations, not unlike those observed in rubeola. This desquamation has not been attended to by Dr Moriarty or Mr Alley, if they have not, by giving the same name to the decrustation which occurs in the last stage, confounded both together. It commences in those places where the eruption first made its appearance, and in this order spreads to other parts. About this period the fauces become sore, the tongue swells, and the eyes appear somewhat inflamed.

The duration of this stage is very various; sometimes it continues from ten to fourteen days, and in other cases it terminates in half that time. When the disease has appeared in its mildest form, the patient recovers immediately after this desquamation, a new cuticle having formed underneath; but, if severe, he has only experienced the smallest part of his sufferings, and the skin now assumes a new appearance, which I have considered as the second stage.

The skin at this period appears as if studded with innumerable minute vesicles, which are filled with a pellucid fluid. These vesicles may be expected, if the patient, at the close of the first stage, complains of increased itching, and sense of burning heat, in those parts from whence the cuticular exfoliations have fallen. They remain sometimes for a day or two, but are most commonly burst, immediately after their formation, by the patient rubbing them, in order to relieve the troublesome itchiness with which these parts are affected. They discharge a serous, acrimonious fluid, which possesses such a very disagreeable odour as to induce nausea in the patient himself, and those who approach near his bed-side. The odour is so peculiar, that it can easily be recognised by any person who has once experienced it.

This fluid is poured out most copiously from the scrotum, groin, inside of the thighs, or wherever the skin forms folds, and sebaceous glands are most numerous. The serous discharge from these minute vesicles form, with the cuticle, an incrustation, which may be considered as the third or last stage.

These

* *Scurf* (furfura); small exfoliations of the cuticle, which take place after some eruptions on the skin, a new cuticle being formed underneath during the exfoliation.—*Willan*, p. 12.

Scale (squama); a lamina of morbid cuticle, hard, thickened, whitish, and opaque. Scales have at first the figure and extent of the cuticular lozenges, but afterwards often increase into irregular layers, denominated crusts.

These crusts are generally very large, and, when detached, retain the figure of the parts from which they have fallen. Their colour is yellowish, but sometimes appears dark and dirty. This period of the disease might be termed, I think, with much propriety, the stage of *decrustation*, in order to distinguish it more fully from the *desquamation* which has been already noticed. From the use of the two last terms indiscriminately, those who have described the disease have introduced into their descriptions a degree of confusion, which has caused its progress not to be well understood. When this stage appears, the fauces become more affected, the eyes intolerant of light, and the tarsi tender, inflamed, and sometimes inverted. The crusts formed on the face, as in other parts of the body, before falling off, divide asunder, so as to leave cracks and fissures, which produce an hideous expression of countenance; and the eyelids are also, from the general swelling of the face, completely closed. The back and hairy scalp are last affected, and, even in very severe cases, these parts are sometimes observed to escape entirely. The patient, whilst in this state, is compelled to desist from every kind of motion, on account of the pain which he experiences on the slightest exertion, and which he describes as if his flesh were cracking. The crusts also fall off in such abundance, that the bed appears as if strewed with the cones of hops. Whilst the eruption is only making its appearance in one place, another part may have arrived at its most advanced form; so that all the different stages of the disease may be present at one time in the same individual. It is attended with typhus through its entire course; but it is very curious to observe, that the appetite for food, in most cases, remains unimpaired, and sometimes is even voracious. This circumstance was particularly remarkable in a patient who laboured under the disease, in its worst form, for the space of three months, in the Royal Infirmary of Edinburgh; for double the usual hospital allowance of food was scarcely sufficient to satisfy his hunger. When the catarrhal symptoms have continued during the progress of the complaint, they are, at this advanced period, particularly aggravated: the anxiety and pain of breast are also very severe, attended with cough, and bloody expectoration, and the patient always feels languid and dejected. The pulse becomes frequent, feeble, and irregular, the tongue black and parched, and at length diarrhoea, delirium, convulsions, gangrene of the surface of the body, and death, supervene. In its mild form, it only goes through the first stage, and terminates, as we have already stated, in a few days, by a slight desquamation. But, when severe, it is often protracted more than two

two months, every stage of the eruption continuing proportionably longer; and when, in this manner, it has run its course, it repeatedly breaks out on the new surface, and passes through the same stages.

Concerning the remote causes of this disease, it is agreed that such an affection has never been noticed, except in those using mercury; and it is necessary to observe, that every preparation of mercury, and every mode of exhibition, are found equally capable of producing the disease. When it first excited attention, it was conceived, on account of its being observed in syphilitic patients under the action of this remedy, to be an anomalous form of lues venerea. But its repeated occurrence, where no syphilitic taint could be suspected, soon removed this mistake; and it then became a question why the disease should appear in so few persons, compared to the great number who are daily using this invaluable medicine.

It was presumed, from its comparative rarity, that those attacked in this manner must be endowed with a peculiarity of constitution, to which the term *idiosynery* has been applied. In such habits, it was supposed that the irritation, which mercury usually produces, proved the exciting cause; and this opinion was supported by the well-established fact, that an eruption immediately shows itself in some persons after the use of certain articles in diet, more particularly the bitter kernels of fruits, cinchona, some species of fish, especially shell-fish, &c. Dr Gregory (who has for many years, in his lectures on the practice of physic, remarked that a peculiar eruption sometimes appears in certain habits from the employment of mercury) supposes that the application of cold to the body, whilst under the action of mercury, is absolutely necessary for its production; and the constant combination of catarrhal symptoms would make me disposed to adopt this opinion.

The disease which bears the most striking analogy to the erythema mercuriale is the *Erysipelas Chinense* of Sauvages, to which those who gather varnish from the Rhus vernix are liable, as will sufficiently appear from the following extract from Du Halde:

'It is necessary to take some precautions to secure the workmen from the bad impression of the varnish; so that whether the merchant maintains them or not, they are obliged to have a large vessel of oil, wherein has been boiled a certain quantity of the fleshy filaments found mixed in hog's fat, and which will not melt with the other part; the proportion is one ounce to a pound of oil.

'When the workmen go to place the shells in the trees, they carry with them a little of this oil, wherewith they rub the visage and the hands; and in the morning, when they have gathered the varnish, and

and return to the merchants, they rub themselves more carefully with it.

'After dinner they wash their bodies with hot water, which the merchant has ready, in which they boil a certain quantity of the following drugs, viz. of the outward rough bark of chesnuts, the bark of the fir-tree, saltpetre in crystals, and an herb which they eat in China, and in the Indies, and is a sort of blits; all these drugs are supposed to be of a cold nature.

'Every workman fills a little bason with this water, and washes himself with it carefully; but instead of the common basons used by the Chinese to wash their faces in the morning, which are of copper, the workmen who gather varnish, rejecting this metal, use those that are made of tin.

'At the time when they work at the trees, they wrap their heads in a linen bag, which they tie about their necks, and leave only two holes to see through; they cover themselves before with a sort of apron made of doe-skin, which they tie about their necks with strings; they have also buskins of the same, and long gloves on their arms.'

'The workmen pay very dear for gathering the varnish, when they do not take the precautions mentioned: The disease begins with a kind of ring-worm, which, in the space of a day, covers the face and the rest of the body, for it spreads in a few hours, and grows very red; soon after, the face begins to swell as well as the body, till the person seems quite covered with a leprosy.

'To heal a man attacked with this distemper, they give him immediately a considerable quantity of the medicinal water that the workmen washed with to prevent these accidents: This water purges violently, and they afterwards make a strong fumigation with the same water, and then wrap him up very close till the swelling is gone down; but the skin is not so soon healed; for it cracks in several places, from whence a great deal of water proceeds: To remedy this, they take of the herb that I have said to be a kind of blits, then dry and burn it, and put the ashes upon the parts affected, which imbibe the sharp humour that proceeds therefrom, and then the skin dries, falls off, and comes anew.—*The General History of China, done from the French of Du Halde*, vol. ii. p. 306. 8vo. London, 1736.

In forming our diagnosis, the only affection with which there is any great danger of confounding it in its first stages is *Rubeola*, and it is only in the first stage that any diagnostic marks are required. The following circumstances are to be attended to in distinguishing them from each other.

1st, The colour of the eruption is very different; for in rubeola it gradually changes from a bright to a dark red, until it has been completed; but this affection assumes, from the commencement, a darker colour, even in mild cases, and seldom acquires a deeper hue during its progress.

2dly,

2*dly*, The rubeolous eruption generally appears first on the face; but, in this affection, the thighs, groin, scrotum, extremities, or where mercurial friction had been applied, soonest effloresce.

3*dly*, Rubeola always terminates by a dry, furfuraceous desquamation; but after that period, in the present complaint, minute vesicles are sometimes formed, which pour out a fluid of an offensive odour, and crusts of considerable size repeatedly fall off. The absence also of some of the characteristics of rubeola, as sneezing, coryza, and epiphora, will assist us in the diagnosis at the commencement.

The surface of the body is more generally affected than in *Erysipelas*; and the vesicles, which are very minute, do not appear (unless in those cases resembling urticaria) until after desquamation. Some have mistaken this disease, at its commencement, for *Scarlatina*; but the colour of the eruption is much more florid, and the affection of the fauces, which, in that disease, is one of the first symptoms, does not take place in erythema mercuriale until the period of desquamation. There remains, as yet, another affection of the skin, which it seems necessary to point out its difference, namely, the venereal eruption; but there cannot be a probability of confounding them, if we reflect that the latter always appears in distinct circular blotches, unattended by any febrile symptoms.

These are the only diseases which bear the smallest degree of resemblance to the present, and it is only when the eruption first breaks out, that any degree of nicety is required in marking the distinction.

I should not have considered it necessary to draw any diagnosis between it and *Pemphigus*, if the very accurate Dr Willan had not published, as an instance of the latter affection, what appears to be a well-marked case of erythema mercuriale. I shall quote it in his own words.

'Pemphigus, or the vesicular fever, is a rare disease in this country. The solitary instance of it, noted in July, was a young woman, about twenty years of age, teacher in a school at Walworth, and of a weakly constitution; she had taken some *mercurial* remedies, for a glandular swelling, three weeks before her eruptive complaint appeared. It began with a violent heat and itching at one of her elbows; the other was soon after affected, when both arms swelled up to the shoulder; and, within two days, they were covered with vesications. The vesicles soon broke, and discharged an acrimonious lymph, which blistered where it fell. Similar vesicles arose in a day or two on the face, the scalp, the trunk of the body, the limbs, the palms of the hands, and the soles of the feet. They were *small*, and close

close together, so that, after they were broken, nearly the whole cuticle was detached. The fever, and the eruptive stage of the disorder, lasted, on the whole, about eight days; during that time, the patient was weak, irritable, and tremulous, her pulse being generally 132; she had no appetite, got but little rest, and was sometimes delirious. Her face was scabbed all over, as in the confluent small-pox. Before a new cuticle was formed on the trunk of the body, there was a thin incrustation, which gradually peeled off in dry yellowish scales; but a fresh discharge and a new incrustation repeatedly took place. The skin of the legs was red and tender, and appeared as if studded with miliary pustules; which breaking, discharged their lymph, and were succeeded by others. At the end of the third week, the skin of her fingers and toes came off entire, together with the nails. Three weeks more elapsed before the cuticle was restored, so that she could stir out of her bed. I saw her on the first of October, free from complaint; her nails were then renewed; her hair, which had at first partly fallen off, was become thicker. The skin of her neck, arms, and legs, appeared rough, papulated, and scaly, as in a slight kind of the dry tetter; her eyes remained weak and tender, as they had indeed been from the commencement of the disorder.'—*Willan's Reports of the Diseases in London, particularly during* 1796, 7, 8, 9, and 1800. 12mo. Lond. 1801.

But pemphigus, in Dr Willan's own arrangement of cutaneous diseases, is a genus of the order bullæ, which he defines in the following words:—" Vesicle (bulla), an elevation of the cuticle, *of a large size*, irregularly circumscribed, and containing a transparent watery fluid." In pemphigus, moreover, the vesicles are succeeded by a black scab.

In its advanced stage, it certainly has some resemblance to *Lepra*, but differs from it in many particulars, and especially in being an acute disease, always attended with fever, and in being diffused, instead of being collected, in scaly patches, nearly of a circular form. Professor Hensler of Kiel, in his classical work on leprosy, has described a case under the title of tyriasis, which seems, in many respects, to partake both of the nature of the lepra tyria, and of our erythema. It was the case of a young woman in Hamburgh, whom he unfortunately saw but once, and the description in his notes is therefore imperfect. " Her whole appearance was swelled, the cuticle of a dirty white colour, dry, brittle, and loose upon the skin, which, to the touch, seemed soft and anasarcous. Here and there it was even cracked, and exuded a little fluid. The epidermis was covered with numerous scaly crusts, resembling lichens in miniature, and, upon the whole, it looked as if it was covered with powder." Of her previous and subsequent history he was only able to learn the following circumstances. On the supervention of this eruption, decided

decided symptoms of phthisis pulmonalis, for the cure of which we are not told what remedies she used, had completely disappeared, and never returned. The eruption had been three times almost entirely removed, once by very large doses of cicuta and corrosive sublimate; a second time, as all antimonial and *mercurial remedies seemed only to aggravate it*, by tincture of cantharides; and a third time, when the disease had reached its greatest height, by arsenic, which, although given in very small doses, only $\frac{1}{16}$ of a grain three times a-day, seemed to promise a cure, when suddenly, after being continued 14 days, it produced poisonous effects, and the patient was with difficulty saved. During this period, a general warm sweat took place; whereas, at all other times, her skin was arid, and did not perspire, and the crusts which remained desquamated rapidly. The skin of the breast and upper extremities remained free from crusts until within a few days of her death. On the brow, upper eye-lids, and nose, it had rather a whitish colour; on other parts it had a pale reddish hue. The hairy scalp was covered with a thick, very ill-smelling crust, which separated repeatedly, slowly, and painfully, but was speedily renewed. Her upper eye-lids were swelled, tense, and stiff; the Meibomian glands were affected, and she had intolerance of light, with frequent watering of the eyes. Her lips and gums always retained their natural colour. No knots resembling swelled glands were ever observed; and her nails never dropped off. When visited the day preceding her death, the foetor from her body was insupportable; she seemed as if her cuticle had been peeled off, and she had been covered in some places with flakes of snow. Of all the cases of lepra or elephantiasis which I have met with (if, indeed, it belong to either), this differs least from the erythema mercuriale, and will therefore serve to point out the distinction between them.

I have been thus particular in giving a diagnosis, as it is proper to attach some degree of importance to an early knowledge of the nature of the eruption; for, in most of the cases which I have had an opportunity of witnessing, the comparative mildness or severity of the disease was proportioned to the length of time which the mercury was continued after its appearance. In our prognosis we should therefore take that circumstance into consideration. We may also sometimes foretell the degree of severity which the disease may afterwards assume, by observing the colour of the eruption, for it is found that the nearer it approaches to a dark purple, the more severe and longer of continuance will be the progress of its different stages. The more troublesome the itching, the more copious in general is the serous discharge; and those parts which feel most itchy first exude, on account of the minute vesicles being burst by the continued friction. The season of the year and the constitution of the patient are likewise to be attended to, and, as happens in other febrile diseases, its symptoms are modified by the nature of the prevailing epidemic.

The disease seldom assumes its advanced stages if the exciting cause be removed, and a proper mode of treatment adopted.

Since this disease is solely occasioned by the use of mercury, under one form or another, it must be obvious that the first step in the treatment should be the immediate discontinuance of its use. And, connected with this part of the cure, it may be remarked, that in large hospitals, and particularly those appropriated to venereal cases, we ought immediately to remove our patient from such wards as may have their atmosphere vitiated by the breathing of persons charged in general with mercury; for although they may not produce what has by some been termed a mercurial atmosphere, yet they cannot but generate such a state of it as must prove highly noxious. With the view of removing the itchiness and uneasiness of the skin, which now occurs, and also as means of cleanliness, we may employ tepid bathing. The proper temperature of the bath would seem to be from the 78th to the 84th degree of Fahrenheit; for within this range they will produce in general the desired effect, without endangering the aggravation of the symptoms, which, from inattention to this point, has in some instances occurred. Where, however, these means are found ineffectual in removing the disease, a strict adherence to the administration of such remedies as are known to alleviate the febrile symptoms must be observed. With this intention, emetics, as tartrite of antimony, or ipecacuanha and diaphoretics, particularly those from the neutral class of salts, as citrate of potash and acetite of ammonia, are properly employed. In this stage of the complaint, however, antimonial medicines should be very cautiously used; for although they are very advantageously employed in most diseases where diaphoresis is indicated, yet, in this affection, from the very irritable state of the bowels, they are scarcely admissible; nor can we with safety correct their action on the intestinal canal by means of opium, which is found rather injurious at this period. The mineral acids, ripe fruits, &c. may also be allowed, at the same time cautiously observing their effects on the bowels. The temperature in which the patient is kept should be somewhat higher than is generally recommended in febrile cases, both on account of the catarrhal symptoms, and from his being in general extremely sensible to the effects of cold applied to the surface; but, at the same time, advantage is always derived from a constant renewal

newal of the air which surrounds him. Having remarked the readiness with which the bowels are affected from slight causes, it will be evident, that when purgatives are required, those of the most lenient kind only will be advisable; as oleum ricini, sulphas magnesiæ, &c. Whilst we attend to the system in general, we must not neglect the local treatment, wihch consists chiefly in a continuance of the tepid bathing, and great attention to cleanliness. Applications of different kinds have been tried in this stage of the eruption, as solutions of sulphate of zinc, acetite of lead, sulphur ointment, and decoctions of oak-bark, but without any good effect. Sprinkling with starch, from its common employment in erysipelas, has been by many used, and this, by superseding the use of more irritating applications, may not have been without its benefit. To allay the cough and soreness of the fauces, mucilaginous mixtures, with the addition of a small quantity of opium, may be used. And although Mr Alley has recommended blisters to the back or breast, yet the danger of the blistered parts falling speedily into a state of mortification should, in most cases, forbid their application. The transition from the first to the second stage of the disease is by no means so well marked as to point out when we should change our first plan of treatment. But, as the fever is always found to assume more strongly the typhoid type as the incrustations become general, it will serve also to direct us in the remedies we employ. With the view of obviating the debility, which is generally very great, bark has usually been prescribed; but from its invariably disagreeing with the stomach, or producing diarrhœa, it cannot be given in sufficient quantity. In some instances, the cold infusion, conjoined with aromatics, has been best retained; and we may now also add some opium, without any dread of those unpleasant effects which are experienced from its use in the first stage. Wine is the best remedy at this period of the disease, and is highly relished by the patient. Porter may also be used with advantage, and diluted alcohol, in moderate quantity, may be employed with the same intention. The thirst being now urgent, large quantities of diluents will be necessary; as whey, light broths, and nourishing drinks of every kind. In this stage, tepid bathing can seldom be had recourse to; on account of the extent of surface which is left raw by the repeated decrustation, the body is unable to bear the stimulus of heat, and the patient usually falls into a state of syncope on its application. All, therefore, we can do in such cases is to employ tepid ablution, which, as means of cleanliness, is indispensably necessary. To relieve the ophthalmia tarsi, the unguentum oxidi zinci will in general prove sufficient. And that distressing symptom, which

 some

ſome deſcribe as if their fleſh were cracking, is beſt removed by the linimentum aquæ calcis, which is perhaps preferable to all other applications, and ſhould be liberally applied as ſoon as cruſts appear.

Conſiderable difference in opinion has ariſen concerning the name by which this diſeaſe ſhould be diſtinguiſhed, and the place which it ſhould occupy in noſological ſyſtems. According to the opinion entertained of its nature, it has been called, by Dr Moriarty, lepra mercurialis, and by Dr Spens, erythema mercuriale; while Mr Alley thinks the unſyſtematic and ambiguous appellation of mercurial diſeaſe preferable to either. This difference of opinion ariſes partly from the imperfection of our noſological ſyſtems, and partly from claſſing the diſeaſe from whatever appears the ſtrongeſt analogy, inſtead of reducing it analytically to its claſs, order, and genus, in that ſyſtem which we prefer. This diſcuſſion, contrary to cuſtom, I have intentionally poſtponed to the laſt, that, in elucidating it, I may take advantage of every thing known with regard to the diſeaſe. If we adopt Cullen's ſyſtem of noſology, it is evident, from being attended with fever from the very beginning to the termination, it muſt be claſſed among the pyrexiæ. It is not, however, ſo eaſy to determine to which of the orders of this claſs it belongs, certainly not to the profluvia, or hæmorrhagiæ, or febres. It would be equally excluded from the remaining two orders, if Dr Cullen's definitions of them were to be rigidly adhered to; from the phlegmaſiæ, becauſe the attendant fever is typhoid, and the blood is not ſizy; and from the exanthemata, becauſe the diſeaſe is not contagious. But Dr Cullen himſelf admits that theſe definitions are faulty, and he has in ſeveral inſtances deviated from them. All his exanthemata are not contagious, and ſome of his phlegmaſiæ are accompanied with typhoid fever. Among the phlegmaſiæ, erythema is the only genus to which it can be referred. Of the exanthemata, ſome ariſe from ſpecific contagion; others do not: to the former family our eruption does not belong; and from all the individuals of the latter, except eryſipelas, it is diſtinguiſhed by the ſmallneſs of its papulæ, and its very general diffuſion. But of the diffuſed inflammations of the ſkin, I am inclined rather to conſider it as belonging to the exanthematic than to the inflammatory; for the affection of the ſyſtem is not ſymptomatical of the external inflammation, but the external inflammation is ſymptomatical of the affection of the ſyſtem. Therefore, if we were to follow Dr Cullen's ſyſtem, it muſt be conſidered as a ſpecies or variety of eryſipelas. But, in Dr Willan's highly improved noſology of the ſkin, it will conſtitute a ſpecies or variety of the 7th genus of his 3d order, exanthemata,

exanthemata *; and therefore, of the various names which have been given to this affection, I have preferred that of Erythema Mercuriale.

* *Rash* (Exanthemata) consists of red patches on the skin variously figured, in general confluent and diffused irregularly over the body, leaving interstices of a natural colour. Portions of the cuticle are elevated in a rash, but the elevations are not acuminated. The eruption is usually complicated with a general disorder of the constitution, and terminates in a few days by cuticular exfoliations.

Willan. Def. iv.

VIII.

Second Essay on the Analysis of Animal Fluids. By John Bostock, M. D. Liverpool.

In my former essay † I endeavoured to ascertain a definite character for the three primary animal fluids, albumen, jelly, and mucus, and to point out tests by means of which their presence might be detected with facility and precision. I now propose to offer some observations upon the method to be employed in the analysis of those compound fluids, of which the three substances above mentioned form a principal part. I shall arrange my remarks according to the order adopted in my former paper, beginning with the consideration of the albumen.

My first object was to discover some method by which the exact proportion of this substance might be ascertained in any fluid of which it formed a component part. The application of caloric, as appears from my former experiments, affords a very accurate test of the presence even of the smallest quantity of albumen; but I found that it was not possible, by this agent, to separate it from the water, or other substance, with which it is combined. When a solution containing $\frac{1}{10}$ of its weight of pure albumen was kept for some time at the boiling temperature, the whole fluid assumed an opake and semi-gelatinous appearance; but the water still remained so far attached to the solid matter, that it scarcely passed at all through a filter of bibulous paper: a part of it was not transmitted, even after it had lain upon it for several days, and was beginning to exhibit marks of putrefaction. When albumen exists in that state of concentration in which it is found in the white of the egg, *i. e.* composing about 15 parts in the 100, it is capable, as we know, of becoming so completely concreted as to resemble a solid substance, and, if it

 be

† See this Journal, vol. i. p. 257.

be divided into ſmall pieces, it may be digeſted in hot water, without its figure or conſiſtency being affected.

It appeared a ſubject of ſome importance to aſcertain the degree of dilution of which albumen admits without loſing this property, as, by this means, ſome general idea might be formed of the proportion of it in any compound fluid, merely by the application of caloric, in thoſe caſes where we may not have it in our power to enter upon a more minute examination. I found that the white of the egg, after being mixed with half its weight of water, ſtill retained the power of becoming ſo far coagulated, that the figure of its parts, when divided by a knife, was not altered; but that when an equal weight of water was added to the white of the egg, though it was rendered completely opake by heat, yet it ſtill retained ſome part of its fluidity, ſo that it might be ſlowly poured from one veſſel to another. In the former caſe the albumen compoſed ſomewhat leſs than $\frac{1}{10}$ part of the weight of the fluid, and in the ſecond about $\frac{1}{13}$.

I had next recourſe to the oxymuriate of mercury, which I had before found to be, as it were, the appropriate coagulator of albumen. I experienced, however, the ſame kind of difficulty in this caſe, as in the employment of caloric. Notwithſtanding the delicacy with which the oxymuriate of mercury detects the moſt minute portion of albumen, I found the coagulation to be ſo incomplete, that the fluid continued to retain a conſiderable degree of opacity, after being paſſed through a filter, and to be ſtill coagulable by the application of heat, even when it indicated an exceſs of the oxymuriate. The entire ſeparation of the albumen ſeemed, however, to be attained by the union of both theſe methods, *i. e.* by ſubjecting the fluid to the boiling temperature, after the addition of a requiſite quantity of the oxymuriate of mercury. That we may be aſſured that a ſufficient quantity of the metallic ſalt has been employed, it is neceſſary that it be added a little in exceſs; a circumſtance which may be eaſily aſcertained, by obſerving whether the filtered fluid poſſeſs the power of precipitating a freſh ſolution of albumen.

The precipitate produced by the joint operation of caloric and the oxymuriate of mercury is a compound of albumen and the metallic ſalt; ſo that, before we can aſcertain the quantity of the former, it will be neceſſary to learn in what proportion they are diſpoſed to combine with each other. But this point, ſimple as it may appear, is not unattended with difficulty; it is not eaſy to collect and detach from the filter a ſubſtance of this peculiar texture; and much nicety is requiſite in the ſubſequent drying, ſo that all the moiſture may be completely expelled, and yet that the ſubſtance ſhould not experience any commencement of decompoſition.

compoſition. Making the experiment with the requiſite precautions, it appeared to me that albumen, when coagulated by the addition of the oxymuriate of mercury, unites itſelf to between $\frac{1}{1}$ and $\frac{1}{2}$ of its weight of the ſalt. If this eſtimate be confirmed by more extenſive experiments, it will be eaſy to calculate, with tolerable accuracy, the quantity of albumen in any compound animal fluid, by employing a ſolution of the oxymuriate of mercury of a known ſtrength, and obſerving what quantity it is neceſſary to ſaturate a given quantity of the body under examination. If, for example, we find that 100 grains of the fluid require 60 grains of a ſolution containing $\frac{1}{10}$ of its weight of the oxymuriate of mercury, it will follow, that it contains 10.5 grains of albumen.

Before I leave the ſubject of albumen, I ſhall make ſome remarks upon the uncoagulable part of the white of the egg. I found it very generally to conſtitute about $\frac{1}{4}$ of the weight of the whole ſolid contents, as ſtated in my former eſſay. A ſolution of this ſubſtance, in about 100 times its weight of water, was not affected by the addition of the oxymuriate of mercury, or the decoction of galls, but a ſingle drop of the aqua lithargyri acetati threw down a copious precipitate. I gradually evaporated the fluid, and occaſionally ſtopped the proceſs when it was nearly completed; but I did not obſerve any tendency towards gelatinization, or the exhibition of any cryſtalline appearance. I concluded, therefore, that it conſiſted altogether of mucus.

In the courſe of my experiments on albumen, particularly thoſe made during the ſummer months, I have obſerved, that this ſubſtance is leſs diſpoſed to become putrid in its natural ſtate than when diluted with a greater proportion of water, and that a ſolution of the mucilaginous part, formed by waſhing the coagulated albumen, was ſtill more ſubject to decompoſition. In ſome inſtances, where I permitted a diluted ſolution of the albumen ovi to become putrid, I was forcibly impreſſed with the reſemblance of its odour to that of pus; whereas the putrid mucilage diſcharged the uſual nauſeous ſmell.

With reſpect to the ſaline ingredients of the albumen ovi, they ſeem to exiſt in very minute proportion. I was never able to detect any viſible indication of ſaline matter by the evaporation of the water in which coagulated albumen had been waſhed; a conſiderable precipitate was indeed produced by the addition of the nitrate of ſilver; but I concluded, from its appearance, that at leaſt the greateſt part of the effect depended upon the coagulation of the animal matter, though ſome part of it might be due to the preſence of the muriate of ſoda.

The albumen ovi exhibits slight alkaline effects upon the appropriate test papers; and, by means of the oxalic acid, a very minute trace of lime may be detected, which probably exists in combination with the phosphoric acid. In order to ascertain the quantity of alkali, I formed a very diluted alkaline solution of a known strength, and observed how much acetous acid was necessary to neutralize a given weight of it. With the same acetous acid I neutralized a portion of the white of the egg, and, making the necessary calculations, I estimated that 100 grains of the albumen ovi contain no more than $\frac{1}{17}$ of a grain of alkali. This alkali has generally been supposed to be soda, and as this salt is more frequently present in the different parts of the animal body than potash, we may conclude, with some plausibility, that it is soda which exists in the albumen ovi. It has been supposed to exist in the pure or caustic state; but I am not aware of any method by which this circumstance can be ascertained. I added the carbonate of soda to a solution of albumen ovi, in considerably greater quantity than that indicated above, yet the addition of the sulphuric acid produced no visible effervescence. I think it must therefore remain undetermined, whether the alkali exist in the pure or carbonated state.

The method of ascertaining the exact quantity of jelly in any compound fluid is, upon the whole, more easy. Isinglass affords us the means of obtaining jelly in a state of almost perfect purity; by forming a solution of this substance, and an infusion of galls of a known strength, by adding them to each other until they are neutralized, and collecting the precipitate, we can ascertain the respective proportions necessary to produce the neutral compound. As the precipitate formed in this case subsides slowly, it is more convenient, after the mixture of the jelly and the galls, to filter the compound, and to add a little of the filtered fluid to fresh solutions of jelly and galls respectively; from observing in which of the solutions a precipitate is produced, we are enabled to determine which ingredient exists in excess, and to correct the deficiency in a subsequent experiment; this process must be repeated until the filtered fluid produces no precipitate with either of the reagents. By proceeding in this manner I am led to conclude, that the compound formed by the union of jelly and tannin consists of somewhat less than two parts of tannin to one of jelly; as we always have it in our power to ascertain the quantity of tan that we employ, we may, by an easy calculation, deduce the amount of the jelly in any fluid under examination.

I have not yet been able to fall upon a method for directly determining the proportion of mucus in a compound fluid, in consequence

consequence of the facility with which goulard decomposes the different ingredients, both animal and saline, which are always to be suspected in those substances that contain mucus, even in a state the nearest approaching to purity. Muriate of soda is, I believe, always present wherever we have mucus; and the goulard, which so readily and completely precipitates the mucus, likewise decomposes the common salt. The nitro-muriate and the muriate of tin, and the nitro-muriate of gold, all cause a considerable precipitation in a solution of saliva; but the supernatant fluid remains opake, as if it still contained some animal matter; and, in consequence of the muriatic acid which enters into the composition of these salts, we are not able afterwards to search for the muriate of soda, by applying the test of the nitrate of silver. The nitrate of silver itself, although it scarcely produces any effect upon a solution of vegetable gum, which is when added to saliva, throws down a very copious precipitate, partly of a dense powder, and partly of a flocculent matter: This, I apprehend, proceeds from its acting both upon the mucus and the muriate of soda. The nitro-muriates of tin and of gold do not decompose common salt, but they precipitate albumen as well as mucus, and, on this account, cannot be employed. The only way of proceeding that I have been hitherto able to employ is to discover the quantity of albumen and of jelly by the methods mentioned above, and after deducting their weight from the whole of the solid contents, to consider the remainder as mucus; but here we are necessarily confounding the mucus and the salts. After this statement, I need not add that the subject still requires farther elucidation.

I have attempted, in a few cases, to apply my ideas respecting the analysis of animal fluids to the actual examination of some substances, and I shall now proceed to detail my experiments. I must premise that, in the two first analyses, the small quantity upon which I was obliged to operate prevented me from determining the proportion of the ingredients as accurately as I could have wished. I have nevertheless inserted them, as these fluids are not at all times to be procured.

The first set of experiments which I performed were upon the fluid discharged, by puncturing a tumour formed on the spine in the disease which is usually called *spina bifida*.

1. The fluid was colourless, slightly opake, and gelatinous, of a specific gravity, scarcely differing from that of water, and insipid.

2. It did not affect either litmus or an infusion of mallows.

3. A hundred grains of the fluid were slowly evaporated; a residuum was left of 2.2 grains only.

4. When kept for some time at the temperature of boiling water,

water, its opacity was ſlightly increaſed, but it did not exhibit any tendency to coagulation.

5. A ſaturated ſoutlion of the oxymuriate of mercury, when firſt added, produced but little effect; after ſome time, however, an inconſiderable precipitate was thrown down.

6. Infuſion of galls produced a precipitate in ſmall quantity.

7. Aqua lithargyri acetati produced a copious denſe precipitate.

8. By the addition of the nitro-muriate of tin, the fluid was rendered conſiderably more opake, and, as if approaching to coagulation, after ſome time a precipitate was formed.

9. The reſiduum from No. 3. was partly diſſolved by being digeſted in hot water.

10. The water from No. 9. produced a copious precipitate with nitrate of ſilver.

11. It alſo produced a perceptible precipitate with oxalic acid.

12. It alſo produced a ſlight precipitate with the infuſion of galls.

13. A quantity of this fluid, being evaporated very ſlowly, left cubical cryſtals of common ſalt in conſiderable quantity.

From No. 3. we learn that 97.8 parts in 100 conſiſt of water. From 4. and 5. we learn that it contained a little albumen. The quantity was too ſmall to be collected and meaſured by weighing; but, from the viſible effect produced by heat and the oxymuriate of mercury, I ſhould conceive it could not be more than $\frac{1}{100}$ of its weight. From No. 6. and 12. and by comparing 6. with 5. we learn that it contains a minute quantity of jelly. From 7. and 8. eſpecially by comparing them together, we learn that it contains mucus. By comparing 7. and 8. and from 10. to 13. we learn that it contains the muriate of ſoda in conſiderable quantity; and from 11. that it contains a very ſmall trace of lime. The compoſition of the fluid will therefore be nearly as follows:

Water	97	8	
Muriate of ſoda	1	0	
Albumen	0	5	
Mucus	0	5	These proportions are in ſome
Jelly	0	2	meaſure conjectural
Lime			a very minute quantity
	100	0	

The next fluid that I had an opportunity of examining was the *liquor pericardii*, which was obtained by opening the body of a boy who had died ſuddenly, in order to aſcertain the cauſe of his death. The whole quantity collected was about half an ounce;

ounce; it was nearly of the colour and appearance of the ſerum of the blood.

1. A quantity of it was ſlowly evaporated, and a reſiduum was left, amounting to $\frac{1}{11}$ of the whole.

2. A quantity of the fluid was kept for ſome time at the heat of boiling water; it became conſiderably opake and gelatinous.

3. A copious precipitate was produced by the oxymuriate of mercury.

4. After the fluid was ſaturated with the oxymuriate of mercury, it produced no precipitate with the infuſion of galls.

5. The nitrate of ſilver produced a precipitate which indicated both animal matter and the muriate of ſoda.

6. A quantity of the coagulated fluid, No. 2. being dried in the temperature of boiling water, was afterwards waſhed with boiling diſtilled water.

7. The water from No. 6. gave no precipitate with the oxymuriate of mercury, nor with galls, but a pretty copious one with the aqua lithargyri acetati.

The ſmall quantity of the fluid which I was able to obtain prevented me from proſecuting the analyſis with more minuteneſs; from theſe experiments, however, we may form ſome idea of its compoſition. From the 1. we learn that it contains 92 of water; from No. 2. and 3. that it contains a conſiderable quantity of albumen, which I ſhould eſtimate at ſomewhat more than $\frac{1}{20}$ of its weight. No. 4. and 7. ſhow that it contained no jelly. No. 7. that it contained mucus; and No. 5. that it contained common ſalt, but the proportion of this latter appeared not very conſiderable. The conſtituents of the liquor pericardii will therefore be,

Water	92 0	
Albumen	5 5	
Mucus	2 0	The proportion of theſe ſubſtances is ſomewhat conjectural
Muriate of ſoda	0 5	
	100 0	

The next analyſis that I attempted was that of the ſaliva; this fluid, in its natural ſtate, is mixed with ſuch variable proportions of water, that it is almoſt impoſſible to fix any ſtandard which can be conſidered even as the average quantity. It is, however, convenient, in obſerving the effects of reagents upon it, to have it in a more diluted ſtate than it uſually occurs; and I accordingly united it, by rubbing in a mortar, with a quantity of diſtilled water, until, by evaporation, 100 grains of the mixture

ture were found to contain two grains of solid residuum. Upon this mixture the following experiments were performed.

1. The fluid was still opake, and there was an appearance as if some flocculent matter were suspended in it.

2. No effect seemed to be produced by exposing it to the boiling temperature.

3. When the oxymuriate of mercury was added, no immediate visible effect was produced, but, after some hours, a light flocculent coagulum separated and fell to the bottom, aving the fluid nearly transparent.

4. A portion of the fluid, left for a few days without addition, gradually suffered a quantity of matter to separate from it, as in No. 3.; but the separation was less complete, and it was much longer in taking place.

5. A quantity of the fluid being passed through a filter of bibulous paper, was rendered perfectly transparent.

6. The oxymuriate of mercury being added to a quantity of No. 5. a very slight precipitate only was produced after some time.

7. The addition of the infusion of galls to No. 1. caused a precipitation of white flakes; but, after filtration, the galls produced no effect.

8. The filtered fluid, No. 5. produced a copious precipitate with the aqua lithargyri acetati.

9. It also produced a considerable precipitate with the nitro-muriate of tin.

10. And with the nitrate of silver.

11. Equal weights of the fluid, before and after filtration, were separately evaporated, and the amount of the residuum being ascertained, the quantities left were to each other nearly as 12 to 8.

12. The diluted saliva, both before and after filtration, slightly reddened a paper stained with litmus.

From these experiments we may draw the following conclusions: From No. 3. it would seem that the fluid contains albumen; but it appears from Nos. 1. 2. 4. 5. and 6. that the albumen is not soluble in water, but in that state in which it is found after coagulation. From this we learn that it constitutes only 0.8 of a grain in 100 grains of the fluid. From No. 7. we learn that there is no jelly; from 8. 9. and 10. that there is a quantity of mucus and muriate of soda; and, from comparing these with each other, we are led to conclude, that the last substance exists only in small quantity. The composition of the diluted saliva will therefore be nearly as follows:

Water

Water	98	0	
Coagulated albumen	0	8	
Mucus	1	1	} The proportion of these is partly conjectural
Salts	0	1	
	100	0	

It will, I conceive, be admitted, that the albumen in this saliva existed in the coagulated state. This I consider to be decidedly proved from the effects of heat, by its gradual, spontaneous deposition, and by the ease with which it was separated by filtration. Still, however, the oxymuriate of mercury and the galls showed that it was albumen. The difficulty of uniting saliva with water, and the effects of filtration, were noticed by Dr Fordyce *; but he imagined that the whole of the animal matter was removed by the process. The saliva that I employed manifested slightly acid properties: How far this may be the case in general, I am unable to decide. Haller thinks that, in a state of perfect health, the saliva is not acid; but, at the same time, he quotes a number of authors who are of a contrary opinion †. M. Hapell de la Chenaie informs us, that the saliva of the horse is alkaline ‡.

The quantity of water contained in the saliva, as discharged from the mouth, is very various. Haller estimates it at about $\frac{4}{5}$ of the whole; but Dr Fordyce supposes that $\frac{1}{11}$ only consists of solid matter. If we take the estimate of Haller, which is sanctioned by Fourcroy § and Thomson ‖, the constituents of saliva will exist in the following proportions:

Water	80	0
Coagulated albumen	8	0
Mucus	11	0
Saline substances	1	0
	100	0

The quantity of the saline ingredients in my analysis is confessedly conjectural; they have been stated by Haller to be $\frac{1}{100}$ of the whole. I have not been able to satisfy myself respecting the nature and proportion of the salts which compose this residuum: it has been said to consist of the muriate of soda, and the phosphates of lime and of soda ‖.

* De Catarrho, p. 17.
† El. Phys. lib. xviii. sect. 2. § 10.
‡ Mem. of Med. Soc. for 1780-1, p. 325.
§ Systeme, ix. 366.
‖ Chemistry, iv. 613.

MEDICAL

MEDICAL BIOGRAPHY.

I.

Dr CURRIE.

LATELY, at a premature age, but at the height of reputation, died Dr James Currie; a man whofe abilities were an honour to his country, whofe death was a lofs to the world. If fplendid talents, unblemifhed integrity, and the moft active philanthropy, can confer immortality on the memory of a man, the name of Currie will live for ever in the records of fame. Whether we contemplate him as an author, as a phyfician, or as a man, we fhall have equal fubject for praife, equal caufe for admiration.

His perfon was confiderably above the middle fize, his limbs were turned according to the fineft proportions of nature, his countenance was characterized by an expreffion of mildnefs, and his eyes fparkled with intelligence. In his demeanour gentlenefs and dignity were moft happily blended, and the charm of his manner was irrefiftible.

The prepoffeffion induced by his appearance and addrefs was amply confirmed by a nearer acquaintance. His voice was mufical and impreffive; his difcourfe always interefting, and often uncommonly animated. No one ever quitted his company without regret, or left him without having derived inftruction of the daily improvements in fcience: none efcaped his rapid glance; at one view his comprehenfive mind could appreciate their relative importance, deduce their numerous confequences, and point out their various applications. Nor did the lefs important productions of tafte or fancy elude his obfervation: upon every topic, therefore, whether ufeful or elegant, whether connected with good or private improvement, his information was accurate and extenfive.

He was gifted with an ample fund of wit and humour; an imagination which could inveft the moft trite and unimportant fubject with the charms of novelty, which perpetually delighted us with new applications of terms, with new combinations of ideas. But the keennefs of his wit is not fo much to be extolled as his forbearance in its ufe: never did it ruffle the ingenuous bofom of modefty, or call up a blufh in the cheek of innocence.

To

To the moſt acute diſcrimination of character he added the moſt happy talent of delineating its ſlighteſt ſhades. By a ſingle epithet he could convey the moſt diſtinct and accurate images, and one of his ſentences not unfrequently ſpoke more than volumes.

From a man of ſuch colloquial powers, however we might have lamented, we could not have been ſurpriſed at a ſtudied diſplay of talent, or a dictatorial aſſumption of importance. But ſuch failings were totally foreign to the liberal mind of Currie. Though perſuaſion hung on his lips, and conviction waited on his arguments, yet was he more ready to hear the opinion of others than to propoſe his own; more deſirous of beſtowing applauſe than of exciting admiration. No man, however, was leſs avaricious of knowledge, or communicated his opinions and diſcoveries with greater freedom. Few men have poſſeſſed in ſo eminent a degree the faculty of diſcovering upon what particular ſubjects the information of thoſe with whom he converſed was moſt extenſive, and, certainly no man ever made a more generous uſe of this talent. To draw forth the ability of others, and to diſplay their information to advantage, was to him a ſource of the greateſt pleaſure. He rendered us more pleaſed with ourſelves, at the ſame time that we could not but admit his ſuperiority. We were indeed proud to acknowledge his aſcendance; the admiration excited by his talents was not an extorted tribute, but a willing homage.

If the ſtrength of his genius and the endowments of his intellect were calculated to excite admiration, the virtues of his mind and his moral excellence could not fail to captivate eſteem. He was dignified without pride, unſuſpicious without credulity, candid without imprudence, and generous without oſtentation. To feelings the moſt acute was added the moſt unwearied benevolence. Not content with the inert philanthropy which is occupied in bewailing thoſe miſeries which it ſhould relieve, or deprecating thoſe evils which it ſhould prevent, he was always actively employed in conferring benefit, or in alleviating misfortune. Even when ſtruggling with that diſeaſe which was ſoon to terminate his exiſtence, he has repeatedly forgotten his own miſery to relieve that of others, has repeatedly haſtened to ſnatch another from that grave which was already open to receive himſelf.

That acute ſenſibility which taught him to feel for others induced him to reſpect himſelf. He was ever prompt to repel inſult, but prone to forget injury. It may with juſtice be ſaid, that he had a bad memory for his friends, but not for his enemies. That cheerfulneſs, which was ſo conſpicuous in his diſpo-

 ſition,

ſition, never deſerted him even under the accumulated diſtreſs of his long illneſs. With him it was perpetual, proceeding not from momentary impreſſions, but from the innate conſciouſneſs of rectitude.

The talent for obſervation, which is an indiſpenſable requiſite in the character of an accompliſhed phyſician, was his in a remarkable degree. The clearneſs of his perception, and the accuracy of his judgment, enabled him at once to ſeize the leading features of diſeaſe, to determine its character, and apply its appropriate remedies. As his conception of diſeaſe was diſtinct, ſo was his mode of practice decided. It is no inconſiderable evidence in his favour, that thoſe who commenced his acquaintance as a phyſician clung to him ever after as a friend.

It were needleſs to expatiate on his character as a friend, as a huſband, or as a father. Thoſe affections, which can extend through the wide ſphere of human nature, muſt neceſſarily be uncommonly ſtrong at the centre. The man who contemplates all his fellow-creatures with the eye of benevolence muſt feel acutely towards thoſe whom the ties of conſanguinity have endeared, or whom ſimilar inclinations and purſuits have linked with him in the ſacred bond of friendſhip. Let it not be objected to this ſketch that it is clothed in the unqualified language of panegyric. Thoſe who know the original muſt acknowledge the faintneſs of the reſemblance. Thoſe who are acquainted with his works may commend with warmth; thoſe who know himſelf muſt praiſe with enthuſiaſm.

To inveſt a human being with the attributes of perfection would be more than abſurd; it would be preſumptuous. That Dr Currie had his failings muſt be allowed, but they were the failings of a great mind; they were not of that prominent kind which decide the character, but of that lighter caſt which gently ſhade the glowing tints of excellence. His frailties have left no traces behind them, they ſleep with him in the grave; but his virtues will be for ever freſh in the remembrance of poſterity. "Quicquid ex illo amavimus, quicquid mirati ſumus, manet, manſurumque eſt in animis hominum, in æternitate temporum, fama rerum."

Beſides ſome detached pieces, the principal works of Dr Currie are, Memoirs of Dr Bell (printed in the Mancheſter Memoirs); Med. Reports on the Effects of cold and warm Water; and the Life of Burns.

The life of Dr Bell was compoſed at the deſire of the philoſophical ſociety of Mancheſter, and during the convaleſcence of from a dangerous illneſs. An illneſs, however, which would ſeem rather to have increaſed, than to have impaired, the faculties of his mind. This tribute to the memory of his friend would have done honour to the pen of Tacitus.

The reports on the effects of cold water, as a remedy in fever, were written to recommend a practice of which Dr Currie may in ſtrict juſtice be conſidered as the author. It is true, that in the records of the ancients, and in the writings of the moderns, we occaſionally meet with an account of this practice. But thoſe who employed it did ſo empirically, or without any fixed principles. It remained for Dr Currie to aſcertain its mode of action, to trace its conſequences, and to lay down rules for its application. This he has effected in the moſt maſterly manner. Had Currie not lived, or had he forborne to write, this gigantic remedy might ſtill have lurked in obſcurity, or might have been productive of infinite miſchief, in place of univerſal advantage. At preſent it is morally impoſſible that any one who has read the medical reports can undeſignedly miſapply this remedy.

To arreſt the progreſs of fever, to circumſcribe the range of death, to exterminate diſeaſe, and to nip contagion in the bud, though preſent to our dreams of felicity, would ſeem denied to our waking hopes. As far, however, as theſe objects will admit of attainment, we may expect them from the remedy which Dr Currie has recommended to our notice. He has taught us to diveſt the jail-fever, the ſmall-pox, and the ſcarlet-fever, of moſt of their terrors. It is a ſingular circumſtance in the hiſtory of the latter diſeaſe, that ſo ſhort a time ſhould have elapſed between the diſcovery of its nature and the final perfection in its treatment. A late celebrated coloſſus in medicine gravely propoſed that the diſeaſe ſhould be rendered milder by inoculation; a meaſure, if it could be effected, pregnant with miſchief, and deſtitute of benefit. It is not improbable, that ere long the propoſal may be read, when the complaint is ſcarcely known but by report.

From the analogy with meaſles, and from the caſe of Dr Currie himſelf (related in the 2d volume of the Reports), it is not improbable that the tepid and even the cold affuſion may prove a powerful auxiliary remedy in every diſeaſe in which the temperature of the body is much and preternaturally increaſed. The thermometer is now become as indiſpenſable to the phyſician as to the natural philoſopher. That we owe this additional and valuable guide through the labyrinths of diſeaſe to Currie alone, will ſcarcely be denied even by the voice of envy, or whiſper of detraction.

Though few will be hardy enough to controvert the efficacy of the cold affusion in many febrile diseases, we must lament that the apathy of many has forbidden them to recur to its application. This frigid indifference in private practitioners may be explained, and can scarcely excite surprise: but the same neglect in those intrusted with the lives of our brave defenders must create a stronger emotion.

The reports on the effects of cold water constitute one of the most elegant as well as useful works, in our own or in any language. With a happiness almost peculiar to himself, the author has contrived to decorate a medical work with all the graces of a most finished style. Indeed, all his writings are in some degree emblematic of his own mind, in which the most refined taste and exquisite judgment were united to manly vigour and philosophical accuracy. The distinguished excellence of the style is, however, one of the least recommendations of this invaluable work. The importance of the doctrine, the perspicuity with which it is delivered, the ingenuity and consummate skill with which it is applied, and the astonishing success resulting from its practice, all entitle Dr Currie's book to rank among the few which have produced a new era in medicine. Nor is our admiration confined to the new and important facts with regard to the application and powers of cold and tepid water. Interspersed with these we find the most comprehensive and enlarged views of diseases, with the most important hints with respect to their treatment, the most judicious criticisms on prevailing systems of medicine, with the most enlightened efforts towards their improvement. To dwell on this theme would confer infinite pleasure, but the task would be endless. Suffice it to observe, that the Medical Reports contain an invaluable mine of knowledge, and that they should be in the hands of every student and practitioner, inscribed with this injunction, 'Nocturna versate manu, versate diurna.'

With the life of Burns few biographical compositions can compare, and it is excelled by none. Nor is the attempt to pourtray individual excellence or peculiar character of easy attainment. Of those who figure in the page of history, the excellence of most is adventitious, and the lustre of all is derived from the reflected splendour of the events in which they were engaged. We seldom follow them into the shade of retirement, seldom contemplate them in the vale of solitude. If, amidst the brilliant succession of public events, our attention is called to the rugged worth of a Cincinnatus, or the milder virtues of an Antonine, we contemplate them with cold approbation, and turn from them without regret. To represent characters such as these requires indeed ability: but, blended as they are with more dazzling

dazzling matter, we ſeldom pauſe to admire the portrait, or examine the accuracy of the reſemblance. To rivet our attention to an individual unconnected with public life, to mark the ſtruggles of his genius as he emerges from the gloom of obſcurity, to diſplay the various features of his character, to trace the hidden ſprings of conduct, to delineate his excellence in glowing colours, and to touch with lenient hand his failings—this taſk demands the pencil of a maſter: Such a pencil was that of Currie. Under his magic touch the vices of Burns are ſoftened down into blemiſhes, and his blemiſhes mellowed into beauties. Though rigidly correct in his own conduct, our author was always ready to extenuate the faults of others. Though the luſtre of genius could not miſlead his judgment, he dropped a tear over its frailties, and veiled with pious hand its errors. The misfortunes which imbittered the life of the Scottiſh bard, have been tardily compenſated by the honours paid to his memory. The laurels which encircle the grave of Burns wave over the never-fading flowers planted by the kindred hand of Currie.

This feeble attempt to deſcribe departed worth, though it may alleviate the ſorrow of an individual, is inadequate to the merits of the man whom it would fain commemorate. The vigour of his mind continued to the laſt, and his brilliant talents were only extinguiſhed by the hand of death. It was an affecting ſpectacle to contemplate his mind ſuperior to the devaſtations committed in his form, and towering above the ruins of its earthly fabric. He who could have viewed this ſcene unmoved muſt indeed have been a ſtoic. To ſuch a man as Currie, a biographer cannot long be wanting. To deſcribe his brilliant career, however, would require no common pen. The pleaſing but melancholy taſk ſeems naturally to devolve on one who was dear to him as a friend, and who has already emulated the fame of a Politiano and a Guicciardini.

C. E. B.

1ſt November, 1805.

THE INQUIRER, N° IV.

What are the chief diagnoſtic ſymptoms of hydrocephalus internus, and of the diſeaſes which ariſe from worms in the inteſtinal canal?

In no claſs of diſeaſes are the difficulties in forming an accurate diagnoſis greater than in thoſe of children. Even the exanthemata, which have a fixed character, which frequently prevail epidemically, and whoſe ſymptoms are the objects of our ſenſes, are ſometimes confounded with other diſeaſes. Miſtakes of this kind are ſtill more to be dreaded in a diſeaſe like the hydrocephalus internus, where no viſible marks are met with, and which often attacks children who are incapable of expreſſing their feelings. The diſeaſe with which, in its early period, it is moſt frequently confounded, is the diſorder ariſing from worms in the inteſtinal canal; and the celebrated Fothergill owns that three caſes, which he had conceived to be hydrocephalus internus, had been cured ſimply by the uſe of anthelmintic remedies.

In the proſecution of the preſent inquiry it is not intended to enter minutely into the hiſtory of the various ſymptoms of the two diſeaſes under conſideration, but merely to point out the leading features by which they are characterized, and to attend particularly to thoſe from which an accurate diagnoſis may be drawn. It will therefore be proper to give a ſhort account of the moſt uſual phenomena in each, and then to point out thoſe which particularly enable us to diſtinguiſh them.

The ſymptoms of hydrocephalus internus vary conſiderably, particularly on their firſt attack. The diſeaſe is not confined to any particular age, but moſt frequently attacks children under 12 or 14 years of age. It begins ſometimes ſuddenly, without any previous warning, in the form of a common fever; or its progreſs is ſlow, like a chronic diſeaſe, and its attack is firſt announced by ſome affection of the head. In the firſt caſe it uſually affects the healthieſt, ſtouteſt, and moſt lively children, rarely under two or three years of age. It does not confine itſelf to any particular conſtitution, although there have been inſtances of ſeveral children of the ſame family dying of it. An attentive obſerver will often ſuſpect its approach ſeveral days previous to the attack, from a tottering or ſtumbling on even ground, and from a peculiar walk of the child, where the limbs do not ſeem to be lamed, but refuſe to perform their natural

natural office, the child lifting them up high, and taking long steps, without complaining of any uneasy sensation. These appearances are soon followed by the true morbid affections, such as the feverish state, intolerance of light, and pain of the head; the child frequently exclaiming, Oh! my head, my head! Vomiting now comes on; there is constant restlessness and drowsiness, which, usually in the course of four or five days, is changed into complete sopor, during which the child, from time to time, utters a short piercing scream, expressive of great pain, without being able to assign any reason for it. It is even sometimes difficult to ascertain whether there is any pain in the head, although, in most cases, it may be presumed that there is, from the child frequently reaching his hand towards the head and eyes, as if to remove something away from them. One arm often appears weak and unable to perform the usual voluntary motions, and a similar numbness sometimes affects one side of the body. If the patient is roused during this state of stupor or drowsiness, the very moment he awakes he again sinks into sleep, and he cannot be kept long awake; he answers correctly, but slowly, and always with monosyllables: he will take food if offered, but is extremely peevish and fretful when disturbed during his sleep to take any medicine. If the patient opens his eyes in this stage (which seldom happens), the pupils are found unusually dilated, frequently in different degrees; sometimes there is strabismus, and always an aversion to light: total blindness often follows later in the disease, and then the eyes remain always open. If the patient lies still for a while, he may be observed to sigh deeply, or to draw his breath alternately, slowly and quickly. He always lies in a horizontal posture, with the head low, and never rises up. The bowels are at this period, and also later, so costive, that even drastic medicines have no effect. In the course of a few days the drowsiness and stupor pass into a state of complete coma and insensibility; the pulse, which had hitherto been quick, becomes not only irregular, but also much slower than in the natural state. The slowness of the pulse continues from 8 to 14 days, till the last period of the disease, when it again increases in frequency, and becomes so quick that it cannot be counted; the cheeks acquire a hectic flush, and the patient is usually carried off in a general convulsion. The duration of this form of the disease is commonly about 14 days or three weeks, and, in very young children, the progress is still more rapid.

When the disease is more of a chronic nature, it is preceded for two or three weeks by a slight pain of the head; the child continues to go about, but gradually loses his liveliness and spirits; so that it is not eafy to fix the precife beginning of the difeafe: he foon takes to bed, and by and by, though rather later than in the preceding fpecies, he falls into the comatofe ftate, which is foon followed by the other fymptoms already enumerated.

In the laft period of the difeafe there appears a white rafh of fmall and almoft imperceptible veficles, about the fize of a millet feed, filled with a thin tranfparent fluid, principally over the forehead, breaft, and temples, and this is is confidered by fome writers as a certain mark of approaching death.

Notwithftanding the many fymptoms here pointed out of the prefence of a watery fluid in the cavities of the brain, it is not to be underftood that any one of them fingly is to be confidered as fufficient to mark its exiftence; but it is only from their combination that we can draw a pofitive conclufion.

The marks of the prefence of worms in the human body are often obfcure and equivocal, as feveral of the fymptoms by which they are commonly indicated may alfo arife from very different caufes; it alfo not unfrequently happens that worms are difcharged by patients who have never fhowed any marks of having been affected by them; their evacuation, either by the anus or mouth, being the only circumftance which can remove every uncertainty with regard to their prefence. Certain morbid phenomena, however, offer themfelves, which, when carefully obferved and contrafted together, at leaft inform the phyfician of the probability of their exiftence.

In perfons affected with worms, the natural colour of the face is altered, fometimes becoming red, fometimes pale, fometimes faturnine, and frequently changing fuddenly: the eyes lofe their natural vivacity, are ufually directed to one object, become languid and dull, and the pupils are evidently dilated, the noftrils are affected with an infupportable itching, and the alæ nafi and upper lip are evidently fwelled. There are frequent and violent pains in the head, efpecially after eating: the mouth is ufually filled with faliva, and the breath is remarkably fetid: the fleep is difturbed and uneafy, and frequently the patient is obferved to grind his teeth: the pulfe is firm, quick, and intermitting; the abdomen becomes fwelled and hard, and there is generally naufea and vomiting; fometimes there is no appetite, at other times it is preternaturally increafed: the belly is affected with fevere pain, and the patient complains of a feeling of tearing or pricking diffufed over the whole abdomen, increafing when the ftomach is empty, and becoming eafier, or even difappearing entirely, after taking food. The patient waftes away, and becomes quite emaciated, notwithftanding the quantity he eats; he is frequently affected with a tenefmus, or a difagreeable itching

ing at the anus; and, lastly, general listlessness, anxiety, and languor, pervade every action.

Although the symptoms enumerated may appear sufficiently satisfactory, yet they so rarely appear in any regular order or connexion, and worms are so frequently discharged in cases in which they were not suspected to exist, and have so often been sought for in vain in children supposed to have died from them, as to render it necessary to contrast particularly the leading symptoms, in order to mark still more clearly their distinction.

In the *first* place, then, in hydrocephalus internus, the symptoms continue uninterrupted for some time, particularly the drowsy state and the headach. Where worms are the cause of the disorder, their duration is not so long, and there are frequent intermissions of weeks or months, during which the child complains, from time to time, of pain in the belly, which is generally swelled and hard. This last affection always occurs in hydrocephalus internus, except when it is complicated with worms.

2. Spasmodic affections and general convulsions are much more frequent attendants of worms, and seldom occur in the early stage of hydrocephalus, unless the children have been previously subject to them. In the first case they are usually of short duration, but in the latter they continue often without ceasing before death; and it is a rare circumstance that a child dies in convulsions from worms, without being affected with some other disease.

3. In the disorders from worms, although the pupils are dilated, it is not attended with any aversion to light, which is a constant symptom in hydrocephalus internus.

4. The very obstinate costiveness, which does not yield even to the strongest purgatives, is a constant symptom in hydrocephalus internus; whereas an opposite state, or that of chronic diarrhœa, is one of the most unequivocal symptoms of worms.

5. In worms there is almost constantly the itching of the nose, which we never observe in hydrocephalus internus, while the tottering and unusual manner of walking is universally confined to the latter.

J. H. W.

PART II.

CRITICAL ANALYSIS.

I.

Description and Treatment of Cutaneous Diseases, Order I. II. and part of III. By Robert Willan, M. D. F. A. S. 4to. 1798, 1801, 1805. Johnson.

This department of medicine has long been in need of cultivation. From the times of the Greek and Arabian physicians a perpetual confusion has prevailed in the descriptions and appellations of cutaneous eruptions, which has not only retarded the investigations of their nature and peculiarities, and of the mode of treatment adapted to each, but has contributed to render the communication of improvement almost abortive. The same diseases have been described again and again as new and unknown to preceding writers, until their synonimes have been multiplied without end, and involved in the utmost perplexity; and remedies, which were recommended for one variety of disease, have been erroneously administered in others, and thence discarded as hurtful or inefficacious. Obscurity again has subsequently arisen from the opposite extreme. The difficulty of obtaining clear ideas of such an infinite variety of eruptions, has led to the use of a few indefinite general terms, under which almost all the chronic species are comprised without discrimination; and hence discrimination in the exhibition of remedies is impracticable.

The labour of unravelling this intricacy, and affording definite notions of the diseases in question by means of a systematic arrangement, and thus, at least, of facilitating the path for farther investigation, is the useful task which the author has enjoined himself. Difficulties, indeed, will necessarily occur in the diagnosis of cutaneous affections, in consequence of the slight shades of difference which exist between different species, the varieties of their appearance in different stages of their progress, and their occasional

occasional combination, and even actual transition or conversion one into another. And these circumstances, as well as the general similarity of treatment, may perhaps suggest doubts as to the essential difference of many of the genera here distinguished, and a probability that the experience which may arise out of this arrangement will lead to a still farther simplification. Convinced, however, of the importance of such an arrangement, founded upon simple and obvious resemblances, we apprehend that we cannot better fulfil our duty to our readers than by occupying a few pages with a retrospective analysis of those parts of the system which appeared prior to the commencement of our Journal.

In forming his arrangement wholly upon external appearances, Dr Willan is necessarily led to separate some *genera* which would be ranged together in a system of "natural orders," and to connect others which, in such a system, would be separated. Although greater and essential analogies are thus, in many instances, overlooked, yet a practical facility of distinction is obtained with greater certainty than by the other method, as is well illustrated in the science of natural history by the artificial system of Linnæus. Dr W. divides the class of cutaneous diseases into eight orders, characterized by the different appearances of pimples, scales, rashes, &c. as follows:

Ord. I. Papulæ.
Strophulus (*red gum, tooth eruption, &c.*
Lichen (*spring eruption, scorbutic pimples, &c.*
Prurigo (*gratelle, or universal itching of the skin.*)

Ord. II. Squamæ.
Lepra (*leprosy of the Greeks.*)
Psoriasis (*dry or scaly tetter.*)
Pityriasis (*dandriff.*)
Icthyosis (*fish-skin.*)

Ord. III. Exanthemata.
Rubeola (*measles.*)
Scarlatina (*scarlet-fever.*)
Urticaria (*nettle-rash.*)
Roseola (*rose-rash.*)
Iris (*rainbow-rash.*)
Purpura (*purple or scorbutic-rash.*)
Erythema (*red-rash.*)

Ord. IV. Bullæ.
Erysipelas (*St Anthony's fire.*)
Pemphigus (*vesicular fever.*)
Pompholyx (*water-blebs.*

Ord. V. Vesiculæ.
Herpes (*ringworm, shingles, wild-fire, &c.*
Varicella (*chicken-pox and swine-pox.*)
Miliaria (*miliary eruptions.*)
Eczema (*heat eruptions.*)
Aphthæ (*thrush.*)

Ord. VI. Pustulæ.
Impetigo (*running tetter.*)
Ecthyma (*large inflamed pustules.*)
Variola (*small-pox and cow-pox.*)
Scabies (*itch.*)
Porrigo (*scald-head, honeycomb scab, &c.*)

Ord. VII. Tuberculæ.
Phyma (*boils, carbuncles, &c.*)
Verruca (*warts.*)
Molluscum (*small, soft wens.*)
Vitiligo (*white smooth tubercles.*)
Acne (*stone-pock; red, tuberculated face, &c.*)
Lupus (*noli me tangere.*)
Elephantiasis (*Arabian leprosy.*)
Frambœsia (*yaws.*)

Ord. VIII. Maculæ.
Ephelis (*sun-spots.*)
Nævus
Spilus (*moles, and other original marks.*)

The parts already published contain an account of the genera belonging

belonging to the firſt and ſecond orders, and the two firſt genera of the third order only. We ſhall paſs briefly over thoſe which are of trivial importance.

The term *papula*, which deſignates the firſt order, has been uſed by medical writers in various ſignifications; ſome applying it to puſtules of various ſorts; and others including under it wheals, *acores*, *vari*, &c. Dr Willan defines the term "a very ſmall and acuminated elevation of the cuticle, with an inflamed baſe, not containing a fluid, not tending to ſuppuration." Def. V. page 15. With this limitation it will include only three genera, ſtrophulus, lichen, and prurigo.

The STROPHULUS is a papulous eruption peculiar to infants; the author has obſerved five varieties of it: 1. S. *Intertinctus*, the red gum; 2. S. *Albidus*, a variety of the former, ſometimes called white gum. Theſe appear occaſionally in the ſtrongeſt children, unconnected apparently with conſtitutional diſeaſe. If ſuddenly repelled, however, they have been obſerved to be followed by diarrhoea, vomiting, and ſpaſmodic affections of the bowels. They require little treatment, except daily ablutions of the ſkin in tepid water, and the warm bath, in caſe of repulſion. 3. S. *Confertus*, tooth-raſh, or rank red gum. 4. S. *Volaticus*, characterized by ſmall circular patches of from ſix to twelve papulæ, which, in about four days, turn brown, and begin to exfoliate. Succeſſive patches often continue to appear at a ſmall diſtance from each other, ſpreading gradually over the face, body, and limbs, for the ſpace of three or four weeks, ſometimes attended with a quick pulſe, white tongue, and fretfulneſs; but often without any appearance of internal diſorder. A gentle emetic, or ſome laxative medicine, followed by decoction of cinchona, is uſeful. 5. S. *Candidus*, conſiſting of large ſhining papulæ, ſucceeds ſome of the acute diſeaſes of infants, but is of ſhort duration.

Gen. II. LICHEN. The term *lichen*, which was originally employed by Hippocrates to expreſs an eruption of papulæ, was uſed by the later Greek authors in a more extenſive and indefinite ſenſe. Pliny, all the tranſlators of the Greek writers, and ſeveral modern authors of credit, have uſed the term impetigo as ſynonymous with lichen; but this is not warranted by the definition of impetigo given by Celſus. By Sauvages, Lorry, Mercurialis, &c. the word lichen has been applied to other eruptions, which have ſtill leſs affinity with the *papular* diſeaſe than with impetigo. In conformity to the original ſenſe of the word, Dr Willan defines lichen "an extenſive eruption of papulæ affecting adults, connected with internal diſorder, uſually terminating in ſcurf, recurrent, not contagious." P. 40. He deſcribes five varieties of it.

1. L.

1. L. *Simplex.* An eruption of papulæ, preceded by symptoms of irritation, commencing on the cheeks and chin, and extending downwards, accompanied with an unpleasant sensation of tingling; the cuticle separates in scurfy scales. Its duration is various. It occurs chiefly in summer and autumn, in weak and irritable habits, attacking women more frequently than men. It passes often into the dry tetter, as was observed by Galen. The diagnosis of this species is sometimes very difficult. It is often mistaken for measles, scarlatina, and other diseases of the order Exanthemata: but by attending to the definitions of *papula* and *exanthema*, which are previously given, Dr W. affirms that such errors may be avoided. It would seem, however, to require an unusual accuracy of *tact* to be able to avoid those errors in all cases, where we are left to this one circumstance of discrimination, that the elevations of the cuticle, which constitute papulæ, are "acuminated;" those which take place in exanthema are "not acuminated," (Vide Def. V. and VI. p. 13.) The most difficult distinction, however, is that of the lichen from scabies, or itch, which the author defers till he comes to treat of the latter in the order of *Pustulæ*.

2. L. *Agrius* is also preceded for several days by febrile symptoms which are often relieved on the appearance of the eruption. The papulæ are distributed in clusters, or large patches, are of a strong red colour, and surrounded by a diffusive inflammation or redness to a considerable extent; and are accompanied with itching heat and a painful tingling. A strong sensation is produced by the heat of the bed, by washing, especially with soap, by great exercise, or by drinking wine. If it be suddenly repelled by improper applications or exposure to cold, a violent disorder of the constitution constantly ensues. By much rubbing or scratching, cracks and ulcerated surfaces are produced, which are not readily healed by medicinal applications. The complaint is usually observed in those who have undergone long-continued fatigue, watching, and anxiety.

3. L. *Pilaris.* A modification of the first species; the papula appearing only at the roots of the hair.

"For the lichen simplex and L. pilaris but little medicinal treatment is necessary. It is sufficient that patients avoid heating themselves by much exercise, or by stimulants, and take a light diet, with mild cooling liquors, and some gentle laxatives occasionally." P. 53. Strong external applications are for the most part improper. "The L. agrius often requires a more active mode of practice. It is useful to give at intervals two or three moderate doses of calomel as a purgative; and afterwards, for some weeks, the vitriolic acid, three times a day, in

the

the infusion of roses, with a decoction of Peruvian bark," P. 54. A mild cooling unguent, such as the rose pomatum, will allay the troublesome heat and itching.

4. L. *Lividus.* So called from the colour of the papulæ. It seems to be a modification of purpura, or petechiæ sine febre. It is readily cured by nourishing food, exercise, bark, with vitriolic acid, or tincture of muriated steel.

An eruption, similar to the L. lividus, often occurs as one of the secondary symptoms of syphilis. In this case, however, the papulæ are smaller, more numerous, and more generally diffused; they seldom become scurfy, never disappear spontaneously, but they assume a pustular form in clusters, and end in ulcerations, only to be healed by a mercurial course.

5. L. *Tropicus*, or prickly heat. A papulous eruption almost universally affecting Europeans settled in tropical climates; of which Dr Willan has given a long account from Dr Winterbottom and others, and from the writings of Bontius, Drs Hillary, Clark, Mosely, and Cleghorn.

The third and last genus of the papulous eruptions Dr W. denominates Prurigo; a term which is employed in the same sense by Pliny, and by Ingrassias, Mercurialis, Hasenreffer, and others. "The symptom of itching," Dr W. observes, "is common, in a greater or less degree, to most diseases of the skin; but there are some cases in which it occurs as the leading circumstance, and is, at the same time, accompanied with an eruption of papulæ, the colour of which scarcely exceeds that of the adjoining cuticle, and, with other appearances, sufficiently particular to constitute a distinct and independent genus of disease." 71. As this is the only definition which the author has given of the genus Prurigo, it is probable that he considers the colour of the papulæ as the most essential characteristic of it, especially in distinguishing it from the preceding genus Lichen. He describes three varieties, which generally affect the whole skin, besides several local varieties.

1. P. *Mitis* is a disease of the spring or beginning of summer, and mostly affects young persons. It is characterized by soft and smooth elevations of the cuticle, somewhat larger than the papulæ of the lichen, retaining the usual colour of the skin, and accompanied, not with tingling, but with an almost incessant itching. When the tops of the papulæ are rubbed off, a clear fluid oozes out of them, and gradually concretes into thin and minute black scabs. In plate VII. we have a very accurate representation of these black spots, surrounded by a circle of red, very much resembling the bites of insects. When persons affected with it neglect washing the skin, or are uncleanly in their apparel,

apparel, the eruption grows more inveterate, and at length, changing its form, often terminates in the itch. Pustules arise among the papulæ, some filled with lymph, others with pus; the acarus scabiei begins to breed in the furrows of the cuticle, and the disorder becomes contagious."

Frequent bathing, or washing with tepid water, persisted in regularly, even though some aggravation of symptoms should at first be occasioned by it, is the simple remedy for this species. When it has become pustular, and lost its original characteristics, the remedies of the itch of course become necessary.

2. P. *Formicans* is much more obstinate and troublesome than the preceding. It affects adults at all seasons, and its duration is from four months to two or three years. The itching is incessant, and almost intolerable, and is complicated with various other sensations. "They sometimes feel as if small insects were creeping on the skin; sometimes as if stung all over with ants; sometimes as if hot needles were piercing the skin in divers places." This complaint is not often obviously connected with a disorder of the stomach, yet it occurs most frequently in those of sallow complexions and weak habits, and seems to be excited by grief, watching, fatigue, and poor diet, as well as by want of cleanliness. It is never, like the former species, converted into the itch, but occasionally terminates in a non-contagious pustular disease, the impetigo. It is commonly, however, confounded with the itch by practitioners, and deemed contagious.

It is extremely difficult to relieve the prurigo formicans either by external or internal remedies; and Dr W. observes, that he has experienced many disappointments from the inefficacy of medicines recommended on the best authority. "Antimonials and preparations of mercury, given separately or combined, produced no beneficial effect; the former, indeed, very generally aggravated the complaint. Neutral salts, and other remedies, administered as diaphoretics, were attended with as little success. The diet-drinks usually employed in cutaneous diseases contributed to allay the troublesome sensation of itching; but as little difference was perceptible in their respective effects, perhaps more may be attributed to the watery vehicle than to the virtues of the impregnating ingredients. Vitriolic acid, sulphur, æthiops mineral, and cinnabar, I tried in a variety of cases for a considerable length of time, without observing any permanent advantage from them.

"Fixed alkali seemed to answer better than any of the above remedies. I employed the natron præparatum of the London Dispensatory, sometimes alone, sometimes in combination with sulphur; at the same time, an infusion of sasafras, or the tops of juniper,

juniper, was drunk freely. Under this course, the disagreeable symptoms were gradually alleviated, and the complaint disappeared in a month or six weeks. The oleum tartari per deliquium, with a small proportion of the tincture of opium added to it, was equally efficacious." P. 81.

Frequent purgatives, Dr W. has generally found to be injurious.

"With regard to external applications, it may be observed that mercurial and sulphureous ointments proved of little service: that decoctions of white hellebore, so much commended by the ancients, were without effect; as also lime-water, or solutions of white vitriol, and corrosive sublimate. It is necessary to keep the skin free from sordes, by frequent washing with warm water. The itching, however, is not always allayed by this means; whence I was induced to employ some of the medicated baths recommended by authors, and observed considerable advantage from those prepared with alkalized sulphur. Sea-bathing also, in some cases, removed the complaint." P. 83.

3. P. *Senilis* differs from the preceding rather in its peculiar inveteracy than in its symptoms. Those who are affected with it in a high degree, the author observes, have little more comfort to expect during life, being incessantly tormented with a violent and universal itching. The state of the skin in the P. senilis is favourable to the production of pediculi, especially of that variety termed body-lice. "Varietas capitis durior, coloratior, vestimentorum laxior, magis cinerea." Linn. They are produced in this disease notwithstanding every attention to cleanliness or regimen, and multiply so rapidly that the patient endures extreme distress from their perpetual irritation.

"The remedies mentioned under the article of P. formicans are of no avail in the present complaint. A warm bath is the only application which allays the itching and irritation; but its effects are, in general, merely temporary. Somewhat more advantage is experienced from baths of warm sea-water, or of the sulphureous waters at Harrowgate, &c. The latter should, at the same time, be taken internally, and, on the whole, I think it may be considered as the best remedy for this complaint with which we are yet acquainted." P. 87.

A long and useful account of some pruriginous affections, which are merely local, follows; as P. podicis, preputii, pubis, pudendi muliebris. On the subject of the latter, Dr W. has inserted an excellent communication from Dr John Sims.

The second number comprises the second ORDER, which is characterized by the appearance of *scales*, arising from a morbid

state

ſtate of the cuticle, and includes four genera, Lepra, Pſoriaſis, Pityriaſis, and Icthyoſis.

The LEPRA, or leproſy of the Greeks, is diſtinguiſhed by "ſcaly patches of different ſizes, but having always nearly a circular form." In this country Dr Willan has obſerved three varieties of it, which he deſignates by the trivial names of *vulgaris*, *alphos*, and *nigricans*; of each of theſe he gives a minute and copious account, of which we can only give a ſlight outline.

1. L. *vulgaris* is characterized by orbicular or oval patches, covered with dry ſcales, and ſurrounded by a red border, which enlarge nearly to the ſize of a crown piece. The eruption is attended with no pain or uneaſineſs, except a ſlight itching, when the patient is become warm in bed, and a tingling from ſudden changes of temperature. It generally commences about the knee or elbow, and gradually extends itſelf, but ſeldom appears except where the bone is neareſt to the ſurface. It often continues for years, and ſometimes for life, not apparently connected with any diſorder of the conſtitution. But a regular mode of diet, with an appropriate medicinal courſe, though it acts very ſlowly on the lepra, will at length accompliſh its cure. The only occaſional cauſes which Dr W. has been able to aſcertain, are, expoſure to cold and moiſture, and the accumulation of ſordes on the ſkin. It is not contagious. The author gives an ample detail of the accounts of this diſeaſe, to be found in the writings of the Greek and Arabian phyſicians.

2. L. *Alphos*. "The ſcaly patches in the alphos are ſmaller than thoſe of the L. vulgaris, and alſo differ from them in having their central part depreſſed or indented:" they do not exceed the ſize of a ſilver penny. This ſpecies ſeldom attacks the trunk of the body, and never appears on the face. It is probably the ſame with the white alphos of the Greeks, and the white morphea of the Arabians. It ſeems to originate from the ſame cauſes as the preceding.

3. L. *nigricans* differs from the L. vulgaris chiefly in the livid colour of the patches, which are nearly the ſame as to form and diſtribution. The ſcales are more eaſily detached than in the other forms of lepra, and the ſurface remains longer excoriated, diſcharging lymph, often with an intermixture of blood, till a new incruſtation forms, which is uſually hard, brittle, and irregular. It was poſſibly compriſed by the ancients under the terms melas and black morphea; though theſe terms ſtrictly expreſs certain appearances of the elephantiaſis.

Dr Willan's obſervations on the remedies of lepra are diſcriminating and uſeful. "Liniments compoſed of tar, or ſome mercurial preparations," he ſays, "are much uſed in the prac-

1 tice

tice of the present times; but frequent bathing or washing is the external remedy most essentially necessary for the two first species of lepra;" especially in the sulphur-waters of Harrowgate, &c. or in baths prepared with a solution of alkalized sulphur and marine salt.

" Bathing in sea-water may be mentioned as a certain auxiliary in the cure of lepra. It is usual, and seems proper, first to use a bath of warm sea-water till the skin be softened, and the scaly incrustations removed; after which a cure is soon obtained, especially in young persons, by bathing in the open sea." But, to prevent a recurrence, this must be persevered in for several summers.

" A simple warm bath, along with moderate friction, likewise contributes to remove the scales, and to produce a soft red skin, which, in time, regains the usual colour and texture. This plan is sufficient, in slighter cases of lepra, without the use of internal remedies. If the disease affect the extremities only, bathing of the whole body is not necessary; it may be enough to apply steam or warm water frequently to the disordered parts.

" Of the mercurial preparations applied externally, a watery insolution of sublimate, and the unguentum hydrargyri nitrati, (Ph. Lond.), seem most efficacious in removing the leprous crusts, and softening the cuticle. I do not, however, think the latter preferable to the tar-ointment which Dr Willis has so justly recommended."

" For the lepra, when confirmed and inveterate, a variety of internal remedies have been employed, or recommended by medical writers, respecting some of which I have had occasion to remark,

" *1st*, That antimonials, sulphur, and nitre, have not alone any considerable efficacy.

" *2dly*, That decoctions of emollient herbs, of guaiacum-wood, sarsaparilla, mezereon, or of elm-bark, which have been recommended as specifics, by no means deserve that character.

" *3dly*, That calomel, hydrargyrus calcinatus, pilulæ hydrargyri, or mercurial frictions applied so as to produce salivation, do not remove the disease. The only preparation of this mineral, which makes any impression upon the lepra, is the sublimate or hydrargyrus muriatus. The spirituous solution of it in small doses, continued for a length of time, will be found very useful; and its operation is promoted by giving, at the same time, an antimonial, and some of the decoctions above mentioned.

" *4thly*, That the nitrous and marine acids, lately recommended in obstinate cutaneous eruptions, have been given in the lepra during three or four successive months, without any manifest advantage. I have often, however, experienced the most beneficial effects in this disease from a medicine of an opposite quality, the caustic alkali, or aqua kali puri of the Dispensatory. The dose of it is about 30 drops, which may be given thrice a-day, in a cupful of any mild fluid."—P. 138, et seq.

Dr W. has seen no advantage from the tinct. of cantharides; but he is of opinion that the tinct. of black hellebore, if the dose be regulated so as not to disorder the bowels, has some efficacy. He introduces a communication from Dr Crichton on the use of the solanum dulcamara in lepra, which is said to have effected a cure, in Dr C.'s practice, of 21 cases in 23. He employed the following decoction:

℞. Stipitum Dulcamaræ unciam i.
Aquæ puræ libram iss. decoque ad libram i.; et liquorem frigefactum cola.

Dr Crichton ordered two ounces of this decoction every morning, noon, and evening; but afterwards increased the quantity, till the pint was consumed daily.

"None of the remedies above mentioned are applicable to the cure of the lepra nigricans. This form of the disease requires, in the first place, a regular and nutritive plan of diet, with moderate exercise: it may be afterwards wholly removed by the use of bark, and the mineral acids, sea-bathing," &c.

The second genus of this order is the Psoriasis, dry or scaly tetter. The Greek physicians have described two different diseases under the title of Psora, viz. ψωρα ἑλκωδης, ulcerated Psora, and ψωρα simply, or sometimes leprous Psora, which is a scaly disease. Dr Willan refers the former to the pustular order (gen. impetigo), and adopts the term Psoriasis for the scaly Psora. "The disease to be thus entitled is characterized by a rough and scaly state of the cuticle, sometimes continuous, sometimes in separate patches of various sizes, but of an irregular figure, and, for the most part, accompanied with rhagades or fissures in the skin. From the lepra it may be distinguished, not only by the different form and distribution of the patches, as formerly stated from the Greek writers, but also by its cessation and recurrence at certain seasons, and by the disorder of the constitution with which it is usually attended." It is synonymous with the Psora or Scabies sicca of Mercurialis, Platerus, Hafenreffer, Etmuller, and Hoffmann; and with the impetigo of Sennertus, Willis, Lommius, Plenck, &c. Dr Willan describes several striking varieties of the Psoriasis, which, however, he observes, might be all comprised in a connected detail; these are P. *guttata*, *diffusa*, *gyrata*, *palmaria*, *labialis*, *infantilis*, and *inveterata*.

 The

The baker's itch, and a similar eruption peculiar to washerwomen, rank under P. diffusa.

The scaly tetter is not contagious in any of its forms. It is most frequently seen in sanguineo-melancholic habits, and sometimes is connected or alternates with arthritic complaints, as was remarked by Galen. The circumstances to which patients have generally referred the complaint are, eating too great a quantity of acid fruits, food of difficult digestion, or some improper mixtures of food, as of milk and fish, the unseasonable use of the cold bath, and large draughts of cold water taken when the body has been heated by exercise. Dr Falconer, "whose observations on the lepra Græcorum are more directly applicable to the present disorder," affirms that he has been able, in numerous instances, to trace the cause of these eruptions to the last-mentioned circumstance.

The psoriasis is one of the most frequent cutaneous diseases in this kingdom; and Dr Willan acknowledges with Willis, that it is sometimes a disease of unconquerable obstinacy. With respect to the treatment recommended by Dr Willis, the author observes, *1st*, That bleeding and purgations are seldom admissible; *2d*, That antiscorbutics, as they have been called, are not of any material use; *3d*, That decoctions of guaiacum, sarsaparilla, &c. cannot alone be depended upon for the cure of psoriasis, but are useful auxiliaries to other medicines in some stages of the P. diffusa, palmaria, and inveterata; *4th*, That the chalybeate waters, which have been called specifics, do not seem to be more efficacious than the sulphureous waters; *5th*, That chalybeate medicines, especially ferrum præcipitatum, are perhaps occasionally useful where the eruptions occur in chlorotic habits; and, *6th*, From many experiments cautiously made, he is assured, that *mercurial preparations eventually rather aggravate than diminish the complaint:* an important observation, considering the indiscriminate use which is made of mercury for diseases of the skin.

"The three first species of Psoriasis, (viz. P. guttata, diffusa, and gyrata), when they appear in a sudden eruption, attended with febrile symptoms, may be advantageously treated by administering in the evening an emetic dose of ipecacuanha, and the following day two or three grains of calomel, or some other gentle purgative; afterwards by the use of fixed alkali, either in its concrete or liquid form, by a light moderate diet, by frequently washing with tepid water, and by abstinence from fruits, acids, and fermented liquors, the above disorders may be brought to a conclusion within two or three weeks. But should the scaly patches, through neglect at their first appearance, or from an unhealthy state of the constitution, have enlarged

ged confiderably, and fpread over the greater part of the body, a more elaborate plan will be neceffary. This confifts of the free ufe of antimonials, of the warm bath, with repeated friction, and of the mineral waters formerly mentioned. The decoctions of elm-bark, farfaparilla, dulcamara, &c. have alfo their fhare of utility.

"The P. inveterata requires the fame plan of treatment as the lepra vulgaris and alphos. A portion of mezereon root forms an active ingredient in the decoctions employed for the cure of thefe diforders."

In the P. palmaria, Dr W. recommends the ufe of oiled filk gloves, to be worn during the night, and as much as poffible during the day; the internal remedies being alfo employed. In the P. labialis, the lips fhould be almoft conftantly covered with fome mild unguent or plaifter: all acrid applications are detrimental.

Several fyphilitic eruptions affume the forms of lepra and pforiafis, of which good reprefentations will be found in the coloured engravings.

The third genus, Pityriasis, is a difeafe of little confequence, but fhould be known, becaufe it has been miftaken for a fyphilitic eruption, in confequence of its brown colour. It confifts of irregular patches of fmall thin fcales, which repeatedly form and feparate, but never collect into crufts, nor are attended with rednefs or inflammation, as in the lepra and fcaly tetter. No remedy is decifively beneficial. Its caufes are unknown. It fometimes continues for five or fix years.

The remaining genus, Icthyosis, or fifh-fkin eruption, is a rare difeafe, and its caufes and cure feem to be equally unknown. It is characterized by "a permanently harfh, dry, fcaly, and, in fome cafes, almoft horny texture of the integuments of the body, unconnected with internal diforder." The author relates or refers to a few cafes given by other writers.—See Philof. Tranfact. N° 424, and the fequel, vol. 49th, for 1755.

Under the denomination of icthyofis *cornea*, he defcribes fome cafes of horny rigidity of the integuments, or horny excrefcences, which have been faid to appear on different parts of the body. See Phil. Tranf. vol. 48th, part 2. p. 580.; and an account of a girl, whofe body was nearly covered with horny excrefcences, *ibid.* N° 176. It may be added, that a horn fimilar to thofe here defcribed, and a drawing of the woman on whom it grew, are preferved in the Britifh Mufeum.

Twelve excellent coloured engravings are given to illuftrate the difeafes of this order.

Having extended our analyfis of the preceding orders to a

great length, we ſhall be compelled to contract our account of the firſt part of Order III. which has lately appeared. It includes only the two firſt genera, meaſles and ſcarlet fever.

I. Rubeola, or Meaſles. Dr Willan gives an ample and accurate account of the progreſſive ſymptoms of meaſles, of which he deſcribes three varieties, R. vulgaris, R. ſine catarrho, and R. nigra. When the diſeaſe is epidemical, he obſerves, a few caſes occur in which the eruption goes through its different ſtages, without any cough, difficulty of breathing, or inflammation of the eyes; without much alteration in the pulſe, or any febrile ſymptoms. This variety of the complaint does not ſeem to emancipate the conſtitution from the power of the contagion, nor to prevent the acceſſion of the rubeola vulgaris at a future period. It is not eaſy, he adds, to collect from authors, who have mentioned ſome recurrence of the meaſles, under what circumſtances it happened. But, after an attentive obſervation of more than twenty years, he has never met with any individual who had the febrile rubeola twice.—See the author's Reports on Diſeaſes in London, p. 106. and 207.) With repect to R. nigra, he ſays, "I never ſaw the R. vulgaris intermixed at an early period with petechiæ; but it ſometimes happens, about the 7th or 8th day, that the ruſh becomes ſuddenly black, or of a dark purple colour, with a mixture of yellow, (repreſented by a plate). This appearance has continued ten days, and in ſome caſes longer, without much diſtreſs to the patient." Dr W. ſubjoins ſome ſatisfactory obſervations relative to the "putrid meaſles," deſcribed by Sir William Watſon (Med. Obſ. vol. iv.), as having occurred at the Foundling Hoſpital in 1763 and 1768. From the evidence which he adduces, as well as from the ſymptoms enumerated by Dr Watſon, and from the names which he at different times applied to the diſeaſe in the hoſpital-books, as from the accounts of contemporary writers, it is obvious that theſe epidemics were the ſcarlatina anginoſa or Maligna. Sir William refers them to the morbilli maligni or epidemii of Morton. But Morton maintained expreſsly that the meaſles and ſcarlatina are the ſame diſeaſe.

II. Scarlatina. To this diſeaſe, which was, during the ſpace of two centuries, the moſt fatal epidemic of Europe, and which has been the ſubject of much diſcuſſion, under an infinity of names, Dr Willan has appropriated nearly three-fourths of the *Part* before us. He has given a full and minute account of all the regular and anomalous appearances connected with the diſeaſe in its different forms, and has traced its progreſs through the different countries of Europe, in which it has ſucceſſively raged, with much reſearch and diſcrimination, amid the confuſion fion of titles under which it has been defcribed. Of its origin, as of that of the meafles, no trace is to be found in the writings of phyficians. The fymptoms of fcarlatina maligna, indeed, do not feem to differ materially from the "peftilential ulcers of the tonfils," defcribed by ancient authors, as peculiar to Egypt and Syria. Rhazes and others obferve that meafles of a highly red colour are more dangerous than thofe which are moderately red. But Ingraffia, a Neapolitan writer, is the firft author of modern times who has defcribed the fcarlatina. (See his Treatife de Tumoribus Præter. Nat.) The difeafe was known at Naples before the year 1500 by the name of Rofalia. A Dutch phyfician has defcribed a contagious fore throat, which raged near Amfterdam in 1517.—A fimilar complaint fpread through Lower Germany in 1564-5, and was epidemical in Paris a few years after. The garrotillo of the Spaniards, which was very deftructive during forty years in the fixteenth and feventeenth centuries appears to have been a variety of fcarlatina. It was afterwards, feveral fucceffive times, at Leipfic, and other places on the continent, defcribed as a new difeafe under different denominations. Sydenham and Morton firft treated of it in England. It is mentioned by Sir Robert Sibbald, in 1680, as having lately appeared at Edinburgh. In the Edinburgh Medical Effays, vol. iii. p. 27. it is defcribed, under the proper terms "fcarlet fever and angina," as an epidemic in 1733. Huxham defcribes it, as a "febris anginofa," 1734, and fubfequently, "febris miliaris rubra," febris anginofa miliaris," &c. The modern accounts of it, fince the time of Dr Fothergill and Dr Cotton, are well known. Dr Willan concludes his very complete literary hiftory of the difeafe with this inference, "That no Britifh author has yet defcribed any epidemical and contagious fore throat, except that which attends the fcarlet fever."

The author defcribes three varieties of fcarlatina; 1. S. *fimplex*, 2. S. *anginofa*, and 3. S. *maligna*. He mentions alfo a fourth form of the difeafe, viz. the fcarlet ulcerating fore throat, without any efflorefcence on the fkin. "It is truly fingular," he obferves, "that the flighteft of all eruptive fevers, and the moft violent, the moft fatal difeafe known in this country, fhould rank together, and fpring from the fame origin; but experience decides that thefe are merely varieties of one difeafe." P. 281. The author's experience alfo tends to confirm another practical inference, that fcarlet fever never attacks the fame individual twice. Among two thoufand patients, whom he has vifited in it, he never faw fuch a repetition. Dr Withering, it may be added, "believed it to be as great an improbability as a repetition of the fmall-pox."

We cannot at present follow the author in his description of the variety of appearances belonging to the different forms of the disease. His account of the diagnostic marks of the efflorescence in scarlatina and measles is particularly worthy of attention. "It is much more full and spreading in the former disease than in the latter, and consists of innumerable points and specks under the cuticle, intermixed with minute papulæ, in some cases forming continuous, irregular patches, in others coalescing into an uniform flush over a considerable extent of surface. In the measles the rush is composed of circular dots partly distinct, partly set in small clusters or patches, and a little elevated, so as to give the sensation of roughness when a finger is passed over them. These patches are seldom confluent, but form a number of crescents or segments of circles, with large intervening portions of cuticle, which retain their usual appearance. The colour of the rash is also different in the two diseases, being a vivid red in the scarlatina, like that of a boiled lobster's shell; but in the measles a dark red, with nearly the hue of a raspberry." P. 260.

In the simple scarlatina, without any affection of the throat, moderate and equable temperature, with light diet and cooling drink, seems to be all that is necessary for its cure.

In the S. anginosa Dr W. recommends the early use of emetics, but has not found it necessary to repeat them so often as Dr Withering has advised. He condemns any endeavour to excite perspiration during the first six days of the disease by antimonials, camphor, aromatics, &c. Before the decline of the efflorescence "they not only fail to produce their usual effect, but often increase the heat, anxiety, and restlessness, they were intended to relieve." It has been ascertained, indeed, by Dr Currie, that where the heat of the skin is much greater than natural) and in scarlet fever it rises higher than in any other disease) the only effectual mode of exciting perspiration, is to *reduce* the external temperature by cool or cold applications. Hence the rapid and salutary effects of the cold affusion. But this practice has not been resorted to in this disease in London. We are happy, however, to find that, during the last autumn, when 52 boys and 19 girls were attacked with scarlatina in the Foundling Hospital, Dr Stanger had recourse to washing with cold water and vinegar. "Most of the patients were repeatedly washed with cold water and vinegar mixed in about equal proportions. Its effects in cooling the skin, diminishing the frequency of the pulse, abating thirst, and disposing to sleep, were very remarkable. Finding this application so highly beneficial," Dr Stanger adds, "I employed it at every period of the fever, provided the skin were hot and dry."

Dr

Dr Willan and Dr Stanger have both lately uſed the oxygenated muriatic acid, which appears to them to be very ſalutary. The doſe for adults is half a drachm by meaſure, for children 10 or 12 drops. Care ſhould be taken that it be accurately prepared. Dr Willan quotes Dr Sims for the uſe of vitriolic acid, and Dr Withering for the uſe of diuretic medicines, eſpecially fixed alkali; but he ſubjoins no opinion reſpecting theſe deduced from his own practice. At the decline of the efflorefcence, if the fever alſo declines, and is not ſucceeded by a cough, Peruvian bark, mineral acids, wine, and nutritious diet, obviate the debility, and contribute to prevent the acceſſion of dropſy. The nitrous fumigation is preferred to ſharp gargles for keeping the throat clean in the more malignant ſpecies. Bliſters are here detrimental, and the cold affuſion inapplicable. Early emetics are adviſed, and cordials, bark, and wine, as the diſeaſe advances.

Dr W. concludes with ſome uſeful obſervations on the neceſſity and importance of adopting and enforcing proper meaſures for preventing the ſpreading of this diſeaſe.

We have been thus ample in our analyſis of this original work, from a conviction of the neceſſity of reſorting to ſome common ſtandard of arrangement and nomenclature in cultivating a knowledge of this tribe of diſeaſes, and from a belief that this ſyſtem is well adapted to that end. It is equally diſtinguiſhed for accuracy and originality of obſervation, as for learning and reſearch. In the practical application of it, indeed, much difficulty will be found; but this ariſes, perhaps, more from the nature of the morbid appearances in queſtion, than from over-refinement in the arrangement before us: and to be accurate in the practical diſcrimination of thoſe appearances will require, at any rate, much habit, and a greater nicety of obſervation than the majority of practitioners are accuſtomed to employ. It is to be regretted that the work proceeds ſo tardily. The plates, which, in the parts already publiſhed, are 24 in number, are excellent ſpecimens of the facility of conveying accurate notions of cutaneous eruptions by the pencil.

II.

II.

A Treatise on Febrile Diseases, including Intermitting, Remitting, and Continued Fevers; Eruptive Fever; Inflammations; Hemorrhagies; and the Profluvia; in which an attempt is made to present, at one View, whatever, in the present State of Medicine, it is requisite for the Physician to know respecting the Symptoms, Causes, and Cure of those Diseases. By ALEXANDER-PHILIPS WILSON, M. D. F. R. S. Ed. Physician to the County Hospital at Winchester, Fellow of the Royal College of Physicians, Edinburgh. 4 vols. 8vo. Winchester, 1799, 1800, 1801, 1804.

THESE volumes are the result of several years application, preparatory to a course of lectures on Febrile Diseases, which the author delivered in Edinburgh in the summer of 1796. An infirm state of health having obliged him to discontinue them, he conceived that his labours might still be rendered useful to others, by filling up a deficiency in the medical literature of this country, the want of a complete treatise on febrile diseases, in which every fact known with regard to them should be collected and systematically arranged. To preclude the necessity of consulting original writers on these diseases, is accordingly the avowed object of this work, and, in a great measure, it is adapted to attain this purpose. In another point of view, it must be considered as an useful index to those practical authors whose writings are to be found in this country; and although we must regret that he has not taken advantage of the industry and abilities of a Hufeland and a Reil, who have trodden nearly the same path, it would be uncandid not to state that he seems to have neglected no source of information to which he probably had access. If Dr Wilson had contented himself with merely increasing the value of a favourite systematic author by a farther accumulation of facts, we should have thought our duty discharged by allowing him the credit due to his industry; but he claims more particular attention by the peculiarity of their arrangement, the original views which he takes of them, his investigations of their relative importance, and the proposed improvement of their classification.

Of a work of such extent as the present we cannot attempt any detailed analysis, and shall therefore chiefly confine ourselves to to some observations on the general conclusions which he has deduced from the examination of so many facts, and more particularly to his nosological arrangement; for perfectly do we agree with our author in his reply to those who had censured him for ascribing too much importance to nosology.

"Let those who slight the labours of the nosologist recollect that it is his province to point out the symptoms which distinguish one disease from another, and to arrange diseases in such a way as may best show their affinity, and consequently assist the memory in recollecting their modes of treatment. The anatomist detects the changes induced by internal diseases; but of what use would this knowledge prove, did not the nosologist point out the means of ascertaining the presence of such morbid states previous to death. In vain might the chemist and botanist supply us with medicines, did not the nosologist enable us to distinguish the cases in which they are useful.

"By far the greater number of mistakes I have witnessed in practice have originated from the neglect of nosology. It often happens that an opinion, at first maintained on no other account than its singularity, becomes current among those who are unable, or will not be at the trouble, to think for themselves. Many exclaim against nosology, but cannot tell why. The truth is, an accurate knowledge of it is acquired with difficulty, and the indolent are glad of an apology for neglecting it altogether."

So far do we differ from our brother critics, that we are inclined to blame Dr Wilson for having disappointed us, by relinquishing his original philosophic plan of concluding his work with a detailed view of the nosology of febrile diseases.

We cannot enumerate the contents of these volumes in a manner more advantageous to our readers than by transcribing his arrangement and definitions of febrile diseases.

ARRANGEMENT OF FEBRILE DISEASES.

CLASS I.—*FEBRES IDIOPATICÆ.*

"Prægressis languore, lassitudine, et aliis debilitatis signis, pulsus frequens, calor auctus, sine morbo locali primario.

ORDO I.—*FEBRES INTERMITTENTES ET REMITTENTES.*

"Febres idiopathicæ, paroxysmis pluribus, apyrexiâ, saltem remissione evidente, interpositâ, cum exacerbatione notabili, et plerumque cum horrore redeuntibus, constantes.

"SPECIES 1. *Tertiana.*—2. *Quartana.*—3. *Quotidiana.*

ORDO II.—*FEBRES CONTINUÆ.*

"Febres idiopathicæ, sine intermissione, sed cum remissionibus et exacerbationibus, parum licet notabilibus, perstantes.

SPECIES

Species 1.—*Synocha.*

"Calor plurimum auctus, pulsus frequens, validus, et durus, urina rubra, sensorii functiones parum turbatæ.

Species 2.—*Typhus.*

"Morbus contagiosus, calor parum auctus, pulsus parvus debilis, plerumque frequens, urina parum mutata, sensorii functiones plurimum turbatæ, vires multum imminutæ.

Species 3.—*Synochus.*

"Morbus contagiosus, febris ex synochâ et typho composita; initio synocha, progressu, et versus finem, typhus.

"*Varietas 1ma. Synochus Simplex.—2da. Synochus Petechialis.—3tia. Synochus Miliaris.—4ta. Synochus Aphthosus.—5ta. Synochus Erysipelatosus.—6ta. Synochus Vesicularis.*

ORDO III.—*EXANTHEMATA.*

"Morbi contagiosi, cum febre idiopathica incipientes; definito tempore, apparent papulæ, sæpe plures, exiguæ, per cutem sparsæ.

"Species 1. *Variola.*—2. *Varicella.*—3. *Rubeola.*—4. *Scarlatina.* 5. *Pestis.*—6. *Urticaria.*

CLASS. II.—*FEBRES SYMPTOMATICÆ.*

"Morbi locales primarii, calore aucto, pulsu frequente.

ORDO I.—*PHLEGMASIÆ.*

"Febres symptomaticæ, pulsu duro; quibus est pro morbo locali, vel inflammatio externa, vel dolor topicus simul læsâ partis internæ functione.

"Species 1. *Phlogosis.*—2. *Ophthalmia.*—3. *Phrenitis.*—4. *Cynanche.*—5. *Pneumonia.*—6. *Carditis.*—7. *Peritonitis.*—8. *Gastritis.*—9. *Enteritis*—10. *Hepatitis*—11. *Splenitis.*—12. *Nephritis.*—13. *Cystitis.*—14. *Hysteritis.*—15. *Rheumatismus.*—16. *Odontalgia.*—17. *Podagra.*—18. *Arthropuosis.*

ORDO II.—*HÆMORRHAGIÆ.*

"Febres symptomaticæ, quibus est pro morbo locali, sanguinis profusio absque vi externa.

"Species 1. *Epistaxis.*—2. *Hemoptysis.*—3. *Hemorrhois.*—4. *Menorrhagia.*—5. *Hæmatemesis.*—6. *Hæmaturia.*

ORDO III.—*PROFLUVIA.*

"Febres symptomaticæ, quibus est pro morbo locali, excretio aucta naturaliter non sanguinea.

"Species 1. *Catarrhus.*—2. *Dysenteria.*

The intelligent reader will readily perceive wherein Dr Wilson's arrangement differs from Dr Cullen's, and in the introduction

tion he has given the reasons why he considers these differences as improvements. On many occasions this actually seems to be the case, but on others it is by no means so evident. Even the propriety of his primary division of fevers into idiopathic and symptomatic may be doubted on account of the difficulty of ascertaining in practice to which of these classes particular instances are to be referred, more especially as the distinctive characters given of them by Dr Wilson do not universally apply. According to him, in the one set of diseases, the fever is the primary complaint, in the other it is the consequence of some local affection; in the one the fever is not at all proportioned to the local affection, in the other it is, and varies in kind as the local affection varies; and in the one the treatment is conducted upon different principles from what it is in the other. The last character drawn from the difference in the treatment would be of importance in framing natural families of diseases, but is inadmissible in artificial systems, contrived for the purpose of recognising diseases previous to their treatment. The two other differences would, however, be sufficient to distinguish them, if they were constant, and always capable of being ascertained; but, if we were disposed to cavil, we might object to Dr Wilson's arrangement, as excluding from the exanthematous diseases inoculated small-pox and cow-pock, in both of which the local affection precedes and is the cause of the fever. But other difficulties attending this division of fevers have not escaped Dr Wilson himself. Thus, when treating of inflammations, he observes, that inflammation may be combined with fever in three ways: the inflammation may supervene on the fever, as in the exanthemata; the fever may be produced by the inflammation, as in the true phlegmasiæ; or a phlegmasia, that is, an inflammation with the fever occasioned by it, may supervene on simple fever. In the last case, the fever precedes the phlegmasia a considerable time, and the first is, according to Dr Wilson, readily distinguished by the appearance of the inflammation not aggravating the fever; but when the phlegmasia supervenes soon after the commencement of the fever, the diagnosis our author confesses to be difficult.

"The truth is, that, in the true phlegmasiæ, both sets of symptoms, especially if the seat of the inflammation be internal, appear together. It is impossible to say which appear first, and it is evident, that if any degree of the local affection produces a corresponding degree of fever, the one cannot appear unattended by the other

"But, if such is the case, it may be asked, How do we determine which is the primary affection? To this question the following circumstances readily afford an answer. The causes which induce fever do do not at the same time induce inflammation. In 19 cases out of 20 inflammation does not supervene on fever, and when it does, it generally arrives from causes different from those which induced the fever. But if, on the other hand, inflammation, that is, such as attends the phlegmasiæ, be excited, fever is the constant attendant, and its degree is proportioned to that of the local affection.

" Besides, as we succeed by local remedies in relieving the inflammation, we find that in precisely the same degree the febrile symptoms abate. If the inflammation be not terminated by resolution, but run on to some of the other termination, the febrile symptoms are still found to correspond exactly to the changes which take place in the local affection; and so constant is this correspondence, that we can determine, from the state of the febrile symptoms alone, in what way the inflammation is terminating, although the termination be induced by means whose action is wholly confined to the inflamed part.

" If, then, fever is not necessarily attended with the inflammations which appear in the phlegmasiæ, if such inflamations are universally attended with fever, the degree and state of the inflammation regulating those of the febrile symptoms, the conclusion is, that in the phlegmasiæ (and the same mode of reasoning applies to the other symptomatic fevers) the local affection is the primary complaint."

But if the difficulty be thus great in forming the diagnosis of inflammations, it is still greater with regard to hemorrhagies and the profluvia, in which the fever not only precedes the local affection, but is so far from being induced by it, that, in the case of hemorrhagies, it is removed by it; or, to use the words of our author, " when the fever has been considerable, it generally continues till the blood ceases, or nearly ceases, to flow." But although we do not, in the present state of our knowledge, approve of making so ambiguous a character the basis of his primary division of febrile diseases, still many of his observations connected with the inquiry are ingenious, and his remarks on the propriety of proceeding in a systematic arrangement from the simple to the compound diseases, appear to be well founded.

The first volume contains the intermittent and remitting fevers. When treating of the proximate cause of fever, Dr Wilson gives an abstract of the Brunonian doctrine, to which he seems, to us, to allow more merit than is consistent with the numerous contradictions and imperfections he has pointed out in it. But having lately stated our sentiments on this subject, we shall not now resume it, farther than by requesting our readers to contrast Dr Brown's genuine doctrine with the following, which, in our opinion, is erroneously said to be a modification and improvement of it by Dr Wilson.

RECAPITULATION.

" I.—*Excitability* is that quality of the living solid which distinguishes living from dead matter.

" II.—*Excitement* is a ſtate of activity.

" III.—*Atony* is a ſtate of inactivity, that is, of debility, in which every part of the ſyſtem is preternaturally ſenſible to the action of ſome agents, and preternaturally inſenſible to that of others; and watchfulneſs is the conſequence.

" IV.—*Agent* is any thing capable of occaſioning a change in the ſtate of the living ſolid.

" V.—Agents are either *Stimuli* or Atonics.

" VI.—*Stimuli* are thoſe agents which produce excitement.

" VII.—Excitement is either *moderate* or *exceſſive*.

" VIII.—*Moderate excitement* is that which is followed by *Exhauſtion*.

" IX.—*Exhauſtion* is a ſtate of inactivity, that is, of debility, in which thoſe parts of the ſyſtem on which the animal functions depend become uniformly leſs ſenſible to the action of all agents; and ſleep, that is, a ſuſpenſion of the animal functions, is the conſequence *.

" X.—*Exceſſive excitement* (VII.) is that which is followed by atony. (III.)

" XI.—*Atonics* are thoſe agents (V.) which produce atony.

" XII.—The ſyſtem in general is either in a ſtate of *health* or *diſeaſe*. Prediſpoſition to general diſeaſe is a ſtate that cannot be defined.

" XIII.—*Health* is either a ſtate of moderate excitement (VIII.) or exhauſtion. (IX.)

" XIV.—*General diſeaſe* is either a ſtate of exceſſive excitement (X.) or atony. (III.)

" XV.—Atony is to be removed by induc ng moderate excitement.

" XVI.—Exceſſive excitement is to be remored by changing exceſſive into moderate excitement.

" XVII.—General diſeaſe includes infinite varieties, from the greateſt exceſs of excitement to the extreme of debility.

" XVIII.—Simple fever is the only general diſeaſe, and may be defined, Exceſſive excitement or debility of all the functions, without any local affection.

" XIX.—All other diſeaſes are either local, or general and local.

" XX.—The laws of excitability are changed in fever. This change is ſufficient to account for the phenomena eſſential to fever, without ſuppoſing any change induced on the fluids.

XXI.—The proximate cauſe of fever, therefore, is a change in the laws of excitability; in conſequence of which, the ſame agents no longer produce the ſame effects.

" XXII.—In ſimple fever, then, there are only two indications of cure; the one to moderate excitement, the other to remove atony. (XV. XVI.)"

The

* " The sleep which is not the effect of and proportioned to the preceding excitement is not natural, and is the consequence of a morbid affection of the brain. It is a local disease, produced by compression, by various substances applied to the brain, such as opium, tobacco," &c.

" Debilitatem absolutam vocamus eam realem vigoris canalium, et solidorum imminutionem ; relative autem debilia fieri solida alicujus partis intelligimus, cum crescente sanguinis impetu, et in eadem ratione crescente solidorum aliarum partium vigore, in canalibus, et solidis ejus partis vigor solitus remanet, qui idcirco aucto sanguinis momento resistere nequit.

" *Prop.* III.—Data eadem partis cujusdam debilitate, non solum coacervatio, et semistagnatio sanguinis fiet in ipsius partis sanguineis vasculis, ut demonstratum est, verum etiam canales laterales lymphaticos, et adiposos ipsius partis sanguis ingredi debet.

" *Prop.* IV.—Ex majori collectione sanguinis in vasculis sanguineis alicujus partis, et ex ingressu ipsius in canales tam lymphaticos quam adiposos, et ex ejusdem sanguinis per ipsos, atque sanguineos canales lentissimo motu inflammatio morbosa in eadem parte oriri potest.

" *Prop.* V.—Ex majori sanguinis in parte quacumque inflammatione, inflammatio pinguedinis circumpositæ, et in ea parte existentis, exorietur.

" *Prop.* VI.—Ex enata inflammatione in aliqua humani corporis parte major sanguinis, et humorum quantitas in eamdem partem influit, atque ideo tumor necessario major fieri debet."

We have given the demonstration of his first proposition as an example of his manner, while the enunciation of the others will serve to exhibit his theory in all its parts. If any one object to the absurdity of the chemical opinions involved in it, it must be remembered that Vacca wrote in 1765 ; and to show that his theory was not an idle hypothesis, but led to a rational and approved method of cure, we must request our readers' indulgence while we make one more quotation.

" Si humores inflammata parte collecti, et effusi quiescentes diu maneant, corrumpuntur, et suppurationem vel gangrænam producunt, aut durescunt, et scirrhus supervenit. Ut igitur ea mala evitentur, necesse est ut fluida stagnantia resorbeantur, et circulatorio motu rursus in gyrum circumagantur. Quod ut fiat, vigor partis inflammatæ solidis reddi debet ; cum jam demonstraverimus, stagnationes inflammatorias ex partis ipsius debilitate nasci. Vigor partis inflammatæ augeri potest, vel immediate et directe, vel indirecte et mediate. Immediate augetur applicando eidem parti medicamenta roborantia. Indirecte autem roborantur partes, vim, qua fluida contra ipsas agunt, infringendo."

The profluvia and hemorrhagies, together with phthisis pulmonalis, do not occupy one-half of the fourth volume ; but our author has altogether omitted the genus of catarrh, if we except the very slight notice taken of it in the preface. The reasons he has advanced for this omission are quite unsatisfactory. The want of an accurate history of epidemic catarrh especially constitutes

ſtitutes a real and important defect in the work; and although it might be adviſable to compriſe the whole in four volumes, that object ought to have been attained by condenſing every article more or leſs, and not by paſſing over any altogether in ſilence. But even this condenſation, although our author's ſtyle would have permitted it to be very conſiderable, with great advantage to the work, was not abſolutely neceſſary, for ſufficient room would have been gained by the omiſſion of the appendixes to the third and fourth volumes, conſiſting of our author's experimental inquiries into the circumſtances influencing the urinary depoſitions which appear in febrile diſeaſes, and into the manner in which tobacco and opium act on the living animal body. That theſe inquiries are important and highly creditable to Dr Wilſon's ingenuity and talents is unqueſtionable, but we conſider them as altogether miſplaced in the preſent work. Had they been original, they ought to have been publiſhed as ſeparate eſſays; but they have been before the public for ſeveral years, and are in the hands of many of our author's readers, and therefore, in a compilation like the preſent, in which the ſpace allotted to each article ſhould be nearly in proportion to its relative importance, they ought to have been merely referred to, or their general reſults extracted in the ſame manner as the publiſhed experiments of any other author. From experience we know how difficult it is to avoid typographical errors, but we cannot conclude our remarks without expreſſing our regret at their frequent occurrence in theſe volumes. As a whole, however, this work does infinite credit to the induſtry and judgment of Dr Wilſon, and we ſhall rejoice if a ſecond edition ſhould give him an opportunity of ſupplying the deficiencies, and correcting the errors, which ſomewhat detract from its merit.

III.

The Modern Practice of Phyſic. By EDWARD GOODMAN CLARKE, M. D. Author of the Medicinæ Praxeos Compendium; of the Royal College of Phyſicians, London, and Phyſician to the Forces, &c. &c. 454 pp. 8vo. London. 1805.

WITH the crowd of compendiums, epitomes, and manuals, written to ſatiſfy the preſent taſte for acquiring ſuperficial knowledge without much trouble, the volume before us is ſcarcely to be confounded. In many reſpects it reſembles the author's Medicinæ Praxeos Compendium, but in a form conſiderably

derably enlarged. To the character of each disease, from Cullen's Nosology, are added the symptoms, causes, diagnosis, prognosis, and most improved method of treatment, written in a plain and perspicuous style; and while our author's former work will still continue to be a favourite with candidates for medical degrees, this will probably become popular with another class of readers.

IV.

The Edinburgh Practice of Physic, Surgery, and Midwifery: preceded by an Abstract of the Theory of Medicine, and the Nosology of Dr Cullen; *and including upwards of six hundred Authentic Formulæ, from the Books of St Bartholomew's, St George's, St Thomas's, Guy's, and other Hospitals in London, and from the Lectures and Writings of the most eminent Public Teachers. With 20 quarto Plates.* A new edition, in five vols. Vol. I. and II. Medicine; III. and IV. Surgery; and V. Midwifery. 8vo. London. 1803.

This work, voluminous as it is, will not detain us long; but we think it our duty to expose the manner in which it has been manufactured. The first edition of this *Edinburgh* Practice consisted of *London* formulæ subjoined to the articles Medicine, Surgery, and Midwifery, reprinted from the third edition of the Encyclopedia Britannica. In this state it formed one volume, and was a cheap, useful, and consistent system. But the speculation having succeeded, the publishers have thought proper, with the view of increasing their profits fivefold, to swell out to five volumes a systematic work, originally compendious, by awkwardly interpolating detailed cases, and long extracts from diffuse writers, and have thereby converted it into an expensive, comparatively useless, and incongruous compilation.

The whole performance, as it now stands, is beneath criticism; but there is one misrepresentation in the preface which we cannot suffer to pass in silence. It is there falsely insinuated, for good reasons, no doubt, that Dr Monro was the author of the article Medicine so unblushingly plagiarised from the Encyclopedia Britannica. This misrepresentation is perfectly inexcusable, as the article is not anonymous.

V.

V. & VI.

Osservazioni Mediche sulla Malattie Febrile dominante in Livorno, per servire d'Istruzioni ai Signori Medici destinati al servizio del nuovo Spedale provisorio di S. Jacopo. Del Dottore GAETANO PALLONI, Prof. onorario dell' Universita di Pisa, e Medico commissionato dal Regio Governo d' Etruria presso la Deputazione di Sanitá di detta Citta. 8vo. Livorno. 1804.

Parere Medico sulla Malattia Febrile che ha dominato nella Citta di Livorno, l'Anno M,DCC,CIV. Del Dottore GAETANO PALLONI, &c. 12mo. Livorno. Avrile, 1805.

WHILE the medical philosophers of the new world ascribe the fever which depopulates their cities to local causes, and deprecate the idea that it can be exported in their ships, we have lately seen kindred epidemics for the first time visit the shores of Spain, and of the Mediterranean. The subject is too interesting to us, to our colonies, and to our commerce, not to excite us to seek with avidity every information which may enable us to prevent the introduction of such a calamity into these kingdoms, of recognising it when introduced, and of checking its progress. It was, therefore, with the most heartfelt gratitude, that, from the zeal of the learned Fabbroni of Florence, we received these interesting memoirs; and we cannot better express our opinion of the value of the gift, than by communicating to our readers, and to the nation at large, the greater part of their contents, without presuming to intermix them with any of our opinions.

The first of these pamphlets was written, during the prevalence of the fever, for the instruction of the physicians appointed to attend a provisionary hospital, the second after the health of the city was restored; and both may be considered as official documents, constituting the most perfect history we yet possess of any of the late epidemics of the south of Europe.

SYMPTOMS OF THE DISEASE.

From the most perfect state of health, without any or a very slight predisposition, the patient is surprised with an attack of fever; a sense of coldness, more or less intense, along the spine,

 and

of all the
of the neck.
of putrid
mental faculties
appearance of ac-
at one time
or small,
repeated, is
of the state or

from the fifth to
convulsions com-
whole limbs.
of a matter ex-
resembling
in great quan-
few drops distil
in great quan-
The secretion
the surface of
or blackish
with red colour,
; the eyes
for breath and
and delirium ap-
pear ;

pear; the extremities get cold, the pulfe intermits, and convulfions terminate the life of the patient on the fifth or eighth day at fartheft.

When the difeafe is not fo violent, and the termination is favourable, the paffage to the fecond ftage is much eafier, and fweatings, turbid urine, with a copious fediment, and abundant bilious ftools, at firft black, and afterwards yellow, are the ways by which nature attempts a crifis. In this cafe, towards the feventh day, the patient appears tranquil and lightened, but the jaundice ftill manifefts itfelf, and renders the convalefcence longer and more difficult. Not only the yellow colour, but a profound melancholy and ftupidity, an extreme proftration of ftrength, and fuch an irritability of the ftomach, that it cannot receive the fmalleft quantity even of the lighteft food, or water itfelf, without vomiting it, along with a large quantity of vifcid, green bile, conftitute the convalefcence from this difeafe in extreme cafes. In fome examples thefe fymptoms have been protracted beyond the fixtieth day.

In many the fever was fo moderate, and the naufea fo flight, that the difeafe was only recognifed by the intenfely yellow colour of the urine, and the jaundiced look of the eye.

In others the difeafe manifefted itfelf with extraordinary fymptoms, fuch as hydrophobia, double vifion, and enlarged appearance of the objects feen, hemorrhagy from the ears, phlyctenæ, and fwelling of the parotids. In fome the jaundice was completely wanting, and others were jaundiced without manifeft fever.

The difeafe was violent and rapid in the young, the robuft, and plethoric, and flower and lefs fevere in the weak, the old, and in females. To pregnant women it was almoft always fatal, and children moft frequently recovered. Intemperance of every kind, and efpecially excefs in wine and fpirituous liquors, predifpofed to the difeafe, and to a more fpeedy and inevitable death.

Generally fpeaking, a fatal termination could be predicted at the commencement of the difeafe, from the violence of the febrile attacks, and the occurrence of very fevere pains in the thorax, knees, and legs, extreme agitation, fudden proftration of ftrength, and conftant vomiting of black matter. The fooner the yellow colour appears on the fkin, the greater is the danger. Dyfpnœa, ifchuria, and hiccough, are generally fatal fymptoms in every period of the difeafe. On the contrary, the abfence of violent fymptoms at the commencement of the fecond ftage, vomiting occurring rarely, or merely of mucus, a moift fkin, the late appearance of jaundice, abundant fecretion of urine, and much ſediment in it, eaſy, looſe, and bilious ſtools, and, laſtly, the abſence of every nervous ſymptom, are the moſt certain ſigns of a favourable iſſue.

APPEARANCES ON DISSECTION.

Externally, the body, eſpecially its upper half, had a livid yellow colour, variegated with grangrenous marks and ſtreaks, particularly in the epigaſtric region and right hypochondrium. The noſtrils were filled with black blood, and from the mouth exuded a quantity of very fetid black matter, reſembling that which was vomited before death. The muſcles, on being cut, were found to be ſoft, and of a blackiſh colour. In one or both cavities of the thorax a reddiſh black fluid like bile, mixed with blood, was extravaſated. The lungs, but eſpecially the right lobe, were gorged with blood, ſo that when cut they reſembled liver, and were marked, particularly on the poſterior ſurface, with gangrenous ſpots. The pericardium contained a larger quantity than uſual of a yellowiſh fluid. The coronary veſſels were turgid with blood; in other reſpects the heart was natural. The omentum was almoſt entirely deſtroyed, and alſo the fat in the reſt of the body ſeemed as if melted away and deſtroyed. The external ſurface of the ſtomach, liver, and inteſtines, had a livid yellow colour, indicating the inflammation and gangrene, which had occupied all the viſcera. The diaphragm was livid and inflamed, where it is in contact with the liver. The liver was ſoft and ſphacelated, and, on being cut, had the colour of having been boiled; its concave ſurface was moſt affected with gangrene; the gall bladder was corrugated, and for the moſt part contained a very ſmall quantity of glutinous bile of a blackiſh colour; but in ſome inſtances it was exceſſively diſtended with a ſimilar fluid. The ſpleen was in general in a natural ſtate, except that it was turgid with black blood. The ſtomach was gangrenous, eſpecially its internal coat, was filled with a black matter ſimilar to that vomited, and had its whole vaſcular ſyſtem turgid with blood. The inteſtines were mortified throughout their whole length, and the ſmall ones, in particular, were filled with a mephitic vapour. The kidneys manifeſted ſymptoms of inflammation, and the urinary bladder was empty, and marked with gangrenous ſtreaks.

The veſſels of the brain and its membranes were generally injected with blood, and ſometimes there was a ſlight extravaſation of a yellowiſh fluid in the ventricles.

Theſe morbid appearances were found in a greater or leſs degree in the bodies of all thoſe who died in this epidemic, even in thoſe who did not ſurvive the attack more than twenty-four hours.

METHOD

METHOD OF CURE.

Having described the symptoms of this epidemic, and the appearances on dissection, Dr Palloni treats of the curative means employed, under the title of Clinical Observations. He divides the disease into three varieties, according as it commenced; *1st*, With symptoms of vascular irritation; *2d*, With gastric symptoms; and *3dly*, With symptoms of debility. In the first case, blood-letting from the arm and hemorrhoidal veins was found to be of great service; in the second, emetics, when administered at the commencement of the attack, for, in an advanced stage of the disease, they were always very hurtful. The third variety was combated from the first by the same medicines which were adopted in the last stage of the other two.

After having diminished the vascular irritation, if it exist, and emptied the bowels as soon as possible, our author advises us to endeavour to excite diaphoresis by warm lemonade, in which a little tartrate of antimony is dissolved, as a copious perspiration, induced on the second or third day, frequently cut the disease short, as if by enchantment. If the disease proceed, he advises the free use of diluting liquids, and extols much the effects of nitric acid, with which the treatment may be begun, in those cases which commence with symptoms of debility. Calomel was given with advantage, in doses of ten grains every three hours, in the beginning of the disease, and in robust, plethoric habits; while, in debilitated and scorbutic constitutions, and in an advanced stage of the disease, when hemorrhagy, black vomit, and other signs of dissolution, have supervened, mercury, he thinks, can only increase the disease, and hasten its termination; and, in these cases, nitric acid appeared to him admirably adapted to the indications.

In a disease where the vital forces sink so rapidly, tonics might seem to be indicated, but experience proved the contrary. In cases of the greatest extremity, on the appearance of hemorrhagy from the mouth or nose, the pulse, which could not before be felt, would return, and recovery commence, and abortion, or a copious flooding in women, would frequently recal them, as it were, from death to life. When extreme prostration of strength, black vomit, and hemorrhagy, suggested the use of corroborants, the simple or camphorated decoction of cinchona was given with advantage in the form of clyster.

Blisters also did more harm than good. Sometimes the lymph contained in them was of an intensely green colour, like the expressed juice of succory, and so acrid as to inflame the skin beneath, and cause it to become rapidly gangrenous. Sinapisms to the lower extremities were adopted with greater success.

It was the character of this disease particularly to affect the liver, and to alter the secretion of bile, in a specific manner, assimilating it to its own nature, determining it to the skin, so as to be succeeded by excoriation and desquamation, as if it had been burnt, and rendering it so caustic as to corrode the internal membrane of the stomach and duodenum, and to destroy the vitality of every part with which it comes in contact, and of the fluids with which it mixes. Accordingly, every thing which acts directly upon the liver, so as to increase its vital reaction, and prevent the absorption of bile, was useful; such as frictions of oxygenated mercurial ointment, frequent clysters, and, where there was any indolent turgidity of the liver, blisters. To correct the diminished secretion of urine, which always accompanies this disease, the digitalis purpurea was well adapted.

The fifth and seventh days were the most commonly fatal, although there were many examples of persons dying in twenty-four or forty-eight hours, or in three days, while others have survived thirteen or fourteen days, or even longer. The period when reconvalescence commences required the greatest attention; mild laxatives, saponaceous pills, a weak infusion of polygala, and the use of oxygenated mercurial ointment, had the best effects.

HISTORY OF ITS PROGRESS.

The disease began in Leghorn about the middle of the month of August, and terminated about the middle of December. Its progress may be divided into three distinct periods; the first, extending from its commencement to the 20th of October, was characterized by the small number of deaths, which were daily from one to six at most, by the slow progress of the disease, and by its being limited to two or three streets. The second, from the 20th of October to the 20th November, was distinguished by the greater number of victims, which increased to 26, by the more rapid progress of the disease, and by its diffusion through various parts of the city. The third period, from the 20th of November to the middle of December, was marked by the gradual diminution of the disease, and its total cessation.

In the first and second periods, the sick had more or less distinctly the symptoms enumerated in the history of the disease, while those of the last period had but a slight resemblance of it. The disease assumed a rheumatic appearance, was milder and slower in its course, and did not declare itself until the ninth day. Recoveries were very rare during the first period, much

more

more numerous in the ſecond, and frequent in the third. Of 164 patients admitted into the hoſpital of St James, 56 died; and in the whole city, containing 60,000 inhabitants, the number ſcarcely exceeded 700.

A very rainy and irregular ſummer was ſucceeded by an autumn rather warm and dry. In the very beginning of November the rainy ſeaſon commenced, and the ſouth wind ſet in, which prevailed until almoſt the end of December, interrupted, however, ſeveral times by ſome days of ſtrong ſouth-weſt winds, or north winds accompanied with intenſe cold. During all this time, the diſeaſe ran its courſe without ſeeming to be influenced by the variations of the ſeaſon, or of the atmoſpheric temperature. It was at its height during the prevalence of the ſouth wind and of the rains; it proceeded during the intenſe and dry cold, and began to decline, and at laſt ceaſed, during the ſame rainy and ſoutherly conſtitution of the weather under which it had reached its height.

The diſeaſe began in the worſt ventilated and moſt unhealthy part of the city. Surrounded on all ſides by lofty buildings, defended from every wind, filthy from the offals of fiſh and butcher-meat, and filled with ſtagnant putrid exhalations, it ſeemed as if it were contrived to be the ſeat of ſuch a diſeaſe; and yet its progreſs was ſlow and almoſt inſenſible, the deaths not amounting to more than one or two a-day for about a month.

The ſmall number of ſick, and the circumſtance of Leghorn being ſubject, by its local ſituatution, to diſeaſes of a malignant and bilious nature, cauſed the diſeaſe to paſs for ſome time unobſerved, or at leaſt rendered its nature doubtful and diſputed. It then made ſome progreſs, but always ſlowly and difficultly, along certain narrow ſtreets and lanes, ill ventilated, with high, confined, and filthy houſes, crowded with inhabitants of the pooreſt claſs. From this time the ſame intercourſe between theſe ſtreets and the reſt of the city continued; the individuals of thoſe families in which the diſeaſe exiſted daily mixed with thoſe of the healthy in all parts, and the exchange and communication of goods and effects continued free and uninterrupted.

With regard to the important ſubject of the manner in which this fever was propagated, Dr Palloni ſtates it to be the reſult of his reſearches, that it was never communicated from one individual to another by goods or any other infected ſubſtances, but only by the approach of the healthy to the ſick; and even to this there were innumerable exceptions, ſo that a particular prediſpoſition ſeemed to be neceſſary to receive the infection. Of the prieſts who attended the ſick only one died; of the numerous

practitioners

practitioners of the healing art, only three. There were many examples of wives ſleeping with their ſick huſbands without being infected, of numerous families in which only one was infected, of children ſucking their mothers, till within a few minutes of their death, with impunity. But, beſides this particular prediſpoſition, it appeared to be another eſſential condition for receiving the infection, that the perſon from whom it was received ſhould be ſituated in a cloſe, filthy room, filled with confined and impure air. Hence, among the poor in that part of the city where it raged, many of the ſame family and houſe died, while, in the other ſtreets, it was confined to one houſe, or one individual of a family. Hence in the hoſpitals no one attendant periſhed, and hence the diſeaſe was not communicated in them to patients labouring under other diſeaſes.

Dr Palloni is of opinion that it is eſpecially with the tranſpiration that certain deleterous principles emanate from the bodies of the diſeaſed, capable of exciting the ſame diſeaſe in others, who reſpire or abſorb them in particular circumſtances, and that theſe principles are eaſily deſtroyed by the contact of pure and renewed air; but that mephitic, ſtagnant air, in which they are accumulated, becomes an excellent conductor, and facilitates its communication.

There cannot be adduced a ſingle inſtance in which the infection was conveyed by ſubſtances which had been in contact with the ſick, and there were many examples of individuals and whole families having continued to inhabit the room, or to ſleep in the very bed, in which a patient had died. Not one of thoſe employed to clean the houſes of the ſick were attacked, nor did any of thoſe who buried the dead fall a victim to the diſeaſe.

Conſiſtently with theſe well-eſtabliſhed facts, and ſince, even in the city of Leghorn itſelf, the diſeaſe was ſo partial, ſo limited, ſo ſlow, nay, even ſo difficult to be communicated, it is no wonder that it did not extend to the ſmalleſt diſtance beyond Leghorn, although the commerce continued uninterrupted, and the French garriſon, ſeveral of whom had contracted the diſeaſe, removed to Piſa when the diſeaſe was at its height, and 8000 of the inhabitants emigrated to Piſa and the neighbouring country. Of theſe ſeveral already infected died of the diſeaſe, but in no inſtance did they communicate it to thoſe around them.

Dr Palloni therefore infers,

1. That the epidemic of Leghorn, in its ſymptoms, progreſs, and appearance, was analogous to the *typhus icterodes* of Sauvages and Cullen; but that, in the ſlight degree of contagion which it exhibited, in its comparatively ſmall mortality, and in having in

1 general

general required the antifthenic method of cure, it differed fomewhat from the peftilential difeafes defcribed by thefe authors under that name, and approached to the fpurious and lefs contagious fpecies defcribed by Anderfon, Jackfon, and others.

2. That, for the reception of the infection, a particular predifpofition in the individual, and actual communication with the fick, in a fmall apartment, and in a confined and impure atmofphere, were neceffary.

3. That the contagious fomites were eafily deftroyed by the contact of pure air.

4. That the contagion was never conveyed by goods of any kind. And,

5. That the difeafe was very limited in Leghorn, and did not extend beyond it.

Dr Palloni concludes this very interefting publication with ftating, that, notwithftanding the mildnefs of the difeafe, and the difficulty of its propagation, the fame precautions were employed as if it had been the oriental plague, and that fo long a time has elapfed fince the city was reftored to perfect health, that the keeping up the cordon any longer, for preventing any communication with the reft of Tufcany, would not only be unneceffary, but unjuft and cruel.

To give greater authority to his ftatement, Dr Palloni has fubjoined the atteftations of all the principal medical men of Leghorn.

VII.

A General View of the Writings of Linnæus. By Richard Pulteney, M. D. F. R. S. The fecond edition, with corrections, confiderable additions, and Memoirs of the author. By William George Maton, M. D. F. R. S. &c. &c. To which is annexed the Diary of Linnæus, written by himfelf, and now tranflated into Englifh, from the Swedifh Manufcript in the poffeffion of the Editor. 4to. pp. 595. London. 1805.

The infeparable connexion of natural hiftory with medicine, independently of the circumftance that many of the writings in queftion relate to fubjects ftrictly medical, would render any apology for briefly introducing this volume to the notice of our readers

readers unneceſſary. The value of the writings of Linnæus can only be ſufficiently eſtimated by comparing the ſtate and progreſs of natural knowledge, during the ſhort period which has elapſed ſince their completion, with the unimproving ignorance that prevailed on theſe ſubjects during the many centuries that preceded it. Within that ſhort period the knowledge of nature has been diſſeminated with incalculable rapidity; and the perfection to which it has attained has been limited only by the phyſical difficulties which exiſt to the exploring of diſtant and inhoſpitable climates. The readineſs with which naturaliſts, educated in other ſyſtems, and habituated to other language, adopted the arrangement and nomenclature of Linnæus, is another deciſive teſt of the obvious facilities and advantages which reſulted from the latter.

In republiſhing the work of his friend, Dr Maton has amply availed himſelf of the great opportunities of information which have fallen to his lot; and, by means of the numerous and valuable additions (which have extended the original ſmall work to its preſent ſize), he has put into our hands a very complete view of the ſtate of Linnæan ſcience and literature up to the preſent time. The poſſeſſion of ſuch an authentic ſource of information as Linnæus's own Diary has enabled him to adduce many new particulars connected with the purſuits and writings of the great naturaliſts, which, together with ſeveral judicious alterations in the order of detail, have converted the biographical ſketch given by Dr Pulteney into a comprehenſive chronological account of the principal occurrences of his public life.

The acuteneſs and indefatigable activity of the mind of Linnæus, which were conſpicuous on all occaſions, and of which he ſeems to have been fully * ſenſible himſelf, were particularly evinced in the formation of the great vegetable ſyſtem, which muſt be conſidered as his *chef d' œuvre*. His firſt work, which does not appear to have been publiſhed (the original manuſcript is now in the hands of Dr Smith), was a little catalogue of his botanical obſervations, entitled *Spolia Botanica*, and dated 1728. In this the plants are arranged according to the ſyſtem of Tournefort and he had not then conceived any notion of reforming the claſſification of vegetables. About a year afterwards "he read, in the Leipſic Commentaries, a review of Vaillant's treatiſe on the ſexes of plants, by which his curioſity was excited to a cloſe inveſtigation of the *ſtamina* and *piſtilla*; he obſerved that theſe

* The following, among numerous self-commendations of this sort, occurs in his Diary. "In the year 1765, he worked at the 12th or last edition of the *Systema Naturæ*, and, the whole of the autumn, on the *Clavis Medicinæ, which would have employed the most learned men for an age.*"

these parts of the plant were of essential importance, and that they varied as much as the petals. Hence he formed the design of constituting a new sexual method." *(Diary.)* In three years from this time, this method, comprehensive as it is, and erected on such a multitude of observations, was so completely matured in his mind, that the plants collected in his journey through Lapland were arranged, according to the sexual plan, in the catalogue entitled *Florula Lapponica*, which he published on his return in 1742. The *Flora Lapponica*, it may be observed, was not published till five years afterwards, and the *Lachesis Lapponica*, containing a general account of the journey, never appeared. Dr Pulteney, more than once, laments that this work was, in all probability, lost for ever to the world: but we have the pleasure to find it stated by the editor, that the manuscript is in the possession of Dr Smith, and that a translation of it will shortly be published.

In his analysis of the great monument of the genius and industry of Linnæus, the *Systema Naturæ*, Dr Pulteney had given short generic characters of the subjects comprehended under the first four classes of the animal kingdom only. Dr Maton has now extended the catalogue of these characters through the two remaining classes, the *Insecta* and *Vermes*: he has also annexed to each order, through the whole of the animal kingdom, abbreviated characters of the new *genera*, which have been formed in consequence of the numerous discoveries of modern naturalists. But the great additional value which this edition possesses, is in its accurate references, not only to all the editions of the works of Linnæus, but also to all the works of succeeding writers, whose researches have contributed in any degree to the extension or improvement of the system, or to the enlargement of the boundaries of natural history.

It is a matter of some interest to observe the numerous additions which have been made to the large catalogue of objects detailed by Linnæus, and the rapidity with which they have been collected and ascertained. This rapid accumulation of knowledge relative to the productions of nature, heretofore unknown, is to be attributed partly, no doubt, to the more general diffusion of science among those who are led to distant countries, but in a great measure also, as the editor justly remarks, to that peculiar facility of accurate discrimination which the Linnæan system itself has introduced. The class *Mammalia*, as left by Linnæus, contained about 230 *species*. Since that time eight new genera have been constructed, and the species are now increased to 600 in number. In the class *Aves* a considerable extension has been made, particularly by the labours of Dr Latham, on whose scientific works the editor bestows a well-merited eulogium. Dr

Latham

Latham has ventured so far to alter the Linnæan arrangement as to constitute four new orders; and he has increased the number of species to considerably more than 2,500, of which 500 at least were first described by himself. In the last edition published by Linnæus (the 12th), this class comprehends about 930 subjects only.

On the topic of *Insects* (a branch of natural history which, before the time of Linnæus, was nearly without method), a writer of considerable ingenuity and industry has lately appeared, whose generic distinctions are considered by many naturalists as preferable to those of Linnæus; we mean Fabricius. He has invented a new arrangement, in which the *instrumenta cibaria*, or different parts and appendages of the mouth, are chosen as the chief basis of discrimination. Dr Maton is not disposed to recommend this new method; on the contrary, he is of opinion, that "Villers has rendered great service to entomology, and to Linnæan scholars in particular, by reducing the species of Fabricius to a conformity with the *Systema Naturæ*; and that thus no small part of the confusion which would otherwise again have taken place in this branch of natural history, has been prevented." * It must indeed be universally allowed that the change of a nomenclature, which has become the common language of the learned throughout the world, can only be countenanced on the supposition that the arrangement with which it is connected abounds in defects, or that the adoption of a new system will be attended with permanent advantages, that will more than counterbalance the impediments which must for a long period necessarily ensue from the attempt. The species of insects described by Gmelin amount to nearly 11,000.

The class of *Vermes* has also been much extended by the labours of various naturalists, to whose works the editor refers. The discoveries of Muller have not only multiplied the species of animalcules, but rendered it necessary to constitute a new order for them, which has been designated by the title of *Infusoria*. This order, as it stands in the 13th (or Gmelin's) edition of the *Systema*, contains 13 genera, the characters of which are here detailed, and 129 species; it includes, however, the Linnæan genera of *Vorticella* and *Volvox*. In the edition just alluded to, considerably more than 6000 *vermes* are described.

In the catalogue of the vegetable kingdom, with the exception of the class *Cryptogamia*, the discoveries of future inquirers were not likely to give rise to any considerable changes, except in the number of plants described, the consequent formation of new genera, and the occasional transference of some of the species to different genera, according to new relations, which might be ascertained.

* This book is entitled "*Caroli Linnæi Entomologia, &c. &c. curante et augente* Carolo de Villers," and was published at Leyden in 1789.

certained. Changes of this sort have, in fact, been extremely numerous. In the last edition published by Linnæus, the number of species amounts to above 7,800; the subsequent edition by Gmelin comprehends at least 17,000 species. In the class *Cryptogamia*, the curious and important researches of Hedwig have thrown considerable light on the fructification of the *Musci* and *Algæ*, which led him to propose an alteration in the distribution of these orders; and his arrangement has been more or less followed by most botanical writers of the present period. In regard to the *Fungi*, the later editors of Linnæus, assisted by the labours of Schäffer, Bolton, Bulliard, and others, have been enabled to improve the distribution of that order very materially; and an entirely new arrangement has recently been attempted by Dr Persoon (see *Tentam. Dispositionis Method. Fungor. Lips.* 1797), of which, however, Dr Maton has not given any abstract.

These alterations of the *Systema Vegitabilium*, being founded on physiological investigation and progressive discovery, are justly considered by the editor as legitimate and necessary reformations; but he appears to doubt the propriety of adopting those changes which affect the general *classification* of Linnæus, especially the reduction of the number of classes to 20, in the manner practised by Prof. Thunberg, Gmelin, Withering, &c., and probably by Dr Willdenow, in the edition now publishing. Facility of investigation is the great object of classification; and we have some reason to apprehend that the student of botany meets with greater obstacles to his research in the classes of *Monæcia*, *Diæcia*, and *Polygamia*, than in almost any other portion of the system; and that the incorporation of these three classes with the others, according to the number of *stamina* in the respective genera, would tend in part to remove those impediments to botanical study. Perhaps the proscription of the class *Gynandria* is not so defensible. The plants of the first order at least constitute a natural assemblage of such peculiar appearances, that the student, after having seen one, is scarcely under the necessity of examining the parts of fructification, in order to ascertain their place in the system. Dr Maton refers his readers to a dissertation on the subject of these innovations in Usteri's *Annalen der Botanik* for 1792, p. 20.

With regard to the distribution of *mineral* substances in the *Systema Naturæ*, the editor acknowledges that the 3d volume, in which it is contained, "from the highly improved state of mineralogical knowledge at the present day, has ceased to be of any utility, except so far as it shows the use made by Linnæus of the materials to which he was limited, and as i illustrates the progress of system." In the edition of Gmelin, [illegible]ed, that volume

is

is no longer the work of Linnæus, but of Werner; and Dr Maton readily fubfcribes to its fuperior utility. He has given the outlines both of the Linnæan and Gmelinian fyftem, and abbreviated generic characters of the fubftances according to each method.

After a more ample analyfis of all the papers of Linnæus in the tranfactions of learned focieties, and in the *Amœnitates Academicæ*, than appeared in the former edition, Dr Maton concludes the volume with fome obfervations on the honours which were paid to him on his perfon, character, and habits, and with fome account of his family. The Diary occupies about 70 pages. It is curious on account of the detail of facts relative to a life of fuch importance as that of Linnæus, and alfo as a fpecimen of that fort of biography, of which the writer and the fubject are united in one individual. Like many other men of fuperior talents, Linnæus appears to have been fully confcious of his powers; and the fuperlative felf-eulogy, which he has not fcrupled to employ, but too clearly evinces that his *foibles*, "if, as the editor remarks, "it be neceffary to record them," were vanity and a love of diftinction. But thefe, perhaps, have ever been the leading motives of mankind to all great undertakings. "And who will charge this great man with having arrogated to himfelf merit that did not juftly belong to him, or with having difputed the pretenfions of others, becaufe they interfered with his own?"

It is always interefting to difcover the efficient caufes of the peculiar bias of great minds; and it may not be impertinent to ftate, before we conclude, that the circumftances which gave rife to Linnæus's predilection for that fcience, by the ftudy of which his genius enabled him to immortalize his name, and to confer a moft important benefit on mankind, are diftinctly traced. He dates his love of botany in the Diary nearly from his cradle, having "almoft lived" from that time in his father's garden. But the bent appears to have been particularly decided by a circumftance which occurred fo early as the age of four years. "He was fcarcely four years old when he accompanied his father to a feaft at Möklen, and in the evening, it being a very pleafant feafon of the year, the guefts feated themfelves on fome flowery turf, liftening to the paftor, who made various remarks on the names and properties of the plants. The child paid the moft uninterrupted attention to all he faid and heard; and from that hour never ceafed haraffing his father with queftions about the name, qualities, and nature of every plant he met with."

Dr Maton has prefixed to the work fome well-written me-pairs of his worthy and learned friend, the author of the original work, as well as two excellent portraits, the one of Linnæus, the other of Dr Pulteney.

VIII.

Observations on the Utility and Administration of Purgative Medicines in several Diseases. By JAMES HAMILTON, M.D. Fellow of the Royal College of Physicians, and of the Royal Philosophical Society, and senior Physician to the Royal Infirmary of Edinburgh. Edinburgh. 1805. 8vo. P. 320.

No rule of health is more generally assented to than that which inculcates regularity in the alvine discharge. There is none, perhaps, more generally overlooked; and to this neglect the physician has too often occasion to refer the origin or aggravation of many complicated ailments. In most diseases, the state of the bowels claims much of our attention, and is seldom indeed disregarded by the physician in his clinical inquiries, for no indication is more familiar than to obviate costiveness. But, with a few exceptions, there prevails in the minds of modern practitioners a cautious reserve in the administration of purgative medicines to any extent beyond what that more simple indication may seem to require. The older physicians, though much less reserved in the employment of purgatives, were yet fettered in their practice by the theories of the humoral pathology, and the doctrine of concoction, which dogmatically determined the periods of evacuation, and the kind of purgative fitted for the occasion. It was common to purge freely at the decline only of acute disorders, when the concoction of the humours was supposed to be completed. In other diseases, the cure was intrusted almost entirely to purgatives, and these often of a very drastic kind. The theory of diseases is now founded on the pathology of the living solids, whence has sprung the doctrine of debility, which, in its turn, embarrasses our practice; and thus the fear of still farther depressing the vital energies has, in these times, contributed to limit the use of free purging in many cases, in which experience, undebauched by theory, might perhaps have sanctioned the practice. Satisfied in general, by keeping the bowels as nearly as possible in a natural state by gentle laxatives, or by clysters, it must be acknowledged that, excepting in the few

 cases

cases where constipation from obstruction or torpor of the bowels forms very palpably the chief part of the disease, the curative indications of modern practice do not often lead to the repeated administration of purgatives. Yet the benefit derived from purging in some tropical fevers, and in many of the diseases of infancy, together with the pathology of morbid irritations, seemed well calculated to relieve practitioners from those apprehensions, which the Cullenian and Brunonian doctrines had engendered, and gradually to lead to a freer and more unreserved exhibition of purgatives in other diseases, in those especially where tonics, and antispasmodics have so often disappointed their hopes, and in which the trains of morbid actions are certainly aggravated, and perhaps kept up by, or associated with, intestinal irritation, or with primary affection of some other of the abdominal viscera.

Accordingly, of one disease of this class, which has very generally resisted the tonic plan of treatment, we have already, by the insertion of Dr M'Mullin's paper on chorea in the first number of this Journal, had an opportunity of laying before our readers a few cases most happily and speedily cured at the Royal Infirmary of Edinburgh, by the repeated exhibition of powerful purgatives only, a practice first introduced by the enlightened author of the volume now before us. We well knew the value of that communication, because we had witnessed more than once the success which attended the new plan of cure, contrasted with the failure of the old method; and were assured, therefore, that we discharged our duty to the public, in giving it an early place in a work professedly undertaken to circulate and to preserve improvements in the healing art. We now, therefore, sincerely rejoice that Dr Hamilton, notwithstanding his acknowledged unwillingness to appear in the character of an author, or, as he too modestly in our opinion, has said, to obtrude himself on the public, has been induced to give a full exposition of the peculiarities of his practice, derived from matured experience, and explained and supported by the most unquestionable proofs and illustrations. In these, indeed, our author has been singularly fortunate. Few practitioners have enjoyed such opportunities of collecting accurate and extensive information. For upwards of thirty years Dr H. has officiated as physician to the Royal Infirmary of Edinburgh, to George Heriot's Hospital, and to the two Maiden Hospitals. In the course of this extensive experience, his observations on the utility of purgative medicines in certain diseases were amply confirmed, while confidence was acquired in that practice he now ventures to recommend to the public. The number, authenticity, and apposite application of the cases adduced

adduced as proofs or illustrations of the utility of the observations delivered in the text, cannot fail, we think, to satisfy the most scrupulous; for these cases are not the finished pictures too often dressed up by an author from imperfect notes, to serve a particular purpose. The greater number are taken from the sick journals of the Royal Infirmary, in which the daily reports of the physician are recorded at the patient's bed-side, before a crowd of intelligent students. Cases of this description, which, in their progress, cannot be perverted to particular purposes, and which cannot afterwards be altered by any retrospective emendation of the practitioner, possess, it is justly remarked by Dr Hamilton, an authenticity peculiar to themselves, and, in the establishing of medical facts, may be produced as an authority that cannot be controverted. Other cases, in farther illustration, are added from the author's private practice, and a few communicated by his friends. Experience, indeed, seems all along to have been the guide of Dr Hamilton, and to have suggested those innovations in his practice which are now with so much candour submitted to the judgment of the professional public. Practical, however, as his observations are, sanctioned by his own respectable authority, and confirmed by such authenticated proofs, he solicits only the unprejudiced attention of the reader to the rules he has laid down, and refers the rest to the impartial decision of experience.

In delivering some general introductory observations on purgative medicines, our author takes occasion to remark, that modern physicians have two objects in view in the administration of this class of remedies; the one to empty the bowels simply by laxatives, the other to promote an increased secretion of fluids into the cavity of the intestines, or, in other words, to induce purging. Without approving the distinction thus made between laxatives and purgatives, inasmuch as the same medicines, according to the dose in which they are employed, are calculated to produce the one or the other effect, he wishes it to be understood that the medicines employed by him in the diseases of which he is to treat, from experience of their superior usefulness, are purgative ones, while, at the same time, he avoids their full effect of purging; and this consideration, he thinks, obviates the objection made to the employment of purgative medicines, that they reduce the strength of a patient already too much weakened. But, in the diseases of which he is to speak, the sole intention being to bring off the contents of the bowels, which are out of the course of circulation, and are already in a manner extraneous to the body, purgative medicines, given under such limitation, can hardly be ſuppoſed capable of inducing debility; we might as well, Dr H. adds, expect it from emptying the urinary bladder.

We would not willingly cavil with a writer for whom we feel ſo much reſpect; but we cannot avoid making two remarks in this place. And, *firſt*, we muſt obſerve, that if the remedies employed do no more than bring off the contents of the bowels, which are, in a manner, extraneous to the body, they ought, in the terms even of Dr Hamilton's explanation, to be deemed rather laxatives than purgatives. But the deſire of avoiding the haſty objection which has been urged againſt the employment of purgative medicines has inadvertently, we imagine, led Dr Hamilton to make this obſervation. For the practice which is afterwards recommended in ſome diſeaſes, as in chorea, for example, does much more than unload the bowels; the remedies employed are truly purgative; and ſuch continued evacuations would aſſuredly, in a ſyſtem not diſeaſed, induce very conſiderable debility. One or two purgatives given occaſionally, and at intervals, would, we apprehend, in moſt caſes, be ſufficient to bring off the contents of the bowels which are out of the courſe of the circulation; but conſtant evacuations, kept up for days and weeks together by very powerful draſtic medicines, muſt be attended with an increaſed ſecretion of fluids into the cavity of the inteſtines, as indeed manifeſtly appears from the liquid and diſcoloured ſtools noticed in many of the hiſtories related in the Appendix.

We remark, in the *ſecond* place, that objections drawn from any reaſoning *à priori*, or from a knowledge even of the general effects of any claſs of remedies, muſt yield to experience in particular caſes. And thus, although the general effects of purging be confeſſedly debilitating, we have little to fear in thoſe caſes where experience has diſcovered their uſefulneſs. Debility is itſelf an effect of diſeaſe, and, when the diſeaſe is removed, the ſtrength and vigor of the ſyſtem will return. Have we not often ſeen the debility which attends ſome of the complaints of infancy removed, as well as the diſeaſe of which it was a ſymptom, by evacuating the bowels by calomel? And nauſea and anorexia, with all the depreſſing ſymptoms of dyſpepſia, how often alleviated by a briſk purgative? Not to mention here the experience of Dr. Hamilton in other caſes. If we would follow out this practice on general principles, we muſt calculate the whole effects of our remedies. Sometimes we empty the bowels ſimply; at others we promote an increaſed ſecretion of fluids by purgative medicines. In ſome caſes it appears ſufficient to unload the bowels of their contents accumulated by long retention, and

thereby

thereby relieve the ſyſtem from the effects of this local irritation; but in others, and eſpecially in thoſe in which a freer and more continued purging becomes neceſſary before the ſymptoms yield, we bring off not only the contents of the bowels which are out of the courſe of circulation, we eliminate alſo the ſecretory organs which terminate in the inteſtinal canal, the obſtruction, torpor, or deranged actions of which may have been a chief cauſe of the morbid actions of other parts of the ſyſtem. We are ſurely authorized to make this inference from caſes in which the purging is continued for three weeks, to the extent of three or four ſtools daily, with progreſſive relief of the morbid ſymptoms, with improved looks and ſtrength, and at length by the perfect cure of a complicated diſeaſe *. In other caſes, we find the cure advancing, with the diſcharge of fetid, fluid ſtools, of a bilious appearance, or black and greeniſh colour.

We believe the biliary organs to be not unfrequently intereſted in ſome of thoſe caſes in which a free uſe of purgatives has been found ſo advantageous. The biliary ſyſtem is often deranged in the diſeaſes of infancy and of childhood, in which purgative medicines are eminently uſeful, when they ſucceed in producing copious bilious dejections, as our own obſervation has more than once taught us. But, for proof of this remark, we have only to refer our readers to ſome of thoſe diſeaſes claſſed by Dr Hamilton under the title of *Maraſmus*, and particularly to the caſe of Malcolm Morriſon, publiſhed in the 4th number of the Appendix. This child, beſides being affected with many of the ſymptoms of acute hydrocephalus, ſuch as pain of the forehead, dilated pupils, frequent ſcreaming, picking of the noſe, hot ſkin, and frequent pulſe, complained of *pain of the right ſide*, near the falſe ribs, attended by a hard, dry cough, and the fæces were of a *gray colour, and clayey conſiſtence.* This caſe was ſucceſsfully treated by remedies, purgative in the ſtricteſt ſenſe of the word, daily adminiſtered for upwards of three weeks.

We have only to add, that we have ſeen caſes very like to this; and in one inſtance, which terminated fatally, on diſſection the liver was found inflamed, and the gall bladder and ducts loaded with dark-coloured bile. The many hiſtories of ſuppoſed hydrocephalus, recorded as cured by a very free uſe of calomel, reflects conſiderable light on the etiology and treatment of ſuch caſes.

We would be ſorry, indeed, to miſtake the indications, or to miſinterpret the practice of Dr Hamilton in the ſeveral diſeaſes of which he has treated in the volume before us. We may be wrong, but at preſent it appears to us, that the purgative

* Caſe of chorea.—*Appendix.*

gative plan of treatment here recommended is not altogether limited to the discharge of the accumulated contents of the bowels which are out of the course of the circulation, and in a manner extraneous to the body. And we cannot help thinking that, in some cases at least, part of the usefulness of purgative medicines arises from their emulging the biliary and other secretory organs not unfrequently obstructed in chronic diseases, and on the freedom of which the natural actions of the chylopoetic viscera, and well-being of the whole system, so much depend. Should we even be mistaken in this opinion, it must at least be prudent to keep in mind, that, whatever our intention may be, it is not so easy to limit the effects of purgative medicines; and that such a continued course as, in these diseases, appears necessary to evacuate the bowels, will very commonly also increase the usual secretion of the intestinal fluids.

After these introductory remarks to which we have just referred, Dr H. proceeds to deliver, in distinct chapters, his observations on the utility and administration of purgative medicines in *typhus fever*, *scarlatina*, the *marasmus of childhood and early youth*, *chorea Sancti Viti*, *chlorosis*, *hæmatemesis*, in *hysteria*, and *some chronic diseases*. And, under the same titles, the reader will find, in a copious Appendix, a variety of cases illustrating the practice recommended in the context.

1. In *Typhus*.—Clinical observations seem first to have suggested to Dr Hamilton the utility of purgatives in this disease. Antimonial medicines were, some years ago, much more frequently employed in fever than they are now; and during the prevalence of a typhus fever of more than usual malignity at Edinburgh, in the year 1781, and which seemed to be imported by the Jamaica fleet, which arrived in Leith Roads in a very sickly state, Dr H. having frequently employed, in the worst cases, a powerful antimonial, the calx antimonii nitrata, which sufficiently answered his expectation, remarked that it was beneficial only when it moved the belly. "The stools were black and fetid, and in general copious: on the discharge of these, the low delirium, tremors, floccitatio, and subsultus tendinum, which had prevailed, abated in some cases; the tongue, which had been dry and furred, became moister and cleaner; and a feeble, creeping pulse acquired a firmer beat." Hence he was led to substitute a medicine simply purgative for the antimonial, and to avoid the unnecessary debility produced by vomiting and sweating. More extended experience confirmed this judicious inference, and gradually led to the early employment and repetition of purgatives in typhus. The full and regular evacuation of the bowels relieves the oppression of the stomach, and mitigates the other

other symptoms of fever. Glysters, the effects of which are limited to the rectum, are inadequate to this good purpose. It is necessary to relieve the whole extent of the intestines by purgative medicines, which at once carry off the load of feculent matter and vitiated secretions. "The object to be attained is the complete and regular evacuation of the offensive feculent matter collected in the bowels, in the course of fever; within this limit the practice is safe and salutary. Of this I am assured, that I have had much satisfaction in the prosecution of it; and have not, in a single instance, had occasion to regret any injury or bad consequence proceeding from it." As the intention of Dr H. in this practice is simply to unload the bowels, and to preserve them in an open state during the course of fever, daily purgatives are not necessary; it is sufficient to give them occasionally, carefully avoiding their full effect of purging, which, by increasing the secretion of fluids, might lower the strength of the patient. Thus managed, we observe, in the cases related in the Appendix, the gradual abatement of the febrile symptoms, and the return of the powers of the system, keeping pace with the free and regular evacuation of the bowels. Useful, however, as this practice is, it is not exclusively employed by Dr H. in the cure of fever. Emetics and glysters, however, are seldom or never now used by him; and, for some years past, he finds wine less necessary than he formerly thought it was. The purgatives employed are calomel alone, or combined with jalap, jalap and its compound powder, aloes, the neutral salts, and infusion of senna.

2. In *Scarlatina.*—Scarlatina, scarlatina anginosa, and cynanche maligna, Dr H. is inclined to consider as varieties only of one and the same disease, depending upon the varying nature and constitution of scarlatina, and upon extrinsic and contingent circumstances. As some doubt, however, may be entertained with regard to cynanche maligna, he speaks of it at present as a distinct disease, and considers it separately from scarlatina. The practice in scarlatina recommended by different writers, or followed by different practitioners, is very various, and, to the young and inexperienced physician, must appear embarrassing and contradictory. Scarlatina, however, is a disease of varying type, which assumes appearances very different in different epidemics, and even in different individuals, during the prevalence of the same epidemic. The general indications must therefore vary with the circumstances of the case; and the reader cannot fail to be gratified by the judicious and instructive reflections of our author. The usual prejudice, the fear of inducing debility, has deterred many from the administration of purgatives in this disease

ease. But the benefit experienced from these medicines in typhus led Dr H. to the employment of them also in scarlatina. Costiveness, too, he had remarked to be a common occurrence in this disease, while the contents of the bowels are generally more changed, and unnatural in their appearance, than in typhus itself. In the treatment of scarlatina he has accordingly experienced the best effects from the judicious administration of purgatives: The limits within which they are employed are the same as in typhus. They are useful not only in mitigating the fever, and relieving the symptoms of oppression and debility during the course of the disease, they are advantageously persevered in also towards the close, with the view of obviating or removing that common and sometimes fatal consequence of scarlatina, dropsical swelling. "I have never," says our author, "witnessed sinking and fainting, as mentioned by authors, and so much dreaded by them; neither have I observed revulsion from the surface of the body, and consequent premature fading, or, in common language, striking in of the efflorescence, from the exhibition of purgatives. Accordingly, in treating scarlatina, I have confided much in the use of purgative medicines; and no variety of the disease, as occurring in different epidemics, or in the course of the same epidemic, has hitherto prevented me from following out this practice to the extent which I have found necessary."

In *Cynanche Maligna* also, Dr H. recommends the exhibition of purgatives. The very objections brought against their use appear to him arguments in their favour; the intention being to free the stomach and bowels from an acrimonious feculent mass, the irritation arising from which aggravates all the symptoms of the disease, and induces that exhausting diarrhœa or dysentery so much to be apprehended in cynanche maligna. Though his opinion of the utility of purgatives in cynache maligna be thus decidedly pronounced, Dr H. most ingenuously acknowledges that his experience in that disease has been limited, and cautions his reader that, in giving this opinion, he has departed from the rule which he had formed to himself. "It is a theoretical opinion," he adds, "and not so fully supported by experience, as to enable me to deliver it with confidence." But it is an opinion well authorized, we think, by his very extensive experience in scarlatina and scarlatina anginosa.

In the Appendix, N° 3. we are presented with a very interesting narrative of scarlatina, as it affected the children in George Heriot's Hospital in autumn 1804, and with other histories confirming the utility of purgatives in that disease.

3. *In the Marasmus of childhood and early youth*—The observations and reflections delivered in this chapter are of a very in-

teresting

tereſting nature. Under the title of Maraſmus, our author has arranged a variety of ſymptoms which are often obſerved to affect the young of both ſexes.

"A ſluggiſhneſs, and laſſitude on ſlight exertion, depravity and loſs of appetite, waſting of the muſcular fleſh, fulneſs of the features, and paleneſs of the countenance, ſwelling of the abdomen, an irregular and generally a coſtive ſtate of the bowels, a change in the colour, and odour of the fæces, fetid breath, ſwelling of the upper lip, and itching of the noſe, mark the beginning of the diſeaſe.

"When theſe ſymptoms have continued for ſome time, they are followed by alternate paleneſs and fluſhing of the countenance, heat and dryneſs of the ſkin, feeble and quick pulſe, thirſt, fretfulneſs, increaſing debility, and diſturbed ſleep, during which the patients grind or gnaſh their teeth, and are ſubject to involuntary ſtarting, and twitching of different muſcles."

This deſcription muſt be familiar to every practitioner. Various combinations, and many anomalous varieties of ſuch ſymptoms, occur in infancy and early youth, and, imitating often other diſeaſes, occaſion much perplexity in our diagnoſtics. They are commonly referred to the preſence of worms in the bowels; ſometimes to meſenteric obſtruction, and not unfrequently have ſo cloſely reſembled hydrocephalus, as to be miſtaken for that diſeaſe. But we are particularly indebted to Dr Hamilton for an obſervation of ſtill higher importance, that the diſeaſe in queſtion may, on ſome occaſions, give riſe to hydrocephalus, by impairing the vigour of the conſtitution, and by favouring ſerous effuſion into the ventricles of the brain. "This conjecture," he adds, "merits the greater attention on this account, that the ſymptoms of hydrocephalus reſemble thoſe of incipient and even of confirmed maraſmus, and have been removed by the diligent exhibition of purgative medicines. The truth of this obſervation has been repeatedly confirmed in my private practice, and it affords an additional reaſon for the exerciſe of watchful attention to prevent the confirmed ſtate of maraſmus, which may, in more inſtances than we are aware of, have been the forerunner, if not the cauſe, of hydrocephalus."

For the truth and importance of this remark, we muſt refer our readers to the caſes in the Appendix, and eſpecially to that communicated by Mr Ben. Bell, a caſe which was conſidered by the moſt experienced practitioners in conſultation as one of hydrocephalus, and actually treated as ſuch, but ineffectually, when pains in the bowels ſuggeſted the exhibition of a purgative, the relief obtained from which encouraged the repetition, till the ſymptoms and diſeaſe diſappeared. Caſes very like to this

have

have come within our own obſervation; and, as we have already remarked, the number of ſuppoſed caſes of hydrocephalus, recorded as cured by the free exhibition of calomel, confirm this view of the ſubject. But Dr H. is alſo inclined to think, that maraſmus may lay the foundation of epilepſy. It is certain at leaſt that convulſions are not unfrequently a concomitant, or one of the fatal terminations of maraſmus. Amongſt theſe alſo might be enumerated various obſtructions of the abdominal viſcera and aſcites, obſtructions eſpecially of the liver and of the meſenteric glands. The opinion entertained by Dr H. of this diſeaſe is ſimple and ſatisfactory. Worms, though ſo conſtantly ſuſpected in theſe caſes, are not, in this country at leaſt, ſo uniformly met with, as to ſupport the opinion that the diſeaſe proceeds from this cauſe. Every phyſician will acknowledge how often this notion has diſappointed him; and we are well aſſured that the ſymptoms uſually attributed to worms often originate in other ſources of inteſtinal irritation. Our author's doctrine is, "that a torpid ſtate, or weakened action of the alimentary canal, is the immediate cauſe of the diſeaſe; whence proceed coſtiveneſs, diſtention of the bowels, and a peculiar irritation, the conſequence of remora of the fæces. I have accordingly been long in the habit of employing purgative medicines for the cure of this maraſmus; the object is to remove indurated and fetid fæces, the accumulation perhaps of months; and as this object is accompliſhing, the gradual return of appetite and vigour mark the progreſs of recovery."

Many other important obſervations are given by our author on this diſeaſe, for which the original muſt be conſulted. The purging plan muſt be actively purſued, and the doſes and repetition of the medicines muſt be determined by the effects and by the appearance of the evacuations, which Dr H. recommends to be daily inſpected.

4. *Chorea Sancti Viti.*—The practice recommended by Dr H. in this diſeaſe, we have already had an opportunity of introducing to the acquaintance of our readers. It conſiſts in the active exhibition of purgative medicines. And certainly when we conſider the almoſt uniform failure of the old method of treatment, and the very great ſucceſs which has attended the one now propoſed, we muſt acknowledge our obligations to Dr Hamilton for the improvement.

A compendious but excellent hiſtory of the diſeaſe, and ſeveral judicious reflections, which we will not here mutilate by attempting to abridge, precede the modeſt and candid ſtatement of thoſe circumſtances which inſtructed Dr Hamilton in the propriety of changing his practice, and which gradually led

to

to thoſe views, and that method, the utility of which has now been confirmed by repeated experience. Coſtiveneſs is a prominent feature in this diſeaſe; and it may be inferred from the ſucceſs which has attended the exhibition of purgatives, that the phenomena of chorea Sancti Viti are induced and continued by the irritation of feculent ſordes accumulated in the primæ viæ. In the early ſtage of chorea, while the inteſtines yet retain their ſenſibility, and the accumulation of fæces is not ſo great, gentle purgatives repeated as occaſion may require, will readily effect a cure, or rather prevent the full formation of the diſeaſe. "In the confirmed ſtage more ſedulous attention is neceſſary. Powerful purgatives muſt be given in ſucceſſive doſes, in ſuch manner that the latter doſes may ſupport the effect of the former, till the movement and expulſion of the accumulated matter are effected, when ſymptoms of returning health appear. Whoever undertakes the cure of chorea by purgative medicines, muſt be decided and firm to his purpoſe. The confidence which he aſſumes is neceſſary to carry home to the friends of the patient conviction of ultimate ſucceſs. Their prejudices will otherwiſe throw inſurmountable obſtacles in his way. Half meaſures, in inſtances of this kind, will prove unſucceſsful; and were it not for perſeverance in unloading the alimentary canal, the diſeaſe would be prolonged, and recurring would place the patient in danger, and thus bring into diſcredit a practice which promiſes certain ſafety."

This confidence in our practice, and this perſeverance in the uſe of purgatives, it is of the greateſt conſequence to attend to, and therefore are much inſiſted on by Dr H. The torpor of the inteſtines in chorea is in many caſes truly aſtoniſhing. The caſes detailed in the Appendix are ample proofs of this. Thus we find 50 grains of the aloetic pills, taken in 24 hours, hardly ſufficient to occaſion one ſtool in a girl of 10 years old. On another day, the ſame child took 70 grains of the pilula ex aloe et colocynthide, beſides an ounce of Rochelle ſalt. And two days thereafter Dr H. found it neceſſary to preſcribe an ounce and a half of Rochelle ſalt, beſides ſix ſcruples of the compound powder of jalap, to be taken in the courſe of 24 hours; and this practice was almoſt daily repeated for ſix whole weeks, when a cure was at length obtained. But this was the moſt obſtinate caſe of all that have been cured by Dr H. For, by the practice here recommended, "chorea is ſpeedily cured, generally in 10 days, or a fortnight from the commencement of the courſe of purgative medicines."

This practice, ſince it became known, we may add, has been equally ſucceſsful in the hands of other phyſicians. Amongſt the

the cafes in the Appendix are two communicated by Dr James Home, the Profeffor of Materia Medica, and one of the Clinical Profeffors in this Univerfity.

5. *Chlorofis.*—The obfervations contained in this chapter have gratified us exceedingly. The concife hiftory of chlorofis is more than defcriptive. It has the ftriking refemblance of a picture, fo admirably is every feature delineated. Nor are the reflections of our author on the pathology of this difeafe, and on the various opinions which have been entertained of its caufes, lefs worthy of approbation. Having examined and refuted, to our fatisfaction, the different theories of chlorofis, in order to prepare the reader for the candid confideration of what he has to propofe, Dr H. concludes thefe general obfervations by the following very juft reflection, which we quote in his own words. " It would have been fortunate if medical inquirers had always followed the progrefs of difeafes ftep by ftep, and viewed them as a whole, from the firft deviation of health to their termination. A contrary procedure has often betrayed us into confufion and error. It is not the febrile ftate that arifes in marafmus; it is not the involuntary convulfive motions that appear in chorea, that conftitute either difeafe. Thefe are only fingle features, but, being prominent ones, they have abforbed the attention of practitioners; while the interrupted action of the ftomach and bowels, and the conftipated ftate of the latter, the common origin of both difeafes, and the fupporter of their various fymptoms, have been almoft altogether overlooked."

" In like manner, in chlorofis, the cacochymia of the juices, and that of the peculiar ftate of the genitals affecting the whole fyftem with flaccidity and laxity, are evidently founded on the appearances which the difeafe exhibits when it is fully formed, and from which appearances alfo it has its name; when, at the fame time, the hiftory of its incipient ftate has been little regarded."

" The flighteft attention to the general hiftory of the difeafe," Dr H. continues, " evinces that coftivenefs precedes and accompanies the other fymptoms. Coftivenefs induces the feculent odour of the breath, difordered ftomach, depraved appetite and impaired digeftion. Thefe preclude a fufficient fupply of nourifhment at a period of growth when it is moft wanted: hence palenefs, laxity, flaccidity, the nervous fymptoms, wafting of the mufcular flefh, languor, debility, the retention of the menfes, and fufpenfion of other excretions, ferous effufions, dropfy, and death."

On this view of the fubject, our author proceeds to explain fome circumftances connected with the difeafe, and then to ftate for the foundations of that practice he is about to recommend, from experience of its superior usefulness.

The constipated state of the bowels suggests the administration of purgatives in chlorosis; they have accordingly been employed by physicians. But the experience of our author has led him at length to trust to these medicines as to the principal means of cure. The method of administering purgatives in chlorosis is nearly the same with that recommended in chorea. "As in chorea, so in chlorosis, the quantity of feculent matter accumulated is often very great, and the movement of it a task of no small difficulty."

"Of course, the same attention and assiduity in the exhibition of purgative medicines, which I have pointed out to be necessary in chorea, are equally demanded in chlorosis. The practitioner who is not aware of this, and who, yielding to the importunity of his patients, or to the caprice of their relations, does not steadily pursue this plan of cure, will be disappointed, his abilities will be called in question, and his practice vilified and neglected."

6. *In vomiting of Blood.*—A variety of hæmatemesis (not dependent on any organic affection), which attacks females from 18 to 30 years of age, and which has commonly been deemed vicarious of the menses, is the case considered by Dr Hamilton in his 6th chapter. He rejects the common opinion entertained of this disease, as suspended menstruation is not its necessary concomitant; this variety appearing sometimes when the menses are regular. Under the usual routine of practice, this disease is of very uncertain duration. But since Dr Hamilton received the hint from Dr Gasking of Plymouth, which suggested the administration of purgatives, his success, "he assures us," has been so uniform, that he now lays it down as a certain position, that the proper exhibition of purgative medicines affords sure and effectual means of removing the hæmatemesis here spoken of.

"The purgatives which I have used in these cases have never excited vomiting; and, what may be thought singular, I have never been able to ascertain the presence of blood in the fæces.

"The fæces which are brought off are copious, unnatural in colour, consistence, and smell, as they generally are after long remora, the consequence of obstinate and protracted costiveness."

7. *In some Chronic Diseases and in Hysteria.*—"I have not ascertained," says our author, "in how many various diseases purgative medicines may be employed with advantage; but I believe

believe the range of their utility is greater than is commonly imagined."

The purging mineral waters are resorted to by valetudinarians, from experience of their efficacy; and, in similar cases, Dr H. has found benefit from the administration of ordinary purgatives. A few cases from the records of the Infirmary are given in the Appendix. We are presented also with two cases of hysteria successfully treated by purgatives. But his general observations on this disease are for the present withheld. "I may perhaps," he adds, "offer a future publication on the utility of purgative medicines; but my professional avocations do not permit me to come under a positive obligation to do so."

We shall now conclude our account of these truly valuable observations, by expressing our hope, that no circumstances may interfere to disappoint the expectation thus raised of future communications from one whose judgment and candour, and long experience, so eminently qualify for extending our knowledge respecting the operation of those medicines to which he has paid so much attention.

PART

PART II.

MEDICAL INTELLIGENCE.

Second Report of the Board of Health.

THE uncertainty in which we remain respecting the poisonous matter which excites the plague, or other similar diseases, necessarily throws a degree of obscurity over any measures that may be adopted for its destruction. Some have relied upon ventilation, some upon fumigation, as the only remedy or security; some again have rejected both; some have advised that the houses and furniture of a whole city should be subjected to quarantine; while others, observing how entirely the disease has in certain instances ceased, although no means had been employed for its extirpation, have hastily concluded that all measures of this kind were nugatory and troublesome, and ought to be laid aside.

In considering a subject of this kind, it is obvious, that we must not risk the lives of our fellow creatures, through a confidence in any speculative opinions which want the sanction of experience. But even experience itself, which should be our surest guide, has been appealed to in support of doctrines totally opposite to each other. Fully impressed with a sense of these difficulties, we have endeavoured, in the following observations, to select from the practice of infected places, what has been employed with the greatest appearance of success; and to correct the inartificial, or sometimes prejudicial directions of antiquity, by the discoveries and improvements of later times.

In the zeal of individuals, and sometimes of the magistrate, to destroy more completely all sources of infection, it has been proposed to burn clothes, furniture, and even houses, in which the plague has been; but whenever this measure has been attempted to be carried into effect, it has been defeated by its own severity. For, by giving occasion to concealment, or to the secret removal of such articles, there is reason to think more harm has been produced, than if no precaution whatever had been taken. On this subject, therefore, as well as in the separation of sick, moderate measures are not only more easy to be executed, but afford, in fact, a greater security to the public.

Exposure to free ventilation in the open air, certainly dissipates and renders inert the poison of the plague, but the length of time required is considerable, even on the supposition that forty days were always

always ſufficient for that purpoſe. Muratori indeed, ſays, that he, with ſome other reſpectable authorities, thinks 20 days may be long enough. Lib. 1ſt. chap. 9. p. 71.

The purification of goods in lazarettos has been almoſt entirely truſted to ventilation. Moſt of the articles of merchandiſe do not admit of waſhing, and nothing ſatisfactory in the way of fumigation has been introduced into practice.

But where other modes of purification are admiſſible, not only the time neceſſary for deſtroying infection may be much ſhortened, but the ſecurity thus obtained may, in many inſtances, be rendered much more perfect than could be done by the moſt protracted expoſure to the open air.

We therefore adviſe, that every article of apparel, bed-clothes, or houſehold-furniture, that has been expoſed to infection, and that will bear waſhing or ſcouring, ſhould be immerſed in water, previous to its removal from the infected chamber; and it ſhould be ſuffered to lie in the water till it can be boiled, and waſhed or ſcoured, which ought to be with as little delay as poſſible. All ſuſpicion of infection would thus be deſtroyed in a very ſhort time.

From on board ſhips, theſe things may be attached by a line, and thrown over into the water, where they ſhould remain an hour, or longer, before they are boiled and waſhed.

Some things, which perhaps would not bear boiling, might be fulled.

Waſhing machines, and fulling mills, are recommended, as particularly proper for the purpoſe of cleanſing infected goods without riſk to the perſons employed.

Such things as have been very near the perſon of the ſick, as linen, bed-gowns, bed-clothes, &c. and indeed every ſuſpicious article, ought to be removed only with a pair of tongs, or forceps, without handling.

Wherever the above directions can be put in practice, we recommend them in preference to all other modes of purification. But there are ſome articles, viz. mattraſſes, feather-beds, bolſters, and pillows, which either could not be put into water, or not, without great inconvenience, or not without much previous handling, by which a great riſk of infection would be incurred. For ſuch, therefore, ſome other mode of purification ſhould be uſed, or at leaſt in the firſt inſtance. With this view, recourſe has been had to fumigations.

In looking into the general practice on this ſubject, if implicit faith were to be given to all that is ſtated, it would ſeem as if fumigations, of almoſt any kind, would deſtroy the poiſon of the plague. Odoriferous woods and gums, ſweet herbs and flowers, aromatics, ſulphur, pitch, amber, aſſafœtida, arſenic, antimony, orpiment, and numerous other ſubſtances, have been recommended. The ſpeculative grounds upon which they have been employed may eaſily be gueſſed, but there are no ſatisfactory experiments to aſcertain their reſpective merits. Sulphur is conſidered as holding the firſt place, and

and probably with reason. Sulphur reduced to powder, and mixed with saw-dust, or powdered charcoal, in the proportion of one part of sulphur to two or three parts of saw-dust or charcoal, should be put in small quantities in earthen pots, and these again should be set in iron pots or braziers, in number according to the size of the apartments; or sulphur and nitre, mixed in the proportion of seven parts of the former to one of the latter, make a good fumigation; the nitre must be well dried. The goods to be fumigated ought first to be exposed to a stream of air, within the infected chamber, for 24 hours, in order to lessen the risk of the expurgators, and should then be disposed on lines, or otherwise, in the manner most favourable for receiving freely on all sides the elastic fumes and vapour. The windows and other apertures should then be well secured, and fire having been set to the fumigating materials, the operator must immediately retire, and the door must be shut. The room having continued to be closed up for 24 hours, the clothes should then be taken out, and exposed to a free current of air for other 24 hours; at the expiration of that time, such things as have been only slightly exposed to infection may be considered as purified; the things under circumstances of stronger suspicion, instead of being discharged, should again be submitted to a repetition of the same process, and not considered as purified till the expiration of 24 hours from the time of their second fumigation.

The lines upon which the clothes have hung may, for further security, afterwards be burnt.

If possible, the fumigation should always be performed in the infected house, without which one of the principal objects in view would be lost. But if, from want of accommodation in the confined parts of a town, or from any other cause, that cannot be done, it may become expedient to provide a public place for these purposes. We recommend the following plan:

That it should consist of,

1st.—An airing and sorting-room, where the goods should remain exposed to the air six hours, during which time an inventory should be taken, and a duplicate delivered to the owner.

2d.—A fumigating chamber, with lines and proper utensils.

3d.—A ventilating house, or shed, with an addition of fires placed in different parts of the room, in number and size proportionate to the said house, furnished likewise with lines, and admitting a free current of air.

The whole should be enclosed with a double fence.

A superintendant, clerk, and servants, would be necessary for this establishment; and they should be prohibited from all intercourse for 20 days, subsequent to their latest exposure to infection.

It is a circumstance of no small importance to determine what should be done with the bed or matrass on which an infected patient has been lying, and which may therefore be supposed in an especial manner to have become impregnated with whatever it is that constitutes the infectious matter of the plague, or other epidemical contagious diſeaſe. After duly conſidering the danger to be feared, and the difficulties to be overcome, we have concluded the beſt ſecurity would be obtained by firſt fumigating theſe articles in the infected room, then tying them up, and carrying them in carts appropriated to the conveyance of ſuſpected goods to a houſe of purification, to be baked in an oven erected for that purpoſe, for 12 hours: they ſhould afterwards be freely expoſed to the air for 14 days.

In caſes of extraordinary ſuſpicion, or where the things are of little value, it might be adviſable to deſtroy them, the magiſtrate finding others in their place.

Wooden furniture may be firſt fumigated, and afterwards ſcoured.

Rooms ſhould be fumigated for 24 hours, then aired for other 24 hours, and afterwards ſcoured, and white-waſhed, or painted, eſpecially the parts which have been moſt expoſed to infection.

The fumigation with ſulphur, as above deſcribed, is at once the moſt efficacious and the cheapeſt; we therefore recommend it to be uſed in preference to all others. But, as the utmoſt caution is neceſſary in conducting the ſulphuric fumigation, it is adviſable that ſuch fumigation ſhould not be attempted but by thoſe who have been previouſly inſtructed in the proceſs, and appriſed of its danger; for it does not admit of the preſence of any living creature, as the fumes of the ſulphur would inſtantly prove fatal. Therefore other fumigations have been uſed in the apartments of the ſick. In place of the elaborate receipts of the older phyſicians, modern chemiſts have ſhown, that although the vapour of the vitriolic acid be inconſiſtent with animal life, yet the vapour of nitrous and marine acids may be employed with ſafety and convenience. Dr Carmichael Smyth has directed the fumes of the nitrous acid to be uſed in the wards of hoſpitals full of ſick; and M. Morveau Guiton has employed the fumes of the muriatic acid in the ſame way; but it muſt not be forgotten, that even allowing theſe acid vapours to poſſeſs all the virtues attributed to them in the diſeaſes againſt which they have been employed, it would be unphiloſophical, and contrary to the principles of juſt reaſoning, to infer that they muſt have the ſame virtues in other diſeaſes. Such is the ſubtile nature of all the poiſons generated in animal bodies, that we are totally ignorant upon what their properties and powers depend, and cannot, upon general principles, apply to one of thoſe poiſons which we have learned of another. We are led to make theſe obſervations, becauſe the language commonly uſed on this ſubject may lead to ſerious error. Contagion and infection are terms which expreſs the mode in which the poiſons are ſuppoſed to be applied to ſound perſons; but, by a common figure in language, they are often uſed to expreſs the figure itſelf, and ſuch poiſons go by the name of contagious and infectious, and what deſtroys contagion in one caſe, it has been inferred would deſtroy it in another; but there is no foundation for this broad concluſion. For example's ſake, we will ſuppoſe it

proved

proved that the acid of nitre or of common ſalt would deſtroy the poiſon of the jail fever; we cannot from thence infer that it would deſtroy that of meaſles, ſmall pox, or the plague. Having premiſed the above reflections, we have no heſitation in recommending trial to be made of the vapour of the nitrous or muriatic acid in the apartments of the ſick, provided none of the precautions reſpecting ventilation, change of apparel, &c. recommended above, be neglected.

The nitrous acid vapour is diſengaged from nitre by adding to it vitriolic acid; and in like manner the muriatic acid vapour, by adding vitriolic acid to ſea ſalt.

Nitre reduced to powder, and vitriolic acid, in equal quantities, mixed in ſmall pots, and diſperſed through the wards of an hoſpital, diſcharge copiouſly the fumes of the nitrous acid, and the diſcharge is more rapid if the pot be placed in hot ſand.

Sea ſalt a little moiſtened	15 parts,
Acid of vitriol (of the ſpecific gravity of 1.7)	12 parts,

mixed in pots of a moderate ſize, which may be put in a ſand bath or not, at pleaſure, produce the acid fumes of the ſea ſalt in the manner recommended by M. Morveau Guiton.

At Woolwich, in the military hoſpitals, they have uſed a fumigation of the oxygenated muriatic acid, made in the following manner, under the direction of Mr Cruickſhanks:

Manganeſe in powder	2 parts,
Common ſalt	4 parts,
Vitriolic acid (the ſpecific gravity of which in our Pharmacopœia is 1.85)	3 parts,
Water	1 part.

To a ſmall quantity of the mixture of manganeſe and ſea ſalt (ſuppoſe three ounces) the whole of the water (which, for that quantity, would be half an ounce) is added, and, to this put in a ſmall pot, (large enough to prevent any riſk from the ebullition of the materials) the vitriolic acid (in due proportion) is added at intervals, which will keep up for a day a diſcharge of the oxygenated muriatic vapour; the ſmell is not unpleaſant, and the vapour gives no annoyance either to the ſick or their attendants. Any of the three preceding modes of fumigation may be uſed in the apartments of the ſick, and every one may uſe his own judgment in deciding to which he will give the preference.

In the expurgation of houſes, it may ſerve, by way of example, to give, as an extreme caſe, the ſteps we would recommend in the purification of an hoſpital that had been uſed for the reception of perſons ill of the plague.

Every door and window ſhould be open for ſome time previous to the expurgators entering upon their buſineſs, that they may run as little riſk as poſſible. In the apartments, ſuch articles of linen apparel, bed-clothes, &c. as remained, ſhould directly be put in water, afterwards to be boiled. The bedſtead, beds, and other articles not admitting of this, ſhould be placed favourably for fumigation. The pots with the fumigating materials of ſulphur, &c. ſhould be properly diſpoſed, and the windows and doors, except one, being all ſhut, fire ſhould be ſet to the pots. The door, left open for the retreat of the perſon that ſet fire to the pots, ſhould be ſhut as ſoon as he has made his eſcape, and the fumes ſhould be confined in the apartment for 24 hours; every apartment muſt undergo the ſame proceſs. The houſe ſhould afterwards be whitewaſhed with quick lime and water, and the floors ſhould be waſhed with a copious ſtream of water, for which purpoſe even the common fire-engine might be extremely uſeful.

It has been doubted how far the purification of any town ought to be extended; and univerſal purification of every houſe, and of all their contents, would not only be impracticable, but we have no reaſon to think it would be neceſſary. Thoſe houſes only ſhould be obliged to undergo purification in the manner above deſcribed, which have either held perſons who have been ill of a peſtilential diſorder, or which have received things ſuſceptible of infection from tainted places; likewiſe the purification of goods can only be neceſſary when they have been expoſed to the touch or exhalations of the ſick, or have beeen in contact with infected ſubſtances. Therefore the things contained in trunks, wardrobes, or ſtore-rooms, may be exempted from quarantine, even though perſons ſhould have died in the houſe, provided they have been locked up and ſealed by the magiſtrate, previous to the diſeaſe having entered the houſe.

The following obſervation is taken from Dr Ruſſel's hiſtory of the plague.

"In large commercial towns it may be matter of deliberation, whether it would not be a prudent meaſure for the merchants to ſhut up their warehouſes, depoſiting the keys with a proper magiſtrate; this, in many caſes, would render the purification of merchandiſe, as practiſed with infinite labour at Marſeilles, unneceſſary, and might contribute to a ſpeedier re-eſtabliſhment of commerce, becauſe ſuch merchandiſe, accompanied with authentic certificates, would certainly be leſs liable to ſuſpicion than ſuch as had remained in open warehouſes all the time of ſickneſs, and might therefore be exported with more ſafety."—And again, "Goods of a more ſuſpicious kind, which have not been thus ſhut up, might be ſent to the lazaretto to be aired, or perhaps be fumigated in the warehouſe."

The whole of the above regulations ſhould be conducted under the inſpection and direction of the magiſtrates. And where the parties are unable to defray the expenſe of purification, it ſhould be paid by the public.

An inventory ſhould be taken, and a watchman or guard placed at the infected houſe, till the purification is completed, and any loſs that may happen ſhould be made good by the public, from rates levied on the neighbourhood.

All perſons employed for the purpoſes here deſcribed, or for any other purpoſe by which they have been expoſed to infection, ſhould be obliged to go into a warm bath, and afterwards perform a quarantine of 20 days, before they are reſtored to ſociety.

What we have ſubmitted muſt be conſidered rather as a ſketch than a detailed plan of purification and expurgation; yet if the general principles of deſtroying the poiſon by ventilation, waſhing, and fumigation, be kept in view, it will not be difficult to adapt them to all caſes that may occur. JA. HERVEY, *Sec.*

Board of Health, April 30. 1806.

Vaccine Pock Inſtitution, Broad-Street, Golden Square.

GENERAL Quarterly Court, November 5.:—*Reſolved*, That, according to the experience of the medical eſtabliſhment of this inſtitution, it appears that the inoculation for the cow-pock affords ſecurity againſt the ſmall-pox equally with variolous inoculation, and that the new practice poſſeſſes all the advantages already ſtated to the public.

Reſolved, That, in order to give a further proof to the public, and to afford an inducement for information adverſe to the new practice, the following propoſal be made public, viz.

That, in future, every patient who ſhall be vaccinated at this inſtitution, on diſcharge, ſhall receive a certificate, ſtating, that ſuch patient has gone through the cow-pock, and engaging, that if hereafter the ſaid patient ſhall take the ſmall-pox, he or ſhe ſhall be entitled to the ſum of five guineas, to be paid from the funds of this inſtitution, at the firſt general court, after the proofs have been given, according to the rules of the medical eſtabliſhment.

Drs Pearſon, Nihel, and Nelſon, *Phyſicians.*
Tho. Payne and John Heaviſide, Eſqrs. *Treaſurers.*
T. Keate, T. Payne, and T. Forreſter, Eſqrs. *Conſulting Surgeons.*
J. Gunning, J. Conſt. Carpue, and J. Doratt, Eſqrs. *Surgeons.*
F. Rivers, E. Brande, and P. D. Bruyn, Eſqrs. *Viſiting Apothecaries.*
WILLIAM SANCHO, *Secretary.*

THE friends and pupils of Deſſault and Bichât have opened a ſubſcription at Paris to erect a marble monument, and ſtrike off a medal, to the memory of thoſe illuſtrious ſurgeons.—Prof. Kurt Sprengel, of the Univerſity of Hallé, is engaged in writing a Hiſtory of Surgery.—Prof. Loder of Hallé, formerly of Iena, is preparing for the preſs a Series of Anatomical and Surgical Obſervations, including a deſcription of ſome remarkable pathological facts, with drawings of the moſt intereſting preparations in his valuable collection. This ſplendid work will be entitled *Obſervationes Academicæ*, and the text will be in Latin.—Prof. Soemmering, who has been invited by the Elector of Bavaria to Munich from Frankfort, has juſt finiſhed another part of his Deſcription of the Senſes, comprehending the organ of hearing.

ing, and illuſtrated with many beautiful plates of the ear. This diſtinguiſhed anatomiſt is now engaged in preparing a work on the tongue and the organ of taſte. We take this opportunity of expreſſing our ſatisfaction at having diſcovered that our remarks on the inconvenience ariſing from the text of theſe ſplendid faſiſculi being publiſhed only in German, are incorrect; for we have ſeen a copy of that on the eye, with the text in Latin, entitled "Icones Oculi Humani." Dr Edmondſton will ſhortly publiſh "An Inquiry into the contagious nature of Ophthalmia; with a hiſtory of the ſymptoms and treatment of ocular Inflammation in general."—Dr H. S. Jackſon has in the preſs "Practical Reflections and Conjectures on the febrile epidemic Diſeaſes of Gibraltar, with compendious obſervations on Fevers in general, particularly the Yellow Fever of tropical climates; forming the ground-work of a new inquiry, on ſyſtematic principles, into the nature, tendency, and treatment of all the commonly ſuppoſed contagious, malignant, and epidemic fevers."

Extract of a Letter from Geneva, November 3. 1805.

"When Pacchioni's account of his diſcovery was read to the National Inſtitute of France, Biot and two other members were named for the purpoſe of repeating the experiments on which the diſcovery was ſaid to be founded. This they did, and made their report accordingly. Biot read his report not long ſince at the Society of Natural Hiſtory at Geneva. He concluded that Pacchioni, as well as the Engliſh experimentaliſt, had been deceived, and that, if the experiment be made with every previous precaution neceſſary to exclude the preſence of ſea ſalt, no muriatic acid will be found in the reſult.

Premiums propoſed by the Univerſity and Imperial Academy of Wilna in the year 1805.

CLASS OF MEDICAL SCIENCE.

PREMIUM I.

Beſides the diabetes mellitus of medical authors, are there any other diſeaſes peculiar to man, which, according to accurate obſervations, produce in different organs a ſecretion of a ſaccharine nature, and ſufficiently abundant, that its diſcharge finally occaſions conſumption? and what are theſe diſeaſes?

The prize conſiſts of 100 Dutch ducats.—Eſſays will be received till the 1ſt of September 1806.

The antients were not unacquainted with a ſpecies of conſumption accompanied with a prodigious loſs of urine, inſupportable thirſt, and an extraordinary dryneſs of the ſkin; ſymptoms which almoſt always terminated in a general dropſy, or in fainting-fits, which proved mortal. The Grecian phyſicians conceived that this diſeaſe reſembled much the effects produced by the bite of a venomous ſerpent,

pent, called dipsas (coluber dipsas Linn.) and for this reason they distinguished this disease by the name of dipsas or diabetes.

It is now more than a century since it was observed that the urine produced in this singular malady had, in almost every case, the smell, and likewise, in some measure, the sweetness of honey; hence they gave the name of diabetes mellitus to this species of diabetes, in order to distinguish it from another much more rare, called diabetes insipidus.

Afterwards it was ascertained by chemical analysis, that the urine in the case of diabetes mellitus contained a considerable quantity of saccharine matter. The gradual decay and consumption in the patient were attributed to the continual and abundant loss of this matter which appeared to constitute the nutritive principle in the aliment.

These discoveries have scarcely tended to diminish the almost certain mortality of persons attacked with this disease. Physicians, indeed, consoled themselves in some degree, by supposing that the diabetes was a malady so rare, that the greater part of experienced practitioners had never once met with it; and, nevertheless, the Academy well knows, that one of its members alone has had opportunities of observing this disease more than 15 times, which to him appeared to be more prevalent in warm climates than towards the north. There is then reason to believe, that very often physicians are not aware of this disease, and one example observed by Dr Rollo, where the urine of the patient attacked with an unknown consumption, without being more abundant than in other complaints, was charged with a prodigious quantity of a saccharine principle (three ounces to the pound of urine), seems to demonstrate, that the superabundance of urine is not an essential or pathognomonic symptom of the disease called diabetes, and that it is possible that it may have proved fatal to patients, the nature of whose consumption was unknown, more frequently than is supposed.

But, from observations on the vegetable kingdom, it appears that trees sometimes experience a malady analagous to diabetes. Many fruit-trees are observed to emit gum; and if, on the one hand, the remarks of the gardener show that cherry-trees, plumb-trees, subject to this exudation, are evidently exhausted and perish by a species of consumption, on the other, chemistry has discovered that gums in general, and thick fluids, which issue from clefts in the bark of certain trees, as the ash (fraxinus excelsior) which furnishes manna, the birch (betula alba) contain a quantity, more or less considerable, of a saccharine principle. The leaves even of several trees, shrubs and plants, appear to suffer a similar discharge. Hence they are so often observed to be covered with small insects, which appear to be attracted by this same sweet and saccharine principle, which they seek for with avidity. The ants, which yield nothing to them in this respect, assemble in a body upon the same leaves, and by irritating the insects, which they disperse, oblige them immediately to give up the mellifluous matter which they have just extracted from the surface of the leaves tainted and attacked, as it would appear, by a ſpecies of diabetes. Theſe conſiderations induce us to think that diabetes mellitus is not, perhaps, the only diſeaſe in which man is quickly deprived of the nutritive juices he derives from the vegetable kingdom. We are aſtoniſhed at a propoſition of Hippocrates, which ſtates, that in conſumption, the ſweet and ſaccharine ſavour of the unctuous matter in the ears of patients is a ſign of ſure and ſpeedy diſſolution: this ſtriking obſervation, which at ſo remote a period, would ſcarcely have been expected, has but once been confirmed after the lapſe of ſo many ages; and it would appear that the natural diſguſt which accompanies ſuch reſearches, and the inattention of many phyſicians to them, as requiring too conſtant application, were the principal cauſes why animal chemiſtry has been ſo long neglected.

And, nevertheleſs, many circumſtances appear to promiſe us an ample collection of facts from a more ſerious examination into theſe objects. For the preſent age, it was reſerved to ſubmit to the niceſt analyſis, not only the products of nature when in health, but alſo when diſeaſed. We are already in poſſeſſion of many very uſeful reſults derived from the chemical analyſis of humours generated in the human frame by diſordered, unhealthy ſecretion. We are not ignorant that we ought to be upon our guard not to conſider this alteration of the fluids as primitive, and as the cauſe of diſeaſes, of which it is commonly only a conſequence; but, in ſpite of this truth, it muſt be agreed, that there are circumſtances in the life of man where the ſecretion of fluids undergoes a conſiderable change without being apparent, and where this alteration produces either waſting, concretions, or effuſions, which may be conſidered as primitive diſeaſes. The diabetes mellitus appears to be one of theſe. But are there not other analogous complaints in which a ſaccharine matter, combined with other liquids, eſcapes in ſufficient abundance to deprive the human body of theſe alimentary principles, before they have become perfectly animalized? The ſweat called, hypothetically, *colliquative*, which is not peculiar to the decay produced by ulcerations of the viſcera, is it not, in ſome ſpecies of conſumption (tabes), analogous to the urine in the diabetes mellitus of authors? The obſervation that this ſame ſweat, collected by the help of a ſponge or napkins, diffuſes, in a ſhort time, a ſmell of vinegar, ſeems to ſhow that it alſo contains principles capable of vinous fermentation; as the water of patients attacked with diabetes furniſhes alſo a conſiderable quantity of carbonaceous principle, and even of alcohol. In ſome rare caſes, a commencement of cryſtallization obſerved upon the ſkin of perſons ſubject to copious ſweats, the viſcous and almoſt gummy nature of theſe in other complaints, their ſpecific or ſometimes acid odour, as in miliary fevers, and in diſeaſes incident to puerperal women, all point out the probability of the object in queſtion. But there are other complaints which heighten this probability much: Does not too great a ſecretion of milk (galactirrhœa) affect nurſes with conſumption? The flux called cœliac (fluxus

cœliacus)

cæliacus) furnishes a whitish matter, which, for a long time, physicians supposed to be chyle, although it often exceeds considerably the quantity of that which the aliment, consumed by the patients, could have furnished. But would not this matter be found to be endowed with the same principles as the urine of persons attacked with diabetes? Does not the consumption called pituitous by physicians, because, on examination after death, the lungs were not ulcerated so as to have furnished the thick and white matter, the copious expectoration of which exhausted, and was the cause of death to the patient, belong to the same class of diseases? Does Leucorrhoea of long duration, and very copious, furnish the same saccharine principles, since it weakens the patient much more than that of a fluid simply mucous would seem capable of doing? In order to obtain a solution of these problems, the Imperial University of Wilna submits the above question to the competition of medical gentlemen.

PREMIUM II.

What are the true characteristics and principal causes of that disease which, though not peculiar to Poland alone, is nevertheless called Plica Polonica? Are there any means of treating it with more success than by the method hitherto known and employed? and what are these means?

The prize is 100 Dutch ducats.—Essays will be received till the 1st September 1807.

The plica (Plica Polonica) is not endemial alone in that country, the name of which it bears, but also exists in other provinces; while neither its true origin is yet determined, nor the cause, nor a method of cure sufficiently satisfactory.—We are even not without works which treat of this disease, and, lately, it has been much elucidated by an author of merit.

Nevertheless, with all our knowledge of it, the plica still prevails in many provinces, and though the method of cure employed in our time has in some cases succeeded, yet in the greatest number it has been otherwise. Therefore, the Imperial University of Wilna have determined to propose the above question, in order to contribute, on its part, towards the extirpation of an evil so prevalent in the provinces. If, on the one hand, most European physicians are deprived of the opportunity of personally observing this singular malady, and consequently of contending for the premium announced, on the other, the number of medical men who have it in their power to trace this endemic disorder, and to try different methods for successfully combating it, is so considerable, as to induce us to expect much from their patriotic zeal and experiment.

PREMIUM III.

What are the principal diseases of vegetables? and what is the true analogy between these diseases and those of animals?

The prize consists of 100 Dutch ducats.—Essays will be received till the 1st of September 1808.

The known works of nature constitute but two classes, essentially differing

differing from each other; the first of which contains bodies organized and susceptible of excitement; the second, bodies destitute of all organization, consequently deprived of the faculty of reacting when excited by external powers. According to this simple and natural division, vegetables and animals belong to one family, differing only in their organization, and in its effects, when excited by external agents. These beings, endowed with an unknown vital principle, undergo the same changes; they are engendered by individuals of their own kind; separated from these, they vegetate; they are nourished by preparing within themselves their nutritive juices; they grow, they ripen, they engender by the same law by which they themselves were engendered; and, arrived at old age, they insensibly quit their connexion with external agents; are no longer subservient to their impulse, but decay, and at last return to that chaos of amorphous and unorganized matters from which they sprang. But these living beings, subject to the same laws of nature, equally suffer by the disproportionate action of external causes, many derangements, which necessarily impair their functions. This state of disease presents more or fewer phenomena, external symptoms, the observation of which constitutes the science of their sufferings, or of their pathology. So long as the physiolgy of man was confined to the simple observation of the functions of his own body and of its parts, its progress was slow, and it was necessary to sustain the structure of this science by the help of a great number of hypothetical pillars, dangerous in medicine. Scarcely had the attentive dissection of other animals, and the examination of the divers functions of their parts taken place, than the physiology of man also made rapid strides in the most interesting discoveries. The same has taken place in pathology; and the examination of diseases to which other animals are subject, and that of their principal causes and effects, has infinitely contributed to the more perfect knowledge of those diseases which afflict the human body. Why, then, should we longer delay the most thorough examination of the principal diseases of the vegetable world, the analogy of which with animals and with man himself appears in many points to be so decided? We know, for example, that the wounds of trees present the same phenomena as those of animal bodies; that their nutritive juices escape by wounds they receive, as blood flows, from those inflicted on a living part of the human body, and that, when this dangerous discharge is once stopt, a scar is formed, and the injured parts are regenerated by the same laws which contribute to the preservation of animals.

We observe trees attacked with caries, gangrene, shrivelling, or atrophy, chlorosis, parasitic insects, &c. like the human body itself, and should we still doubt for a moment the utility or the necessity of an exact examination of the diseases to which these living beings are subject, and so often sacrificed? The University, therefore, thinks that the question above proposed merits the attention of all those who feel an interest in the perfection of the pathology of the human race.

Account

Account of Diſeaſes treated at the Public Diſpenſary, Carey-Street, from 31ſt Auguſt to 30th November, 1805.

ACUTE DISEASES.

	No. of Caſes.		No. of Caſes.
Quotidiana	1	Rubeola	2
Ephemera	2	Variola	7
Synochus	5	Varicella	2
Typhus	1	Scarlatina	1
Ophthalmia	1	Eryſipelas	2
Cynanche tonſillaris	7	Pertuſſis	5
Pneumonia	10	Catarrhus	71
Peripneumonia notha	5	Dyſenteria	10
Gaſtritis	1	Cholera	3
Enteritis	1	Febris poſt Partum	2
Rheumatiſmus	7	—— Infantium	4

CHRONIC DISEASES.

	No. of Caſes.		No. of Caſes
Cephalæa	9	Hæmatemeſis	1
Hemicrania	3	Hyſteria	4
Vertigo	2	Melancholia	2
Aſthma and Dyſpnœa	8	Epilepſia	2
Catarrhus Chronicus	47	Hemiplegia	5
Hœmoptyſis and Phthiſis	13	Rheumatiſmus Chronicus	29
Aſthenia	28	Pleurodyne	3
Dyſpepſia	41	Lumbago	5
Hepatitis Chronica	2	Hydrothorax	3
Icterus	2	Aſcites	4
Enterodynia	8	Anaſarca	8
Colica Saturnina	2	Tympanites	1
Tænia	1	Rachitis	1
Aſcarides and Lumbrici	7	Scrofula	2
Tabes Meſenterica	3	Syphilis	4
Diarrhœa	6	Strophulus	2
Phyſconia	1	Aphthæ	1
Nephralgia	2	Prurigo	3
Dyſuria	4	Lichen	3
Pyuria	1	Pſoriaſis	2
Hæmorrhois	4	Porrigo	1
Prolapſus Uteri	2	Impetigo	7
Menorrhagia	3	Scabies	5
Leucorrhœa	7	Herpes Chronica	1
Dyſmenorrhœa	1	Ecthyma	3
Amenorrhœa	6		

The weather during the month of September was regular, dry, and warm; in October it became moderately cold, with an almost constant north-east wind, but with little rain; and during the present month there have been frequent thick fogs, together with occasional frost, and some heavy rains.

The small-pox is still very prevalent, but does not appear to be increasing. It will probably follow its usual course, and gradually become less general as the winter approaches *. It is chiefly the very severe cases which apply to a public institution, and the majority of those in the foregoing list were of a very unfavourable sort: the eruptions on the face were small and numerous, and attended with a diffuse erythematic redness; but on the body and extremities they were few in number, small, acuminated, and never fully maturating; the extremities were generally cold, and the patients exceedingly restless and uneasy. In one of the cases, several large purple spots were intermixed with the scattered and imperfect pustules on the third day of the eruption; hemorrhagies from the mouth and bowels succeeded, and the patient died on the 8th day.

The instances of cholera and bilious diarrhœa were but few; a circumstance which (cool as the season has been) may be considered as tending to confirm the observation, that these complaints do not originate from the use of the summer fruits; but that the *heat* is the common source of the fruit and the bilious diseases.

Of nearly 470 cases which the preceding list comprehends, about 200, or somewhat more than 2-5ths, are diseases of the lungs. Catarrhal coughs, indeed, have prevailed through the greater part of the year; but during the month of November, and especially in the third week, when there occurred some severe frosts, accompanied by thick fogs during the day, the number of these complaints suddenly and rapidly increased. In that week almost all the asthmatics, who have been for some years annual applicants at the Dispensary, appeared at once; and their complaints seemed to be more severe than usual. The cases of pulmonary inflammation were not of the acute pleuritic species; and instances of what has been called *peripneumonia notha* have been more numerous than is usual at the beginning of winter. In one case the latter disease was rapidly fatal; the rest yielded to blisters (with the internal use of antimonials and squills), without the use of the lancet. This disease, in fact, as it now appears in London, will not bear blood-letting: those on whom it is employed almost invariably die. Such, indeed, is the general state of the human constitution in this metropolis, that diseases of a high inflammatory type are comparatively rare, and powerfully debilitating remedies are inadmissible in any complaints, in the same degree in which they are most advantageously adopted in the country.

It may be collected from the observations of Sydenham, that in the autumn, or towards its close, a continued or remittent fever frequently appeared among the diseases of that season. He gives no name to this fever, but considered it as allied to, and deriving its character from, some

* See Sydenham on the Epidemic Constitution of 1661, &c.—*Willan's Reports of Diseases in London*, 18.1.

some previous or more prominent epidemic, such as the dysentery, tertian or quartan intermittent, &c. It was at this season that the dreadful plague of 1665 occurred, and in September destroyed 8000 persons in a week *. Dr Fothergill has also noticed the presence of a continued or remittent fever about the same period of those years to which his observations are directed †. And, according to the later observations of Dr Willan, the synochus, or mild fever of the summer months, was usually succeeded by a typhus, which prevailed to a considerable extent. For example, during the period comprehended by our present Report, and in the same district, he noticed, in 1798, about 40 cases of malignant fever; in 1799, no less than 54 cases; and in 1800, above 80. The almost total absence of fever of this description, in the autumnal months of the last and of the present year, is therefore the more remarkable, and the circumstances to which this diminution of so great an evil can be attributed become interesting objects of inquiry.

It is usual, in the discussion of these topics, to hear a great deal assigned to some occult and undiscoverable qualities of the atmosphere, which are supposed to exist at certain intervals, and to produce all epidemics, whether contagious or not. These qualities, however, are purely imaginary, and beyond the cognizance of our senses? and it would, perhaps, be more rational to endeavour to trace a connexion between the existence of the epidemic diseases, and the *obvious* conditions of the atmosphere, upon which much unquestionably depends. Perhaps it may be affirmed, without hazard of contradiction, that those years in which the temperature never continues long in extreme heat or extreme cold, in which it is generally moderate throughout every season, and in which vicissitudes are frequent, but not great, are most favoured in this island with general good health, and most free from all epidemics. The few records of the seasons, and the diseases connected with them, which we possess, seem to afford results, on the whole, tolerably uniform. That a hot and droughty summer is productive of numerous and dangerous diseases is well known to physicians; and that a continued frost through the winter is also extremely detrimental to health (contrary to the popular opinion), and even excites the most malignant fevers, has been shown by Dr Heberden ‡ from indubitable evidence. And it may be observed that the winter preceding the great plague before mentioned was distinguished by a frost of remarkable intensity. The coincidence of the state of the seasons in 1751 and 1752, as described by Dr Fothergill, with that of the years 1804 and 1805, is extremely great as to every variety of the condition of the atmosphere: and a similar absence of epidemic diseases, and a general prevalence of good health, is also particularly recorded. It was not so, however, in the hot and droughty summer which succeeded in 1754, when diseases of the stomach and bowels prevailed to a great extent, and in the autumn a dangerous remittent fever was also very prevalent. A register of the weather and diseases, continued with unremitting attention for some years, would be the only means of elucidating this important subject.

November 30. T. B.

* Sydenham, ibid. † Observ. on the Weather and Diseases, 1751, &c.

‡ Philos. Trans. for 1796.

On the Present State of Vaccine Inoculation on the Continent.

[Extract of a Letter from Dr Henry Reeve, dated Vienna, 10th October 1805.]

"The vaccine inoculation is universally adopted throughout Germany, France, and Switzerland. With regard to the first and the last of these three countries, I can speak from the result of my own observation, and from inquiries made in most of the principal towns. In the beginning of last year, the small-pox was very prevalent at Lausanne, and proved fatal to several persons. Although it was spread in almost every quarter of the town, not one of those who had been previously vaccinated was affected by it, notwithstanding many of them lived in the same rooms, and even slept in the same beds, with those labouring under small-pox. A few instances of the inefficacy of vaccination were talked of, and exaggerated into some sort of importance; but all these cases, amounting only to four in number, on inquiry were most decisively and satisfactorily proved to have been either cases in which the cow-pock inoculation had produced no effect, or in which a spurious, irregular disease took place. These are the only examples of suspected failure that I have heard of on the continent, and, since that time, the public confidence in Switzerland has been restored. The medical men at Lausanne have formed a committee for inoculating the poor *gratis*; and, moreover, they have offered a handsome pecuniary reward to any person who shall show themselves affected with small-pox, either by contagion or by inoculation, after having been once inoculated with cow-pock matter, and having had this disease in the regular progressive way. A case of this sort was considered as well worth the price; but the reward has never been claimed, and all the clamour has ceased. At Bern, Neuchatel, Basle, &c. the cow-pock has superseded the small-pox, and it is only in the accounts from England that I hear of the ravages of this terrible malady. Since I have been at this place, I have continued my inquiries. My friend Dr De Carro has obliged me with a written document on this subject; it is in itself completely satisfactory. If any additional testimony were necessary, I could add, that it corresponds in every respect with all that I have been able to learn, and it may be looked upon as perfectly authentic. I send you enclosed a copy of Dr De Carro's letter.

"Dear Sir, *Vienna, October* 9. 1805.

"It is with the greatest pleasure that I comply with your wishes in giving you a short account of the actual state of vaccination in Germany, while, at the same time, I give my opinion upon the disrepute into which it seems to fall in England, of which the public newspapers, and the private account from Norwich, which you read to me yesterday, afford a melancholy example. It would be both useless and difficult to enumerate all the various institutions which have been formed in Germany for the progress and success of vaccination. I know

know none of its ſeveral governments which have not encouraged, and, as far as poſſible, ordered its adoption. Every eccleſiaſtical court, and each individual clergyman, has taken ſome ſteps about it. Several crowned heads, among whom are the Emperor of Auſtria and the King of Pruſſia, have ſubmitted their own children to this beneficial operation: innumerable books, ſermons, catechiſms, popular dialogues, &c. &c. have been publiſhed; copperplates and wax figures, repreſenting the true vaccine puſtule, have been diſtributed, where they were ſuppoſed to be neceſſary; and, for theſe laſt three years, I do not know one ſingle line of any conſequence that has been written againſt the cow-pock. Some few works, publiſhed againſt it previouſly, are now entirely forgotten, and, though there are ſtill ſome practitioners careleſs in promoting vaccination, I know none publicly hoſtile to it, and Germany has neither *Goldſons* nor *Moſeleys*. From the unanimity, and from the excellent meaſures taken for inſtructing the under claſs of country ſurgeons, barbers, &c. we really do not now hear any more of blunders in inoculation, and no ſuch thing is to be found in our innumerable periodical and polemical works as *caſes* of *ſmall-pox* ſubſequent to cow-pock, nor even ſuſpicions of the inefficacy of the latter. In my own practice, which began the 10th May 1799, on my eldeſt ſon, and which has ſince been very extenſive, and in the innumerable reports which have been ſent to me from thoſe to whom I have ſent vaccine matter, I declare, upon my honour, that I have not met with any accident which could in the leaſt diminiſh my complete faith in the Jennerian method; and, indeed, you can appeal to the teſtimony of the whole city of Vienna, to which my conſtant attention, with regard to vaccination, is ſufficiently known. My care in minutely examining any of thoſe reports, which are almoſt inevitable on the appearance of eruptive diſeaſes in children previouſly vaccinated, has been as great as thoſe I have taken, and ſtill take, in the diffuſion of cow-pock matter.

"What I have ſaid of Germany I might repeat of the preſent ſtate of vaccination in India, where I have had the good fortune to introduce it by the way of Bagdad, Baſſora, Bombay, &c. after every attempt to forward the matter by ſea, by Dr Jenner himſelf, and the moſt celebrated vaccinators in England, had failed. Some of my letters on the oriental vaccination have been publiſhed; I have written an account of it in my *Hiſtoire de la Vaccination en Turquie, en Grece, et aux Indes*; the Eaſt India Company and the Governor of Bombay have publicly acknowledged their obligations to me by preſents. As the principal phyſicians and ſurgeons of Bagdad, Baſſora, Bombay, Madras, Goa, and Colomba, in the iſland of Ceylon, do me the favour to continue their communications by every poſt, I can affirm, upon their authority, by private and public documents, by letters from bramins themſelves, which I have ſhown you, that the progreſs of vaccination in the Britiſh ſettlements is truly aſtoniſhing. Dr Milne, now at Goa, has inſpired among the Portugueſe of that ſettlement ſuch confidence in the vaccine preſervative, that nothing can ſurpaſs the

the eagerneſs with which thoſe people make uſe of it. Dr Milne has deſcribed to me ſeveral of his excurſions, made in the environs of Goa, which can be compared to none but thoſe of Dr Sacco in Lombardy, who goes from one town or village to another, and the children are all aſſembled and called together *en maſſe*, to be vaccinated, by the ringing of the church-bell.

" How, then, to account for the caſes adverſe to the efficacy of cow-pock in England, when we ſee ſuch invariable ſucceſs in other countries *with the matter ſent from England*? Surely ſuch inſtances muſt be owing to errors now unpardonable in a country which gave birth to Dr Jenner, to that man who is as great by the importance of his diſcovery, as he is by the manner in which he publiſhed it. If Engliſh vaccinators follow his precepts as faithfully as we do on the continent, and as Britiſh and Indian phyſicians do in Aſia, none of thoſe fatal events will occur. In the year 1804, two children only died of the ſmall-pox at Vienna, and even they did not belong to the town: one caught the diſeaſe on the Danube in coming from Suabia, the other was brought with the diſeaſe from a diſtant village to the Foundling Hoſpital. This year we have been leſs fortunate here, ſix or ſeven children have already died of ſmall-pox. But that number is quite inſignificant, when compared with the yearly mortality before the introduction of the cow-pock. None of theſe children had been vaccinated *.

" If, my dear Sir, this letter can be of any uſe to re-eſtabliſh a belief in a remedy ſo precious to mankind, and ſo honourable to your country, you may diſpoſe of it in any manner you think moſt proper.

" Believe me, with the greateſt eſteem, yours very truly,

To Dr Reeve, Vienna. J. De Carro, M. D."

* Vaccination was introduced into Vienna in 1801. Its effects in decreaſing the deaths by ſmall-pox are evident from comparing the deaths ſince that period with the medium of the preceding ten years, as ſtated in Dr Marc's Medical Annals.

	Total Deaths.	*Small-pox.*	
1791—1800	14,600	835	or one in 17 ½.
1801	15,181	164	93.
1802	14,522	61	238.
1803	14,383	27	532.
1804	14,035	2	7017.

TO CORRESPONDENTS.

We have received communications from Dr Macleay, Oban; Mr Collins, Swanſea; Dr Anderſon, Madras; Mr Henry, jun. Mancheſter; Dr Torrence, Thurſo; Dr Gillum, Bath; Mr Paton; and Dr De Carro, Vienna.

The following publications have alſo been ſent for analyſis: Mr Chamberlayne on Cowhage; Mr Ware on Cataract; Mr Cooper on Cataract; Berthollet on Chemical Affinity; Theſaurus Medicaminum, 3d edit.; Mr Luxmore's Manual of Anatomy; the London Diſſector; Boyer on the Bones; Dr Jones on Hæmorrhagy; Mr Parkinſon on Gout; Prof. Reil on the Education of Empirical Practitioners; Fabbroni on the Analyſis of Cinchona; Mr Young on Cancer; Dr W. Hunter on the Diſeaſes of Laſcars; and Arguments in favour of a gradual Inoculation of Cow-pock, by R. Gillum, M. D.

. No. VI. *will be publiſhed on Tuesday the 1ſt of April, 1806.*

THE

EDINBURGH MEDICAL AND SURGICAL JOURNAL.

APRIL 1. 1806.

PART I.

ORIGINAL COMMUNICATIONS.

I.

Case of Abscess in the Abdominal Muscles, which terminated fatally. By CALEB CROWTHER, M. D. Wakefield.

ALICE HURTHWAITE, aged 15, was admitted into the Dispensary on the 11th of June 1805, labouring under violent pain in the right side of the abdomen, about the middle of the external oblique muscle, accompanied with great thirst, increased heat, frequent shiverings, a quick pulse, nausea, and vomiting. The account which she gave of herself was, that she was seized suddenly with the pain on the 1st of June, and with difficulty walked a few hundred yards from the place where she was in service to her mother's cottage. Of her own accord she took some opening medicine that produced a good deal of purging, which still continues. She feels most easy when the abdominal muscles are relaxed, the knees being brought towards the chin. She does not recollect having received any injury on the abdomen, and has previously enjoyed good health. She is tall, and rather thin. I ordered the abdomen to be fomented with flannels wrung out of hot water, and eight leeches to be applied to the pained part. She was directed to take 10 drops of Tinct. Opii, when the pain became urgent, and one scruple of P. Cretæ comp. cum Opio, in case the purging should continue to be violent.

12th. She experienced relief from the fomentation and leeches, and continued free from pain for about an hour after their application. The purging ceased without the use of the astringent, and the Tinct. Opii was rejected by vomiting. The other symptoms as before. The fomentation and leeches to be repeated. I was at this period desirous of using the warm bath, but the cottage did not afford convenience for heating the water.

13th. She found but little relief from the application of the leeches and fomentation. She felt pain on pressure upon the part affected, but neither tumour nor hardness were perceptible. The urine was very high-coloured, the bowels costive, the other symptoms as before. I ordered a blister to be applied to the part affected, a common enema to be administered, and the saline mixture to be taken in a state of effervescence.

15th. The pain in the abdomen ceased as soon as the blister rose, and she has since felt in every respect better. The skin is cool, and the pulse about 90 in a minute, and of moderate strength; urine turbid. Ordered to continue the saline mixture.

18th. She began on the 15th, in the evening, to feel much pain in the region of the liver, betwixt the shoulders, and in the calves of the legs, and to-day these pains continue to be very urgent. The pulse is very quick, the skin is hot; she has frequent rigor, alternating with flushings in the face. Singultus sometimes occurs; thirst is urgent; the stomach retains nothing but the effervescing mixture; the bowels are rather loose; the countenance is very languid. I ordered her to take six drops of Tinct. Opii with each dose of the mixture, and to rub half an ounce of it into the thighs.

20th. She appears to-day in every respect worse; she gets some disturbed sleep after the frictions and opiate mixture, but does not at all appear refreshed by it. The nausea continues; the tongue and mouth are covered with aphthæ. I ordered her to continue her medicines, and to dissolve in her mouth frequently a small quantity of an electuary, consisting of borax and honey.

21st. She continues to grow weaker; the pains in the region of the liver and between the shoulders have been very urgent; the tongue is dry and red, but the white aphthous crust lining the mouth has disappeared. She takes nothing but balm tea, and a little milk or weak mutton broth occasionally. I ordered a blister to be applied between the shoulders, and a pill, with half a grain of opium, to be taken with a dose of the effervescing mixture every three hours. The opiate frictions to be continued, the electuary to be omitted.

23d. The right leg and thigh have become œdematous, and she complains of pain in the part of the abdomen first affected, but nothing unusual is to be seen or felt there; the urine is plentiful, and not so turbid. She sleeps the greatest part of her time; the sickness continues. I ordered her to take her medicines only every four or five hours.

26th. The œdema has increased, and the skin continues hot and dry; in other respects much the same as before. To omit the opiate pills, and, instead thereof, to take two of the following with each dose of the mixture every four hours.

℞ P. Ipecac. comp. ʒ iv.
Calomel pp. gr. iv.
Conf. Cynosbt. q. s. ut ft. pil. N°. xxxij.

30th. The left leg and thigh have become œdematous. She voids about a quart of clear straw-coloured urine in 24 hours. The bowels are very loose, owing probably to the calomel. She has perspired a good deal; the skin is cooler, but the pulse is very rapid and weak; thirst considerable; no appetite; frequent nausea, as before. Ordered to omit the pills, and to take two of the following with each dose of the mixture.

℞ Pulv. Ipecac. Comp.
— Opiat. ana ʒ ij.
Conf. Cynosbt. q. s. ut. ft. pil. N°. xxxij.

5th July. The pains about the region of the liver and between the shoulders still continue, and she now again experiences much pain in the part of the abdomen first affected. The œdema continues; the urine is scanty; she has for the three last nights had a good deal of difficulty of breathing, and she has her head much raised by pillows. She has hectic paroxysms, sometimes once, sometimes twice, or even three times, in 24 hours. The pulse is very quick and irregular. She gets some disturbed sleep after taking each dose of her medicine, but she still labours under diarrhœa. Ordered to continue her medicines, and to take one ounce of Mist. Cretac. after every loose stool. The stomach and bowels have all along been too much disordered to bear the operation of squill or digitalis.

The powers of life continuing to decline very fast, and the effusion of water to increase, so as to leave not the most distant prospect of recovery, I saw her again only once before the time of her decease, which took place on the 19th.

APPEARANCES ON DISSECTION.

The body was opened on the 20th. On cutting transversely through the oblique muscles, on the right side of the abdomen,

 an

an abſceſs of an irregular oval form, about three inches in diameter, was diſcovered between the external and internal oblique muſcles, ſituated, as nearly as could be aſcertained from the putridity which had already taken place, and the confuſion of parts, in the centre, between the linea ſemilunaris, the ſpine of the ilium, and the termination of the loweſt falſe rib. The diſeaſe extended in the lower part of the muſcle to their inſertion in the groin. In the internal oblique muſcles were diſcovered two holes, through which the matter had paſſed on to the peritoneum. It had not penetrated into the inteſtines, which were found in a natural ſtate, but had paſſed over the peritoneum to the convex ſurface of the liver, where it eroded the peritoneum, and formed in the liver two holes with jagged edges. A conſiderable ſpace of the convex ſurface of the liver was ſuperficially ulcerated. The interior parts of the liver were perfectly ſound. A quantity of purulent matter was found lying on the little omentum, but, as there did not appear to be any diſeaſe in the circumjacent parts, it is probable that this effuſion had not taken place long before death. On opening the thorax, a conſiderable quantity of water was found in each cavity of the cheſt, as well as in the pericardium. The cellular membrane in the lower extremities was loaded with water.

A few days after the death of this patient, her mother called upon me to ſay, that about a fortnight before our patient was taken ill, ſhe fell from a ladder into a cellar, and hurt her body, ſo as to experience much pain for a day or two; but both mother and daughter had entirely forgotten this circumſtance when interrogated by me on my firſt attendance; this is one proof, beſide many others, of the great difficulty we often experience in obtaining from the poor a correct hiſtory of the prediſpoſing cauſes of diſeaſe. The diſſection illuſtrates well the progreſs of the diſeaſe. On the application of the bliſter to the abdomen, the pain ceaſed, not in conſequence of any good effect having been produced by the bliſter; but from the inflammatory action of the part having ceaſed, after the formation of the purulent matter. From the time of my firſt attendance until a few days after this period, my patient paſſed the greateſt part of her time in an armed chair, the hind feet of which were reclined ſo as to form an angle with the floor of about 45°. Her feet reſted upon the front rail of the chair, and her head and ſhoulders were ſupported by pillows. In this poſition her knees approached her chin, and, owing to the relaxation of the abdominal muſcles, ſhe felt the moſt eaſy. It was owing to this poſition that the purulent matter, after penetrating through the abdominal muſcles, deſcended over the peritoneum to the convex

1 ſurface

furface of the liver, and there occafioned a train of fymptoms not readily to be accounted for without the affiftance of the diffection. The mufcles were much difeafed at their termination in the groin, and the œdema of the right leg commenced in all probability from the deftruction of the lymphatic veffels there, in confequence of fome of the purulent matter infinuating itfelf between the mufcles, and paffing into the groin. The prefence of purulent matter in the fyftem, and the gradual finking of the vital powers, afford a ready explanation of the fymptoms occurring in the laft ftage of the difeafe.

Had this patient applied for medical aid immediately after the accident, fhe might, I have no doubt, have been very readily cured.

Cafe of Syphilitic Ulceration of the Skin, accompanied with Caries of the Tibia.

On the 4th December 1808, I was fent for to vifit A. B. æt. 19, whom I found labouring under hectic fever, accompanied with very frequent cough and copious expectoration, the urine being high-coloured, and depofiting a copious lateritious fediment; the pulfe 120 in a minute. He had great thirft, was very reftlefs, and had profufe nocturnal perfpirations. The countenance had a melancholy afpect; the appetite was very bad. On the tibia of the left leg there was an ulcer about one inch and a half long, which had deftroyed the periofteum, and rendered the bone carious. The probe paffed readily into the numerous cavities of the denudated bone. From the previous hiftory of the difeafe, it was evident that this ulcer was of fyphilitic origin. For fix or eight months prior to the ulceration, a node had made its appearance on the tibia, attended with fevere nocturnal pains, which gradually increafed in fize until the integuments burft. The ulcer had been dreffed daily with mild digeftive by the furgeon who attended him. He was taking two of the following pills every night at bed-time,

℞ Hydrarg. Calcinat. gr. iij.
P. Opii puri gr. vj.
Confect. Aromat. q. f. ut fi. pil. N° xij.

and Decoct. C. Cinchon. ℥j. thrice a-day, with a few drops Tinct. Opii and nitric acid.

I ordered the pills to be continued, a pint of Decoct. Guaiaci, with 40 drops of nitric acid, to be taken, at divided intervals, daily. The ulcer to be dreffed with lint focked in Tinct. Myrrhæ,

 and

and a warm linſeed poultice. The dreſſings to be changed thrice a-day.

Dec. 8th. I found my patient this day aſtoniſhingly better in every reſpect. The pulſe was natural. The hectic fever and its accompanying ſymptoms had vaniſhed. The cough and expectoration had nearly ceaſed. The ulcer put on a healing appearance, and the appetite returned.

He was ordered to continue his medicines, and, in the courſe of about a week, was ſufficiently recovered to be able to ſuperintend his buſineſs. He continued gradually to recover until the 12th January 1804, when the ulcer healed, and he was in perfect health. The leg has ſince continued ſound; and he is, at this day, ſubject to no complaint, except occaſionally to nocturnal pains in the bones.

This was the moſt ſpeedy cure of a chronic diſeaſe which I ever recollect to have witneſſed; indeed, unleſs I had myſelf attended the patient, and ſeen the rapid recovery, I ſhould have had much difficulty in attaching credit to it. It appears that the lint and the poultice abſorbed the purulent matter from the ulcer as it was ſecreted, in conſequence of which the hectic fever ceaſed. From the carious ſtate of the tibia I fully expected that an exfoliation would have taken place.

II.

Remarks on the Internal Uſe of Tincture of Cantharides in Gleet and Leucorrhœa; illuſtrated by Caſes. By JOHN ROBERTON, Surgeon, Edinburgh, and Member of the Royal Medical Society of Edinburgh.

MUCH diſpute, controverſy, and error, would be prevented in medicine, as well as in the other departments of ſcience, if ideas were expreſſed with more perſpicuity of language, and the ſubjects of inquiry deſcribed with more preciſion than is uſually done. The truth of this remark is well exemplified in what authors have ſaid concerning the medical properties of cantharides, which has been with equal ardour condemned as the moſt pernicious, or praiſed as the moſt ſalutary of ſubſtances; and perhaps with equal judgment alſo, ſince the one approved, without underſtanding in what circumſtances, or why it was uſeful, and the other rejected, without inquiring why it had been unſucceſsful. This, like every other moſt powerful agent, when injudiciouſly or raſhly employed, muſt have very pernicious

cious effects; but, when rationally and deliberately used, the effects may be as conspicuously salutary.

In the consideration of every inflammatory disease, it is of the utmost importance to distinguish accurately between inflammation, properly so called, and its consequences; wherefore we venture thus to distinguish gonorrhœa and gleet, or blenorrhagia.

GONORRHOEA, an active inflammation affecting the yard, with a puriform discharge from the urethra.

GLEET, an atony of the yard, the effect of active inflammation, or other debilitating causes, accompanied with a glairy discharge from the urethra *.

These two conditions, in principle and in practice, are completely analogous to the states of active and passive inflammation as distinguished by Cullen, and the other most correct systematic writers; nor is there any rule of medical practice more firmly established than that, in the first, strong stimulants are as hurtful, as they are beneficial in the second.

Accordingly, we need not be surprised that one person, using the very active substance of cantharides in the gonorrhœa, as above defined, should meet with chagrin and disappointment; while another, who used it in gleet, which was also named gonorrhœa, should, as we do, from undoubted experience of its superior efficacy, recommend it to the notice of practitioners as a most valuable addition to the resources of the healing art.

We might have suspected, from the relation of the contradictory effects which this substance is described to have produced, what was the source of the error; but if this suspicion is corroborated by the facts contained in the writings of those who have prescribed it; if gonorrhœa has been confounded, both in name and in practice, with gleet; if, where cantharides have been unsuccessful in removing discharges from the urethra, these have been gonorrhœas, but, where successful, gleets; in fine, if positive experiment prove that, by inducing gonorrhœa, it cures gleet, will not this point be established, that gonorrhœa, being confounded with gleet, is the cause of the opposite sentiments of writers with regard to the effects of cantharides in certain discharges from the urethra?

In the same manner we may, I presume, reconcile the difference of opinion with regard to the use of the corrosive muriate of mercury in gonorrhœas.

4 That

* It seemed unnecessary to express these definitions in such a manner as to suit both sexes, since the mind can easily make allowance for the difference of structure, and perceive that the facts signified are equally applicable to both.

That the word gonorrhœa was employed to ſignify the diſcharge from the urethra in both the conditions above pointed out, the ſlighteſt attention to authors will amply ſatisfy any one; indeed the word etymologically denotes a flow of ſemen, and has been applied indiſcriminately to all diſcharges from the urethra; it is only in the advancement of ſcience that the neceſſity of words preciſely defined becomes urgent.

Dr Greenfield relates many caſes of gonorrhœa, which he and others cured by means of cantharides; but if we examine the hiſtories of the affection which they treated, we ſhall be convinced that they are thoſe of gleet; and the phraſes, violent gonorrhœa, virulent, painful, &c. which other writers employ to deſignate the affections in which the cantharides were unſucceſsful or hurtful, ſhow that thoſe were diſcharges accompanied with active inflammation, or real gonorrhœas. Laſtly, I have not only the teſtimony of authors, but have found by indubitable experiment, that cantharides induce active inflammation, with puriform diſcharge, before gleet is remedied: How, then, could they but fail in their attempts to remove active inflammation, uſing a moſt inflammatory ſubſtance?

On examination of the facts, we firmly believe that thoſe pernicious effects which have ſucceeded the uſe of cantharides, and which have excited ſuch horror and averſion to its exhibition in diſeaſe, have, as in the inſtance of gleet and gonorrhœa, principally originated in the want of diſcrimination between inflammatory action and its conſequences.

Previouſly to my employing cantharides in gleet, I had not conſulted authors on the ſubject; nor am I aſhamed to confeſs it, ſince the lifetime of any individual would not be ſufficient ſimply to read over, far leſs to examine, the merits and doctrines of one-twentieth part of the books written on the powers of particular medicines: beſides, when we conſider how uſeleſs the moſt of them are, a man has not much reaſon to regret that he is not endowed with dull perſeverance enough to pore over them. Having ſince, however, examined the works of authors on this ſubject, I am happy to find that the experience of ſome of the moſt eminent medical men has found cantharides as efficacious a remedy for gleet as I have done; among theſe I may reckon Bartholine, Hoffman, Liſter, &c.

When I firſt employed cantharides in gleet, I only knew that the ſubſtance was a powerful ſtimulant taken internally, and produced powerful effects on the urinary organs; and as all pain indicates a certain degree of inflammation, I thought that, in inveterate gleets, where there is both general debility and exhauſtion, with torpor and atony in the parts of generation, this ſubſtance

ſubſtance might have conſiderable influence in reſtoring both the general and local activity; and the experiment, when made, exceeded in ſucceſs my utmoſt hopes.

In order to demonſtrate the truth of this aſſertion, I ſhall relate one caſe ſelected out of many; averring that, when exhibited with due caution, the cantharides effect the cure without vomiting, ſtrangury, or any of thoſe alarming ſymptoms which we have been taught to dread as the inevitable conſequences of their adminiſtration.

S———d, aged 55 years, a ſmall meagre man, on the 20th April 1804, mentioned to me that he laboured under an uncommonly ſevere gleet, but at the ſame time ſaying that he had no hope of cure, as the moſt eminent practitioners of England and Scotland had already preſcribed for him in vain; but, as the effects of it were now very ſevere, he requeſted that I would deviſe ſome method of relief, as, to uſe his own phraſe, life was become a burthen to him. I inquired minutely into his caſe, and found that he had been affected with a diſcharge of this nature from the urethra for about 20 years, which he attributed to the effects of a bad cuſtom originally commenced at ſchool, and ſince aggravated by repeated claps.

Such was his ſituation, that, beſides a continual diſcharge from the yard, emiſſion ſucceeded the moſt trifling erection, and ſtraining at ſtool had the ſame effect, which was followed by all that languor and depreſſion of ſpirits which gave origin to the celebrated aphoriſm, "Poſt coitum omne animal triſte."

Though married, connubial enjoyment was beyond his faculties; but this was not his only misfortune; headachs, loſs of appetite, lumbago, incontinence of urine, in fine, general emaciation and debility, threatened the ſpeedy termination of his life.

On inquiry, I found that all the moſt common means had been employed to remove his complaints; accordingly, to make him undergo a repetition of the ſame was neither conſonant to my own feelings, nor to the ſtate of my patient. I therefore preſcribed as follows:— .

℞ Tinct. Cantharid. ʒiſs.
Sp. Lavend. Comp. ʒj.
Aq. f.———— ℥vij miſce.

Cujus cap. coch. magn. mane et veſp.

This having no effect, the doſe was increaſed on the 23d to ʒij.; this likewiſe had no effect, and, on the 26th, was augmented

mented to ʒijſs. which, though taken in the courſe of two days, an increaſed doſe was ſtill neceſſary.

On the 28th ℥ſs. was preſcribed, with the above quantity of water; and this being all taken, without having as yet produced any evident effect, was, on the 30th, increaſed to ℥j. of the tincture, which was conſumed in four days, and at this ratio he continued to the 8th of May. Between the 8th and 10th, he took ℥ſs. per diem; but inflammatory ſymptoms of the urinary organs appearing for the firſt time, the doſe was diminiſhed to ʒij. in die, and ſo on to the 17th; and whenever the ſigns of inflammation commenced, the glairy matter of the gleet aſſumed the appearance, in ſome meaſure, of laudable pus, accompanied with cordee and ſevere erections. There was yet no degree of ſtrangury; but, what was remarkable, the erections were not now followed by thoſe emiſſions, languor, ſadneſs, and ſudden impotence, which had been ſo certain conſequences of that ſtate.

The diſcharge from the urethra having now the form of the matter of the moſt inflammatory gonorrhœa, it was deemed unneceſſary to perſiſt in the uſe of the remedy; and, unequivocal inflammation being indicated, it ſeemed prudent, on the 18th, to employ what are reckoned ſedatives, for the purpoſe of mitigating the ſymptoms. Accordingly, a ſolution of one ſcruple of ſulphate of copper in ſix ounces of water was adminiſtered as an injection, to be uſed three or four times a-day; and, contrary to my expectation, the cure ſeemed to be complete in the courſe of four days from this date.

January 1806. Has remained perfectly well, and has become a father ſince I laſt ſaw him; thus affording an indubitable proof of the cure having been complete.

Having for ſeveral years found the cantharides a very uſeful remedy in gleet, I became imperceptibly acquainted with the phenomena that ſucceeded its admiſſion into the ſyſtem. I had uniformly obſerved that it rendered the mind more cheerful, ſtrengthened the circulation, promoted the animal functions, appetites, and evacuations, and greatly mitigated that ſenſe of general debility, as well as of pain and feebleneſs in the loins and joints, of which thoſe, who have long laboured under this affection, ſo much complain. Theſe are the firſt effects; but, in a ſpace of time longer or ſhorter, according to the ſtate of the patient, the diſcharge begins to be inſpiſſated, pain attacks the urethra, erections are frequent, and even accompanied with ſome degree of cordee; but theſe erections are not, as formerly, of ſhort duration, ſucceeded by languor, debility, depreſſion of of spirits, and spontaneous evacuation of seminal fluid, but precisely resemble the erections in gonorrhoea, and the matter discharged is puriform, often, after erection, mixed with semen, particularly during the night. While my mind was impressed with these facts, some obstinate and very inveterate cases of leucorrhoea came under my care; and reflecting that the constitutional symptoms of leucorrhoea are precisely similar to those of gleet, the matter discharged of the same appearance and consistence, and as the gleety discharge evidently depends on the debilitated state of the mucous membrane of the urethra, so does the leucorrhoeal on that of the mucous membrane of the vagina; in short, that all the circumstances were as completely similar as the structure of two sexes would admit, it appeared to me very probable that cantharides might also remove leucorrhoea, by invigorating the general system, and producing a change in the action of the mucous membrane concerned, as happened in gleet; and the event confirmed my opinion.

Mrs L——n, aged 25, a little woman, mother of several children, who were all dead-born, or died a few hours after birth; her general appearance indicated languor and debility; her eyes peculiarly dull and heavy; pulse feeble. I learned that she had laboured under fluor albus for five years and a half, and the attack commenced about two months before the birth of her first child. She has, during that time, employed those remedies that are usually prescribed in such complaints, but, notwithstanding, her complaint had gradually increased in violence, and was at length intolerable.

She said she had learned from other medical gentlemen that a complete cure was scarcely to be expected by her; but she begged, nay, would undergo almost any degree of suffering, to obtain alleviation. Her pain of back was excruciating, her appetite impaired, and she could, so far from walking, not even stand or sit without the utmost uneasiness. The discharge per vaginam too was so copious and incessant, that, though she used cloths, &c. she was always afraid of being in company, lest marks on the floor should discover her condition; in addition to all which, she was frequently attacked by paroxysms of hysteria.

The discharge was of a glairy appearance and consistence.

During the whole time of the affection, the menstruation has been regular and natural, and, what is worthy of remark, the fluor albus evinced itself much worse during pregnancy than at other times; showing us, I would venture to allege, that the particular state of the mucous membrane alone has no small share in promoting the disease.

The

The patient ſays the fluid was not in uniform quantity, but that an unuſually great diſcharge was always preceded and announced by an excruciating pain in the region of the kidnies, on which occaſion ſhe always had the diſtinct ſenſation of ſomething flowing, as it were, downwards from the loins, and the cloths applied to the parts were found wet with the diſcharge. Is there not reaſon to conjecture that the mucous membrane of the urethra is equally affected with that of the vagina?

As, in other caſes, I had been accuſtomed to uſe the tincture of cantharides with great ſucceſs, I preſcribed

℞ T. Cantharid. ʒiiſs.
Aq. font. ℥vj. m.

One table-ſpoonful to be taken thrice a-day.

12th October. Cantharides mixture repeated, with ʒiv. and aq. font. ℥vj. and again repeated, in the ſame quantity, on the 16th.

17th. She felt ſlight pain in the uterine region, extending down the vagina, particularly on making any exertion. The diſcharge was now ſomewhat thicker and whitiſh.

19th. Cantharides mixture repeated; in the evening the pain became very troubleſome, even when ſitting, and the diſcharge was much thicker and whiter. I now preſcribed, as an injection,

℞ Sulph. Cupri. ʒſs.
Aq. font. ℥vj. m.

To be thrown into the vagina thrice a-day.

20th. Diſcharge and pain almoſt gone; when I deſired her to take two tea-ſpoonfuls of the cantharides mixture every three hours till the pain ſhould return; but, before ſhe had taken a ſufficient quantity to produce this effect, the diſcharge reſumed almoſt its former violence.

21ſt. Diſcharge conſiderably diminiſhed, attended with ſlight pain.

22d. No pain, although ſhe has taken, within the laſt 24 hours, ʒiv. of Tinct. Cantharid.: The diſcharge now leſs by more than two-thirds than it was previouſly to the exhibition of the cantharides. I now ordered the injection to be omitted, and the following increaſed doſe of tinct. cantharid. to be uſed:

℞ T. Cantharid. ℥j.
Aq. font. ℥vj. m.

To be uſed as the former mixture.

23d. After taking one doſe of the laſt mixture, ſhe was, for the firſt time, ſenſible of pain in voiding urine. This was the period

period for the return of the menses, which accordingly appeared, but she was at the same time seized with a fever, and species of cynanche tonsillaris, that had raged epidemically in the town for some weeks. Tinct. cantharid. and injection now intermitted, as the fever, &c. continued to the 1st November.

2d November. Fever gone; throat getting better, after one of the tumours had suppurated and burst. Menstruation still continuing, and of an alarming quantity.

Prescribed this day

℞. Acidi Nitrici, ℥ij.
Aq. font. ℔ij. m.

One wine-glassful thrice a-day, till the flooding stops.

7th. Flooding ceased; the discharge of the fluor albus considerably abated.

9th. Discharge much aggravated. General stimulants were now prescribed, because the system was much reduced by the fever, &c.

12th. Discharge much diminished.

13th. Discharge entirely gone; the general health much improved.

17th. Discharge returned in a slight degree, and of the same appearance and consistence as before the use of the tinct. cantharidis.

21st. After earnest persuasion on my part, she was prevailed on to recommence the tinct. cantharid. in small doses.

22d. Great sickness during the night, and inflammatory symptoms, with a puriform colour in the discharge, came on before morning.

℞ Camphor,
Gum. Mimosæ Niloticæ ana scrup.
Alcohol q. s. ut fiat massa pil. divid. in xv partes equales.

One of these pills was directed to be taken an hour after each dose of the tinct. cantharidis mixture, which was to be taken thrice a-day.

23d. Cantharides continued. Very great pain this day, but as it has never become so severe as on the 21st, she has used none of the camphor pills.

24th. Discharge entirely gone. Cantharides continued in smaller doses, but sufficient to maintain what Mr John Hunter would probably call the suppurative stage.

25th. Pain of head; no return of the discharge.

℞ Supertart. Potassæ, ℥j.
Solve in Jusc. bov. ℔j.

To be taken presently. Cantharides continued.

26th.

26th. ℞ Tinct. Cantharid. ʒv.
Aq. font. ℥vj.

On the evening of this day, after having fatigued herſelf by walking, and having alſo neglected to take tinct. cantharid. ſince morning, the pain in the uterine region abated, and the diſcharge returned in a ſlight degree.

27th. Cantharides to be taken during this day till the pain return. Pain and conſiderable difficulty in making water came on this night at bed-time, with nearly a complete ceſſation of the diſcharge.

28th. Cantharides continued, and one of the camphor pills to be taken. Diſcharge ſlight.

29th. Cantharides continued. Diſcharge not entirely gone, but nearly ſo.

30th. Diſcharge entirely gone. Cantharides continued, and quantity laſt mentioned repeated. Conſiderable uneaſineſs, or rather pain, in making water. Partial ſickneſs this day and yeſterday, with headach. Supertart. Potaſſ. as above, which relieved theſe ſymptoms.

1ſt December. Very early this morning there was an almoſt imperceptible diſcharge. Cantharides continued, and injection.

2d. Uneaſineſs extending along the vagina and uterine region ſtill kept up by the uſe of tinct. cantharid. Injected two or three times ſince yeſterday, but no return of the diſcharge.

3d. The pain in the region of the kidnies, which is wont invariably to indicate the returning diſcharge, was felt this morning, but not followed by the diſcharge, or even the ſmalleſt appearance of matter per vaginam; in other reſpects as yeſterday. The menſtruation not having returned at the regular period, there is reaſon to ſuſpect the intervention of pregnancy; I have therefore ordered the doſe of the cantharides to be diminiſhed, but the injection into the vagina to be continued.

4th. Had a violent attack of hyſteria this morning, occaſioned by mental agitation. Such an attack never happened before during the complaint, without its being ſucceeded by an uncommonly copious diſcharge, of which there is no appearance. Medicines to be continued as laſt preſcribed.

5th. No diſcharge; uneaſineſs of the parts gradually abating.

6th. A repetition of the hyſteric paroxyſm from a ſimilar cauſe.

7th. Early this morning the diſcharge reappeared, of a puriform nature, and continued to augment all this day. Pain from the cantharides almoſt gone. Cantharides to be taken in increaſed doſes, and the injection ſtill to be uſed.

8th. Diſcharge gone, pain of the parts returned. Remedies as laſt directed, but in diminiſhed doſes.

10*th.*

10th. No difcharge, pain gone. General health much better than fhe thinks it ever was fince fhe laboured under this affection; is not oppreffed with that defpondency from which fhe felt very difagreeable in her former pregnancies.

14th. No cantharides taken fince the 10th. Pain and difcharge gone. Complains of ficknefs in the mornings, lofs of appetite. Formerly, when pregnant, fhe had none of the ufually concomitant fymptoms of that ftate, except the ceffation of the menfes, and the increafe of fize; at which time, too, the difcharge per vaginam was fignally augmented.

20th. Previoufly to this date fhe had ufed the injection very irregularly. During the afternoon of yefterday fhe had been walking, failing, and dancing a good deal. Suddenly awoke this morning, with violent palpitation of heart and agitating mind, from a dream. Slight return of the difcharge. Injection to be ufed more regularly. Cantharides to be repeated in fmall dofes.

22d. Vomits the cantharides immediately on taking it, and difgufted with it. Her common food is loathfome to her, and excites fevere ficknefs and vomiting, but no pain in the ftomach or cheft. The fame occurs on rifing in the morning. Some difcharge, though fcarcely perceptible. Cantharides difcontinued for fear of injuring the fœtus. Injection ufed once a-day.

1ft January 1806. Difcharge has continued as on the 22d ult. She danced and fatigued herfelf a good deal this evening, but this was fucceeded by no augmentation of the difcharge, as on the former occafion, when fhe had been failing and dancing. Could the expofure to the cold fea-air produce any difference in the refult? For on the 1ft January fhe fatigued herfelf much more than on the former occafion.

5th. Says the difcharge is ftill perceptible. I afked her what it was, compared to what it had been? She replied emphatically, "It is not the ten thoufandth part of what it formerly was; and I feel myfelf as well in my general health as ever I was in my life, except that my bones and joints are ftill fore from the exertion of the firft day of this year."

I may mention that cantharides feems formerly to have been ufed fuccefsfully in leucorrhœa, though the nature of the affection which this medicine removed does not feem to have been underftood by thofe who employed it. Dr Greenfield, for example, had adopted a notion that almoft all fuch difcharges as thofe of leucorrhœa and gleet depended on ulceration of the bladder, and that cantharides were an infallible remedy for fuch ulcers; juft as, in our own times, fome promulgate that almoft all affections of the organs of generation, nay, even of the head,

The diſeaſe generally appears without any very evident previous ſymptom. Its preſence is generally announced by a degree of itchineſs, redneſs, and heat, in the ſkin of the part, ſucceeded often by a veſicle, and the part is more or leſs inflamed and ſwelled. Under the veſicle, which contains a white, thick mucus, the head of the worm may be often diſcovered. It not unfrequently happens, however, that the worm cannot be found for ſeveral days after ulceration. Sometimes a ſmall ulcer is the firſt thing obſerved; at other times, tumour of the whole limb, with much inflammation. The worm ſometimes, at firſt, appears like a hair, ſeveral inches long, and becomes thicker as it is extracted; but it generally has a ſharp point, and is all of the ſame thickneſs. It may often be felt and traced with the fingers, like the ſtring of a violin, under the ſkin, where it excites no very ſenſible uneaſineſs, until the ſkin becomes affected from the animal perforating it.

When removed from the body, the worm exhibits no appearance of life, although extracted at one operation; but it is ſaid that, on being ſubjected to different ſtimuli, it has afforded ſigns of vitality. The length of the worm is, I believe, ſeldom leſs than eighteen inches, or more than ſix feet. Inſtances, however, are mentioned wherein they have exceeded this length *. They are elaſtic, white, and tranſparent, and contain a milky juice. Their diameter is generally about that of a violin tenor ſtring; ſometimes they are ſcarcely half the ſize, and at other times much thicker.

When the diſeaſe appears in parts that are tender, when there is extenſive ulceration, or when the conſtitution is irritable, there is always more or leſs fever, loſs of appetite and ſtrength; and there is an exacerbation of the fever in the evening, which is ſometimes increaſed and kept up by the worm having been drawn too tight. Sympathetic tumours of the inguinal glands alſo ſometimes occur, when the complaint is ſeated in the lower extremities.

Various cauſes are aſſigned for the generation of this inſect. Some of the ancients, as well as the moderns, attribute its production to the drinking of putrid ſtagnant water, containing the ova of the worm. Horſtius, who ſeems to miſtake the diſeaſe, attributes it, as well as others, to ſuppreſſed perſpiration, of an acrid quality, confined in the excretories of the ſkin, which putrifies, and gives riſe to the germ and ova of the inſect.

Another

* In the 6th vol. of the Edin. Med. Eſſays, a caſe is detailed of a boy who had arrived at Bermudas from Guinea, from whom, at different times, above thirty yards of worm had been extracted; an entire worm, from the leg, meaſured three yards and a half.

Another opinion regarding the generation of this worm is, that it is produced from ova deposited in the skin by insects of a certain kind, which are supposed to reside in or near water. The ova thus deposited may be supposed gradually to acquire, from the heat and nourishment of the human juices, life and subsequent growth.

That the last mentioned opinion is by far the most probable and satisfactory in explaining the phenomena of the worm, I shall endeavour to show from observations founded on facts.

1. The disease most frequently attacks parts which are liable to immersion in water, such as the feet and legs; and at the first appearance of the complaint, in any particular station, the lower extremities are, in the first instance, almost always affected *.

2. It prevails in wet seasons, and in damp situations, more frequently than in dry; and the source of the disease may be often traced from those situations which, from moisture, confinement, heat, want of cleanliness, or other causes, may favour the generation of the worm.

Many circumstances concur in rendering it probable that the disease, when perfectly formed, probably after the evolution of the head of the worm, is capable of being propagated by infection †; and also that this infection may exist and be communicated at a period long subsequent to the time of its first appearance, although the disease may have been supposed extinct, and although no probable causes may exist at the time to account for its reappearance ‡. To account for the origin of the disease, several

* It has been observed that Bheesties, or water-carriers in India, who carry the water in a mushuk, or leathern bag, suspended from their shoulders over the back and side, are most subject to the Guinea worm in those parts which come in contact with the mushuk.

† Dr M'Gregor, in his 'Medical Sketches of the Expedition to Egypt from India,' has given a very clear and ample account of the disease as it appeared, in an alarming degree, on board the Minerva transport, employed in that expedition The result of his observation led him to conclude that it was infectious, particularly as it was found that separation of the infected from the sound, and extreme cleanliness, stopped the ravages of the disease.

‡ In the beginning of March 1801, after having been at sea for more than a fortnight, in a vessel from the island of Ceylon, I was attacked with this disease in my left knee. The head of the worm formed an exit first below the patella, and the cure was extremely tedious. More than a month afterwards I discovered another under the skin of the right metatarsus, nearly at the time that the wounds from the former had been healed. The vessel was small, and crowded with soldiers, but none of them had embarked with any signs of the complaint, Several of them were also affected with it before this time, and its prevalence after this became so alarming, that it was found necessary to remove all those affected with it on board of another vessel, notwithstanding which, several fresh instances afterwards occurred of a very serious nature. The infection was probably communicated to me from the soldiers labouring under this disease, whom I regularly dressed every day.

ſeveral cauſes, probably, are neceſſary. Many damp ſituations exiſt in hot countries, wherein the diſeaſe is totally unknown. Confinement, heat, want of cleanlineſs in perſon and habitation, all ſeem to aſſiſt in its production. But the real cauſe of it, like that of many other phenomena, is ſtill much involved in obſcurity.

The means of prevention of this diſeaſe appear to conſiſt in an attention to cleanlineſs of the perſon and habitation, avoiding dampneſs and damp places, taking care to keep the feet and legs covered *, and bathing in the ſea, when convenient, in preference to rivers or lakes. Patients with this complaint ſhould, as much as poſſible, be ſet apart from the reſt, and, when it can be done, removed to a dry and roomy ſituation; and all intercourſe with ſuch patients ſhould be reſtricted.

In the cure of this diſeaſe, many remedies and methods have been employed by authors †. Some remedies have been held as ſpecifics, internal as well as external. It does not appear, however, that any are entitled to this appellation.

When the diſeaſe commences with tumour, common emollient poultices ſhould be applied over the part where the worm is likely to appear; and, according to the degree of inflammation, the other means employed in caſes of phlegmon, ſuch as leeches, fomentations, &c. are to be alſo uſed, until ſuppuration takes place, or until the head of the worm appears through the ſkin. When the worm can be ſeen or found out, it ſhould be laid hold of with the forceps, and pulled very gently and gradually until there be a little reſiſtance, and the worm becomes moderately tight. The reſiſtance is often more or leſs overcome, and the extraction of the worm facilitated, by frictions with warm oil, as well as compreſſion of the limb all round, particularly in the direction of the reſiſtance, and from thence towards the wound. This operation tends alſo in a ſmall degree to obtund the pain which neceſſarily attends the extraction. When as much of the worm has been drawn out as the reſiſtance and the ſufferings of the patient will allow, the end of it ſhould be ſecured by means of a ligature or thread paſſed round it. The thread ſhould then be tied to a piece of ſmall bougie, twiſted lint, or ſmall quill, an inch and a half in length, and, with the ſlack part of the worm, is to be rolled up until it be moderately tight, taking care that it may not be on the ſtretch, which will occaſion fever, and a chance of breaking the worm. A piece of adheſive plaſter, or ſome other dreſſing, is neceſſary to retain it

* Soldiers in India, when off duty, go almoſt naked.

† Some of the ancients, in the extraction of the worm, employed leaden weights, which they appended to the end of the inſect; others rolled it on metallic tubes.

it in its place. Poultices are usually continued for some time, particularly where there is tumour, to promote a discharge and the expulsion of the worm. In many cases, I think, I have found a cataplasm of raw onions, cut very small, or bruised, and frequently changed, in a great degree contribute to the extraction of the worm. It creates less irritation than might be supposed, and is lighter and more convenient than the common poultice *. Of the external use of garlic in this complaint I have no experience.

In general, the extraction should only be attempted once in the twenty-four hours; but when the disease is seated in muscular parts, and when there is no great irritation, the worm may be tightened twice, or oftener, in that period. The length of the animal extracted at once is very uncertain. Sometimes none can be drawn out, at other times nearly a foot. The extraction should be repeated in the same manner, as often as circumstances will admit, until the whole of the worm comes away. The ulcer remaining after the extraction is to be treated as a common sore, care being taken to use sufficient compression along the parts under which the worm was situated. When there are extensive sinuosities, which is never the case if the worm is not ruptured by injudiciously pulling it, or accidentally breaking it by a blow, fall, or other violence, counter-openings are sometimes advisable in superficial parts, to prevent the lodgement of sanies. When there is much discharge, and of a sanious quality, the remedies employed in similar cases, such as bark, opiates, and stimulants, are also to be employed according to circumstances.

Cautious extraction of the worm is particularly necessary to prevent its breaking, which is an accident but too common, particularly in the feet and ancles. When this unfortunately happens, tumour, fever, and tedious suppuration in some other part, are the frequent consequences. Recourse must again be had to cataplasms and warm bathing, until the ruptured end of the worm can be again discovered, either at the former wound, or until it appears in some other part.

The aloe leaf pared on one side, or sliced in two, and applied heated, with the inside next the part, has been long recommended, and is a convenient application. I cannot say, however, that I have seen much advantage derived from it. When this application is tried, it should be changed several times in the day, and applied as hot as the patient can bear it.

* Velschius recommends the use of salt frequently rubbed on the end of the worm, but I never saw it tried.

Soap-berries (*Saponariæ Nuculæ*), bruiſed and made into a paſte with water, and applied over the ulcer when the worm has been broken, tends, I think, to favour its expulſion. If it can be conveniently removed, the application ſhould be uſed daily, accompanied with cataplaſms and fomentations, when there is much ſwelling.

Immerſion of the feet in warm water, when the complaint is ſeated there, is uſeful, and ſhould be repeated daily. Fomentation is almoſt always uſeful. When there is a great deal of tumour of the limb at firſt, and extenſive ſuppurations take place afterwards, it is probable that more than one worm is preſent. Hemorrhage ſometimes occurs in a bad ſtate of the diſeaſe from the ſpreading of the ulcers. In theſe caſes the worm is expelled in a diſſolved ſtate, or diſcharged in decayed portions; to promote which, care ſhould be taken to allow a free exit to the diſcharge by inciſions or otherwiſe, that the wounds may be reduced as ſoon as poſſible to the ſtate of ſimple ulcers.

When the worm can be diſtinctly felt by the fingers under the ſkin, before breaking through, it is adviſable to extract it by means of a ſmall inciſion made over the part where it is moſt ſuperficial, and, as near as can be judged, over its middle. A ligature ſhould then be applied, and the worm extracted double, in the manner before mentioned. By this method, which is practiſed by the Eaſt Indians, much pain and trouble would be ſaved.

The practice of cutting off the extracted part of the worm, and applying freſh ligatures each time, can be attended with no good effects, and can only be ſafe when a very great length of worm has been extracted, and when it has become dry, and is without life.

Mercury has been thought to poſſeſs the power of deſtroying this worm. Of this, however, I am extremely doubtful. Electricity, with this view, has been alſo employed, but I never ſaw it productive of any benefit.

With regard to the remedies uſed internally in the cure of this diſeaſe, I have nothing to offer. Aloes has been long in uſe, and was, no doubt, given as an anthelmintic. With this intention, I apprehend, it can be of little ſervice. The ſame may be ſaid of garlic, which has been ſtrongly recommended as a certain antidote, if given to the extent of two drachms daily. I never ſaw it, however, of the ſmalleſt benefit, after a careful and extenſive trial.

IV.

Cases of Guinea Worm, with Observations. By Mr Paton, Surgeon of the Cirencester.

The Guinea worm is a disease not uncommon among the lascars, and frequently appearing, I understand, in the army in India, affecting both officers and men.

It seldom or never occurs in the ships trading to or from India. At least, in several voyages which I have performed in the ships of the Honourable East India Company, I never had an opportunity of seeing a single case of Guinea worm, until it broke out in the Cirencester during our late voyage homewards; and other surgeons in the service, whom I have consulted, agree in its being a very rare occurrence.

It occurred in the Indian army during its transport from Ceylon to the Red sea; and many observations led Mr M'Gregor to suspect that the disease was infectious, or, in other words, that the Guinea worm spread chiefly amongst the men who lived with those already affected with the insect, which seemed, therefore, to propagate itself from one individual to another.

The origin and propagation of the worm has more commonly by others been attributed to the water of the particular countries where its appearance is common. The subject is curious, but involved as yet in the greatest obscurity. Nor do I pretend, on this occasion, that the observations which are to follow will throw any immediate light upon it. The facts, however, may serve, with others, as data for future investigation. But I cannot avoid remarking, that if the Guinea worm were received into the body from the water used for drink, or in washing, it should be a more common occurrence in our ships; and, on this supposition, it would be difficult to reconcile its very rare appearance with the circumstances of its occasional propagation.

If Mr M'Gregor's conjecture be well founded, we will be at no loss to explain its introduction amongst the crew of the Cirencester, as an infected lascar was received on board at Bombay, in whom the Guinea worm appeared during the passage thence to China. This, however, was the only instance at that time; nor did it reappear and spread amongst the crew till many months after, when we arrived at St Helena on our passage homewards, long after the diseased lascar had been discharged.

Without hazarding any conjecture of my own, I shall here

simply state the facts as they occurred; after which I shall give short notices of the different cases, as extracted from the sick journal of the Cirencester, and a table, exhibiting in one view the progress of the disease, and the order of its propagation amongst the crew.

We sailed from Bombay for China on the 15th August 1804, with 45 lascars in addition to the ship's company, of whom one appeared, in the course of the passage, with a Guinea worm in his left ancle joint. He was discharged on the 5th of January uncured, along with 22 others in good health; the remaining 22 were brought in the ship to England, none of whom ever had the most distant appearance of worms; which, if the disease is infectious, is the more singular, as they messed together during the time they were on board. Twenty-four Chinese embarked at the time the 23 lascars were discharged, and had no appearance of the disease. Seven invalids received on board at Prince of Wales's Island had nothing of it. Of those affected only two were men who had been engaged in India; all the others came from London in the ship.

The last of the Liberty men came on board from Canton in December, after which none of the seamen were on shore until their arrival at St Helena. Sailed from China January 5. Arrived at, and sailed from, Poolopenang in the end of January, and arrived at St Helena April 2, where the worms began to make their appearance, on the 30th of May, in a man who had not been on shore. This disease is unknown at St Helena, and none of the other ships had it on board. At this time there were on board, including passengers, about 200 in all. The number with worms was 26. The principal change in the method of victualling was the substituting a pound of potatoes per man daily for their pease and flour. A good many fish (mackerel) were caught occasionally, and four or five days fresh provision was obtained from the shore. Sailed from the island July 11.

This disease is not uncommon among lascars, and, I understand, frequently appears in the army in India, affecting both officers and men. On the Malabar coast, some years ago, an officer's wife had one in the thigh, which inflamed to a great degree, and required an active antiphlogistic practice and regimen to overcome the inflammation.

The worm is an extraneous body, producing inflammation, and should not be drawn forcibly, but very gently from day to day, and even then very cautiously, merely as if it were to discover whether it be loose or fast; it never comes away with advantage,

vantage, until it becomes of a dead-white appearance, and then the milky fluid it contains can be pressed from one part to another, like as if a little milk had been injected into a fine transparent tube, formed of pellucid membrane. It gives the patient much pain when drawn; and it is of little use to make any thing fast to it, as a little adhesive ointment prevents its retracting, and the piece drawn dries in the course of the day. The inflammation is to be treated in the usual way. I used poultices.

TABLE, exhibiting the Order in which the Guinea Worm spread amongst the Crew of the Cirencester.

1805.	*1st, St Helena.*	Guinea		
May 30	P. Waldstrom	Worm.	Seaman.	Cured July 12. 1805.
June 9	S. Propavo	——	——	—— Aug. 29. ——
14	A. Otkin	——	——	Disch. Sept. 15. ——
17	J. Berry	——	——	Cured July 31. ——
19	J. Fielding	——	——	—— 15. ——
20	J. Melthier	——	——	—— 29. ——
22	J. Martin	——	B. M.	—— Aug. 22. ——
—	C. Gosling	——	Seaman.	—— July 10. ——
24	R. Seal	——	——	Disch. Sept. 15. ——
25	A. Fanassi	——	——	Cured Aug. 7. ——
—	J. Split	——	——	—— 24. ——
27	M. Louffe	——	——	Disch. Sept. 15. ——
July 1	M. Minus	——	——	Cured July 29. ——
—	T. Wilkinson	——	Carpenter.	—— Aug. 10. ——
—	J. Jamison	——	Steward.	—— 27. ——
7	Geo. Baily	——	——	—— Sept. 15. ——
8	J. Peters	——	——	Disch. —— ——
11	J. Roebuck	——	——	Cured Aug. 29. ——
	2d, At Sea.			
13	T. Ward	——	Sail-maker	—— Sept. 5. ——
—	F. Nelson	——	Seaman.	—— Aug. 28. ——
14	J. Price	——	——	—— 22. ——
16	J. Longber	——	——	—— Sept. 2. ——
22	J. Brown	——	Cook.	Disch. Sept. 15. ——
—	C. Churchill	——	Seaman.	Cured —— 8. ——
28	G. Polard	——	Boatswain	Disch. —— 15. ——
31	J. Frederick	——	Seaman.	Cured Aug. 7. ——
Aug. 9	P. Waldstrom	——	——	Disch. Sept. 15. ——

The

The Order of their Messes, with the Number in each.

					Number of People forming the Mess.
May	30.	P. Waldstrom	In the same Mess.		6
July	16.	Isaack Longber			
June	9.	Steph. Propavo	ditto	ditto	9
	14.	Ant. Otkin			
	25.	A. Fanassi			
	—	John Split			
July	1.	Mindar Minus			
	31.	John Frederick			
	17.	John Berry	ditto	ditto	9
	13.	Thomas Ward			
	—	Frederick Nelson			
June	19.	John Fielding	ditto	ditto	8
	20.	John Melthier			
	22.	James Martin	ditto	ditto	8
	24.	Robert Seal			
July	14.	James Price			
June	22.	Charles Gosling	ditto	ditto	10
	27.	Manus Louffe	ditto	ditto	7
July	8.	John Peters			
	11.	Jonas Roebuck			
	1.	Tho. Wilkinson	ditto	ditto	2
	–	Joseph Jamison	ditto	ditto	7
	7.	George Baily			
	23.	George Polard			
	22.	John Brown	ditto	ditto	8
	—	Charles Churchill			

Peter Waldstrom, æt. 30. seaman, St Helena, a German of a sanguine temperament, gives the following account of his complaints.

May 9th. This morning he drew two or three inches of a white, round, slender substance from a small opening, a little above the outer ancle of the left leg. His leg was somewhat swelled and painful 14 days ago; a small vesicle formed, and discharged a little water; it then healed, but has again begun to discharge ichorous matter within these last three days. Finding a small sinus, I enlarged the opening to half an inch.—Curetur Cerato simplice.

June 4th. The white substance, resembling a piece of catgut, has again appeared. I fastened it to a piece of linen rolled to the thickness of a writing-quill, and got three turns.

6th.

6th. To-day, when in the act of turning the roller, the substance suddenly broke about half an inch within the edge of the sore, without any change in its appearance. I laid open the sinus to the bottom, being about an inch. Discharge of a brown colour, turbid and ichorous.

9th. Ulcer looks well; discharge purulent. Some hardness and inflammation over the tendo achillis opposite the wound. Several doublings of the substance have appeared on the outer edge of the ulcer, which have been secured as before.

11th. The substance came away to-day with perfect ease; the end flat, and very soft. About 10 inches in all extracted.

18th. The tumour has discharged a little serous matter by the ulcer. Inflammation almost gone.

19th. Inflammation and swelling returned. Watery discharge from the ulcer continues.—Cataplasm. Emolliens.

20th. Ulcer very dark-coloured.—Cont. Catapl.

28th. Ulcer preserves nearly the same appearance. Inflammation and swelling diminishing.—Cont. Cataplasm.

July 4th. Ulcer granulating at the edges; tough adhesive yellow matter adhering to the bottom; discharge ichorous. Swelling and inflammation gone. A little pain about an inch under the sore, along the edge of the outer ancle.—Curet. Mercur. Precip. Rub.

5th. Ulcer cleaning; discharge somewhat purulent.—Rr. Merc.

12th. Ulcer nearly well. No return of inflammation, but still a little pain, as before. Is at work.

Stephen Propavo, æt. 30, Seaman, St Helena, a Russian, of a sanguine melancholy temperament.

June 9th. About an inch of substance, resembling strong catgut, tinged brownish at the extremity, which is pointed, was found protruded from an opening over the root of the left middle toe, of which I drew out easily four inches with the forceps, and secured it to a roller of linen. When left loose, it retracted near an inch, but without a regular vermicular motion. The foot is œdematous. The foot and leg have been somewhat swelled, and a little painful, for two weeks past. A pustule formed and broke three or four days ago, from the opening of which the worm appeared to-day.—Curet. Cerato simplice.

11th. After getting one turn to-day, the worm became fixed; on using a little more force, a crack was heard, and another turn was got with perfect ease, when it again became immoveable.

14th. Have got from half a turn to two turns daily. To-day found

found it immoveably fixed, and, on attempting to force it, a slight laceration took place, and a small round white body protruded into the lacerated part, which I seized with a pair of forceps, and found it soft as mucus. Desisted from turning.

16th. The worm has recovered its first appearance by the lacerated part having healed. Much foetor from the roller, which I removed and applied a new one; got about one turn of the worm.

JAMES MARTIN, æt. ——, Boatswain's Mate.

June 22d. A worm under the inner ancle was discovered and secured to a roller.

24th. Much pain, swelling, and serous discharge.

27th. Worm immoveable.

30th. Worm broken, but the end in sight.

July 1st. Considerable inflammation and pain.—Catapl. Emolliens.

4th. Swelling gone.—Omitt. Cataplasm.

7th. A tumour forming a little above the opening.—Repr. Cat. The worm has disappeared to-day.

12th. Discharged pus from the tumour by incision. Has much pain in the ancle joint. Swelling diminishing.—Repr. Catapl.

16th. Swelling continues to diminish. Still much pain, which prevented sleep last night.—Cr. Catapl. Opiat. h. s.

26th. A pustule broke yesterday near the inner ancle, from which the worm has reappeared. Swelling nearly gone. To hang loose.

August 2d. A considerable portion of the worm drawn out daily, which dried and shrivelled during the day. It was become much more tender, and has disappeared to-day.

5th. Much inflammation.—Cataplasm. Emolliens.

12th. Inflammation gone. Still a little swelling of the ancle joint, and a few drops of water from the openings where the worms were.

22d. A little pain and stiffness in the tendo achillis when he walks.

ROBERT SEAL, æt. ——, Gunner's Mate.

June 24th. A worm in the fore part of the right ancle joint, Three weeks ago felt a little pain at times in this part, and over the outer ancle. In both places he could perceive under the skin a hard body, like a piece of cord, turning in various directions, and moveable when pressed by the fingers; could, in some places, trace it a little way by the sight, the skin being elevated.

vated. A little itching at times. There has never been either ſwelling or inflammation until three days ago, that a ſmall puſtule roſe and broke, and to-day a ſtrong worm has made its appearance, which was faſtened to a roller.

30th. About five inches on the roller, worm becoming tender. Much pain, incipient ſwelling, and inflammation. Omitted the roller.—Applic. Cataplaſ. Emolliens.

July 5th. Inflammation and ſwelling gone. A little ſwelling and inflammation at the root of the little toe for two days, and a ſmall veſicle formed yeſterday, which broke to-day; and there is a diſcharge of watery matter from a ſmall orifice in the ſkin at the centre of the veſicle.—Cont. Catapl.

10th. Worm getting ſtronger, and bears drawing a little. Sore under the toe diſcharging.—Cont. Catapl.

12th. Inflammation returned laſt night to a conſiderable degree.—Cont.

13th. Found eight inches of the worm detached to-day.

18th. A diſcharge of pus from under the toe, and a worm has appeared, rather tender in its ſubſtance.

22d. The worm broken, and inflammation returning.—Rep. Catapl.

27th. The tumour broke, diſcharged a little pus and water, and another worm has appeared, tender as before. To hang looſe.

29th. Worm again broken. A bliſter under the outer ancle.—Cont.

Auguſt 3d. Inflammation increaſing. Was rather reſtleſs laſt night. Skin hot, tongue white, thirſt, pulſe 86, body regular.

5th. No return of febrile ſymptoms. Still much inflammation.

11th. Bliſter broke ſix days ago, and to-day a hair-like ſubſtance hangs out an inch. Swelling and inflammation almoſt gone.

20th. Worm again diſappeared. Inflammation returning.—Catapl.

September 15th. The inflammation and worm reappeared and diſappeared again and again, and to-day the foot is nearly well.

Frederick Nelson, æt. 34.

July 13th. A worm in the left foot, near the root of the little toe. Says he had much itching a month ago about the knee joint, which gradually deſcended, accompanied by pain, to his foot, where he could feel the worm coiled under the ſkin, where a watery veſicle has formed and broken, and the worm has appeared. Has a little pain on walking, but no ſwelling or inflammation.

15th.

15th. Pain, fwelling, and a little inflammation.—Catapl. Emolliens.

28th. Inflammation diminifhing; worm tender.—Cont. Cataplafm.

29th. The worm has difappeared.

Auguft 5th. Swelling and inflammation returned.—Cataplafma.

10th. Worm appeared, and rather tender. Inflammation diminifhing.—Cr. Catapl.

11th. Extracted feven inches with eafe; its end foft.

13th. Fifteen inches extracted as above. Swelling continues.

20th. Still much pain; fwelling almoft gone.—Om. Catapl.

28th. Only a ftiffnefs of the tendo achillis remaining.

THOMAS WARD, æt. 22, Sail-maker.

July 13th. About a month ago had an itching in his foot, which lafted about a week, when a vesicle formed and broke, and a week ago a worm appeared in each. Has never had pain, fwelling, or inflammation.

24th. The worms hang loofe. The right one broken two days ago. An incipient inflammation.—Catapl. Emolliens.

28th. A tumour forming over the right fhin-bone. The left inflaming; its worm hanging loofe.—Catapl. Emolliens.

Auguft 4th. Right worm reappeared.

5th. Right difappeared again, and ancle fwelling. Left as before.

September 5th. The worm and occafional inflammation have been breaking and returning at times, and he is now quite well.

JAMES PRICE, æt. ——, Seaman.

July 14th. A watery veficle formed and broke outfide the right foot, without any previous affection, three weeks ago; a very tender worm appeared to-day. To hang loofe.

17th. Worm becoming ftronger.

20th. Able to bear gentle drawing by the forceps.

26th.—Inflammation and fwelling taking place.—Catapl.

28th. Worm difappeared. Inflammation and fwelling as before.—Cont.

Auguft 4th. Worm reappeared, and three inches came away; end ragged. Inflammation increafing.—Cont. Cataplafm.

12th. Inflammation diminifhing faft. Very little pain. A veficle on the outer ancle, which difcharged contents ferous.

22d. Swelling and inflammation gone. Veficle well. Is at work.

ISAAC

ISAAC LONGBER, æt. ——, Seaman.

July 16th. The left leg has become ſomewhat ſwelled laſt night.

19th. A veſicle containing water has formed.

27th. The veſicle has healed, and another formed.

Auguſt 2d. The laſt veſicle has not ſkinned over, and there is a ſmall point in the centre formed of pus. No pain.

15th. The veſicle never healed, and to-day an inch of ſtrong worm projects. Slight pain and inflammation. To hang looſe.

25th. Inflammation increaſing.—Cataplaſm. Emolliens.

29th. The worm of a dead-white appearance. A little extracted daily, with very little pain.

September 1ſt. Drew out about five inches to-day.

2d. About 15 inches drawn to-day, with apparently a pointed extremity, but being empty makes it uncertain.

MINDAR MINUS, æt. ——, Seaman.

July 1ſt. A ſtrong worm outſide the calf of the leg. No ſwelling or inflammation even to within ¼ of an inch of the orifice, which was a puſtule two days ago. Allowed it to remain without a roller.

4th. About three inches of the worm ſhrivelled and dry. On drawing it out, it retracts again, unleſs forcibly held.

6th. Applied a roller.

13th. Worm becoming very tender. Found four inches on the roller. Allowed it to remain looſe, with a thread tied to it. No inflammation.

18th. The worm ſo tender, that it has broke and diſappeared.

22d. Leg ſwelling.—Cataplaſm. Emolliens.

27th. Swelling gone. A worm appeared yeſterday, ſo tender, that it broke when wiping the ſore.

29th. No reappearance of worm. No ſwelling. Very little pain.

THOMAS WILKINSON, æt. ——, Carpenter.

July 1ſt. A worm about the centre of the left tibia, ſtrong and firm, of which about five inches are left hanging from the opening. Had an itching three weeks ago, when he could perceive under the ſkin a hard ſubſtance running in various directions, in ſome places convoluted. Ten days ago the leg put on an œdematous appearance, which is now gone, previous to which he received a ſlight bruiſe, which rubbed off a little cuticle, where the worm has come.

7th.

7th. Found the worm broken to-day. Incipient inflammation.—Catapl.

11th. Found three inches more worm detached to-day. Inflammation very extensive. Ulcer two inches in length, foul and fetid. Has been walking much, and working.—Cataplasma Emolliens.

13th. Another small opening close above the other. A piece more worm found loose. Considerable hemorrhagy last night.—Cr.

20th. Inflammation diminishing. Ulcer healing, but matter forming close to the ulcerated part.—Cont. Cataplasma.

25th. The tumour has burst, and discharged pus mixed with serum.

31st. The former ulcer healed, the latter healing. Inflammation almost gone.

August 10*th.* Ulcer nearly closed. Discharge watery.—Asperg. Merc. Prec. Rubro. After another sprinkling, the ulcer healed kindly.

JOSEPH JAMISON, æt. 33, Ship's Steward.

July 1*st.* A very tender worm over the root of the toes of the right foot. Has had an itching all over the foot for three weeks past, and has torn the cuticle in some places by scratching. Had a vesicle several days ago.

6th. Another in the sole of the left foot, very tender, with much inflammation.—Cat. Emol. To use a roller.

10th. Right worm comes slowly; foot inflamed. Very little of the worm got from the leg. Swelling gone.

16th. Right one preserves an uniform strength, and comes slowly. Left one disappeared.

30th. The right one came away whilst turning the roller, with a regular pointed extremity, without giving pain.

August 12*th.* Right foot well. No swelling or inflammation of the other, and the worm has acquired strength to bear drawing a little daily.

27th. A little drawn every second or third day. Last night left about an inch loose, and to day found five inches in his shoe, with apparently a pointed extremity. No swelling or inflammation.

JOHN BERRY, æt. ——, Seaman.

June 17*th.* A white-coloured substance, about the size of large catgut, pointed, projecting from the tendo achillis of the left leg, about an inch of which I have drawn out, with a little pain,

pain, four inches, of a ſerpentine figure; it feels firm beween the fingers. It broke with a loud ſnap when turning, without ſhowing any tendency to break by previouſly elongating. A little milky fluid dropped from it, and it became quite flaccid; a little of the ſame fluid iſſued from the orifice.

Says his ancle was ſwelled 14 days ago, and a veſicle formed, and diſcharged a watery fluid, where the worm has appeared. No appearance of inflammation remaining.—Curet. Cerat. ſimp.

24th. A tumour forming near the former orifice.—Catapl. Emol.

25th. A ſmall quantity of purulent matter diſcharged.

July 4th. A phlegmon forming on the fore part of the leg.—Cat. Emol.

5th. Tumour broke, and diſcharged a little pus with reddiſh ſerum.

6th. Original opening heal. A ſlender worm has appeared at the firſt phlegmonic opening. To be left hanging looſe.

10th. Worm gaining ſtrength.

13th. A worm at the ſecond orifice. To be left looſe.

14th. A tender worm has appeared on the fore part of the ancle joint, where a bliſter has formed. Left it looſe.

16th. Ten inches of the ſecond worm cut off to-day, and left as before.

19th. Five inches of the ſecond got away, with evidently a pointed extremity, reſembling the end which firſt appeared; 18 inches of ſubſtance little thicker than a horſe's hair, and having much the appearance of a wetted ſtrong fibre of flax, found under the dreſſing. Had a febrile paroxyſm yeſterday.—Pulv. Cort. Peruv.

28th. No return of paroxyſm. Worm on the fore part of the ancle joint has diſappeared, and the other was found broken under the dreſſing.

31ſt. The two openings near the outer ancle ſtill diſcharge a few drops of ſerous matter. The one on the fore part of the joint healed. A little pain over the ſhin bone above the ancle.

John Fielding, æt. ——, Seaman.

June 19th. A worm under the outer ancle of the right, and another under the inner ancle of the left leg, where he had watery veſicles and a little ſwelling a fortnight ago, which healed, and have formed and broke again. No pain. Uſed a roller of linen to each.

21ſt. Much pain in the right leg, ſwelling, and ichorous, brown-coloured diſcharge.

27th. Removed the right roller, and found 16 inches of

worm

worm on it, half of which was extracted to day. Fastened a clean roller.

30*th*. Have got six inches more of the right. Left somewhat more painful.

July 1*st*. Three and a half inches more of the right extracted with great ease; it has a pointed extremity, and is not flaccid. Removed the left roller, and found ten inches on it; being very tender, left it loose.

5*th*. The left foot much swelled —Cataplasm. Emolliens.

10*th*. Right foot well. Inflammation of the left nearly gone. Worm disappeared.

15*th*. Foot so far well, that he is doing duty.

ANTONY OTKIN, æt. ——, Seaman, of sanguine temperament.

June 14*th*. About an inch of a rather flaccid worm from a small opening immediately under the left outer ancle, where a watery vesicle formed and broke 16 days ago. Got three turns around a roller of lint. No swelling of the foot. Much pain when drawing the worm. Had no previous pain in the affected part.

17*th*. Immoveable to-day.

24*th*. Worm again immoveable yesterday and to-day. Very much pain on attempting to turn, and the worm very tender.

25*th*. The worm broke on attempting to turn.

29*th*. Much inflammation of foot and ancle.—Catapl. Emol.

July 2*d*. A phlegmon forming a little behind the opening.

10*th*. The phlegmon broke and discharged a little pus yesterday. Says he found about three inches of worm loose on removing his dressing this morning, which he threw away. Swelling and inflammation disappearing slowly.—Cont. Cataplasm. Emolliens.

17*th*. Scrotum and penis much swelled, colourless, and elastic, which he first observed at ten o'clock last night.

20*th*. Swelling of scrotum gone. Swelling of foot nearly gone.

28*th*. The two small openings continue to discharge a little serous matter. No reappearance of the worms.

August 1*st*. A worm has appeared inside the thigh, a little above the knee, where there was a pustule two days ago.

3*d*. Worm broken. No swelling or inflammation of the thigh.

6*th*. Worm reappeared double, and, on drawing, find one end terminates in a fine hair-like substance.

8*th*. A colourless tumour, containing fluid on the right heel.

20*th*. A vesicle discharged under the left outer ancle.

25*th*.

25th. Right heel inflamed. Discharged the tumour by incision; it contained pus.

September 15th. The inflammation disappeared gradually, but a worm appeared at the incised part, with which he was to-day discharged the ship. An irregularly formed substance, approaching to an oval, was discovered, probably adhering to the septum scroti, which gave no pain, except when roughly handled.

JOHN MELTHIER, æt. 18, Seaman.

June 20th. A worm projecting about an inch from under the left outer ancle, preceded by a blister. Had a little pain for some time, and itching. Worm rather tender; fastened it to a roller.

22d. Found the worm broken to-day.

28th. Worm reappeared, and secured to a roller. Another inside the right heel, where a blister formed two days ago, and broke yesterday. The substance of the worm very tender. Let it hang loose.

July 4th. Left worm again broken. Much inflammation.—Cataplasm.

10th. Inflammation very much reduced. Right one getting stronger.

13th. Tumour forming outside the left calf.—Cataplasm. Emolliens.

20th. Can trace the right worm under the skin, and at a little distance from the orifice; can feel it tense when drawn; have got a little daily; it dries and shrivels in the course of one night.

24th. The right came to a pointed extremity to-day. Laid open the tumour, and discharged a little pus floating in serum.

25th. The left worm has not reappeared. Still a little inflammation.

29th. The incision and former openings healed. Can feel a hollow an inch in length, resembling a sinus, near the incision. Is at his work.

CHARLES GOSLING, æt. ——, Seaman.

June 22d. Four inches of worm strong and pointed between the ancle and heel. Cut it off, and secured to a roller. A small pustule appeared 16 days ago, and healed again, from the site of which this worm has protruded.

25th. Found 9½ inches on the roller. Applied another roller.

July 1st. Found the worm broken to-day. Have not been able to extract any since last report. Much inflammation since last night.—Cataplasm.

5th. Swelling and inflammation gone.—Omitt. Cataplafm.
10th. Sore heal. Is at work.

GEORGE BAILY, æt. ——, Gunner's Servant.

July 7th. A veficle about half an inch in diameter, containing a dark watery fluid, formed under the right inner ancle yefterday, which I have difcharged to-day, and find a very minute opening in the centre of the bliftered part, from which half an inch of a hair-like foft fubftance hangs. Says he has had no pain, but an itching for ten days, and has a firm cord-like fubftance under the fkin.

18th. The hair-like fubftance gone. Cuticle again forming. No fwelling or pain.

22d. The place well. The left leg fwelled, pits a little on preffure.

26th. The leg has been inflamed a little for two days, and a puftule formed and broke infide the calf. The opening of the fkin one-third of an inch in diameter, filled with a tough inflammatory incruftation, from the centre of which hangs half an inch of foft hair-like matter.

28th. Drew away the inflammatory exfudation with a pair of forceps, and left a thimble-like cavity. The hair broken.

Auguft 1ft. The right foot has become much inflamed.—Cat. Emolliens.

2d. Both feet inflamed, and a tender worm in each.

4th. A little got daily. The right worm came away with the dreffing, apparently broken. Swelling fpreading up the leg.—Cat. Emol.

5th. A double portion of the right appeared, which, on drawing it, broke.

25th. Has had a little occafional inflammation, which has been relieved by poultices, and draws a little of the worm from time to time; but it is very tender, and breaks frequently.

September 15th. Continued as laft report, and is now quite well.

JOHN PETERS, æt.——, Seaman.

July 8th. A fmall puftule formed and broke on the ancle-joint; a hair-like fubftance hangs out. No fwelling, pain, or inflammation.

12th. Every appearance of worm gone. Difcharge ichorous.

Auguft 6th. Ancle fwelling, fomewhat inflamed.—Catapl. Emolliens.

12th. Swelling and inflammation gone.

20th. Worm reappeared pretty ftrong. Let it remain loofe.

September 15th. The worm has difappeared repeatedly, and he has been from time to time as in the reports above; and at prefent much inflammation of the ancle.

JONAS

JONAS ROEBUCK, æt. ——, Seaman.

July 11*th*. A large inflamed tumour immediately under the knee-joint.—Cataplasm. Emolliens.

14*th*. The tumour broke yesterday, and discharged a little pus mixed in serous matter of a red tinge. The opening is filled with an inflammatory exsudation, hollow in the centre, from which hangs an inch of slender soft matter, like a hair or wetted fibre of flax.—Cont. Cat. Emol.

22*d*. The fibry matter and inflammatory crust separated. A strong worm, which retracts quickly after drawing, has appeared. Several small openings discharging serous matter. A roller.

29*th*. The inflammation diminishing, but much pain in the joint, and a little redness above the knee. Hæmorrhagy last night. The worm retains a uniform appearance, and comes away daily.

August 3*d*. Knee rather more swelled to-day.—Cont. Cat.

12*th*. The inflammation continues, with a large moveable tumour inside the thigh.

18*th*. The tumour contains matter, a little of which is discharged by the opening of the worm.

21*st*. The worm extracted, its extremity pointed, full and firm. The discharge continues. The abscess is above the joint, and the opening on the fore part the tibia, about an inch below the joint.—Cont. Cataplasm.

22*d*. Enlarged the opening. Still considerable discharge.

29*th*. No discharge. A little pain in the joint, and stiffness of the ham.

JOHN BROWN, æt. ——, Ship's Cook.

July 22*d*. A vesicle five days ago, preceded by itching; and a worm appeared yesterday, which, he says, has retracted to-day.

29*th*. Says he observed a slender thread, which broke when drawn to-day. A little itching at times. No pain, swelling, or inflammation.

August 16*th*. Says the worm appears, disappears, or is broken, from time to time. No inflammation. A watery discharge.

September 15*th*. Continued to go on as before. Foot and ancle at present much inflamed and swelled.

CHARLES

Charles Churchill, æt. ——, Seaman.

July 22d. A watery vesicle three-fourths of an inch in diameter, over the foot two days ago; from the centre of which hangs a slender thread. Has had no previous affection.

26th. Worm disappeared. Blistered part healing.

August 30th. Has got a little from time to time. Ancle very much inflamed to-day. No worm in sight.—Cat. Emolliens.

September 8th. No complaint.

George Polard, æt. ——, Boatswain.

July 23d. Says that for six weeks past he has had an itching at times in his right leg and foot, which was always relieved by washing or rubbing. Has also had a pain in the calf, which he supposed to be rheumatic, and wore worsted stockings without relief. Three days ago a vesicle formed and broke, and a soft hair-like substance hangs from the centre from a very minute opening. No swelling, pain, or inflammation.—Curet. Cerat. simpl.

August 4th. The hair has disappeared for some time, and reappeared again two days ago. Feels pain and itching in the other leg.

September 15th. Has been drawing a little of the worm from time to time. Broke it a few days ago. Much inflammation to-day.—Cataplasm. Emolliens.

John Frederick, æt. ——, Seaman.

July 31st. Says a small pustule appeared a little above the knee, inside the left thigh, several days ago, without any previous complaint, from which a pretty strong worm protruded to-day, of which I have drawn out four inches. No swelling, pain, or inflammation.

August 5th. Worm still hangs loose, and the portion last drawn shrivels and dries in the course of the day. No inflammation.

7th. Has produced about six inches of dried worm apparently pointed, which, he says, he drew out with ease this morning.

Azary Fanassi, æt. ——, Seaman.

June 25th. A worm over the centre of the left middle metatarsal bone.

July 3d. Worm broken; foot much inflamed.—Catapl. Emolliens.

10th. Still considerable inflammation.—Cont. Cataplasm.

12th. The worm has reappeared in doublings, and is very tender. Have drawn out and cut away eight inches, and left the end loose.

13*th.*

13th. Two pieces, of about two inches each, found under the dressing. Still much inflammation. A sore forming under the outer ancle.—Cont. Catap.

18th. Sore under the ancle, filled with tough matter. The opening, fore part the foot, healed up. Inflammation much diminished.—Cont. Catap.

22d. Asperg. Ulcus Merc. precip. Rubro. Omitt. Cataplasm.

27th. Swelling gone. No pain. Ulcer healing.—Cont.

August 7th. Foot well.

John Split, æt. ——, Seaman.

June 25th. A worm under the right outer ancle. Used a roller.

July 13th. Worm become very tender. Found only six inches on the roller. Tied a thread to the worm, and left it loose.

14th. The left foot much swelled to-day, with a vesicle in the centre of the fore part. Much pain.—Utat. Catapl. Emolliens.

22d. The right one comes away slowly. Swelling left foot nearly gone. An opening, filled with inflammatory crust, in the centre of where the vesicle was.—Cont. Cataplasm.

24th. A strong worm in the left. Right one also become strong. Both left hanging loose.

August 2d. Left foot swelling. Worms extracted slowly.—Cataplasm.

6th. Right worm as before. Left disappeared. Swelling increasing.

7th. Extracted 12 inches of worm, with a pointed extremity.

15th. Right foot well. Swelling and inflammation of left diminishing.

20th. A little fungus where the left worm protruded.—Apr. precip. Rub.

24th. Only a small ulcer remaining.

Manus Louffe, æt. 56, Seaman.

June 27th. A worm over the right inner ancle. Got $3\frac{1}{4}$ inches, when it broke suddenly with a snap.

28th. Again found the worm, and secured it to a roller.

30th. Removed the roller, and found $5\frac{1}{2}$ inches. To hang loose.

July 2d. Inflammation appearing.—Cataplasm. Emolliens.

5th. Worm become very tender. An orifice formed near the former.

10th. Inflammation and swelling diminishing. There has been

been a little fungus from the last opening, but it is nearly gone. Worm broken.

17*th*. A worm has appeared in the edge of a superficial sore formed some time ago by a hurt, without any previous warning, in the left leg.

20*th*. The last mentioned worm broken; no swelling or inflammation. A small pustule, with a little surrounding inflammation, above the left knee. A worm has appeared under the outer ancle.

29*th*. Swelling of the right diminishing still. The worm under the left outer ancle comes slowly.

August 3*d*. A worm from the pustule over the left knee, and a blister on the outside the right foot. A discharge of pus from the place where the worm broke in the left calf.

6*th*. Worm in the left foot broken. Vesicle under the right outer ancle.

10*th*. Worm in the thigh broken. An ulceration taken place under the left outer ancle; discharge fetid. Right vesicle broken, and a worm appeared. Discharged pus, by incision, from the left calf.

19*th*. Worm appeared in a small pustule under the left knee. The left heel much inflamed, swelled, and painful.—Catapl. Emolliens. The worm again disappeared under the ancle.

25*th*. Right ancle joint inflaming. Worm under the knee continues.

Sept. 15*th*. The worms disappeared and reappeared as above, and he was discharged with one under the knee joint, when a sudden crack was heard, and two more turns got with ease. No particular appearance in the worm. Œdema diminishing slowly. Ulcer of a somewhat spacelated appearance. Discharge watery, of a brownish tinge, with, at times, a little brownish matter resembling coffee grounds. Found 8½ inches on the old roller.

18*th*. Found the worm broken. Find three inches on the roller. Foot very painful. Has always had much pain when in the act of extracting the worm.

25*th*. The œdema continues to diminish; discharge lessening. Seven inches extracted to-day, soft and flaccid, came to an extremity with ease, flat and ragged.—Curet. Cerato simplice.

26*th*. Swelling and inflammation to-day.—Catapl. Emol.

July 3*d*. Swelling gone.—Omitt. Cataplasm. Cont. Ceratum.

7*th*. A blister, with surrounding inflammation, has appeared in the centre of the sole of the foot, which was only slightly painful yesterday.

1 13*th*.

13*th*. Foot well. Is at work.

19*th*. A worm has appeared at the sole of the foot at the place of the former blister. Worm strong, exciting much pain when drawn forcibly. Another near the right outer ancle. No swelling or inflammation. Each projects about an inch and a half not straight, but a little serpentine and stiff.

25*th*. On drawing the left, about an inch came away, hollow in the end, leaving the worm of the same appearance as before. Swelling and inflammation, as before, returning.—Catapl. Emolliens.

2 *th*. Have got very little of the worms, they are becoming flaccid, are allowed to hang loose; much pain when drawn, and are drying and shrivelling.

31*st*. The right worm has disappeared.

August 4*th*. Worm reappeared under the right outer ancle. The one in the sole of the foot disappeared. Let it hang loose.

5*th*. Right worm again broken. Left (in the sole) disappeared.

8*th*. Worm in the sole reappeared double.

11*th*. Worm broken. Both ends project about half an inch each, and tender.

17*th*. Both ends of the worm drawn out; about six inches of the one, and rather less of the other. Extremities soft and ragged.

24*th*. Right foot inflaming.—Cataplasm. Emolliens.

29*th*. No inflammation, pain, or swelling.

September 15*th*. No return since last report.

Peter Waldstrom.

August 9*th*, 1805. A small pustule formed and broke on the lower edge of the right gluteus muscle eight days ago, from which a very tender worm appeared, and has disappeared this morning. There is still a small incrustation on the other leg.

16*th*. The worm reappeared. No swelling, pain, or inflammation. Is and has been at work.

28*th*. The worm has again disappeared, and considerable inflammation has taken place.—Cat. Emol.

Sept. 15*th*. The inflammation went off gradually, and the worm never reappeared.

V.

V.

Case of Encysted Ascites, with Hydatids. By K. Macleay, M.D. Oban.

Some time ago I was called to visit a man named Monro, who lived at the distance of five miles from me. The extreme wretchedness which the economy of his hovel, and the appearance of his wife and five children, together with his own miserable situation, reclining upon a parcel of straw, and labouring under the double misfortune of disease and poverty, exhibited, called up that sympathy which interests the heart in the sufferings of humanity.

Upon inquiry, I found he was in the prime of life, aged about 40, by trade a weaver, and that he had enjoyed uninterrupted good health until 18 months before, when his disorder began. For a considerable period he was incapable of attending his occupation, or providing for his family, and had never thought of applying for assistance till it proceeded to an alarming height. From his appearance I considered his case to be ascites, and, from the violence of the symptoms, a very hopeless one.

On examination, I found the abdomen greatly distended, with evident fluctuation, although not quite so yielding as is generally the case, which I attributed to the excessive enlargement and stretching of the muscles. The legs were somewhat swelled, and retained an impression; a frequent small pulse; tongue and skin dry; thirst urgent, and urine rather scanty; and the bowels costive, and at times much pained. Respiration was so laborious that he could not lie down, but was under the necessity of being supported in a half-erect posture. He was greatly emaciated, his appetite having wholly forsaken him. His countenance was sunk, and his skin of a pale yellow colour, so that death seemed not very distant.

In this state of the case it was useless to prescribe any medicine, and I immediately proposed the operation of Paracentesis as the only means of relieving his distress, and, in some degree, preventing a miserable dissolution; to which, however, he and his friends strenuously objected.

As I was very unwilling to leave the poor man to his fate, I agreed to give him some medicine, hoping that when, its inefficacy would appear, they would consent to the operation. He was consequently ordered a laxative and an anodyne. These were repeated occasionally, and I saw him pretty regularly for ten days thereafter, when the operation was consented to, as his situation became daily more intolerable. I accordingly placed him

him in the ordinary posture, and introduced the trocar, which readily entered, at the usual place, in the left side; but, upon withdrawing the stillet, I was surprised that scarcely an ounce of fluid followed. I introduced a probe through the canula, which met with no resistance, and produced no effect. Disappointed at this want of success, without being able to account for it, I did not well know how to keep up the sinking spirits of my poor patient, who expected relief from the operation; and, as I still believed the case dropsical, from the fluctuation and regular distention of the abdomen, I repeated the operation on the right side, but, to my mortification, with no better success. I was now convinced of its being an encysted case, and as nothing farther could be done to relieve the unfortunate man, I left him, with regret, to sink under an incurable disease.

He died in three days thereafter, and, as the case was uncommon, I requested the liberty of examining the body, which his friends readily gave me.

Upon laying open the parietes of the abdomen, an immense cyst, occupying the whole cavity, presented and concealed the intestines, except a portion of the arch of the colon, which appeared above it in the epigastrium, and towards the left hypochondrium. On both sides of the cyst the wound made by the trocar appeared, and showed that it had entered in the attempt to empty the belly. About a pound of fluid, which seemed to have escaped by these perforations, was collected within the peritoneum, to which there was a slight adhesion of the cyst towards the right ileum. This great bag was distended to the utmost, and, without any irregularity of its surface, evidently contained a fluid readily fluctuating, and, when opened by a longitudinal incision was found completely filled with hydatids. The quantity was so great that it would have been folly to attempt enumerating them, and I therefore measured thirty-five English pints. The size of a great proportion was much beyond what I had ever seen, and exceeded that of the largest orange. In this quantity was included the fluid which surrounded the hydatids, but it was so inconsiderable as not to cover them when carefully collected, measured, and put into a washing-tub.

The cyst was connected to the mesentery above the second lumbar vertebra by a considerable neck. Several of the glands of the mesentery and mesocolon were greatly enlarged and indurated, and the intestines were unusually contracted, as might be supposed from the long-continued pressure of the cyst, the loss of appetite, and consequent emaciation. The liver was small and pushed upwards, and the right lobe partly scirrhous. The other viscera were sound, although somewhat smaller than usual.

I

I was much gratified by the opportunity which the dissection afforded me of ascertaining the nature of the case, which, from the amazing collection of hydatids, was very singular, and of which I now beg leave to transmit this concise statement.

Oban, 6th December, 1805.

VI.

Description of the Koutam-Poulli, showing, contrary to the commonly received Opinion, that it does not afford Gum-Gamboge. In a Letter to Dr J. ANDERSON, Madras, from Dr WHITE, Cananore.

MY DEAR SIR,

MY botanical pursuits having necessarily of late suffered a long stagnation, I have been thereby prevented from endeavouring to supply a variety of commissions and queries, relative to that department, transmitted to me from different quarters.

I had long since consigned to a memorandum-book the following notice of an interesting specimen, but the expectation of coupling it with something equally so has hitherto delayed the communication.

Dr Berry's description of a tree which flowered in the Nopalry at Madras in 1801 suggested to me the indentity of our two trees, and that the differences may have chiefly arisen from the youth of his specimen, aided perhaps by a strange soil and climate;—circumstances which, even in a state of nature, I have frequently found to exert a marked influence in modifying vegetable productions.

I need not observe to you, that the koutam-poulli of the Hortus Malabaricus, or kour-kampoulli of Acosta, of which I am now to treat, has hitherto been described in a manner too general or too vague to give us accurate generic and specific notions of it, much less for enabling us to correct the concomitant error which assigns, for its produce of gum-gamboge, a substance entirely foreign to any quality observable in our tree, as will afterwards appear.

It is not improper previously to remark, that I am partly indebted for the successful investigation of the present subject to a little philological care first applied in tracing the meaning and origin

origin of its indigenous names. Had this been earlier attended to, our inquiries would have aſſumed a more natural, and moſt likely a more ſucceſsful direction. For who would have thought of ſearching for gum-gamboge, a ſubſtance of much acrimony, and frequently of violent efficacy, when taken in ſmall quantities, in a tree whoſe mild juices produce a fruit of ſuch univerſal uſe in food, as to have originally impoſed the eminently appropriate names by which it has been known to the natives from time immemorial. Rumphius, more than 100 years back, drew the attention of botaniſts to this ſubject, and firſt ſuggeſted the great probability of miſtake in the affirmation of gum-gamboge being the produce of the koutam, or kourkam-poulli, of Malabar; but, with that diffidence inſeparable from the true ſpirit of obſervation, he would not hazard a poſitive opinion, ſeeing the chance of deception from a dried ſpecimen, and that brought from a great diſtance.

My repeated opportunities of actual and careful inſpection of the tree upon the ſpot, though entitled to little conſideration, may contribute to render what follows an object of intereſt to you, who are ſo capable of appreciating the nature of all ſuch attempts.

I had made many and vain inquiries for the meaning of khoddam, or coddam, (for it is written both ways, according to European caprice), till, on inſpecting ſome error in orthography or enunciation, and ſubſtituting mutes of analogous powers, I found that koutam ſignifies, all over Malabar, a made-up or mixed diſh of victuals; and koutam-poulli, the ingredient of the ſame. Kourkam-poulli is a name alſo perfectly appropriate, but rather of a more general meaning, as it ſignifies the acid ingredient of any kind of food, literally the eating or meal acid. The Malabar Marum, ſignifying tree in general, when added, completes the indigenous appellative.

Botanical Deſcription of the Koutam-Poulli, or Kourkam-Poulli, of the Malabar Coaſt.

Claſſis Polyandria. Ordo mono-gynia;—of the natural order of pomaceæ.

Calyx.—Four parted diviſions, fleſhy and gibbous, with ſquamous edges, one oppoſite pair ſhort orbicular; the longer oblong and rigid, all placed oppoſite to the interſtices of the corolla, and adhering to it beneath —Permanent.

Corolla.—Four petals longer and larger than the calyx, erect, oblong, coloured, and fleſhy, with a ſquamous contour, ſubequal, plane outwardly, gibbous internally, and thickening to a broad unguis,

unguis, which is clofely glued to the receptacle, and the bafe of the germen.

Stamina.—Numerous filaments, fhort and flefhy, united below, and frequently embracing clofely the hollow divifions of the germen. Anthers large, ftriated, and incumbent, of an irregular fhape.

Piftillum.—Germen globular, with from feven to nine (moft commonly eight) furrows, and as many rounded and fubequal vertical fegments; no ftyle, ftigma plane expanded, radiating into obtufe angles or lobes.—Permanent.

Pericarpium.—An apple, various in fize, from half an inch to one and a half in diameter; fpherical, fometimes approaching to an oval fhape; fegments more or lefs equal, from feven to nine (moft commonly eight) with as many deep furrows between each fegment, enclofes in a pulpy membrane a folid crefcent formed feed, in fhape and fize correfponding to the fegments, and, of courfe, tapering inwardly to unite their edges at the axis of the pome.

This tree, in its natural foil and climate, is one of the moft ftately and beautiful productions of the foreft on the Ghauts, which feems its moft congenial fituation: it fhoots up to the height of 66 or 80 feet, with a ftem naked half-way, and then thickly befet with branches and foliage. But it feldom exceeds half this fize on the fea coaft.

Trunk.—Perpendicular, round, and flightly tapering; bark uniform and fmooth, of a dark-brown colour externally, but of a more vivid brown next the parenchyma, and of a pale yellow, clofe to the wood, from which it very eafily peels off; on incifion there exudes a light yellow juice in moderate quantity, which, by expofure to the air, fpeedily lofes its bright colour, concreting into a fufcous, tenacious mafs of no tafte, and not foluble in the faliva.

Branches.—Proceeding regularly from fucceffive points round the ftem as it rifes; fmall branches in oppofite pairs, crofs-armed, or the plane of each pair regularly croffing the fucceeding one at rectangles.

Leaves.—Petioled, iffuing in pairs; entire, acutely oblong, rigid, fmooth, and finely veined, of a fhining and rather light green; their tafte acid.

Flowers.—Axillary, from the fmall lateral and terminal twigs; feffile moft commonly in fmall clufters, from two to four, with minute flefhy bracts, generally fingle.

The feafon of inflorefcence is March, or the beginning of April. The fruit ripens in May, or the commencement of June, juft before the periodical rains. The apple, as above hinted, contains

contains an abundant and pleaſant acid both in its pulp and membranes.

I have not learned that the wood is applied to any mechanical or domeſtic purpoſes. The ripe fruit, diſcoverable by its dropping, receives a very ſimple management to fit it for the market, as, after ſprinkling them (the large apples being previouſly ſplit open) with a little ſalt, they are ſpread out to dry in the ſun, and, when this is finiſhed, they are laid up in mat bags.

Their great uſe in curries, and other ſimple diſhes of the natives, renders them a conſiderable article of trade from place to place all over India. I have frequently ſeen them imported on the Malay coaſt, and the adjacent iſlands. Southern Malabar, the kingdom of Travancore, and Ceylon, furniſh this extenſive demand.

I have not ſeen the koutam-poulli in the interior of the peninſula, and it is even very rare in Kanara. The natives of this coaſt do not cultivate it with any attention; now and then we meet with a ſolitary individual near a riot's * habitation; he and his neighbours are hereby ſupplied with as much as their families can conſume, and they look no farther. To make up for this, moſt part of the mountains of the Ghauts produce the tree in the greateſt perfection, and the fruit in an abundance ſufficient for any demand.

I have thus finiſhed as circumſtantial a detail of the koutam (erroneouſly koddam or coddam, as I have found from careful inquiry among the beſt-informed natives) poulli-marum of the Hortus Malabaricus, or kourkam-poulli (erroneouſly ſpelled and pronounced carka) of Acoſta, as my obſervations have enabled me to make; and I think that, in future, our ideas will be fixed on this point.

Indeed, it ſurpriſes me that even any confuſion ſhould have exiſted relative to the two trees, cambogia and koutam-poulli. It could ſcarcely have originated with the natives, as they have not ſo much as a name for the former, and its produce, the gum-gamboge, is not to be had in any Malabar bazar;—a clear proof that they are ignorant of its qualities, and that they never made any application of them in their arts or medicine.

Cananore, 4th January 1805.

* A villager, or country man.

THE

THE INQUIRER, No. V.

Obſervations on Secondary Hemorrhage, and on the Ligature of Arteries after Amputation, and other Operations.

I HAVE always been of opinion, that the quicker we produce adheſive inflammation, by which we look forward in amputation to the union of divided parts, the more are we likely to obviate ſecondary hemorrhage. As I conſider this poſition undeniable, even where there may be an exiſting diſpoſition in the veſſels to diſeaſe, it may be productive of ſome good to inquire how far the methods uſually taken in this important operation coincide with the views of the practitioner, who has in contemplation healing by the firſt intention.

The general practice in amputation is to ſecure the blood-veſſels by very broad ligatures, not inferior in their dimenſions to ſome kinds of tape; and it is not unuſual to ſee the femoral artery taken up by ſuch a ligature, including in the courſe of the needle a conſiderable quantity of the contiguous muſcular and other parts.

The ſecurity of blood-veſſels of any importance we are ſtill under the neceſſity of truſting to ligature, which is an introduction of foreign matter into a wound intended to be healed by the adheſive proceſs, the effects of which are undoubtedly at variance with the intentions of the ſurgeon; and on their number, ſize, and diſtribution in the wound, depends, in a great degree, his ſucceſs or failure.

Independent of the obſtacles which ligatures muſt ever place againſt healing by the firſt intention, particularly when of ſuch immenſe dimenſions, and where they are numerous, which often happens, the mode of arranging them uſually adopted by the profeſſion has alſo a tendency to counteract the adheſive efforts of nature, and performs an important part in eſtabliſhing the ſuppurative proceſs in almoſt every part of the wound. The ſurgeon, when the blood-veſſels are ſecured, generally draws the ligatures out at the ſuperior and inferior parts of the wound, ſo that the whole living and recently divided part of the ſtump becomes covered by a foreign body; in fact, he eſtabliſhes a ſeton where he has in view healing by the firſt intention,–a meaſure which muſt conſtitute a decided obſtacle to the accompliſhment of his deſigns; and, beſides the diſadvantages to the healing of the wound, their removal, when it can be attempted with ſafety, becomes more difficult from the point acted on, and the extremity of the veſſels ſecured neceſſarily forming an angle, the ligature is forced, where there is reſiſtance,

ſiſtance, into the contiguous parts, giving riſe at times to pretty conſiderable diſcharges of blood.

The above is a ſhort, but, I believe, a correct view of ſome imperfections in the preſent mode of performing amputation, to which it is the object of this eſſay to call the attention of ſurgeons, by pointing out the impoſſibility of healing by the firſt intention under ſuch arrangements, and to endeavour to remove ſome of the difficulties which obſtruct the adheſive efforts of nature, by a ſimple, ſafe, and, I believe, eaſily practicable deviation from the eſtabliſhed method.

Where the habit and condition of the patient has been favourable to operation, I have moſt unexpectedly ſeen the ſuppurative proceſs interfere with the exertions of men of the higheſt eminence; matter form, the ſtump in ſome inſtances open; a diſpoſition to exfoliation follow, the perioſteum quit its adheſion to the bone; the muſcles retract; the co[illegible]ition of the wound change, and hectic fever ſucceed, from r[illegible]ewed irritation and diſcharge, terminating in the death of the p[illegible]tient; and to thoſe unfavourable changes the improper ſize [illegible] ligatures, joined to their equally improper diſtribution, contr[illegible]buted a moſt important and conſpicuous part.

Let any one, to feel the force of the preceding obſervation, recollect how ſuddenly the diſcharge of pus ceaſes on the removal of the ligatures, and how great it is where even the ſmalleſt of them remains. The irritation and ſloughing, alſo, ariſing from the natural removal of a piece of carious bone, offers a ſtrong leſſon in favour of the propriety of diminiſhing every ſource of irritation as far as poſſible, and decidedly points out large ligatures as the probable cauſe of ſecondary hemorrhage in ſome inſtances, where, under an oppoſite treatment, it would not have taken place.

Although I have, in my operations, been as ſucceſsful as many, ſtill the ſtrong impreſſion made on my mind by my failures, has never been effaced by that ſucceſs, and has excited in me a deſire to obviate their recurrence. To this feeling of regard for my fellow-creatures am I to trace the deviations which I am about to notice. As the ſubject is of importance, and thus early produced for the purpoſe of exciting attention and gaining information, it will, I hope, be treated with the ſpirit of candid inquiry: I ſhall therefore proceed to detail my late practice and ideas of this important part of ſurgery.

In place of ſecuring the blood-veſſels and diſtributing the ligatures in the manner followed in amputation, I have, in one caſe, above the knee, tied every veſſel from the femoral artery downwards, including nothing, if poſſible, but the artery, with a ſingle ſilk thread, and, when this was done, I afterwards, as

 near

near to the knot as poſſible, took off one half of each ligature, ſo that the foreign matter introduced was a mere trifle, compared with what I had been accuſtomed to ſee. There is conſiderable diſadvantage attending the including in the ligature on the artery much of the contiguous parts, as it may interfere with the contractile powers of the arteries exerting themſelves to their immediate and full extent. On cloſing the wound by adheſive ſtraps, inſtead of the uſual arrangements of the ligatures from the ſuperior and inferior parts, I drew each ligature out as nearly as poſſible on a line with the veſſels ſecured; and, provided the edge of the adheſive ſtrap, when applied to bring the oppoſite ſides of the wound into contact, urged the ligature from its direct courſe, it was opened carefully with a pair of ſciſſars in the direction of the wound, ſo that the ligature might be allowed to paſs out on a line with the veſſel it ſecured, by drawing it or them gently into this diviſion of the ſtrap. The next ſtrap was applied ſo as more than to cover and ſupport the extent of diviſion in the preceding one, and, provided it interfered with the direct courſe of the ligatures from their ſource (the veſſels ſecured), the ſame ſteps were taken. In this manner the wound was cloſed, and every ligature drawn out, as nearly as poſſible, on a line with the point to which it was tied; and, although a man of 60, and much weakened by previous diſeaſe, the wound healed with the rapidity of hare-lip. The parts were united in the courſe of ſix days, and, with the exception of the points of ligature, there was no purulent diſcharge. What can prove a greater ſecurity againſt ſecondary hemorrhage than ſuch a union of parts? The great objections that have been ſtated to this mode of ſecuring the blood-veſſels have been founded on the ideas of cutting or injuring them ſo much as to give riſe to ſecondary hemorrhage. This mode of thinking and reaſoning, although plauſible, does not appear to me to be well-founded. A large ligature excites the proceſs of inflammation and ulceration throughout its whole courſe, and much beyond itſelf, in the direction of the artery towards the body. The parts, in place of coaleſcing and approaching each other, which is of material conſequence in favouring the ſupport of the divided arteries, recede very conſiderably on all ſides, ſo that the extremities of the arteries remain unſupported, and, as it were, floating in a ſinus, with ligatures, moſt unneceſſarily large, attached to them, capable of exciting, by undue irritation, exceſſive inflammation in the very ſubſtance of the artery itſelf; a change of action from that of the adheſive diſpoſition, highly dangerous, in my opinion, as being favourable to ſecondary hemorrhage, by its tendency to excite the ſloughing proceſs. The mode of ligature which I have lately tried will

 obviate

obviate ſuch inconvenience, as the parts will be found much more diſpoſed to general union from the cauſe of irritation and inflammation being ſo much diminiſhed, and will prove one great means of obviating, where practicable, in place of promoting ſecondary hemorrhage. Indeed, I really think we are juſtified in aſcribing hemorrhage after amputations, as well as ſome other operations, to the great volume of ligature, the very means adopted to obviate ſuch an occurrence exciting ſuppuration and ſloughing; for it is but fair to conclude, where undue action does follow, that the veſſels ſecured by ſuch ligatures will be more likely to aſſume the ulcerative and ſloughing form of action than others. In the dead body, where the key-ſtone of the fabric is gone, and reſiſtance conſequently become leſs than in the living, you cannot, by a ſingle thread, or any ligature compoſed of ſilk threads, fairly exerted, divide the external coat of the artery, even if you introduce a hard and round ſubſtance into its cavity capable of occupying its diameter. Here certainly, as obſerved, there is leſs reſiſtance than in the living body, where the powers of reparation are coeval with the injury inflicted; and the nature of the ligature, when the change it produces is duly conſidered, will certainly have its influence in retarding or accelerating theſe powers. A broad ligature bruiſes more extenſively than the ſmall, and will conſequently be more likely to produce the diſpoſition to ſloughing. The ſingle thread offers ſomething like the delicate inciſed wound, with its diſpoſition to unite; the broad ligature preſents ſomething like the wound, attended with contuſion and irritation, which ſeldom fail to preſent difficulties to the exertion of the ſurgeon.

The changes which ligatures induce, joined to the natural powers of the artery in repreſſing hemorrhage, have been ingeniouſly and ably treated by Dr Jones, and are worthy of the attention of every medical man. The operation which I have deſcribed was performed before ſeeing or knowing any thing of that valuable tract.

The removal of the one half of the ligature requires perfect ſteadineſs, and a little time; but the time occupied by this part of the operation, as far as my obſervation yet goes, is not to be admitted for a moment into calculation, when contraſted with its advantages. But, if even both parts of the ligature are allowed to remain, this mode of ſecuring the arteries would ſtill have a decided ſuperiority over the general practice. J. D.

VIII.

Case of Teeth and Hairs found in the right Ovarium. By JAMES ANDERSON, Fellow of the Royal College of Surgeons, Edinburgh.

MAY 18. 1804, I was called to visit Mrs A——, immediately after delivery. She was upwards of 30 years of age, much emaciated, and had a hectic appearance, with a pulse rather quick and feeble. I was informed by the midwife who attended her that the placenta had been expelled easily by natural efforts, but she was alarmed because the abdomen, although much softer, was still as bulky as that of a woman in the last months of gestation. Having ascertained that the bulk had no connexion with any thing contained in the uterus itself, I only gave directions that she should be bound up in the usual manner.

She was delivered of her first child, a boy, on the 15th of June 1795, at which time nothing uncommon occurred; her second, a daughter, was born on the 23d December 1797, when she was long and very ill, both at and for two or three months after delivery, and always complained of a severe pain in her right side. In the third month of that pregnancy she was attacked with uterine hemorrhage from over-exertion, which, however, subsided, and she was delivered at the ordinary time. The placenta was partially removed by the midwife, and the remaining part was propelled naturally within 24 hours; but, from that time, her complexion became pallid, and she never has recovered her natural colour. She was afterwards delivered of a son, 17th July 1800, and of another son on the 13th June 1802. During both these pregnancies nothing particular occurred. About the month of August 1803, at which time she conceived her last child, a daughter, she complained much of a pain in the same side, similar to what she felt in her second child, which became particularly severe from the time she was half gone till delivery.

For two months after I first saw her, the hectic symptoms continuing to increase along with her bulk, which had now induced considerable tension of the abdomen, and the presence of a fluid having been distinctly ascertained, it was deemed adviseable to make an attempt to relieve her by the operation of paracentesis. The fluid drawn off weighed four pounds, ten ounces, and had a purulent appearance from the commencement to the conclusion of the discharge, which ceased spontaneously. By its evacuation the size of the abdomen was diminished, but in a trifling degree, and she

ſhe continued very unwell, for a fortnight after the operation, from pains in the abdomen, with occaſional diarrhœa, and an increaſe of hectic ſymptoms. She afterwards got ſo far well as to be able to walk out for ſome months, although the bulk was again increaſing.

January 1805. The ſwelling had increaſed to ſuch an extent, accompanied by painful tenſion, that I was again ſolicited to tap her; but, upon examination, I obſerved a ſlight inflammation and prominence of the umbilicus, to which I ordered poultices to be applied.

In the month of February an abſceſs burſt at the umbilicus, from which a very conſiderable quantity of matter, amounting, upon an average, to half a pound per day, continued to be diſcharged till within a few days of her death, which happened on the 16th September 1805. During this time the abdomen gradually diminiſhed in ſize, and with it the loſs of muſcular fleſh kept pace, down to the loweſt degree of emaciation. The matter was thin, browniſh-coloured, and ſo intolerably fetid that it was neceſſary to apply epithems of charcoal powder, and to uſe every poſſible means to correct it. The diſcharge was moſt readily effected, and indeed took place in a ſtream, as from the point of a ſyringe, when the patient lay upon her back, with her ſhoulders lower than her loins, and applying her claſped hands to the inferior part of the abdomen, drew them up towards the umbilicus.

In the courſe of a few days after the abſceſs burſt, my patient ſhowed me a dozen or two of hairs, from two to four inches long, which had paſſed through the wound, and, from time to time, other parcels of hairs were diſcharged.

APPEARANCES ON DISSECTION.

Before opening the abdomen, a probe was introduced into the umbilicus to aſcertain the direction of the ſinus, which ran towards the right ſide to a conſiderable depth. On opening the abdomen, the right ovarium was found adhering to the peritoneum and umbilicus. It was very much enlarged in ſize, but collapſed, containing only a ſmall quantity of a greyiſh coloured matter, of a granulated appearance, and unctuous to the touch; a very few hairs, and two teeth of the firſt ſet, all looſe within its cavity; there was alſo another, but apparently of the ſecond ſet, firmly fixed in the ſide of the ovarium itſelf. The left ovarium was ſound. And the uterus, although healthy in its appearance, was as ſmall as it uſually is in its virgin ſtate.

Although the circumſtance of hairs and teeth being found in the ovarium has been repeatedly deſcribed, yet it occurs ſo

 rarely,

rarely, that Mr Fyfe, who was so obliging as to conduct the dissection, has only met with one example beside the present; of which there is an excellent preparation in Dr Monro's museum. From the small size of the uterus, it was supposed to have occurred in a woman who had never been impregnated; but this supposition is rendered extremely doubtful by the present dissection. It is remarkable, that wherever teeth are found in the ovarium, hairs are also present, but unlike other hairs they have no bulbs, and they are never fixed in the sides of the uterus, as the teeth commonly are. The intolerably fetid smell, which always accompanies the presence of hairs, is so peculiar as almost to indicate their presence, and it adheres obstinately both to the hairs themselves, and every thing which touches them.

From the circumstances of the case, it is not improbable that these teeth and hairs were the remains of a twin conception with the second child: If this conjecture be correct, all the subsequent impregnations must have occurred in the left ovarium; and as the children born were of different sexes, it completely refutes the absurd opinion once entertained, that the right produced only males and the left only females.

IX.

The Efficacy of Inoculated Small-Pox in promoting the Population of Great Britain. By R. Gillum, M. D. Bath.

The prevention of plague by inoculated small-pox rests on good authority, and was first suggested in a late publication, viz. Arguments, &c. inscribed to the Right Hon. Lord Hawkesbury, by Dr Gillum. This superior advantage is concisely proved by the London bills of mortality: in a period of about 73 successive years, the plague raged in the metropolis no less than six times, including the last memorable plague of 1665. Since inoculation, plague has never once appeared.

It is an observation attested by long experience, that diseases of a very opposite kind or state seldom, perhaps never, prevail together, nor occur at the same time in an individual. Nature, even in her disordered operations, observes a degree of simplicity. Many passages in Sydenham confirm this remark. When the last plague was at its height, small-pox appears to have been extinct, and neither could gain an ascendancy while intermittents prevailed.

The

The essential character of a reigning distemper often depends on the one which immediately preceded: thus, a dryness of the skin was a constant attendant, till profuse perspiration, and eruption of pustules, succeeded. A remarkable difference is observable in diseases following close on each other; for example, soon after the *fatal* plague of 1665, *mild* small-pox was general, and less fatal than any kind witnessed by Sydenham in the course of his whole practice. Did not plague render the small-pox mild, by removing the dry state of the skin, thus allowing the virulence prevalent in the system to be discharged?

To account for the existence of plague in 1665, it is necessary to know the previous distempers. Before the plague, intermittents prevailed for several years, attended with uncommon dryness of the skin, and great loss of strength. It is singular, in all their variety, no extraordinary evacuation of any kind was general. Such a state of the body must consequently be productive of lingering and obstinate complaints: accordingly persons attacked in the spring, were liable to a relapse in autumn. Dropsy, rickets, and madness, were, in some instances, the sequel. The attacks of such intermittents were mostly ineffectual efforts; consequently they weakened the body by their repetition, and probably fixed the cause of these complaints. Noxious matter, not duly carried off, acquired acrimony; the heat of the body, to which it was continually subjected through a lingering distemper, augmented its putrid, and engendered its virulent qualities; at length this noxious matter of itself, or united with a contagion, was dislodged, at a certain season of the year, from the inert parts, where it had gradually collected, and passed suddenly into more sensible and vital parts of the body. Then commenced the plague of 1665, which, by improper treatment, want of nourishment, dread and horror, increased; not ceasing till it proved fatal to 100,000 persons (this account is confirmed by the symptoms of plague and the dissection of dead bodies).

Small-pox was partial some years before this plague; the dry skin, the great loss of strength, were adverse to its appearance, and the renewal of intermittents never failed to put a stop to its continuance. So impoverished was the system, that many persons sunk under the distinct small-pox. In such cases the perspiration, never considerable, stopped; no remedies then in use could restore it, and the patients died in a few hours. Plague was produced, in a great measure, by the retention of matter which the system had not power to discharge by this *suppressed* small-pox.

The reverſe is mild ſmall-pox; for it is a fact, that no ſpecies diſcharges noxious matter ſo completely from the body, though the puſtules are few. Upon this depends its power of preventing plague, exemplified in this effect of inoculation. Inoculation has ſupplied mild ſmall-pox, and conſequently ſaved to the country the multitude of its inhabitants formerly deſtroyed by the plague.

Hence, had inoculation been known and ſeaſonably employed, the plague of London in 1665 might have been prevented, and the lives of 100,000 of its inhabitants ſaved, excluſive of their offspring,

"Et nati natorum, et qui naſcentur ab illis."

The liberal and diſcerning part of the faculty ſurely muſt, upon reflection, admit that, before a *new diſeaſe* is to be propagated among mankind, it is neceſſary to know the tendency and connexion between exiſtent diſeaſes.

Population has been immenſely increaſed by inoculation. Inoculation has long diffuſed happineſs among mankind by the ſecurity it has afforded. Where is the family that will not acknowledge this truth?

Parents, to procure their offspring the ſecurity themſelves enjoy, muſt employ inoculation. No viſionary ſcheme ſhould be admitted to interfere with and defeat the performance of this important duty.

It is a duty every member of ſociety owes to his country and poſterity to promote the inoculation of ſmall-pox, decidedly oppoſing any attempt to deprive mankind of this invaluable Gift of Providence.

Bath, October.

NOTE BY THE EDITORS.

Though we have given a place to this ſingular ſpeculation of Dr Gillum, we are very far from adopting his ſentiments, or participating his fears: On the contrary, we are quite unable to comprehend how the few facts collected from Sydenham can have ſuggeſted that relation between ſmall-pox and plague which is here inſiſted on. When a great city is nearly depopulated by an exiſting plague, while the ordinary intercourſe of ſociety is ſuſpended, we are not ſurpriſed at the diſappearance of ſmall-pox. If, after the extinction of the plague of 1665, Sydenham has remarked, that the ſmall-pox which ſucceeded was, though very general, of a genuine and kindly ſort, deſtroying few in proportion to the multitudes attacked, other circumſtances

circumstances than the antecedency of the plague might be assigned as more natural causes, because more constant in their operation. For our own part, we are satisfied that the disappearance of the plague is to be ascribed to the extension and improvement of the metropolis after its destruction by fire in 1666, to a better police, and to the laws of quarantine, but not to the inoculation of small-pox, a practice not introduced till near a century after the last visitation of plague in this country. Nor has the plague ceased to devastate that very country whence we received the first lesson of inoculation. Inoculation, it is true, has long diffused happiness among mankind by the security it has afforded; but who, before Dr Gillum, ever imagined that the security was against other dangers than those arising from a malignant small-pox? A mild disease was all the security expected, and not always obtained. The cow-pock gives us a higher security; a security against the small-pox itself. And while we continue attentive to the rules of medical police, and to the execution of our quarantine laws, we may consider ourselves equally secure against the plague.

X.

Essay on the External Use of Oil. By WILLIAM HUNTER, A. M. Master of the Asiatic Society of Calcutta, and Surgeon of the Marine Establishment, Bengal. *

THE external application of oil to the human body is of high antiquity, and it was directed to various purposes. Of these, the most ancient, of which we have any account, was for the consecration of kings, of priests, and even of inanimate things set apart for holy uses (1). The practice appears to have been peculiar

---

(1) 1 Samuel, x. 1. Exod. xxviii. 41. xxix. 7. xxx. 23—25. xxxvii. 29. Levit. viii. 12. Psal. cxxxiii. 2. Gen. xxviii. 18. xxxv. 14. The same word, שמן, translated ointment, in Psalm cxxxiii. 2. is rendered oil in Exod. xxix. 7. And, in fact, the holy ointment, Exod. xxx. 23.

* Extracted from Mr Hunter's valuable Essay on the diseases incident to Lascars in long voyages, of the other parts of which an analysis will be found in the present Number.

peculiar to the Hebrews, and from them handed down to Christian princes. It ſeems intended to typify, by its ſoothing qualities, the benign influence of divine grace (2). Of nearly equal antiquity was its uſe, among this people, as an article of luxury (3).

Among the Greeks it was uſed for this purpoſe, with the addition of perfumes, as early as the Trojan war, or at leaſt before the days of Homer. Thus we find Juno anointing her body with perfumed oil, before ſhe adorned herſelf, to faſcinate the mind of her huſband (4). It was alſo conſidered as neceſſary to prepare the body for violent exerciſe, or to relieve it from the fatigue which was the conſequence of it (5). Hence, in

---

23—25, was nothing more than a perfumed oil. The ſpices were pounded ſeparately, then mixed and infuſed in water. The water, thus impregnated, was mixed with oil, which was boiled till the water exhaled. (Maimon. Patrick Comment. on Exodus xxx. 25. Witzii Miſcel. Sacr. l. ii. Diſc. 2. § 56.) In this proceſs, we ſee at leaſt a practical knowledge of elective attractions. Had the mere infuſion of ſpices been expoſed to the heat of boiling water, the eſſential oils would have been volatilized along with the water, and the fragrance entirely diſſipated. But the addition of the fixed oil, by its chemical attraction, retains the eſſential ones, and the watery parts only ariſe in vapour.

(2) The reader may ſee the ſymbolical uſe of oil treated of at large in a curious treatiſe on General Philoſophy, by Theophilus Gale, publiſhed at London in 1676. L. iii. c. 2. ſect. 7. § 5. page 315.

(3) Deut. xxviii. 40. &c. This, among other indulgences, was forbidden to the Jews on the days of expiation; which is alluded to by our Saviour in Matth. vi. 17. Surenhuyſen's Miſchna. vol. ii. page 252.

(4) ——————————ἀλείψατο δὲ λίπ' ἐλαίῳ
Ἀμβροσίῳ, ἑδανῷ, τό ῥά οἱ τεθυωμένον ἦεν. Il. ξ 171.
——————————, and round her body pours
Soft oils of fragrance, and ambroſial ſhowers.
Pope, xiv. 197.

where the reader will find an intereſting note on the antiquity of the practice. See alſo Potter's Antiquities, l. iv. c. 19. and Athenæus, l. xv.

(5) Μετὰ δὲ τούτῳ ἐλαίου γένεσιν, πόνων ἀρωγήν.—Plato Menex. 238.

Communia deinde omnibus ſunt poſt fatigationem cibum ſumpturis, ubi paulum ambulaverint, ſi balneum non eſt, calido loco, vel in ſole vel ad ignem ungi, atque ſudare: ſi eſt, ante omnia in tepidario reſidere; deinde, ubi paulum conquieverunt, intrare, et deſcendere in ſolium;

in every gymnasium, there was an apartment called *elæothesium*, *alipterion* or *unctarium*, appointed for the unctions which either preceded or followed the use of the bath, wrestlings, &c. (6). This application was thought to preserve a due moisture of the body, and suppleness of the muscular fibre (7), and by such operation to conduce towards the prolongation of life (8).

At

---

folium; tum multo oleo ungi, leniterque perfricari. Celsus, l. i. c. 3.

Si nimium alicui fatigato pene febris est, huic abunde est, loco tepido demittere se inguinibus tenus in aquam calidam, cui paulum olei sit adjectum: deinde totum quidem corpus, maxime tamen eas partes quæ in aqua fuerunt leniter perfricare ex oleo, cui vinum et paulum contriti salis sint adjectum.—Ibid.

Ex iis [arboribus] recreans membra olei liquor, viresque potus vini. Plin. Nat. Hist. l. xii. c. 1.

[Axungia] prodest et confricatis membris; itinerumque lassitudines et fatigationes levat. Id. l. xxviii. c. 9.

Oleum quod ex maturis olivis exprimitur, salis expers, ætate medium, moderate candidum est, lenit, omniumque maxime humectat et emollit, lassitudinis optimum remedium, et ob id Græcis *Acopum* appellatum: corpus ad obeunda munera promptius alacriusque reddit. Fernelius. Method. Med. l. vi. c. 4.

It was joined, for this purpose, with the affusion of warm water. Hom. Odyss. x. 306—364.

(6) Encyclop. Brit. vol. viii. page 250. The Athletæ were anointed with a glutinous ointment called *Ceroma*.—Martial, vii. 31. 9. iv. 4. and 19. xi. 48. Juven. vi. 245. Adam's Rom. Antiq.

(7) *Ἀλουσίη ξηραίνει, καὶ καταλισκομένου τοῦ ὑγροῦ, ἀσαύλως δὲ καὶ ἡ ἀπάλειψις. λίπη δ' θερμαίνει καὶ ὑγραίνει, καὶ μαλάσσει.* Hippoc. de vict. rat. l. ii. page 362. ed Foes.

Τρίψις ἐλαίου σὺν ὕδατι μαλάσσει, καὶ οὐ δυνατὸν ᾗ διαθερμαίνεσθαι. Ibid. page 364.

Omni autem oleo, mollitur corpus, vigorem et robur accipit. Plin. l. xxiii. c. 4.

(8) Duo sunt liquores, corporibus humanis gratissimi; intus vini, foris olei, arborum e genere ambo præcipui, sed olei necessarius. Plin. l. xiv. c. 22.

This alludes to the following story: Centesimum annum excedentem, eum [Pollionem Romulum] Divus Augustus hospes interrogavit, quanam maxime ratione vigorem illum animi corporisque custodisset. At ille respondit, intus mulso, foris oleo. Id. l. xxii. c. 24.

The commentator on this passage remarks, Democritus rogatus *πῶς ἂν ὑγιεῖς καὶ μακραίωνες γίγνοιντο οἱ ἄνθρωποι*, intus vino, foris oleo respondit; eadem propemodum sententia qua Pollio. Vid. Rhodigin.

At length, from observing how conducive gymnastic exercises, of which the bath and unctions formed an essential part, were to the preservation of health, one Herodicus, who was born a little prior to Hippocrates, but lived contemporary with him, and was master of a gymnasium, as well as a physician, first applied them expresly to the Hygieine, and to the cure of diseases; whence he is esteemed the inventor of gymnastic medicine (9). The books on regimen, commonly ascribed to Hippocrates, contain several precepts regarding unction. On one of its properties there seems to be some discordancy between the different texts. In most of them it is alleged to warm the body, and fortify it against the influence of external cold. Thus, he advises those of a temperament between the sanguine and phlegmatic, but inclining most towards the latter (10), to anoint rather than wash their bodies (11). And, towards winter, he recommends the body to be prepared for gymnastic exercises by unction; whereas, in summer, he directs that it should rather be covered with dust (12). The same sentiment is repeated by Pliny (13). This effect was esteemed stronger

---

gin. cap. et l. 6. Athen. 2. Alii respondisse ferunt, intus melle, foris oleo.

Lord Bacon tells a similar story of one Joannes de Temporibus, who was said to have attained the extraordinary age of three hundred years. Hist. Vitæ et Mortis Super. excl. aëria. 18. In the same place, he quotes the examples of several nations remarkable for longevity, who use this practice.

Professor Hufeland reckons, among the means of attaining longevity, frequent friction of the whole skin; for which sweet-scented and strong ointments may be employed with great advantage, in order to lessen the rigidity of the skin, and to preserve it in a state of softness.—Art of prolonging life, vol. ii. p. 324.

(9) Plutarch ex Platone, libro de iis qui sero a numine puniuntur. Encyclopedie sur le mot *Gymnastique Medicinale*.

(10) This I take to be the meaning of the following description: Ει δὲ πυρος τῦ ἐλαχιστοτάτου και ὕδατος συγκρησιν λάβοι ὀξύτερον δὲ τὸ πυρ ἤη του ὕδατος ὀλίγον. De vict. rat. l. i. page 351.

(11) Χρίεσθαι δὲ ξυμφορώτερον ἢ λούεσθαι. Ibid.

(12) Προσαγοντα προς τον χειμωνα - - - - - χρίεσθαι - - - - - ἐν ἱματίῳ προσκινησαντα τῇ τε τρίψει, καὶ τῇ πάλῃ ἐν ἐλαίῳ. Ibid. l. iii. page 368. Ἐπειδὰν πλειαδες επιτειλη, - - - - τη τε παλη ἐν κονει, ὅκως ἥκιστα εκθερμαινηται. Ibid. The author here alludes to the heliacal rising of the Pleiades, which, in the time of Hippocrates, must have been about the middle of May. See the dissertations of Mr Wales, and the Bishop of Rochester, annexed to Vincent's Nearchus.

(13) Oleo natura tepefacere corpus, et contra algores munire: Eidemque

ſtronger in old than in recent oil (14); which might proceed either from the diſſipation of its watery parts, or from the abſorption of oxygen. The former ſeems to have been Pliny's idea, as he adviſes to reduce freſh oil to the ſtate of old, by boiling (15). But another paſſage of Hippocrates would lead us to ſuppoſe that he, or the author of the books on diet, aſcribed to him, conceived it to poſſeſs a power of cooling the body (16). Perhaps their idea was, that it guarded the body againſt either extremity of temperature.

In a ſhort time, the external application of oil, for the cure of diſeaſes, became a diſtinct branch of the medical art, called *Jatraliptic Medicine*. It was firſt introduced, according to Pliny (17), by Prodicus, a native of Selymbria, and a diſciple of Hippocrates (18). The volumes which treat expreſsly of its precepts are loſt; but we find the anointing of the body with oil recommended, among other remedies, in various diſeaſes, as fevers (19), puſtular eruptions (20), gout (20), palſy (21), lethargy

---

demque fervores capitis refrigerare. Plin. l. xv. c. 4.—Does he mean by a kind of revulſion?

(14) Vetus autem magis excalefacit corpora. Id. l. xxiii. c. 4.

(15) Si vetuſti non ſit occaſio decoquitur, ut vetuſtatem repreſentet. Ibid.

(16) Ἠμφιέσθαι δὲ χρὴ, τοῦ χειμῶνος, καθαρὰ ἱμάτια, τοῦ δὲ θέρεος, ἐλαιοπινέα. Hip. de ſalubri victus ratione, page 338.

(17) Nat. Hiſt. l. xxix. c. 1.

(18) Not of *Æſculapius*, as ſtated in Encyclop. ſur le mot *Jatraliptc*.

(19) Ungi enim, leniterque pertractari corpus, etiam in acutis et recentibus morbis oportet; in remiſſione tamen, et ante cibum. Celſ. l. ii. c. 14.

Utile eſt etiam [in febribus] ducere in balneum, prius demittere in ſolium, tum ungere, iterum ad ſolium redire, multaque aqua fovere inguina; interdum etiam oleum in ſolio cum aqua calida miſcere. L. iii. c. 6.

Sæpe igitur ex aquâ frigidâ, cui oleum ſit adjectum, corpus ejus (febre lenta detenti) pertractandum eſt, quoniam interdum ſic evenit, ut horror oriatur, et fiat initium quoddam novi motus; exque eo cum magis corpus incaluit, ſequatur etiam remiſſio. In his frictio quoque ex oleo et ſale ſalubris videtur. Ib. c. 9.

Perfricandæ quoque eæ partes (pro quibus metuimus in acceſſione frigoris febrilis) manibus unctis ex vetere oleo ſunt eique adjiciendum aliquid ex calefacientibus. Ibid, c. 11.

Febres cum horrore venientes, perunctis leviores facit (oleum balſaminum). Plin. N. H. l. xxiii, c. 4.

(20)

lethargy (22), tetanus (23), cholera (24), hydrophobia (25), melancholy (26), dropſy (27), profuſe ſweating (28), and pſora, (29).

---

(20) [Axungia] pruritus et papulas in balneo perunctis tollit: alioque etiamnum modo podagricis prodeſt mixto oleo vetere contrito una ſarcophago lapide, &c. Id. l. xxviii. c. 9.

Lenticulam tollunt galbanum et nitrum, cum pares portiones habent, contritaque ex aceto ſunt, donec ad mellis craſſitudinem venerint. His corpus illinendum, et, interpoſitis pluribus horis, mane eluendum eſt, oleoque leviter ungendum. Celſ. l. vi. c. 5.

(21) Unctioni vero aptiſſimum eſt (in Paralyſi) vetus oleum, vel nitrum aceto et oleo mixtum. Id. l. iii. c. 27.

(22) Vetus [oleum] lethargicis magis auxiliare. Plin. l. xxxiii. c. 4.

(23) Utilius igitur eſt, cerato liquido primam cervicem perungere; deinde admovere veſicas bubulas, vel utriculos oleo calido repletos, vel ex farina calidum cataplaſma, vel piper rotundum cum ficu contuſum. Utiliſſimum tamen eſt humido ſale fovere, quod quomodo fieret, jam oſtendi. Ubi eorum aliquid factum eſt, admovere ad ignem, vel, ſi æſtas eſt, in ſole, ægrum oportet; maximeque oleo vetere; ſi id non eſt, Syriaco; ſi ne id quidem eſt, adipe quam vetuſſima, cervicem, et ſcapulas, et ſpinam perfricare. Celſ. L. iv. c. 3.

See a ſimilar practice recommended by Aretæus, de curat. morb. acut. l. i. c. 1.

(24) Si extremæ partes corporis frigent, [in Cholera] ungendæ ſunt calido oleo, cui ceræ paulum ſit adjectum. Celſ. l. iv. c. 11.

(25) Sed unicum tamen remedium eſt, nec opinantem in piſcinam, non ante ei proviſam projicere, &c. Sed aliud periculum excipit, ne infirmum corpus in aqua frigida vexatum, nervorum diſtenſio abſumat. Id ne incidat, a piſcina protinus in oleum calidum demittendus eſt. L. v. c. 27.

(26) Si nimia triſtitia eſt [in inſanientibus] - - - demiſſum corpus in aquam et oleum. Id. l. iii. c. 18.

Aretæus ſays, becauſe the habits of thoſe labouring under melancholy are of a denſe and dry nature, therefore fat ointment, with gentle friction, ſhould be uſed. De cur. morb. chron. l. i. c. 5.

(27) Quin etiam [in Hydrope vehementiore] quotidie ter quaterve opus eſt uti frictione vehementi, cum oleo et quibuſdam calefacientibus. Celſ. l. iii. c. 21.

[In Leucophlegmatia] ſi is vehementior eſt, caput velandum eſt, utendumque frictione, madefactis tantum manibus aqua, cui ſal et olei paulum ſit adjectum. Ibid.

(28) Sudorem prohibere. Id præſtat acerbum oleum, vel roſa, vel melinum, aut myrteum. Quorum aliquo corpus leniter perungendum; ceratumque ex aliquo horum tum componendum eſt. L. iii. c. 19.

Magiſque

(29). In surgery, it was supposed to allay irritation in those who had undergone severe operations (30), to resolve indurations (31), even the exuberant callus of a fractured bone (32), and to remove the pain and swelling attending luxations (33). Of its application to wounds we have an instance in scripture (34).

At length, with the growth of effeminacy and the corruption of manners, various refinements were introduced into the use of baths and of ointments. Pliny accuses the Greeks of having converted their use, which formerly was moderate and salutary; to an article of luxury (35). Yet he thinks it was originally a Persian invention (36). He says the time when the custom was

---

Magisque discutit sudores [nempe vetus oleum]. Plin. l. xxxiii. c. 4.

(29) Oleum insignem habet usum in medicina; *ἔλαιον τῆς ἀγριελαίας sylvestris olivae oleum*, deferente Dioscor. l. i. c. 119. lepras et impetigines sanat, in doloribus capitis utiliter pro rosaceo substituitur, sudores illitu arcet, defluentes capillos cohibet, ulcera manantia, scabiemque abstergit. Gale, Philos. Gener. p. 314.

Hinc adversum flumen subiit classis, et altero die appulsa est haud procul lacu salso, cujus ignota natura plerosque decepit, temere ingressos aquam. Quippe scabies corpora invasit, et contagium morbi etiam in alios vulgatum est. Oleum remedio fuit. Quint. Curtius, l. ix. c. 10.

Arrian says, the lake was formed either by the overflowing of the river, or the influx of water from the neighbouring country. Being a mixture of salt and fresh water, it was eminently liable to putrefaction. See Sir John Pringle's Experiments, Paper iii. Exp. 25. It would thus furnish a nidus, favourable to the generation of animalcules, which might cause this disease. They would be communicated by contact from one subject to another, and oil, by destroying them, might effect a cure.

(30) Tum multo is [cui calculus sectione evulsus] oleo perungendus. Cels. l. vii. c. 26.

(31) Duritias magis diffundit [vetus oleum]. Plin. l. xxiii. c. 4.

(32) Quod ubi incidit [offi fracto superincrevit nimius callus] diu leniterque id membrum perfricandum est oleo, et sale, et nitro. Cels. l. viii. c. 10.

(33) Id [nempe cubitus luxatus] diutius ex oleo, et nitro, ac sale perfricandum [reliquis membris luxatis]. Ibid. c. 16.

(34) Luke x. 34.

(35) Usum ejus ad luxuriam vertere Græci, vitiorum omnium genitores, in gymnasiis publicando. Plin. l. xv. c. 4.

(36) Persarum esse debet gentis unguentum. Illi madent eo, et accersita commendatione, ingluvie natum virus extinguunt. L. xiii. c. 1.

was introduced among the Romans is uncertain; but that, after the defeat of Antiochus, and the conquest of Asia, an edict was issued by the censors, forbidding the sale of foreign ointments. He inveighs against the height to which this luxury had attained in his time, the excessive price of the compositions (whereof he exhibits several formulæ); and complains that private persons, not contented with anointing the whole body, even to the soles of the feet (37), sprinkled the walls of their baths, and mixed the water in bathing-tubs, with these precious ointments. That their use had even reached the camp, where the military standards were perfumed on feast-days (38).

At this time the application of these ointments and perfumes employed as many people as the management of the baths. The person who superintended this department, as well as he who directed unctuous applications to the sick, was called *Jatraliptes.* Under him were the *Unctores*, who applied the ointment; the *Fricatores*, who rubbed or curried the skin with the strigil, or other instruments of a similar kind; the *Dropacistæ*, or *Aliparii*, whose business it was to remove the hair, either by extraction or depilatory applications; and, lastly, the *Tractatores*, who were employed in gently moving, and squeezing, or kneading all the limbs, to render them supple, and at the same time give a pleasing sensation (39). Mr Le Chevalier de Jaucort adds, that they carried depravity so far, that men had those offices performed in the bath by women; for which he gives the authority of Martial (40). Here we may observe, that we sometimes find a remarkable coincidence between the practices of the rude heroic ages, and those wherein vice

---

(37) The ancients anointed their feet with oil, before they put on shoes; and therefore, when they went abroad, they carried a small vessel of it for that purpose. Hesychius. Meursius, tom. v. p. 517.

(38) Plin. l. xiii, c. 1. and 3. The ancients were wont to anoint themselves, and afterwards expose their bodies to the sun, that their skin might the better imbibe the oil. Those who did so were said chromatiari. Thus Persius, Sat. iv. 17.

Quæ tibi summa boni est? Uncta vixisse Patellâ
Semper, et assiduo curata cuticula sole.
Meurs. t. vi. p. 92, Cornut. in Pers.

I, precor, et totos avida cute combibe soles:
Quam formosus eris.—Martial, L. x. Ep. 12.

(39) Encyclop. sur le mot *Gymnastique medicinale.*

(40) ——————— Percurrit agile corpus arte tractatrix,
Manumque doctam spargit omnibus membris.—L. iii. E. 81.

vice and corruption have attained the greatest height. Customs, in which the plain and simple virtue of the first saw nothing to blame, are laid aside, as scandalous, in times of more refinement, and again revived when degeneracy has increased so far as to destroy even the sense of shame. Thus the virtuous Polycaste was not ashamed to bathe and anoint with oil the youthful guest of her father (41).

From the above description of the Greek and Roman baths, we see that they very exactly resembled those still used in Egypt, and in various parts of Asia, of which we have a very minute account from the accurate Alpinus, and an animated and voluptuous picture from the lively Savary. The former mentions the habitual use of unction in those baths (42), and gives several instances of its application, by the Egyptian physicians, to the cure of diseases (43).

The power of oil to destroy vermin was known to Pliny (44); but we owe to the researches of modern physiologists the

---

(41) Τόφρα δὲ Τηλέμαχον λοῦσεν καλὴ Πολυκάστη,
Νέστορος ὁπλοτάτη θυγάτηρ Νηληϊάδαο.
Αὐτὰρ ἐπεὶ λοῦσέν τε, καὶ ἔχρισεν λίπ' ἐλαίῳ. Od. iii. l. 464.
The last fair branch of the Nestorean line,
Sweet Polycaste took the pleasing toil
To bathe the prince, and pour the fragrant oil.—Pope, l. 593.

(42) Eæ [mulieres] etenim sæpissime corpora in iis [balneis] lavant, et mundant ab illuvie, perlotaque variis ornant odoribus, ut recte unguentis oleant. Alp de med. Ægyp. l. iii. c. 15.

Frictio [in balneis] quam volis manuum plerique operantur, et nonullis inunctis oleo sesamino. Ib. c. 18.

(43) In biliosis febribus - - - - balneorum - - - est frequentissimus usus. Corporaque illa in primis in aerem, temperate calidum paululum versari sinunt, in quo exudant, atque cutanei meatus laxantur, mox oleo violaceo, vel nenupharino ab eis inunguntur, &c. L. iii. c. 19.

Sunt qui inungunt per horam ante accessionem [febris] totam spinam dorsi a nucha ad lumbos usque, oleo antiquo, sampsuco, ruta, artemisia, absinthio, spica Inda, mastiche ac thure ebullito, ipsoque calido inungentes, præmissa parva ac levi frictione. L. iv. c. 15.

Primis harum febrium [pestilentium] ita peractis diebus, ad inunctionem totius corporis accedunt, cute quippe leniter perfricata, atque postea calida inunctione inuncta naturæ ad cutim expulsionem eo auxilio maxime adjuvantes; inunctionem vero ex oleo amygdalarum amararum, cum nitro rubro, quod natron appellant, parant. In pueris, ut etiam nuper dictum est, variolis vel puncticulis infectis, hac linitione nullum remedium securius vel præstantius habent. Ibid.

(44) Contra vespas remedio est, olea aspergi [uvas] ex ore. Plin. N. H. L. xv. c. 28.

the discovery that this is effected by shutting up their respiratory pores whereby the air, necessary to oxygenate their blood is excluded, and they die as by drowning (45).

Lastly, We find the anointing of the body with oil, as one of the last pious offices towards the dead, in times of remote anquity (46).

As our present business is with the use of unction among Asiatics, it is desirable to know the opinion of their own physicians on its effects. A compendium of this is contained in the following translation of a passage which I received in manuscript from a Mussulman doctor. I regret that I did not at the time inquire from whence it was taken, which I have not since been able to ascertain. "The practice of inunction in the bath is attended with several advantages. In the *first* place, although the bath is of itself moist, yet, because of its promoting perspiration, and thus dissipating moisture, it may become a cause of dryness. But

---

Oleo quidem non apes tantum, sed omnia insecta exanimantur, præcipue si capite uncto in sole ponantur. L. xi. c. 19.

(45) Mr John Bell relates an experiment which finely illustrates this position. "When we close up the stigmata of an insect, one by one, the parts become in the same proportion paralytic; if we varnish over the stigmata of one side, that side becomes paralytic; if we varnish over the stigmata of both sides, up to the last holes, the insect lives, but in a very languid condition; it survives in a kind of lethargic state for two days, without any pulsation in its heart; if we stop the two highest holes, it dies." Bell's Anatomy, vol. ii. page 167. See the progress of this discovery in the works of Malpighi, Reaumur, and Bonnet.

(46) Καὶ τότε δὴ λοῦσάν τε, καὶ ἤλειψαν λίπ' ἐλαίῳ. Il. xviii. l. 350.

The body then they bathe with pious toil,
Embalm the wounds, anoint the limbs with oil. Pope, l. 411.

——————— ῥοδόεντι δὲ χρῖεν ἐλαίῳ,
'Αμβροσίῳ, ἵνα μή μιν ἀποδρύφοι ἑλκυστάζων. Il. xxiii. l. 186.

Celestial Venus hover'd o'er his head,
And roseate unguents heavenly fragrance shed. Pope, l. 228.

——————— and smooth'd the hero o'er with oils,
Of rosy scent ambrosial, lest his corse,
Behind Achilles' chariot dragg'd along,
So rudely should be torn. Cowper.

The translator gives, from Villoison, the following note on this passage:—"The oil would lubricate, and make the body slide over such impediments as might otherwise tear and disfigure it."

Δμωὰς δ' ἐκκαλέσας λοῦσαι κέλετ', ἀμφί τ' ἀλεῖψαι. Il. xxiv. l. 582.

Then call the handmaids, with assistant toil,
To wash the body, and anoint with oil. Pope, l. 730.

But the oil, entering the pores, prevents this effect, and confers moisture and softness (47). *Secondly*, In consequence of profuse perspiration, certain matters are drawn outwards, and, in passing, through the pores, irritate the skin; whence we see eruptions of pimples (prickly-heat) in the hot season: now the oil, by its unctuous quality, softens the pores, and guards them from injury (48). *Thirdly*, It cannot be doubted that, during the great inanition which takes place while sweating in the bath, part even of the radical moisture of the body is expelled: but the oil which enters the pores retains the radical moisture in its place. Farther, the physicians of that country (probably Greece or Arabia) chiefly use the oil of olives, which prevents the accumulation of morbific matter. Besides, the bath is often used in diseases of the skin proceeding from dryness. The oil, besides correcting this defect, confers a softness on the skin. *Lastly*, the skin becomes hard from any obstruction of the pores, and oil removes that hardness."

The Hindoo physicians repose great confidence in the use of oily friction. In answer to my inquiries on this subject, Mr Boyd, whose knowledge of the Sunskrit language has enabled him to search deeply into their medical records, favoured me with some extracts from the Sushurt, a very old book, and of high authority among the Burhumuns, in which is enumerated a variety of oils and unctuous substances, both from the vegetable and animal kingdoms. The articles of both kinds are no less than seventy-six in number. Among the most distinguished are clarified butter from the cream or milk of various animals, and the oil of Sesamum.

The

(47) Dr Mitchill says, that oil, applied to the skin by friction, is useful when the oily effusion from the exhalant vessels of the skin is too sparingly supplied, or too quickly removed, in consequence of which, the epidermis is apt to become horny, to crack, and to induce disagreeable or painful sensation. Medical and Physical Journal, vol. iv. p. 10.

(48) A medical friend informs me, that one hot season he was in the daily habit of cold bathing, and his body was covered with prickly heat to such a degree as to be almost intolerable. At length it occurred to him, that by rubbing himself with pease-meal, or *besun*, which had been his constant practice while bathing, the skin was deprived of its unctuous defence, and so more affected by the acrid matter of perspiration. He immediately desisted from such frequent use of *besun*, that is, instead of once and sometimes twice a-day, he applied it only twice a-week, but continued the cold bath in all other respects as before: the prickly heat disappeared, and gave him no farther trouble.

The principal virtues for which their use, by way of inunction, is commended are, giving softness and sleekness to the skin, flexibility to the limbs, and stability to the body in general; increasing the secretion of fat and of the seminal fluid; prolonging life; curing madness, epilepsy, fever, œdema, cutaneous diseases, and worms; allaying lancinating pains of the abdomen, and those from bruises, in whatever part; curing the bites of wild animals, and even of serpents.

Besides this long catalogue of simple oils and unctuous substances, the Hindoo books treat of various medicated oils, calculated to answer particular indications.

The declension of arts and of discipline going hand in hand with that of the Roman empire, gymnastics fell into disuse; and the new form which society assumed on the revival of letters, together with the revolution which gun-powder caused in the military art, prevented them from being resumed. The habitual application of oil to the body in health was inconsistent with modern ideas of cleanliness; and our faith in its medical efficacy is greatly diminished. Yet there are not wanting, among the later annals of the healing art, instances of its salutary effect.

Dr Cullen considers the operation of emollients (whereof oily and unctuous substances, whether from the animal or vegetable kingdom, constitute one class) to be rendering lax and flexible the parts to which they are applied. He thinks the direct action of oil, applied externally, is nearly, if not entirely, confined to the cuticle; but that the relaxation produced there is often, by sympathy, extended much farther (50). On this principle we must account for the efficacy ascribed by Murray (51), on the authority of Rosenstein, to oily frictions, in allaying the uneasiness which, on changes of weather, attacks the seat of old wounds and fractures. We have seen before, that Celsus recommended them with a similar intention (52). For the sensibility of a part depends greatly on the tension of its fibres. On the same principle, joined, perhaps, to its power of obtunding acrimony, we must account for the good effects which Professor Hufeland found from its application in a morbid irritability of the male genital organs (53). And the same property must explain a fact mentioned by Dr Blane (54), that, in a case of locked-jaw, successfully treated by Dr Warren, the uneasiness

(50) Materia Medica, vol. ii. p. 116, 117, 120, 126.
(51) Apparat. Medic. Tom. ii. p. 63.
(52) L. vii. c. 26.
(53) Medical and Physical Journal, vol. vi. p. 71.
(54) On Diseases of Seamen, p. 570.

uneasiness arising from the spasm was allayed by constantly drawing a feather wetted with oil over the temples.

But, in considering the external operation of oil, we must take into our account the effect of the friction, by means of which it is applied. This, if extensive and long continued, excites the vessels of the skin, and consequently the whole vascular system, to stronger action. The cutaneous pores are at the same time relaxed by the oil, and by these united causes perspiration is increased. Dr Hufeland accounts in this way for the good effect which anointing the body is said to have had in the early stage of plague; for, says he, "it has been observed that this remedy was only of avail when a great perspiration ensued." (55) The attention of medical men has lately been called to this remedy by Mr Baldwin, who appears to have been led to the trial by a very wild and eccentric theory (56). But, independently of that, its use among the Egyptians in pestilential fevers, described by Alpinus, might naturally have suggested it. Whatever we may think of his reasoning, the facts which he has adduced in favour of its efficacy deserve some attention. And they have received a strong confirmation from the benevolent exertions of Father Lewis in the plague hospital at Smyrna (57).

If

(55) Medical and Physical Journal, vol. vi. p. 71.

(56) Baldwin's Political Recollections relative to Egypt. See also Annals of Medicine, vol. ii. p. 373; and Currie on Water, Appendix, p. 54.

(57) Monthly Magazine, April 1798. American Medical Repository, vol. ii. p. 117. The Sçavans who accompanied the French expedition to Egypt mention the remarkable success which had attended the practice of friction with oil in the plague hospital at Smyrna, and give an abstract of a little work, containing instructions for its application, and proofs of its utility.

The necessity of early inunction, and of continuing the frictions till the perspiration flows copiously, is strongly inculcated. The perspiration may be promoted by drinking an infusion of alder flowers, (probably any diluting and lightly aromatic drink would answer equally well), and several directions are given for the regulation of diet, but nothing else is recommended in the way of medicine. (Memoirs relative to Egypt, &c. New Annual Register for 1800. Head Criticism, &c. p. 161).

Dr Wittman tried the oily frictions, as recommended by Mr Baldwin, in a case of plague, which occurred in Syria. It excited profuse perspiration, but could not rescue the patient from a fatal termination on the sixth day of the disease. It proved more successful with a typhus patient, who derived very evident benefit from its use. Travels in Turkey, &c. p. 487, 512, 536.

If inunction with oils and fats have ever been succeſsful in curing the bites of ſnakes and other venomous animals, or of the mad dog, it muſt be explained in the ſame manner. And, notwithſtanding its inefficacy in the numerous trials made by Fontana on animals, it is difficult to withhold our belief from ſome of the teſtimonies in its favour. Of theſe we find a long liſt in Murray (58), to which we may add thoſe made by Mr Baldwin, apparently with great fairneſs, on rats, with the poiſon of the ſcorpion (59). Murray gives alſo ſeveral inſtances of its failure, and endeavours to reconcile the diſcordant evidence by the want of accuracy in aſcertaining the ſpecies of ſnake which inflicted the bite; a difference in the depth of the wound, or in the nature of the part which received it; the quantity of poiſon infuſed, or the peculiar temperament of the ſubject. And he concludes by declaring the remedy worthy of farther trial.

For the bite of a mad dog, it was recommended by Dr Sims, on the authority of an ancient Greek manuſcript (60); and one caſe is given by Mr Shadwell, where inunction with oil, and forcing ſmall quantities of it down the throat, ſeem to have effected a cure, after the diſeaſe had begun (61).

But perſpiration is not the only excretion increaſed by friction with oil. Dr Cullen informs us, from his own experience, that, when long continued upon the teguments of the lower belly, it remarkably augments the diſcharge of urine (62). And, on this principle, it has been uſed in the cure of dropſy. Among the ancients, we have ſeen above its employment by Celſus in that diſeaſe. And Murray adduces precepts from Ætius, Galen, and Dioſcorides, to the ſame purpoſe (63). He then gives, from modern writers, many inſtances of its efficacy in the cure of aſcites, and lays down the following directions for its application. "The belly of the patient is to be well rubbed, morning and evening, or three times a-day, for one quarter, one half, or a whole hour, with the hand dipped in olive oil. This practice to

(58) App. Medic. ii. p. 57, &c.

(59) Political Recollections.

(60) Memoirs of the Medical Society, vol. ii. p. 1.

(61) Ibid. vol. iii. p. 464. In ſo hopeleſs a diſeaſe, a ſingle ſucceſsful caſe is abundantly ſufficient to juſtify farther trials. But, that expectation may not be raiſed too high, which inevitably leads to diſappointment, it is proper to add, that Mr Shoolbred informs me he has tried this remedy, both in this diſeaſe and in tetanus, as far as it could be tried, by the mouth, by conſtant univerſal frictions, and by gliſters, without the ſmalleſt benefit.

(62) Materia Medica, vol. ii. p. 126.

(63) Appar. Med. vol. ii. p. 51.

to be continued for some weeks, or a month. Thus, after some days, a copious flow of urine is excited, the belly becomes open, and the swelling of the body subsides, with a return of the natural strength. A swelling of the feet remaining disappeared under the same treatment (64)." Dr Donald Monro found the best effects in anasarca, from rubbing the belly, the legs, and the feet, morning and evening, with oil (65).

From what has been said, we may draw the following conclusions:

1. That the application of oils, and other unctuous substances, to the skin, serves to guard the body against the inclemency of the weather, particularly cold and moisture.

Dr Sparman says, the ointment of soot and grease, with which the Hottentots smear their bodies, defends them so much from the action of the air, that they require very few clothes. And Dr Currie, with a similar intention, recommends the use of inunction to Europeans in warm climates, especially after warm bathing, to defend the body from the chilling effect of evaporation (66). He adduces the example of savage nations, who compensate in this way for the defect of clothing; and observes that the ancients were accustomed to anoint their bodies, before the exercise of swimming, to mitigate the shock of immersion (67). In the moist climate of Bengal, the practice of inunction is more frequent than in the northern and western parts of Hindoostan, where the air is drier.

2. It may prevent too profuse perspiration in hot weather, which is one cause of debility. It seems to be with this view that Hippocrates, in a passage quoted above, recommends, in summer, the wearing of clothes imbued with oil; and we see that the Asiatic physicians entertain the same idea. Murray is of

(64) Ibid. p. 55.

(65) Treatise on Chemistry and Materia Medica, vol. ii. p. 299.

(66) Medical Reports on Water, &c. p. 204, &c. He quotes the following passage from Lord Verulam: "Inunctio ex oleo, et hyeme confert ad sanitatem, per exclusionem frigoris, et æstate ad detinendos spiritus, et prohibendam exolutionem eorum, et arcendam vim aeris, quæ tunc maxime est prædatoria. Ante omnia igitur usum olei, vel olivarum vel amygdali dulcis, ad cutim ab extra ungendam, ad longævitatem conducere existimamus. Hist. vitæ et mortis. Operatio super exclusionem aeris. § 20, 17."

(67) Medical Reports, &c. p. 112. He gives the authority of Horace.—L. ii. Sat. 1.

——— Ter uncti
Transnanto Tiberim, somno quibus est opus alto.

And Hieron. Mercurial. de arte gymnastica, L. iii. c. 14.

of the same opinion (68). Dr Cullen says there is no just foundation for this (69); but the only argument which he produces against it, viz. "the general practice of the ancients, as well as of Asiatics in modern times," may only prove that a diminution of perspiration, which, though perhaps very considerable, will be compensated by other secretions, is attended with no bad effects on the system. Dr Currie says, that unguents of a proper consistence may retard excessive sweating, yet not obstruct moderate and necessary perspiration; and, being themselves evaporable, they may keep up a coolness that shall diminish the necessity of the natural discharge (70). The real state of the fact can only be ascertained by statical experiments.

3. May it serve as a protection from contagion? Mr Baldwin thinks that persons so prepared may attend their friends in the plague, without the apprehension of danger (71). And a similar

---

(68) Claudendo poros, sæpe nocet; in morbis præcipue, qui miasma pro causa habent. App. Med. vol. ii. p. 51.

(69) Materia Medica, vol. ii. p. 127.

(70) Currie, l. c. p. 205.

(71) The French sçavans in Egypt say, that in one year, in which the plague carried off a million of people in Egypt, there was no instance of an oil-porter being attacked by it. And they give numerous histories of inunction having preserved from the disease. (Memoirs relative to Egypt, &c. New Annual Register for 1800, p. 163.) The translator remarks on this passage, that, during the great plague in London, the tallow-chandlers enjoyed a similar exemption. Dr Wittman says the merchants of Cairo positively affirm that the oil-sellers, water-carriers, and tanners, are not subject to plague (p. 531). He also adduces several instances which fell under his own observation, wherein he thinks that oily frictions proved effectual as a preventative (page 487, 492, 512). Captain Francklin informs me, on the authority of Mr Thornton, a respectable merchant of Constantinople, that the same enviable security is enjoyed by the oil-sellers in that city, and that the wearing of shirts dipped in oil (the *ἱμάτια ἐλαιόπινα* of Hippocrates) had been found useful in the prevention of the disease. Mr Eton says, the plague is unknown to those nations who are accustomed to rub their bodies with oil. (Survey of the Turkish Empire, p. 267), Dr Mitchill quotes a similar exemption from pestilential fever, enjoyed by the tallow-chandlers of Philadelphia in 1793, and by those of New-York in 1795 and 1796; (Trotter's Med. Naut. vol, ii. p. 304), and, thinking he has sufficient evidence that the matter of contagion is a peculiar modification of nitrous acid, he explains, on that principle, how oily substances arrest the noxious effluvia, and how a person may *shield himself from pestilence by unction with grease.* (Ibid. p. 291, 295).

similar practice is hinted at by Dr Monro Drummond (72). If the practice has any effect in this way, it is by obstructing one channel of contagion, that by the skin. But the experiments of Mr Seguin and Dr Currie make it rather improbable that contagion is ever conveyed in this way, while the epidermis is sound (73). At any rate, it is evident that, without other precautions, this must be unavailing.

4. May nourishment be thus conveyed? Dr Cullen says, the absorption of oils from the surface is never in considerable quantity (74); and from the experiments related by Dr Currie (75), we must conclude that when the body is immersed even in watery fluids, much less is absorbed than had been supposed. The relief to thirst experienced from that practice must therefore be accounted for by the diminution of perspiration, and the sympathy of the vessels of the mouth with those of the skin. It is also worthy of remark, that Alpinus, in his minute account of the process used in Egypt for fattening the human body (an art which, it seems, is there reduced into a system, and of which the bath is a principal instrument) does not mention unction as applied to that purpose (76).

5. It is worthy of trial in the incipient stage of plague, and, combined with internal exhibition, in the bites of venomous animals, of the mad dog, and in tetanus. But we have not yet sufficient grounds of confidence in it to supersede the use of other remedies; and therefore it should be used so as not to interfere with their exhibition.

6. Its utility in dropsy appears to be better founded; and as it does not prevent the giving of proper medicines by the mouth, it ought, in general, to be used as a powerful auxiliary. In this as well as the last instance, it must be remembered, that as much is to be expected from the brisk and long-continued friction as from the oil.

---

(72) Sintne quibus spiramenta linere ita possis ut contra contagionem impune claudas, nescio. Majores profecto nostri, pigmentis se infecerunt, Indique adhuc Americani corpora sic inscribunt, diversisque imaginibus variant; homines utrique sanissimi. De Feb. Arcend. Thes. med. III. p. 149.

(73) Medical Reports, p. 272; and Appendix, 62—63.

(74) Mat. Med. ii, p. 126

(75) L. c. p. 177, 245, 266.

(76) De Med. Ægypt. If we may credit his account, Dr Gregory's maxim, "Neque homo, ut bos ad libitum saginari potest," (Consp. med. 1, 58), is not applicable to the Egyptians.

To

To the preceding excellent Effay on the external Ufe of Oil, the following Extract from Mr Jackson's Reflections on the Commerce of the Mediterranean, printed at London in 1804, forms a valuable addition.

The Effects of Olive Oil on the Human Body.

In the kingdom of Tunis, the people ufually employed as *coolies*, or porters, are, in general, natives of Gereed, or the country of Dates, about 300 miles from the fea coaft. Their drefs is, in general, a wide woollen coat, its natural colour, with fhort wide fleeves over, wrapping round the body, and tied round the waift with a cumber band; they never wear a fhirt, and feldom have either trowfers, fhoes, or ftockings, they have always a fcarlet woollen cap upon the head, and fometimes a coarfe white turban. Thofe coolies that are employed in the oil ftores feldom eat any thing but bread and oil; they fmear themfelves all over with oil, and their coat is always well foaked with it. Though the plague frequently rages in Tunis in the moft frightful manner, deftroying many thoufands of the inhabitants, yet there never was known an inftance of any of thefe coolies who work in the oil ftores ever being in the leaft affected by it. In the fummer it is cuftomary for thefe coolies to fleep in the ftreets upon the bare ground; we have frequently feen, in the night, fcorpions and other venomous reptiles running about them in great numbers, yet we never heard of a fingle inftance where the coolies were ever injured by them; nor do the mufquitoes, which are always very troublefome to other people in hot climates, ever moleft thefe people, though their face, hands, and arms, from their elbows, are expofed, as alfo their legs and feet; any other people, being fo much expofed, would be nearly deftroyed by the mufquitoes. In Tunis, when any perfon is ftung by a fcorpion, or bit by any other venomous reptile, they immediately fcarify the part with a knife, and rub in olive oil as quick as poffible, which arrefts the progrefs of the venom. If oil is not applied in a few minutes, death is inevitable, particularly from the fting of a fcorpion. Thofe in the kingdom of Tunis are the moft venomous in the world.

The ftrength and agility of thefe coolies and porters are almoft incredible; having a great many fhips to load, we employed feveral of thefe people, and have frequently feen one of them carry a load upon his back which weighed half a ton Englifh weight, a diftance of thirty or forty yards.

XI.

XI.

Case of Crural Hernia, in which the Obturator Artery surrounded the Mouth of the Sac. By JAMES WARDROP, Fellow of the Royal College of Surgeons, Edinburgh.

THE following case appeared to me interesting, as it records a variety of crural hernia, which has been met with only in one other instance, so far as I know, and as the knowledge of such a variety must be of considerable importance in a practical point of view.

A female subject was brought into an anatomical theatre in Paris, and, after laying open the abdominal cavity, I observed an unusual looseness of the peritoneum at both the crural rings. On introducing the point of the finger, it passed readily into a sac, which extended below the ligament of the thigh, the common place of crural herniæ. The peritoneum was dissected from the abdominal parietes, and removed from the inside of the pelvis.

In this stage of the dissection, the annexed sketch was made as a memento of the case.

It represents the disease on the right side; (A) the pubes cut through at its symphisis; (B) the abdominal muscles thrown back over the thigh; (C) the iliacus internus muscle; (D) the two psoi muscles; (E) the obturator muscle.

The external iliac artery (F), and accompanying vein (G), take their usual course along the edge of the psoi muscles. About half an inch from the fossa, formed by the insertion of the abdominal muscles into the bones of the pelvis, the artery sends off a branch (H), which is the common trunk of the epigastric and obturator arteries. The epigastric artery (I) takes its usual direction, and passes obliquely, upwards and inwards, along the inner surface of the abdominal muscles. The obturator artery (K) passes downwards and inwards till it enters the thyroid foramen. The veins pass along the inside of the arteries, run parallel with them, and take a similar distribution.

Within the circle formed by these vessels and the bone there is a large lymphatic gland, with vessels passing from it along the inside of the great iliac veins (L). The gland is situated at the mouth of the sac, or rather at the opening through which the hernia passed, called the crural ring.

Another case of the same variety of crural hernia, and the only

only one I have heard of, I had an opportunity of ſeeing diſſected by Dr Barclay; and the preparation is ſtill in his poſſeſſion. The difference between it and the one juſt now deſcribed is in the ſize of the ſac, which, in the former, was much larger than femoral herniæ generally are.

It is evident, that if a portion of inteſtine had become ſtrangulated in this variety of hernia, ſo that an operation was neceſſary, there would have been great danger of wounding the obturator artery, ſuppoſing the operation had been performed in any of the modes uſually recommended. The artery [illegible] formed nearly a complete ring round the mouth of [illegible] the greateſt care muſt have been neceſſary to have di[illegible] portion of Gimbernat's ligament, in order to have preſer[illegible] veſſels.

This mode of diſtribution of arteries, in the natural [illegible] the parts, is by no means unuſual, and has been p[illegible] marked by Prof. Murray of Upſal. Rougemont, the [illegible] of Richter's work on hernia, has alſo obſerved it, b[illegible] never ſeen hernia combined with it. In a conſidera[illegible] tion of the ſubjects which I have ſeen diſſected, the[illegible] this form in the diſtribution of the veſſels. It is then[illegible] bable that the variety of crural herniæ which has now [illegible] ſcribed happens more frequently than medical men [illegible] aware of, and therefore the poſſibility of its occurrenc[illegible] be taken into conſideration in laying down general ru[illegible] forming the operation.

It ought alſo to be remarked, that the relative ſitua[illegible] hernial ſac and obturator artery will always vary in [illegible] to the length of the trunk common to it and the epig[illegible] tery. If the trunk is ſhort, the artery will paſs round [illegible] of the ſac; if it is longer, it will be found on the out[illegible] poſterior part of the ſac. A caſe, where this laſt men[illegible] diſtribution took place, is deſcribed and delineated [illegible] Monro jun.

My friend, Mr William Wood, in a very neat eſſay on cru[illegible] hernia, publiſhed in the form of an inaugural diſſertation, takes [illegible] tice of the caſes which I have juſt now related. Dr Saunders [illegible] publiſhed the ſame caſes in his Theſis on Crural Hernia, [illegible] gave a drawing of Dr Barclay's preparation; but as the circulation of theſe works is confined to the friends of the authors, I have taken the preſent method of making them known to the profeſſion at large.

What relates to the mode of performing the operation, and the improvements which have been propoſed ſince this variety of femoral hernia has been known, are ſo well expreſſed by Mr Wood, that I ſhall conclude with quoting his own words.

" Mr

Edinburgh Medical & Surgical Journal.

Mr. WARDROP'S CASE OF HERNIA

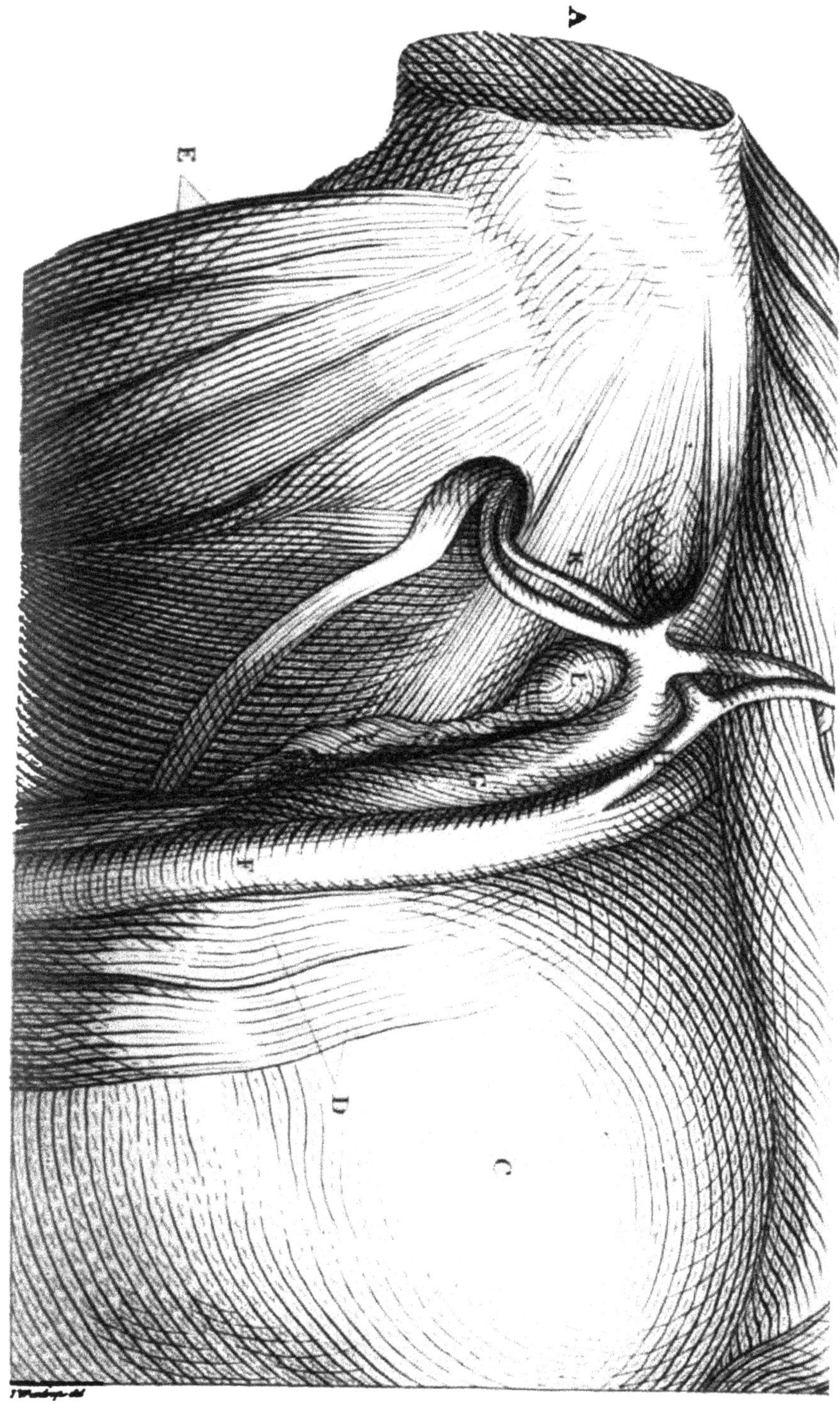

J. Wardrop del.

Published by A. Constable & Co. April 1808.

"Mr Thomson, in reflecting on the danger of wounding the obturator artery with which these two methods of operating is attended, was led to propose another, with a view to avoid that danger; but a similar method, as he afterwards found, had been recommended by the late Mr Else and by Mr Cline, though with a different view. By them it was proposed merely to avoid wounding the epigastric artery in dividing Poupart's ligament. This operation is to be performed in the following manner. A small opening is to be made in the parallel fibres of the tendon of the external oblique muscle, immediately above Poupart's ligament, by separating these by very slight scratches of the knife. Into the opening the point of a curved grooved director is to be introduced, which is to be passed downwards, so as to be brought out at the crural ring. Great care must be taken, in passing the director, to keep its point closely pressed to the fibres of the crural arch, to prevent its getting behind the obturator artery, when it happens to surround the hernial sac. The director will then lie immediately behind the ligament of Gimbernat, which may be divided on it without the risk of wounding any blood-vessel *.

"The only other method of dividing the ligament of Gimbernat, which has, as far as I know, been proposed with the view of avoiding the obturator artery, is the following. The hernial sac being laid open, a curved grooved director is to be introduced into the crural ring, and directed inwards to the symphysis pubis, as recommended by Gimbernat, but on the *outside* of the hernial sac: care must be taken, in introducing the director, to keep its point closely pressed to the ligament of Gimbernat; on it a few of the fibres forming that ligament are to be divided †. The division of a very few fibres will generally be sufficient to allow of the return of the prolapsed parts. This operation differs from that of Gimbernat, in the director being passed on the *outside* of the hernial sac. By this means the director lies between the ligament of Gimbernat and the obturator artery, which will therefore be completely removed from the edge of the knife. One objection to this method of operating is, that in cases in which inflammation has taken place, previous to the performance of the operation, the hernial sac is apt to adhere to the crural ring; so that in such it would be impossible to pass a director between them ‡."

---

* The operation has been performed successfully in this way, in two cases in the Royal Infirmary, by Mr Law.

† Cooper's Lectures on Surgery. Thomson's Lectures on Surgery.

‡ Vide a probationary Surgical Essay on Crural Hernia, submitted to the examination of the Royal College of Surgeons of Edinburgh, by William Wood, Member of the Royal Medical Society, &c. 8vo. Edinburgh. 1805.

CRITICAL

PART II.

CRITICAL ANALYSIS.

I.

Coup d' Oeil ſur les Revolutions et ſur la Reforme de la Médecine. Par P. J. G. Cabanis, Membre du Senat Conſervateur, de l' Inſtitut National, de l' Ecole de Médecine de Paris, &c. &c. 8vo. Paris. 1804.

To all thoſe who practiſe phyſic as a trade, and to thoſe whoſe minds are concentrated within the narrow ſphere of noſological arrangement, the preſent work will appear inſipid and uſeleſs; it will be received, on the contrary, with gratitude and applauſe by men of refined and cultivated minds, by the ſcholar and the philoſophical phyſician. The country where good ſenſe and freedom of inquiry are indigenous will greet the arrival of this ſpecimen of the exertions of a foreigner, who thinks for himſelf, and thinks with that juſtneſs and profound accuracy which delights the mind capable of generalization, unſhackled by the terrors and unſeduced by the charms of novelty.

The object of M. Cabanis is to give a ſketch of the hiſtory of the revolutions of medicine, to characterize each revolution by the circumſtances in which it originated, and by the changes it produced in the ſtate and progreſs of the ſcience; and *laſtly*, to examine whether ſuch hiſtorical deſcriptions cannot furniſh ſome uſeful views relating to its reform and its improvement. In the firſt chapter the author diſcuſſes the degree of certainty belonging to the art of medicine. His ideas on this important ſubject agree ſo completely with thoſe which have been long familiar to us, and which we have endeavoured to illuſtrate in another place, that it is unneceſſary to enlarge farther on that point at preſent.

With regard to the various points of view in which the healing art may be conſidered, M. Cabanis juſtly obſerves, it is not to be confined to the principle of direct utility, to the relief and preſervation of our fellow-creatures, however pleaſing and important

portant that practical consideration must appear to every good man. A scientific knowledge of man comprehends his moral and physical history. The physician gives rules for the preservation of health, he administers remedies against supervening diseases; the moralist regulates our conduct by precepts embracing all the private relations of life; and the legislator determines political duties in the way best adapted to the preservation of social order. It is with the portrait of man in their hands that each of these classes of men is to proceed. The object of their care is a being susceptible of a limited but hitherto unappreciated degree of improvement. A physical education, properly conducted, developes the powers of his organs, creates new faculties, almost new senses, and the distance to which two men of the same original capacity can be removed from each other, by different degrees of moral and intellectual cultivation, is equally immense. The sum of those causes which tend to improve the physical part of our frame prepare the materials, or furnish the instruments, for putting others into a state of activity. All are in a state of contact; medicine is their natural centre. The science of medicine, therefore, may justly claim a considerable influence on the improvement of mankind.

The 2d chapter contains a brief retrospect of the history of medicine from its origin to the present time. It may be sufficient to extract two or three passages which seem best calculated to interest our readers.

The article concerning Hippocrates is particularly interesting; it shows the influence which a strong mind has upon the progress of science, and points out this lamentable truth, that a man of great genius, overstepping the age in which he lives, often leaves nothing behind him but the recollection of something strange and irregular. His name lies dormant till another rivals his predecessor, restores him to public view as a pattern of excellence, and leaves him perhaps again to oscillate between fame and oblivion. It was amidst the games of his youth that Hippocrates received from his parents the first rudiments of medical knowledge; it was at the bed of the sick that he learned to recognise their ailments; and by being an eye-witness to the preparation and the use of remedies, their nature and effects became familiar to him. The true philosophical method of Hippocrates is to be found in his books of Epidemics and of Aphorisms. The former not only present faithful pictures of the most important diseases, but they demonstrate also how observations of that sort are to be made, and how it is possible to lay hold of the most striking features of a complicated fact, without losing one's self and misleading others amidst useless particulars.

The

The aphoristical books have always been looked upon as models, both for the grandeur of the views, and the precision of the style. There we find the true universal method, the only one which is adapted to the exercise of our intellectual faculties, which, in every art or science, arises from observation, and transforms the results of numerous facts into practical rules. That new spirit of investigation, applied to the healing art, was like the bursting forth of light, dissipating the phantasms of darkness, and restoring to the surrounding objects their true form and colour. Hippocrates had courage enough to throw away former errors, and to retain the useful part of the labours of his predecessors: he traced out the only road to solid discoveries, and if his disciples had well understood the principles of their master, they might have laid the foundation of that method of analysis which will hereafter daily create new instruments for the operation of the human mind. To this great and good man his friends, his countrymen, and the world at large, are indebted for much; how he was repaid by them can be presumed from the contents of his letter to Democritus. He therein complains of his professional troubles, of the wrong and partial judgment of which a physician is commonly the object, of the injustice of the public towards those who practise their art with most skill and talents; and he declares, that in the course of a long life devoted to the service of his fellow-creatures, and not without some degree of fame, he had incurred more blame and censure than obtained success and applause.

Among the physicians who have contributed most to the re-establishment of the Hippocratic method, lost in the barbarism of the dark ages, Sydenham holds a very distinguished rank. At the time of his appearing in this country, medicine was buried in a scholastic jargon; the progress of the other sciences was marked only by their baneful influence on the theory of physic. Sydenham, guided by his genius, endeavoured to recal the practice to the rules of experience. Locke was his friend, and the friendship of such a man marks sufficiently the turn of his mind who deserved it. Such, indeed, was the confidence which he placed in the philosopher's judgment, that, in his treatise on acute diseases, he mentions its being approved by his illustrious friend, as a proof of the rectitude of his method. He attacked, with the arms of experience, several dangerous prejudices which existed in his time; he condemned the use of cordials at the beginning of acute diseases, and showed most clearly that the exclusive employment of sudorifics in small-pox, and other eruptive diseases, had been more fatal to mankind than a series of destructive wars. We are indebted to him for the

knowledge

knowledge of thoſe general variations to which epidemical complaints are annually ſubjected, of their relations with the different ſtates of the atmoſphere, and of their independence of thoſe ſtates, often equally evident; of the influence which they have on ſporadical diſeaſes; and, *laſtly*, of the manner in which they are balanced in their ſucceſſion, though the order of that ſucceſſion be not yet ſubject to fixed rules on which perfect reliance can be placed.

Boerhaave was originally educated for the church, but he was afterwards diverted from it by his taſte for the mathematical and phyſical ſciences, which he taught for ſome time in order to gain a livelihood. It was not till late in life, after being already furniſhed with profound and diverſified knowledge, that he began his medical career. His mind had acquired ſtrength, a habit of ſevere diſcuſſion, and great powers of attention; but his tact, exerciſed for the firſt time on new objects, at a period of life, too, when external impreſſions begin to become weak from a diminution of the general ſenſibility, or rather confuſed by their multiplicity, never reached that degree of perfection which renders the treaſures of knowledge and the vigour of reaſon of ſo much avail at the bed-ſide of the ſick. Miſled, beſides, by the temptation, ſo natural and ſo general, of applying whatever we learn to what we already know, and confiding in the vigorous proceedings of geometry, he endeavoured to bring them into a ſcience, ſo unfortunately characterized by the mobility and uncertainty of its rules. Boerhaave had peruſed the writings of every ſect and of every age; he analyzed and commented upon them; he modified and combined their labours, diffuſed over the whole a moſt luminous order, and ſoon brought out thoſe inſtitutions of medicine, and thoſe practical aphoriſms, which form the moſt extenſive and accurate picture that had ever appeared in natural ſcience. Happy would it have been, if the notions of various ſuppoſed acrimonies, and of their neutralizations, if the mechanical and hydrautical hypotheſes, had not ſo often impaired the beauty of the work. It is equally to be regretted that, in more ſtrict adherence to the natural order of the formation of ideas, he ſhould not have begun his expoſitions by collecting and claſſing facts, inſtead of commencing always by ſtating reſults; the writings of that extraordinary man would then have been as great models in the art of teaching and philoſophizing as they are of erudition, perſpicuity, and preciſion.

After the reſtoration of learning, public inſtruction was intruſted to bodies of men, ſlow in their progreſs, and always intereſted, from vanity or policy, in rejecting new ideas, and reſiſting the general advancement of knowledge. During the eighteenth century the progreſs of public inſtruction gained in ſtrength and rapidity : reaſon and common ſenſe ſurrounded the ſchools, beſieged them on every ſide, and crept between the benches. In juſtice to them, it muſt be granted, that they have moſt bravely fought againſt their opponents, but in vain ; for, let them do what they will, their *deſpotical* reign is over !

M. Cabanis proceeds, in the 3d chapter, to give ſome general remarks on the method of teaching medicine. Theſe may be read by the ſpeculative as well as the medical philoſopher, as an inſtance of ingenious and accurate reaſoning, ſuch as is not often met with in medical books. The author has too much good ſenſe to object to the principle of claſſification in general ; it is not only uſeful, but abſolutely neceſſary, in the expoſition of medical facts. Noſological arrangements, however, are ſo liable to abuſe from the raſhneſs with which they are frequently framed, and their incorrectneſs when applied to practice, that it is pleaſing to ſee the well-directed efforts of thoſe who wiſh this pillow of indolence to be ſupplanted by more accurate obſervation and inquiſitive induſtry.

We recommend likewiſe the peruſal of a few pages in which the author attempts to anſwer the two following queſtions : *1ſt*, How does it happen that ſo many well-informed men, who had living pictures of diſeaſes daily before their eyes, could have been miſled by notions which thoſe pictures ſhould, it ſeems, have continually prevented ? *2d*, How is it poſſible for the authors of the moſt wretched theories to have been, at the ſame time, wiſe phyſicians and uſeful practitioners ? The ſubject is the more intereſting, becauſe ſimilar incongruities between theoretical and practical habits occur equally in our moral conſtitution ; and both ſorts of anomalies frequently preſent themſelves in the ſame individual, whenever the imagination is cultivated at the expenſe of the active powers.

In preſenting the following reflections in the author's own words, it would be ſatisfactory to add, that thoſe men who preach reform with moſt eloquence are the firſt to enter the laborious career, in the way not only of precept, but alſo of example.

" Quand on jette les yeux ſur la maſſe entière des faits de médecine, que les ſiécles ont recueillés, l' eſprit ſe trouve comme perdu dans leur nombre, et dans leur diverſité. Que faire alors ? ce que fait un homme qu' on place á côté d' un amas d' objets confondus, et qu' on charge de les diſtinguer et de les claſſer en indiquant, dans l' ordre même de leur diſtribution, les rapports qui peuvent être obſervés entre eux. D' abord cet homme s'arrête ſur les grandes differences ſur celles qui ſont le plus inconteſtable, et, en même tems, les plus facile á ſaiſir ; il en tire ſes premiers moyens de diviſion ; il

revient

revient ensuite sur chacune de ces classes generales. En considerant, avec plus d' attention, les objets qu' elles renferment, il y reconnoît des differences moins frappantes; mais cependant sensibles, qui lui servent á tracer des divisions secondaires. Ainsi, de proche èn proche, il va classer, divisant et subdivisant jusqu' á ce que tous les objets ayent trouvé la place qui leur convient le mieux."

" La science, ou du moins les ouvrages destinés á en presenter le tableau le plus fidèle se reduiroient donc d' un partie á des recueils complets, et bien ordonnés d' observations; de l' autre á des courts exposés théoriques où l' on rendroit compte, 1. De l' esprit dans lequel ces recueils sont et doivent être formées, des resultats les plus directs qui peuvent être tirés de ces differentes observations. Pringle disoit que la médecine étoit depuis les Grecs jusqu' á nous une science, où sur peu de faits l' on faisoit beaucoup de raisonnemens; et qu' il falloit, au contraire, á l' avenir y faire peu de raisonnemens sur beaucoup de faits. Dans cette manière d'elementer l'art de guerir, la seule dont il soit encore susceptible le veu de cet empirique respectable seroit rempli.....Ne seroit ce pas aussi le moyen de raminer la paix, et de l' établir solidement entre les deux grandes sectes, qui divisent la médecine depuis sa naissance, entre les dogmatiques et les empiriques? Les esprits les plus sages de l' un et l' autre part ne retrouveroient ils pas dans ces tableaux tout ce qu' ils s' accordent á desirer dans un bon systême et rien de ce qu' ils se reprochent mutuellement? Et qu' on ne se dise pas que ce seroit couper les ailes au genie, et le reduire á l' emploi servile de copiste, où de faiseur de tables arides. J' ignore d' abord, si, dans les sciences qui demandent avant tout de l' attention et de l' exactitude, il est si necessaire de donner ce qu' on appelle *des ailes au genie*, où si, comme le dit un homme (Bacon) qu' on accuseroit difficilement d' avoir été timide, il ne vaudroit pas mieux attacher du plomb aux pieds. D' ailleurs qu' on se rassure, le genie et le zèle auront encore de quoi s' exercer dans cette grande reforme, ou plutot, la carriere qui s' ouvre devant eux est entièrement neuve, et pour ainsi dire, illimitée; et l' on ne pourroit presque plus delors faire des faux pas réellement dangereux." P. 270.

In the concluding chapters of this book, the author proceeds to treat of the various branches of medical studies. He particularly insists upon the advantage of clinical institutions, as the *sine quâ non* of useful instruction. There, and there only, the student becomes conversant with the essential object of his labours; the teacher can point out and accurately determine what must be examined and recognised in actual practice; and there only the method of observing can be traced in its elements. The Greeks taught practical medicine at the bed of the sick; the Romans and Arabs enjoyed the same advantage; and, among the moderns, the schools of Vienna and of Edinburgh have been the first to avail themselves of that most important part of medical instruction. The philosophical zeal of Joseph II.

 rendered

rendered the school of Vienna superior to every thing which had been before conceived; that of Edinburgh, rendered conspicuous almost all at once by a reunion of eminent men, has not only appeared in the greatest possible splendour, but has, in fact, formed a number of excellent practitioners, many of whom are now rendering the greatest services to humanity in every part of the world.

Among his remarks on the study of the materia medica, M. Cabanis states, with equal reason and force, the absurdity of classing one article under several heads, to make it appear calculated to answer the most different purposes, without specifying the circumstances which, in any particular instance, have determined one certain mode of action instead of another. Observations on the properties of remedies ought not only to be made at the bed-side of the patient, so as to give particular facts instead of generalities, but the various causes apparently operating upon the system along with the drug should be most accurately enumerated. Without that precaution we must ever remain in the dark; no analytical knowledge of the virtues of medicines can possibly be obtained. Our materia medica is already too rich; there is no want of new remedies, but rather of a good method for using those which are already known. Cappivaccius used to tell his pupils, "*Discite meam methodum, et habebitis arcana mea.*"

Moral philosophy is a subject which has not escaped the attention of our judicious physician. Unlike many of his brethren, who, abstracting man from man, fetch all their medical reasoning from the apothecary's shop, without ever suspecting (justly enough perhaps) that there is any thing within themselves but flesh and blood, M. Cabanis points out the great difference discovered by attentive observation between the physical susceptibility and organical habits of the different classes of society. The modes of treatment, often simple and uniform when applied to individuals whose mind or sensibility has received little or no cultivation, become complicated, varied, and difficult, when directed to persons whose moral existence has attained a greater degree of developement. Thus, he adds, the practice of medicine is reduced to a few formulæ only in the country and in hospitals, while it is obliged to multiply, to vary, and to combine its resources in the treatment of patients devoted to study, to business, or to the pleasures of a refined life.

What has been now said of the work of M. Cabanis may be sufficient to satisfy most of our readers, and may perhaps awaken the curiosity of others. Within the limits of a few pages it is impossible to do justice to a treatise in which all the ideas stand

in

in close relation to each other, and in which we have to admire the correctness and splendour of the views, rather than any particular discovery of the author. His book should be read from beginning to end, and considered with attention by men who do not dislike reasoning, because the word sounds heavily in their ears. Such works are not common, but, should any come again before us, we shall deem it our duty to persevere in recalling similar home truths to the recollection of our professional brethren.

II.

Relation Historique et Chirurgicale de l' Expedition de l' Armée d' Orient, en Egypte et en Syrie. Par D. J. LARREY, Docteur de l' Ecole Spéciale de Médecine de Paris; Chirurgien en chef de l' Armée d' Orient, &c. &c. 8vo. Paris. 1804.

THE author of this work was the surgeon-general of the French army in the celebrated expedition to Egypt. His post afforded him abundant opportunities for practical observation, and he seems to have been diligent in availing himself of them, by collecting a number of important and interesting facts, which he lays before the public as the result of his professional labours. The dryness of dull and minute detail in the narrative is relieved by short accounts of the marches and counter-marches of the armies; of the difficulties and dangers they passed, of the hardships they underwent; and concludes with some entertaining remarks on the customs and manners of the inhabitants of that remarkable country. M. Desgenettes has already published the history of the medical department; his colleague, M. Larrey, will suffer nothing by a comparison of his book with that distinguished physician's, which has been so favourably received. The various contents of this surgical history are divided into ten sections, from each of which some curious information might be extracted. So many historical documents, however, relative to this memorable expedition have been printed, that we shall confine ourselves to a general review of the surgical or professional topics treated of; and the more readily, because very few good books or complete medical histories of our victorious armies have been published in our own language. M. Larrey's description of the ophthalmia corresponds with that given by all authors now familiarly known. He obſerved perſons with light eyes were more frequently attacked with this diſeaſe than thoſe with dark-coloured eyes; and that the right eye was more violently affected than the left; for all thoſe who became blind of one eye were ſo on the right ſide. This circumſtance is ſuggeſted by our author to have been owing to the habit of lying down to ſleep on the right ſide, by which means this part firſt receives the impreſſion of the cold and wet ground. Moiſture, and the cold and damp air of the night, are conſidered as the cauſes. The method of cure conſiſted of general and topical blood-letting, warm and emollient fomentations, with the exhibition of acidulating and refreſhing remedies internally. The moſt favourable and complete ſucceſs attended this plan of treatment according to M. Larrey's account, not one man loſt his ſight, or became perfectly blind, out of 3000 men, and upwards, who were affected with ophthalmia. He ſays the Engliſh ſurgeons followed the ſame method of cure which they found deſcribed in the hoſpitals at Roſetta; but it is well known no ſuch boaſted ſucceſs enſued. Many French ſoldiers, who had eſcaped this diſeaſe in Egypt, were ſuddenly ſtruck with blindneſs, more or leſs complete, on returning home; which ſeemed to ariſe from a paralyſis of the organ of ſight, induced by a ſudden change from the hot climate of Egypt to that of France in the coldeſt ſeaſon of the year.

Tetanus, accompanying wounds in Egypt, appeared to be attended by ſymptoms different from thoſe which the author had before obſerved in Europe and in North America. Wounds on the courſe of nerves, or on the joints, were often followed by tetanus, particularly during the ſeaſon when the temperature of the air changes from one extreme to the other, in wet ſituations, in the neighbourhood of the Nile, or near the ſea. Many men were ſeized with this ſpaſmodic affection after the battle of El-Alrich, and after the taking of Yâfa, when the wounded were placed in tents on the wet ground, expoſed to conſtant rain, and in want of many neceſſary articles. Dry and irritable temperaments were moſt liable to be attacked by tetanus, and it generally terminated fatally on the 5th or 7th day. The ſuppreſſion of cutaneous perſpiration by cold ſeemed to have a remarkable effect in increaſing the morbid irritation excited by the local injury. Opium in large doſes proved of great ſervice; bleeding in ſome caſes was uſeful, in others forbidden. Cataplaſms of tobacco leaves applied to the wounds were not followed by any alleviation of the ſymptoms: alkaline medicines were employed with no better ſucceſs: the moxa ſeemed to aggravate the diſeaſe; frictions with oil produced no effect, and mercurial frictions appeared to increaſe

crease the ſymptoms. The uſe of this remedy in the way of friction requires great caution in Egypt, even for venereal complaints. Our author found by experience that the exhibition of mercury in Egypt, as in Europe, was followed by terrible conſequences. Bliſters applied to the throat in triſmus were of no uſe; moxa and the actual cautery, recommended by the father of medicine, were tried with the ſame reſult. When the convulſions are cauſed by the reflux of purulent matter (as M. Larrey expreſſes it), bliſters applied as near as poſſible to the wound, or upon the wound itſelf, bring back the ſuppuration, and the ſymptoms of tetanus ceaſe. Several examples of the ſucceſs of this practice are adduced A young man was ſeized with tetanus 24 days after the amputation of his leg, when the limb was juſt healed; a large bliſter was immediately applied to the ſtump, which produced a copious ſuppuration, and determined a miliary eruption to the ſkin; and, from that moment, the ſymptoms of tetanus abated, and the patient was ſoon cured. The inefficacy of the ordinary remedies, the fatal termination of ſo many caſes, and the unexpected ſucceſs attending the amputation of a wounded limb, in the caſe of an officer attacked by a chronic tetanus, all theſe conſiderations ſuggeſted to M. Larrey the following queſtion: 'Whether it would not be better to amputate the wounded limb, as ſoon as the ſymptoms of tetanus ſhow themſelves, rather than to wait for an uncertain cure, either from the reſources of nature, or from the action of doubtful remedies?' This important queſtion is reſolved in the affirmative by our author, and the following are his reaſons:

'Lorſqu' il eſt bien reconnu que le tetanos eſt determiné par la bleſſure, il ne faut pas heſiter de faire l' amputation dès l' apparition des accidens. On peut s' aſſurer, qu' il eſt traumatique, par la nature de la place, la marche des premiers ſymptômes, et en conſidérant l' époque de leur invaſion, qui ſe fait du cinquième au quinzième jour, au plus tard. Il parait que c' eſt le moment ou la mobilité nerveuſe eſt trés forte. Lorſque la ſuppuration s' établit, la ſtupeur ſe diſſipe promptement, les vaiſſeaux ſe dégorgent, les eſcarres ſe détachent, et les nerfs entrent dans un état de liberté parfaite; alors leur ſenſibilité eſt extrême, et ils ſont ſuſceptibles, par les legères impreſſions, d' une irritation des plus grandes qui ſe propage bientôt dans tout le ſyſtême nerveux. Si dans cette circonſtance la place eſt frapée par un air froid et humide, ou qu' il ſoit reſté des corps étrangers piquant les parties nerveuſes iſolées de leurs eſcarres, le tetanos eſt inevitable, ſurtout dans les climats chauds. On doit enſuite s' attendre à le voir s' aggraver rapidement, en ſorte qu' en très-peu de temps, toutes les parties du membre ſont priſes, et tous les nerfs irrités. - - - - - La ſection du membre, faite dans les premiers

 momens

momens de la declaration des accidens, interrompte toute communication de la ſource du mal avec le reſte du ſujet : cette diviſion, degorge les vaiſſeaux, fait ceſſer les tiraillemens nerveux, et detruit la mobilité convulſive des muſcles, les premiers effets ſont ſuivis d' un collapſus général, qui favoriſe les excretions, le ſommeil, et retablit l' equilibre dans toutes les parties du corps.'—P. 75.

To us this reaſoning does not appear quite ſatisfactory; it is by no means proved that tetanus is occaſioned by a wound, though accompanied by it. The cold and moiſt air of the night is ſtated to have been the remote cauſe of this ſpaſmodic attack, and it ſeems moſt probable. How, then, can the amputation of a limb obviate the effects of a general cauſe, which is acting upon a ſyſtem, the equilibrium of which is deſtroyed by a local injury, either by a wound from a cannon ball, or from a ſurgeon's ſcalpel? The ſeat of the irritation may be changed, but not removed; and, if the ſame remote cauſes continue to operate, there ſeems little to be gained by amputation of the limb. "*Sublatâ cauſâ tollitur effectus*," is an axiom which does not hold good in animal as in mechanical bodies; the cauſes are ſo multiform and various, and the mind is ſo apt to refer to one an effect which depends upon many, whoſe influence is often overlooked or diſregarded. M. Larrey regrets not having it in his power to adduce a greater number of caſes ſucceſsfully treated by this operation performed under ſuch formidable circumſtances. One inſtance only is related of a perfect cure; two others were greatly relieved, but terminated fatally in a few days by the recurrence of the ſpaſmodic ſymptoms, for want of proper means of avoiding the increaſing coldneſs and wetneſs of the night. However, he draws the two following concluſions: 1. That of all the remedies recommended by the moſt able practitioners, he has found by experience the extract of opium (*l'opium gummeux*), combined with camphor and nitre, diſſolved in a ſmall quantity of emulſion, made with ſeeds or ſweet almonds, produce the beſt effects; eſpecially as patients who have a diſlike for other liquids take this medicine with pleaſure, which can be aſſiſted by bleeding, if neceſſary, or by bliſters applied in the manner already mentioned. 2. That amputation timely performed is the moſt certain method of arreſting the progreſs of tetanus, when it depends upon a wound ſeated on the extremities.

In ſpeaking of Yâfa, M. Larrey ſays, he ſhall paſs over in ſilence the horrible conſequences which commonly occur at ſieges. He was a melancholy witneſs of what happened at Yâfa; but it will be remembered that he is an admirer of the bold

bold and adventurous ſpirit of Bonaparte, and now holds the rank of ſurgeon to the conſular guard. Circumſtances oblige him to refrain from recording thoſe tranſactions, which muſt tarniſh the victory of the greateſt hero, and ſtamp the nobleſt exploits with the deteſtable characters of cruel and ſelfiſh ambition. The ſiege of Acre coſt the lives of many ſoldiers, and added about 2000 to the liſt of the wounded. The wounds, in general, were ſerious and complicated. It was neceſſary to perform 70 amputations, two of which were at the hip joint; the firſt on an officer, who gave great hopes of recovery, when he was attacked by the plague, and died; the ſecond on a ſoldier, who died from the conſequences of violent concuſſion from a ball. Out of ſix amputations at the ſhoulder joint, four were completely cured; two died from the effects of concuſſion. Seven caſes trepanned, and five of them cured; two of them were trepanned on the frontal ſinus.

Before the army left Syria, a great number of the ſoldiers were attacked by the plague; it ſeldom attacked the wounded men, and ſcarcely an inſtance occurred of any one being affected by it, whilſt the wounds were in a ſtate of ſuppuration, though many were infected as ſoon as their wounds were healed. This obſervation was made by all the writers on the plague; and it is well known that Europeans who are eſtabliſhed in Egypt and Syria guard themſelves from this peſt, or at leaſt ſeem to be leſs diſpoſed to be affected by it, by means of habitual iſſues. A ſhort memoir, then, is inſerted of the plague, which coincides with the hiſtory given by Deſgenettes and other French writers, and by our countryman Mr M'Grigor, in his valuable work reſpecting the army of the eaſt. Some important remarks are to be found under this article, for which we muſt refer the reader to the original narrative. We paſs by that part to notice another equally curious, and not ſo commonly deſcribed. In paſſing a deſert, before reaching Sſalahhiek, the ſoldiers, tired and thirſty, lay down and drank with avidity of ſome ſoft and muddy water, which they found in ſmall pools at ſome diſtance from each other. A great quantity of ſmall inſects were in this water, and, among them, a ſpecies of leech, which proved a very ſerious enemy to many of the men who quenched their thirſt at theſe places. This little animal reſembles thoſe deſcribed as being common in Ceylon; it is ſometimes long, and, though naturally not larger than a horſe's hair, it is capable of being enlarged, by ſucking blood, to the ſize of a common leech; its colour is black, and its form not particular. The effects of this leech were ſoon perceived by thoſe who had ſwallowed any of them. A violent pricking was firſt

first felt in the throat, accompanied by cough and spitting, slightly tinged with blood, and efforts to vomit. Violent hemorrhagies then took place, difficulty in swallowing, laborious respiration, and constant tickling in the throat, which excited cough, &c. These symptoms increased to an alarming degree, and in some instances proved fatal, without any assistance being given, for want of knowing the cause of the disease, or not being able to apply the proper remedy. Extracting the leech by the polypus forceps was the best means of relieving this complaint, or employing injections and gargles of salt water and vinegar, and fumigations, with tobacco and squills. The Egyptians know that horses sometimes get these insects into their nostrils when they drink at particular ponds; they are informed of this circumstance by the uneasiness of the horse, and by bleeding from the nose, which happens the same day, or the day after. The farriers of that country extract them, with great dexterity, by means of pincers made for this purpose; when they have no instruments at hand, they inject salt water. A similar accident happening to a man was never known before; such instances were now frequent.

After the battle of Heliopolis and the siege of Cairo, the fatal consequences of the wounds made the soldiers believe that the balls of the enemy were poisoned: it was easier to get rid of this erroneous notion than to get rid of the disease. It presented, says M. Larrey, all the symptoms of the yellow fever, as it appeared at St Domingo; and accordingly it is here described under the title of yellow fever complicated with gun-shot wounds. This disease appeared on the 4th of April, and ceased at the beginning of June; it was contagious, and proved fatal to many. The causes were, the bad state of the hospital, the damp rooms, the troops having been encamped in a marshy situation, the excessive fatigue, want of food and proper medicines, &c. The author thinks there is great analogy between the yellow fever and the plague. Mr M'Grigor has run this parallel very closely, and with great plausibility. The 5th section contains some speculations on the pernicious influence of warm climates upon fat people, and some practical remarks on hepatitis, in which the propriety of opening abscesses in the liver is strongly insisted on, and illustrated by cases; and it concludes with an account of a wasting of the testicles. Several soldiers of the army of Egypt, on their return home, complained of the almost total disappearance of their testicles without any venereal disease. This atrophy gradually took place without any pain; it is attributed, by our author, principally to the effects of the hot climate.

Lepra and elephantiasis are common diseases in different parts of Egypt; the use of salted meat and fish, and unwholesome animal food,

food, especially pork and wild-boar, are considered among the causes of these disorders, in conjunction with the dirtiness and negligence of the inhabitants. It was observed, that all the French who lived upon pork for some time suffered inconvenience from it; many were attacked by a leprous eruption. The flesh of hogs is well known to be unwholesome in that country, where they are fed differently from what they are in Europe; and, it is probable, experience of this sort induced the Eastern legislators, Moses and Mahomet, to forbid its use by an article in their respective codes of laws. Lepra seems to be communicated from one person to another by bedding and other means of close contact. Elephantiasis is not contagious: it attacks the legs and scrotum, and is confined chiefly to those persons who work in the rice-grounds, and live in marshy situations. At Damietta great numbers are affected with this disease in different degrees; on the other hand, scarcely any are met with in dry airy places, as on the borders of deserts, or in Upper Egypt. Lepra, on the contrary, rages in these latter places, and was never seen where elephantiasis is common. The same predisposing causes belong to both maladies; but, in elephantiasis, the immediate application of bad air and bad water to the feet and legs may determine the seat of its attack, by injuring the texture of the skin and cellular substance. An enlargement of the scrotum often attends this disease of the legs; these tumours constitute the disorder called *sarcocele*, in the true and strict meaning of the word; it is not uncommon in warm climates, though comparatively rare in Europe. Tumours of this nature grow sometimes to an enormous size, even to an hundred pounds weight; the author removed one weighing six pounds: when cut into, they are found to consist of a fatty brawny substance, of hard consistence in some parts, and soft in others, not very vascular, and endowed with little sensibility: the testicles are sometimes diseased, constituting a complicated malady; but, in general, these parts are in a sound state, attached behind or on the sides of the tumour, the spermatic cord being only increased in length. Women, as well as men, are liable to have tumours of this sort on the organs of generation; a history of a large excrescence on the labia pudendi is given, with a plate, and an account too of a similar disease in the scrotum of a man, which is likewise represented by an engraving. Both these cases were to have been operated on, when orders were received to march immediately, and they were unfortunately obliged to be left to their fate.

During a short interval of peace and tranquillity, M. Larrey began to arrange and put in order the observations that he had made

made from the beginning of the firſt campaigns in Egypt. Theſe remarks are collected together and recorded under the article *Surgery*, a ſeparate and diſtinct part from the hiſtorical narrative, and occupying one ſection of the book. Before noticing this, however, we ſhall ſtop juſt to tranſlate the author's deſcription of the treatment of the venereal diſeaſe. "I remarked (ſays he) that ſyphilis in Egypt was ſeldom attended with violent ſymptoms, and was eaſily cured there; but, if brought thence into Europe, eſpecially into the weſtern countries, it became extremely obſtinate, and very difficult to be ſubdued. I have had proofs of this among the French ſoldiers who came to France with the diſeaſe contracted in Egypt; they could not get rid of it without great difficulty, and after a long time. The treatment which ſucceeded beſt in Egypt conſiſted in the exhibition of mercury internally, combined with tonics and diaphoretics, and aided by vapour baths. Mercurial frictions were hurtful; they did not only not cure the diſeaſe, but produced violent frenzy in ſome patients, and ſpaſms, and convulſions, and profuſe ſalivation, in others.

"In a memoir which I propoſe ſoon to publiſh, I ſhall make known what great advantages I have often derived from the inoculation of gonorrhœa, for the cure of many maſqued venereal complaints, in Egypt and at the hoſpital of the conſular guard."

Almoſt all the wounds from fire-arms received in Syria, on the upper extremities, complicated with fracture, eſpecially of the os humeri, were followed by artificial articulations, although carefully dreſſed and attended. This unfortunate circumſtance was attributed to the continual motion to which the wounded men were expoſed from their leaving Syria till their arrival in Egypt, being obliged to travel on foot, or mounted on horſes or camels: *2dly*, To the bad food and brackiſh water which they were obliged to drink during this laborious journey, and alſo to the bad air of Syria, loaded with effluvia from marſhes. In this campaign, very ſlight wounds on the ſhoulders, without any injury done to the bone, were ſucceeded, in almoſt every inſtance, by partial or complete paralyſis of the wounded limb; a circumſtance which never happens in Europe, unleſs, indeed, the principal nerves are divided or materially injured. On returning to Egypt, where the air is more pure, the motion and feeling of the paralytic limbs were reſtored to many of the wounded by the repeated application of moxa, afterwards applying ammoniac to prevent the inflammation and ſuppuration of the burnt parts. The uſe of mineral waters, and the climate of Europe, completed the cure in thoſe inſtances where the moxa had failed. The unfavourable influence of the atmoſphere, and of the

ſouth

ſouth winds, on the wounds in Syria and in Egypt, was compenſated in ſome degree by the rapid manner in which ulcers and wounds were healed in Egypt during the ſeaſon when the northern winds prevailed.

The application of the trephine on the frontal ſinus has been forbidden by moſt writers. M. Larrey deviated from this precept in two caſes of fracture of the ſides of this ſinus; the trepan was applied without much difficulty, and the operation ſucceeded perfectly well. Several ſingular caſes are related of wounds of the head, jaws, and parts of the throat. Wounds of the cheſt afforded ſome remarkable phenomena, and they were in ſufficient number to offer ſufficient opportunities for new experiments. In one recent caſe Mr L. ſucceeded beyond his expectations: A man was wounded between the fifth and ſixth rib; the wound was about two inches in length, and penetrated into the cavity of the thorax: a large quantity of red frothy blood iſſued out at every inſpiration; his extremities were cold, his pulſe ſcarcely perceptible, his countenance pale, and his breathing ſhort and difficult; in ſhort, he was threatened every moment with ſuffocation. After examining the wound, the lips were brought together and confined by means of ſticking plaſter and proper bandages. As ſoon as the wound was cloſed, the poor fellow breathed more freely, and felt himſelf relieved: he gradually recovered in a ſhort time, without any obſtacle to his cure. Two ſimilar caſes preſented themſelves at the hoſpital of the conſular guard. From the time of Ambroſe Parey down to the preſent day, all authors have adviſed not cloſing the wounds of the thorax, when accompanied by hemorrhage; but experience ſhows that the oppoſite method is preferable; and indeed this practice is noticed by the old writers. The operation of empyema was performed ſeveral times in Egypt with complete ſucceſs, to relieve effuſion of blood in the cheſt; and the author thinks it adviſable to make the opening ſomewhat higher than the ſpot uſually mentioned, becauſe the depth of the cavity of the thorax is diminiſhed by the preſence of any foreign body which irritates and cauſes the contraction of the arch of the diaphragm. This operation failed, in ſome inſtances, by being performed too low down, and the effuſed fluid was diſcovered on diſſection after death.

Some caſes of wounds of the abdomen, combined with injury done to the inteſtines and the bladder, which were perfectly cured, are here detailed. The colon was wounded at its ſigmoid flexure in ſeveral inſtances, and healed without leaving any fiſtula. In ſpeaking of the injuries done to the head of the humerus, without affecting the other parts of the arm, M. Larrey mentions

mentions the removal of the head of this bone, as practised by Mess. Park and White. Sabatier and Chaussier, two of the most distinguished surgeons in France, have lately paid particular attention to this subject: some experiments have been made on animals by the latter. M. Larrey has removed the head of the os humeri and its fractured portion in ten instances, by which measure he flatters himself to have prevented the unfortunate consequences, perhaps the amputation of the limb; and he describes minutely his method of performing this delicate operation.

He next gives an account of a still more formidable operation, which, he says, he has performed three times; this is, *the amputation of the thigh at the hip joint.* We shall extract the account of the mode of performing this operation in the author's own words, and thus forego the necessity of copying his arguments to prove the possibility of it, and to show its absolute utility under particular circumstances.

"Pour executer mon procédé, je mets d'abord le blessé sur le pied de son lit dans une position presque horizontale, et me place en dedans de la cuisse que je dois opérer: un aide vigoreux et intelligent comprime l'artére crurale, à son passage sur la gouttière osseusse du méme nom: ensuite je fais une incision aux tégumens de l' aine sur le trajet des vaisseaux cruraux que je mets au decouvert; je les dissèque avec précaution, et apres avoir isolé le nerf qui se trouve en dehors, je passe entre lui et l' artére une aiguille courbe mousse, de manière à y comprendre l' artère et la veine pour les lier ensemble. J'ai l'attention de porter cette ligature immédiate au dessus de l'arcade crurale, pour la faire au-dessus de l' origine de la musculaire commune, dont la section, pendant l'operation, causeroit, sans cette mesure, des hemorragies mortelles. Aprés avoir fait cette ligature, et placé celle d'attente, je plonge perpendiculairement mon couteau droit entre les tendons des muscles qui s' attachent au petit trochanter et la base du col du femur, de manière à faire sortir la pointe à la partie posterieure ou diamétralement opposée, et en dirigeant le couteau obliquement en dedans et en bas, je coupe d' un trait toutes les parties qui doivent former le lambeau interne, auquel il ne faut pas donner trop de volume. Je fais relever le lambeau vers les parties génitales par un aide, et on découvre aussitôt l' articulation. L'artère obturatrice et quelques branches de la honteuse, sont comprisés dans cette coupe, il faut en faire de suite le ligature. Un seul coup de bistouri suffit pour couper toute la capsule articulaire, et, par une simple abduction de la cuisse, la tête du femur est presque luxée; le ligament interarticulaire se presente, et l' on juge combien il est facile de la couper avec le même bistouri. Je prends ensuite un petit couteau droit, avec lequel je forme le lambeau externe et posterieur, en passant son tranchant entre le bourrelet osseux de la cavité cotyloide et le grand trochanter, et je finis le lambeau par une division dirigée en bas et en dehors, faite à-peuprès au niveau de cette eminence et de manière à donner à ce

lambeau

lambeau une forme arondie ; l' aide qui tient le lambeau bouche l' orifice des artères ouvertes, des quelles on fait la ligature successivement. Il faut les lier toutes, jusqu' aux plus petites, pour prévenir les hemorragies consecutives, et pouvoir reunir les lambeaux. Si les parties qui les forment ne sont point irritées, on peut y faire quelques points de suture entre coupés avec les aiguilées dont j' ai parlé : mais il ne faut point toucher les muscles, il suffit de comprendre dans la suture la peau et le tissu graisseux. On fixe les lambeaux en contact par des compresse graduées, trempées dans le vin rouge, et par un bandage contentif et bien appliqué."—P. 283.

According to this method, M. Larrey has performed the operation three times; the patient was always relieved, and every circumstance, as far as regarded the operation, appeared to go on very favourably for several days; but one of these cases terminated fatally from an attack of the plague on the sixth day after the removal of the limb, and the other two perished during the fatigue and hardship of a forced march.

A memoir upon amputation of limbs wounded by fire-arms, which was the author's thesis on taking his doctor's degree, forms an interesting conclusion to this chapter. The reasoning is supported by numerous facts, and the questions are discussed with a constant reference to multiplied experience.

Among the various topics treated of in the two last sections, the singular exemption of the dogs in Egypt from hydrophobia is mentioned. Such a dreadful malady is never known to attack these animals in that country, which is attributed to their peculiar character and different mode of life.

We shall conclude this article with quoting a general remark from a celebrated French writer, d'Alembert: « Un ouvrage est bon, lorsqu' il renferme plus de bonnes choses que de mauvaises; il est excellent, quand le nombre de ces bonnes choses surpasse beaucoup celui de choses mediocres." If this narrative be estimated by this fair standard, it will be ranked among our best professional works.

III.

III.

A Treatiſe on the Proceſs employed by Nature in ſuppreſſing the Hemorrhage from divided and punctured Arteries; and on the Uſe of the Ligature; concluding with Obſervations on Secondary Hemorrhage; the whole deduced from an extenſive Series of Experiments, and illuſtrated by 15 *Plates.* By J. F. D. Jones, M. D. Member of the Royal College of Surgeons of London. 8vo. pp. 237. London. 1805.

Our curioſity, early attracted by the importance of the ſubjects announced in the title, has been amply gratified by the peruſal of this intereſting volume, which has left upon our minds very favourable impreſſions of the critical judgment of the author, as well as of his talent for experimental inquiry.

Few facts in phyſiology are more curious, or more intereſting to the naturaliſt, than thoſe which belong to the ſubject of animal reproduction: There are few of higher importance to the ſurgeon, for this knowledge points out to him, in many caſes, at once the object and the limits of his art. The proceſſes employed by nature in the reproduction and reunion of ſeparated parts are the faireſt ſubjects of experimental inquiry, and the labours of many ingenious men have accordingly been rewarded by the deriving of new and important facts. The obſervations and experiments of Duhamel, Haller, Troyes, and M'Donald; of Murray, Huhn, and Hunter; of Cruickſhanks and of Haighton, leave, indeed, little to deſire in the departments which they have examined.

From the moſt perfect reſtoration of a loſt or amputated part, to the cicatrization of the ſimpleſt wound, we obſerve a uniformity in the attempts of nature at reproduction, or a ſeries of analogous events, which expound to us the proceſſes of nature in the reproduction and reunion of the bones, and of moſt of the ſoft parts of animals. The proceſs employed by nature in ſuppreſſing the hemorrhage from divided arteries, though perhaps of all the moſt important to be fully underſtood, has not been ſo perfectly explained. Experiments and obſervations, indeed, have not been more neglected here; badly imagined, however, and limited in their direction, by the influence of ſome hypotheſis to be confirmed or refuted, they leave us ſtill uncertain of the truth. Some ſteps of the proceſs have been ſeen or affirmed, while others, equally important and efficient, have been overlooked or denied. Limited obfervation, and the inclination to fimplify the mechanifm of nature, have led to theories founded on fome one or other of the fteps of the entire procefs; and hemorrhage has been fuppofed to be naturally ftopped by an obturating clot of blood, by the contraction and crifpation of the divided artery itfelf, or by the tumefaction or injection of the furrounding cellular fubftance. The limited theories of Petit, of Morand, and of Pouteau, gave rife to other fubordinate hypothefes not more fatisfactory. Diftrufting, then, thefe refults of partial obfervation and of hafty conjecture; to arrive at the truth, it was neceffary again to confult nature herfelf, and by a feries of obfervations and experiments, carried on through every ftage of the procefs, from the firft effufion of blood to the natural fuppreffion of the hemorrhage, and complete cicatrization of the wounded artery, to mark the various changes which take place, and the order in which they fucceed: a tafk which has been undertaken and executed, with equal zeal, ability, and fuccefs, by Dr Jones.

The experiments are numerous, but not redundant; they are well imagined, fkilfully executed, and, to all appearance, faithfully related. The refults are alfo exhibited in 15 neat engravings. The experiments are compared with, and his obfervations are afterwards illuftrated and confirmed by thofe of other eminent phyfiologifts and furgeons: For the error of his predeceffors feems to have been chiefly that of feizing exclufively one ftep of the procefs of nature which they really did obferve, and of haftily concluding that they had nothing farther to look for. So far, indeed, as they did obferve, their obfervation was correct and accurate; but this being limited to fome particular period of the procefs, they differently faw the correfponding fteps of a feries of changes, which really conftitute the procefs of nature in fuppreffing the hemorrhage from divided or wounded arteries.

Dr Jones having examined and freely expofed the defects of Petit, Morand, Sharp, Pouteau, Gooch, Kirkland, and J. Bell, proceeds in the relation of a feries of experiments on the arteries of horfes and dogs, undertaken with the view of afcertaining the procefs employed by nature in the fuppreffion of hemorrhage from *divided* arteries, and the order of the events which conftitute it. In thefe experiments the larger arteries were completely divided; the fuppreffion of the hemorrhage was left to nature, and the condition of the divided veffel was, in the different cafes, afcertained by careful examination, at different periods, after the firft ceffation of the hemorrhage. Though we muft refer to the original for a full detail of thofe experiments, we fhall here quote the following as examples.

EXPERIMENT VII.

'The femoral artery of a dog was divided, and the integuments were brought together, as in Experiment II., the section of the artery being made as high as it was detached. Half an hour after the hemorrhage had completely ceased, the dog was drowned.

'Dissection. A considerable clot of blood was found between the integuments and the artery, covering both of its cut extremities, and adhering to the lower, and to the parts about it: the extremities of the artery were nearly an inch distant from each other: a black cylindrical coagulum was found stopping up the mouth of the upper extremity, and extending at least one third of an inch down from it, and between the vein and nerve. The mouth of this extremity was slightly contracted. The division of the artery appeared to have been made immediately at its connexion with the cellular membrane; this appearance was, no doubt, rendered more complete by the retraction which had taken place. There was an effusion of blood between the artery and its sheath, to the extent of at least two inches: there was also a considerable effusion in the surrounding cellular membrane; but the artery had not the slightest appearance of being compressed by it. On cutting open this part of the vessel, a long and very slender coagulum of blood was found within it, which by no means filled up its canal at any part, nor adhered to the internal coat of the artery. Hereafter I shall call this the internal coagulum, to distinguish it from the external.

About four lines breadth of the inferior portion of the divided artery was detached from the surrounding cellular membrane; its mouth was much more contracted than the upper, and was slightly turned on one side; it adhered to the clot, which filled the wound, and lay over it; and the internal coagulum was very slender and thready.'

EXPERIMENT XVII.

'The carotid artery of a horse was divided just above a ligature, which had been made on it to prevent hemorrhage from that portion of it next the heart, and the integuments were secured by sutures previously passed. The blood flowed too fast at two or three interstices, but these were closed by additional sutures, and the external hemorrhage presently ceased. A very large tumour instantly formed, but its size considerably diminished in the course of twenty-four hours. The animal was killed sixty-six hours after the operation.

'Dissection. The clot, which originally filled the cavity of the wound, and distended the integuments, had nearly disappeared, having been either washed away by the discharge or absorbed. The ends of the artery were separated between one and two inches. The sheath was tinged with blood to the extent of many inches. To the circumference of the cut artery, and just within it, the external coagulum, consisting partly of lymph, partly of blood, adhered. Its figure was conical, and it was supported at the mouth of the artery by its

its intimate connexion with the inner lamina of the ſheath, which, by the retraction of the artery, formed a canal for it; and it derived farther ſupport, on all ſides, from the blood effuſed and coagulated between the inner and outermoſt lamina of the ſheath. The internal coagulum was an inch and a half long, correſponding to the diſtance between the external coagulum and the firſt collateral branch. It completely filled the canal of the artery, and had every appearance of having been formed ſoon after the operation. It was quite detached, and lay two inches above the external coagulum, having, in all probability, ſlipped from its original ſituation in handling the parts previous to the artery being opened. See plate II. fig. 2.'

EXPERIMENT XIX.

'The femoral artery of a dog was divided, and the integuments were brought together in the manner already deſcribed. The animal was killed nine days after the operation.

'Diſſection. The wound was open, but its extent much diminiſhed. Its ſurface was formed of a thick layer of very vaſcular lymph, which, being divided, diſcovered the truncated extremities of the artery half an inch apart. The cellular membrane ſurrounding each extremity of the artery, for the ſpace of an inch, was very much thickened with coagulated lymph. The ſuperior portion of the artery was ſlightly contracted at its extremity, which was completely cloſed, and filled up with lymph. From this cloſed extremity extended, about two lines breadth, a ſmall rounded whitiſh ſubſtance, of the conſiſtence of jelly, which, probably, was the remains of the external coagulum not yet abſorbed. Within this portion of artery we found a ſmall conical coagulum of blood, attached at its baſe to the lymph that cloſed the mouth of the artery, but not adhering to, nor even appearing to touch, any other point of its internal ſurface.

'The inferior extremity of the artery was much more contracted than the ſuperior, its termination being very diſtinctly of the figure of a cone. On cutting it open, we found its mouth completely contracted, and adhering to the lymph that cloſed it. An internal coagulum, ſimilar to that of the ſuperior portion of the artery, was attached to this lymph. The coats of both portions of the artery were very much thickened. See plate I. fig. 4.'

Not one, then, but a variety of circumſtances conſpires in the natural ſuppreſſion of the hemorrhage from *divided* arteries. The divided artery retracts and contracts; the force of the circulation, after the firſt impetuous flow of blood, is gradually weakened and reduced; the blood is effuſed into the cellular ſubſtance, and the ſheath within which the divided artery had retracted; the effuſed blood is here entangled, and the foundation laid for the formation of a coagulum, which fills the ſheath and cellular membrane, and eventually cloſes up the mouth of the artery;

2 and

and this, which is termed the external coagulum, is the firſt complete barrier to the effuſion of blood. "This coagulum, viewed externally, appears like a continuation of the artery, but, on cutting up the artery, its termination can be diſtinctly ſeen with the coagulum completely ſhutting up its mouth, and encloſed in its ſheath."

The next ſtep in the proceſs is the formation of the *internal* coagulum, the clot within the artery, a ſlender conical clot which lies looſe in the arterial canal, and connected with the artery only by its baſe, which, by its circumference, is ſlightly attached to the divided extremity of the veſſel. The formation of this internal coagulum, however, appears to be merely a contingent event in the proceſs, and depends on the ceſſation of the circulation in that part of the artery which lies between the firſt collateral branch and the divided extremity, after that extremity has been cloſed, and the hemorrhage ſtopped by the external coagulum. The figure and ſize of the internal coagulum vary according to the remoteneſs of the firſt collateral branch, and where this goes off very near to the divided extremity of the artery, the internal clot is often not to be found. "The *internal* coagulum contributes nothing to the ſuppreſſion of hemorrhage in ordinary accidents, becauſe its formation is uncertain, or, when formed, it rarely fills the canal of the artery, or, if it fills the canal, does not adhere to the internal coat of the artery."

Soon after, there is obſerved, between the external and internal coagula, a layer of coagulable lymph, poured out by the inflamed veſſels of the cut extremity of the artery, to the internal coat of which this coagulum of lymph is firmly united. And now, by the gradual contraction of the artery, and by the effuſion of lymph, theſe parts become intimately blended together; the canal of the artery is obliterated, and its extremity loſt in the ſurrounding parts. Thus, the *temporary* ſuppreſſion of the hemorrhage is accompliſhed by the retraction and contraction of the artery, and by the formation of the coagula, or clots of blood; *permanent* ſecurity is afterwards obtained by the effuſion, conſolidation, and organization of coagulable lymph. The artery, however, gradually undergoes other changes: "Its obliterated extremity no longer allowing the blood to circulate through it, the portion which lies between it and the firſt lateral branch is no more diſtended and excited to action as formerly, but gradually contracts, till at length its cavity is entirely obliterated, and its condenſed tunics aſſume a ligamentous appearance." "At the ſame time, the remarkable appearances at the extremity of the artery are undergoing a conſiderable change; the external coagulum of blood, which, in the firſt inſtance, had ſtopped the hemorrhage,

hemorrhage, is abſorbed in the courſe of a few days, and the coagulating lymph which had been effuſed around it, and had produced a thickened and almoſt cartilaginous appearance in the parts, is gradually removed, and they again appear more or leſs completely reſtored to their cellular texture."

Such is the outline of the proceſs employed by nature for the ſuppreſſion of hemorrhage from *divided* arteries, as more fully deduced by our author from his own experiments and obſervations, and which he very happily illuſtrates and confirms by a judicious expoſition and criticiſm of ſome of the obſervations of Pouteau, Kirkland, Morand, Gooch, Haller, and others.

Let us conclude, then, with Dr Jones, that "we can no longer conſider the ſuppreſſion of hemorrhage as a ſimple, a mere mechanical effect, but as a proceſs prepared by the concurrent and ſucceſſive operations of many cauſes: Theſe may be briefly ſtated to conſiſt in the retraction and contraction of the artery, the formation of a coagulum at its mouth, the inflammation and conſolidation of its extremity by an effuſion of coagulable lymph within its canal, between its tunics, and in the cellular ſubſtance ſurrounding it."

We now paſs to the 2d chapter of this treatiſe:—"On the means which nature employs for ſuppreſſing hemorrhage from *punctured* or *partially divided* arteries; and on the proceſs of reparation which takes place in thoſe arteries."

The common conſequence of a punctured artery, in man at leaſt, is the formation of aneuriſm; and the experiments of this chapter were originally inſtituted with the view of aſcertaining the manner in which aneuriſm is produced, and with little hope of witneſſing the complete and perfect reunion of a partially wounded artery. But Dr Jones found it very difficult to produce aneuriſms in the arteries of horſes and dogs; on the contrary, he diſcovered that, when the artery was ſimply punctured, the wound often cicatrized by a proceſs of reparation, its canal continuing pervious, and its functions entire; or, when a larger portion of the circumference of the artery was wounded, that either the canal of the artery became obſtructed, or that a complete diviſion took place by laceration or ulceration.

We ſhall take the 6th of this ſeries of experiments as an example of the cicatrization of a punctured artery.

EXPERIMENT VI.

"The carotid artery of a dog was laid bare, and a longitudinal wound made in it with a lancet, without removing it at all from its ſituation or ſurrounding attachments; a profuſe hemorrhage followed; the integuments were ſewed up as quickly as poſſible, and ſoon after they were found diſtended with blood, and the hemorrhage ceaſed.

S "Nine

"Nine days after this experiment the animal was killed, and, on examining the parts, the external wound was found to be very nearly healed. Its surface was formed by a vascular layer of lymph. The artery was injected from the aorta, and the injection passed very readily through it. As it had been wounded anteriorly, I cut open its posterior part, immediately opposite to the wound. The canal of the artery and the injection were very slightly narrowed just at this part; the coats of the artery and the surrounding cellular membrane were very much thickened. On picking away the portion of injection which passed through this part of the artery, the longitudinal wound was seen to be completely cicatrized. There was a collateral branch filled with injection on one side of it, and on the other a very thin lamina of lymph adhering to the internal surface of the artery. See plate V. fig. 3."

But if these animals had been longer preserved, if they had fully recovered their blood and health, if they had been allowed to return to their wonted freedom and exercise, might not these cicatrized arteries have dilated into aneurisms? However this may be, the process of cicatrization, as deduced from these experiments, appears to be this:—The sheath becomes injected with blood; the relative position of the puncture in the artery and in the sheath is altered, so that they no longer oppose each other; a layer of coagulated blood is confined by the sheath over the puncture in the artery, and forms the *temporary* barrier to farther hemorrhage. Lymph is now effused under the coagulum of blood, and the process of reparation is completed in the usual way, till permanent security is obtained.

Though it appears, from Dr Jones's experiments, that the punctured arteries of brute animals may thus be cicatrized, and their functions preserved entire, we are not to flatter ourselves with equal success in the surgery of wounded arteries in man. Although there is such an appearance of cicatrix in a case quoted from Petit, we perfectly agree with Dr Jones, that in the treatment of a wounded artery, "in every case in which it can be done, it is best to tie the artery above and below the wounded part, and to divide it between the ligatures."

Chapter 3d:—"On the operation of the ligature; showing that its immediate effect is to divide the middle and internal coats of an artery which gives rise to the adhesive inflammation."

The experiments contained under this head are novel, and highly interesting. In these, after exposing the arteries, ligatures were passed round them, and tied in the usual way, but, immediately afterwards, loosened and withdrawn; the freedom of circulation was instantly restored, and the blood passed through the artery as before the application of the ligature. Yet, very shortly after, the artery became obstructed, and was eventually cicatrized

cicatrized for ſome way above and below where the ligature had operated, and that as effectually as if the ligature had been ſuffered to remain. The proceſs by which this is brought about ſeems to conſiſt of the following parts: The internal and middle coats of the artery are torn or divided by the ligature, an obſervation firſt made by Deſſault, and confirmed by Mr Thomſon and by Dr Jones; the divided coats inflame; coagulable lymph is poured out ſo abundantly as to obſtruct the arterial canal; above and below this obſtructing coagulated lymph there are formed internal clots, or coagula of blood, as far as the firſt collateral branches, which complete the obſtruction, and at length all this portion of the artery becomes cicatrized, with the circumſtances more fully expoſed by our author in the next chapter, "On the proceſs of adheſion, and the changes which an artery finally undergoes, in conſequence of the application of the ligature."

In the experiments undertaken with a view to the inveſtigation of this proceſs, the ligatures were applied in the uſual manner, and allowed to remain, the artery being, in ſome, divided between two ligatures, and allowed to retract, and, in other caſes, left undivided.

From the whole of Dr Jones's experiments, it appears that the effects of tying an artery properly are,

1ſt, To cut through the internal and middle coats of the artery, and to bring the wounded ſurfaces into perfect oppoſition.

2d, To occaſion a determination of blood on the collateral branches.

3d, To allow of the formation of a coagulum of blood juſt within the artery, provided a collateral branch is not very near the ligature.

4th, To excite inflammation on the internal and middle coats of the artery by having cut them through, and conſequently to give riſe to an effuſion of lymph, by which the wounded ſurfaces are united, and the canal is rendered impervious; to produce a ſimultaneous inflammation on the correſponding external ſurface of the artery, by which it becomes very much thickened with effuſed lymph; and, at the ſame time, from the expoſure and inevitable wounding of the ſurrounding parts, to occaſion inflammation in them, and an effuſion of lymph, which covers the artery, and forms the ſurface of the wound.

5th, To produce ulceration in the part of the artery round which the ligature is immediately applied, viz. its external coat.

6th, To produce indirectly a complete obliteration not only of the canal of the artery, but even of the artery itſelf, to the collateral branches on both ſides of the part which has been tied.

7th, To give riſe to an enlargement of the collateral branches.

A knowledge of the changes which an artery undergoes, in conſequence of the application of the ligature, explains to us, at the ſame time, its occaſional failure, and inſtructs us how to avoid ſome of the cauſes of ſecondary hemorrhage; thoſe, at leaſt, which depend on the improper form and application of the ligature. And, with ſome very pertinent remarks on this ſubject, Dr Jones brings his treatiſe to a cloſe.

It is proved by ſome experiments of Dr Jones, that, to produce thoſe changes in the artery which terminate in the adheſion of its coats and obliteration of its canal, which it is our object to attain by the proper application of the ligature, it is neceſſary that the internal and middle coats of the artery be completely divided by the ligature; and hence that form and mode of application, which are beſt calculated to produce this requiſite diviſion of the internal coats, muſt be preferred. Large flat ligatures are therefore improper; round ligatures, which are ſmall and ſufficiently firm, are preferable; they ſhould be perfectly regular. No part ought to be included in the ligature but the artery. Care ſhould be taken to tie the ligature with ſufficient force, and always as nearly as poſſible in the direction perpendicular to the axis of the artery. The artery itſelf ſhould, in every caſe, be as little as poſſible detached from the neighbouring parts; and, if experience has diſcovered any advantage in the mode of tying and dividing the artery between two ligatures, Dr Jones is diſpoſed to think that this advantage conſiſts in the artery being tied cloſe to the part at which its connexion with the ſurrounding cellular membrane is complete; whereas, when a ſingle ligature is uſed, a conſiderable portion of the artery is detached, and the ligature, perhaps, applied in the centre; or, if applied at the upper end, ſtill there remains a conſiderable portion of detached artery below it.

From the foregoing analyſis, our readers will be enabled to anticipate the general merits of this excellent treatiſe. To us it appears a work of uncommon merit, and we doubt not our judgment will be confirmed by every one who, after an attentive peruſal, conſiders the unuſual labour beſtowed upon it, the great number of facts contained in it, the excellence of the plan by which all thoſe facts are arranged, the preciſe and accurate developement of the moſt important proceſſes, of which very inadequate and confuſed notions had been formerly entertained, and the induſtry and fidelity with which they have been illuſtrated by the ſcattered facts relating to theſe collected from the writings of others.

IV.

IV.

Chirurgical Observations relative to the Eye, with an Appendix on the Introduction of the Male Catheter, and the Treatment of Hemorrhoids. By JAMES WARE, Surgeon, F. R. S. &c. In two volumes. Vol. I. Second edition. 8vo. pp. 527. London. 1805.

THE subjects treated of in this first volume are the ophthalmy, psorophthalmy, and purulent eye of new-born children; the epiphora, or watery eye; the treatment of fistula lachrymalis; the introduction of the male catheter; the treatment of hemorrhoids.

These tracts, we need hardly inform our readers, have already, in another form, been before the public. They are here collected into one view, after having been revised and enlarged by Mr Ware, well known as an eminent practitioner in diseases of the eye. The present, therefore, must be considered, in some measure, as a new book, of which, as a work of practical usefulness, it is our duty to take some notice.

We have no fault to find with Mr Ware's general history of the causes and symptoms of ophthalmia. It is difficult, it is impossible perhaps, to communicate to others all the fruits of individual experience; to delineate all those shades in the character of a disease which the experienced and enlightened practitioner is himself so well acquainted with, and which guides him so accurately in the choice of his means of cure. This is more especially the case in ophthalmic inflammation, of the varieties of which, demanding corresponding varieties of treatment, we have still to regret the want of precise and accurate descriptions. Whoever has had occasion to observe the frequent errors committed by routine practitioners in the misapplication of some of the most powerful auxiliaries, and to compare their failures and blunders with the steady success obtained by the more enlightened and discriminating oculist in the happier choice of his indications and remedies, will acknowledge how insufficient it is, for the purpose of instruction, to enumerate in succession merely all the remedies, general and topical, which may, in different cases, or at different periods, be employed, without attempting some arrangement and description of the varieties of the disease to which the particular modes of treatment are applicable. Such a discrimination of cases would lay a foundation for that precision

precision which we know to be attainable in the treatment of ophthalmic inflammation, but which is generally so little understood. And hence, indeed, arises the equivocal reputation of some of the most valuable remedies.

If the history of ophthalmia given by Mr Ware be too general, if deffective in the description of their varieties, we must allow that he has added to the account of the different remedies some excellent practical observations, which may serve, in some measure, to supply this defect.

There are few external applications more strikingly useful in certain stages of ophthalmia than the vinous tincture of opium, so highly recommended by Mr Ware. But it affords also an example of a remedy which may be easily abused. When prudently used, it not only procures great relief from pain, but greatly assists in dissipating the inflammation itself. The method of using it is, to drop into the eye a single drop of it once or twice a-day. This causes at first a sharp pain, and copious flow of tears. But a remarkable degree of ease commonly succeeds; the inflammation abates, and is often entirely removed after a few applications of the tincture.

The thebaic tincture is used with the greatest effect in the second stage of ophthalmy, after the necessary evacuations have been premised. Used earlier, it is less beneficial, and, in some cases, rather hurtful, especially where the eyes appear shining and glossy, and feel exquisite pain from the rays of light. Even in such cases, however, Mr Ware informs us, the application is sometimes found to succeed; "and whether it will or not, can only be determined by making the trial, which is attended with no other inconvenience than the momentary pain it gives." "When it is found to produce no good effect, the use of it must be suspended, until evacuations, and other proper means, have diminished the excessive irritation; after which it may be again applied, and bids equally fair for success as in those instances in which it never disagreed."

In scrofulous and intermittent ophthalmiæ, where, with no very great appearance of inflammation, the pain both of the head and eye continues violent, and is subject to remit, and sometimes wholly to intermit, Mr Ware has found the internal use of the muriate of mercury very useful, and he now recommends it in preference to all other remedies, even to Peruvian bark. It has often succeeded with him in cases where the cinchona had failed. He has also found the internal use of the muriate of mercury singularly useful in several cases where the ophthalmy followed putrid and nervous fevers. "The inflammation in these cases, though small in appearance, is generally attended

attended with a deep-seated pain in the orbit, which is much increased during the night, with a peculiar dulness in the transparent parts of the eye, and with considerable general debility."

In another variety of ophthalmia, which is accompanied with sneezing and coughing, and in peculiarly irritable eyes, very small doses of opium, or of cicuta, given once or twice a-day, have been found useful.

A topical application, of great efficacy in many cases of chronic ophthalmy, is the unguentum hydrarg. nitrati, or an ointment prepared with the red nitrate of mercury, in the proportion of one-eighth part. This ointment is peculiarly useful where the edges of the tarsi are ulcerated, where the inflammation is kept up by the irritation of the secretion from these parts; in most cases where, from the long continuance of inflammation, the vessels of the eye have become relaxed and weakened, and where specks are beginning to form on the cornea. We have used the application with excellent effect also in more recent cases, after scarification of the conjunctiva of the eyelids, especially in the ophthalmy of scrofulous children, and in that which is a sequela of eruptive disorders.

'It is a question of no small moment,' says Mr Ware, 'and perhaps has not been sufficiently attended to by surgeons, whether a *lotion* should be applied to the eye warm or cold. It has been a usually received opinion, that warm applications relax and weaken those parts to which they are applied; and, on the contrary, that cold applications have a tendency to brace and strengthen them. But though this observation be sometimes just, it is by no means universally true. Weakness is not unfrequently the result of pain; and whatever removes pain in the same proportion contributes to give strength. Weakness, again, is sometimes occasioned by too great fulness, not merely in those vessels which convey red blood, but likewise in the lymphatic vessels, and often also in the glands that are connected with the surface of the body, and the ducts that carry off the secretion of these glands; and whatever tends to diminish the fulness of these parts, or to carry off the substances that are morbidly lodged in them, contributes in the same proportion to increase their strength. In some of these ways, I presume, it is that the application of hot water to the eye is frequently useful, not only when it is in a state of inflammation and pain, but when the ciliary glands are enlarged, and when they secrete an acrimonious or glutinous humour; which humour adhering to the orifices of the ducts, as it passes through them, forms more or less of gum on the edges of the eyelids, and causes them to stick together when they have been long in contact. Weakness, again, is sometimes the result of too great tightness or stiffness in those elastic parts which are formed for a greater or less degree of contractile action; and whatever tends to restore the

power

power of contraction of these parts contributes to increaſe their ſtrength, and promote their uſefulneſs. In this way, I account for the utility of the application of hot water when the eye feels morbidly dry, and alſo when it begins to loſe its power of accommodating itſelf to the view of near objects; a change which takes place in moſt eyes that are not naturally ſhort-ſighted, as perſons advance in life, and which, it is probable, in ſome degree depends on the too great tenſion of the cornea, and its inability to acquire that increaſed convexity which it is neceſſary it ſhould have, in order to enable it duly to refract the rays of light when they come from near objects. Uſeful, however, as hot applications undoubtedly often are, it ſhould not be forgotten, on the contrary, that in thoſe caſes when the weakneſs of the eye is accompanied with a morbid ſecretion of tears, without much inflammation, and ſometimes in thoſe alſo where the lachrymal ſecretion is accompanied with an increaſed acrimonious diſcharge from the ciliary glands, which diſcharge excoriates the edges of the eye-lids, and makes them adhere together when they have been long in contact, as during the time of ſleeping, cold applications, and thoſe which poſſeſs a degree of aſtringency, ſuch as the zincum vitriolatum, ceruſſa acetata, lapis tutiæ, and lapis calaminaris, (and particularly five or ſix grains of the zinc vit. mixed with an equal quantity of the ceruſſa acetat. and four ounces of the aq. flor. ſambuci) have often afforded very eſſential aſſiſtance. But in the compoſition of all remedies for the eye, where inſoluble bodies are employed, whether they be in the form of ointments, or in that of lotions, it is of great importance always to remember, that they ſhould be reduced to an impalpable powder; and, in general, it is deſirable that aqueous mixtures ſhould be paſſed through filtering paper, before they are ſent to be uſed by the patient.'

The applications recommended for ſpecks or opacities of the cornea, which admit of any remedy, are the diluted ſolution of the muriate of mercury, the citrine ointment, the ointment prepared with the red nitrate, and a powder compoſed of one-eighth part of alum mixed with white ſugar, and diviſion of blood-veſſels, where they are obſerved to feed the ſpeck.

There is a very curious change of figure to which the cornea is ſometimes, though very rarely, liable; it loſes its round figure, and acquires a conical, or ſugar-loaf ſhape, in conſequence of which, viſion becomes myopical, imperfect, and confuſed; the apex of the cone is ſometimes obſcured by a ſpeck, without any preceding ophthalmy. The opacity may be removed, but the morbid projection is ſeldom got the better of. The cornea has been punctured, and the aqueous humour evacuated by Mr Ware; after which he has attempted to contract the morbid propenſity by compreſſion, but without any good effect.

The

'The greatest relief I have hitherto given,' he continues, 'has been by the application of a few drops of a strong infusion of tobacco; by a perseverance in the use of which remedy three or four times a-day, the conical appearance of the eye has, in a few instances, been diminished, and the patient's sight greatly mended.'

After a violent ophthalmia, vision is sometimes obscured by a deposition of matter in the anterior chamber of the aqueous humour of the eye. Not unfrequently this matter is gradually again absorbed, as the inflammation is dissipated, or this absorption may be afterwards promoted by stimulating applications to the eye. If, however, the collection of matter is not soon made to disappear, and especially if it rather appears to increase, Mr Ware strongly urges the propriety of discharging it by an incision of the cornea, and even of repeating the operation, if necessary. He cautions us against delaying the operation, as such delay, if continued for any considerable time, may end in the destruction of the cornea, and, of consequence, the irrecoverable loss of sight.

We think, however, that Mr Ware has estimated this operation too lightly; and we believe that there is more danger from such early incision, and evacuation of the matter, than is here insinuated. The eye is still in a diseased state, the internal inflammation is not subdued, if the matter is on the increase; and the incision of the cornea, under such circumstances, is likely to aggravate all the symptoms, and to hasten the total destruction of the eye.

Scarpa decidedly condemns this operation, on account of the dangerous consequences which experience has shown to result from it. He proscribes it altogether, and advises us to trust to the remedies employed for the cure of ophthalmia; if the healthy state of the organ be restored, the matter will be gradually absorbed.

'Il est certain,' says Scarpa, 'que les moins versés dans le traitement des maladies des yeux, se persuaderont que le moyen le plus prompt, le plus efficace de traiter l'hypopion devenu stationaire dans la seconde periode de l'ophthalmie aiguë grave, doit être d' inciser la cornée dans la partie inferieure, afin de donner bientôt issue à la matière contenue dans les chambres de l' humeur aqueuse, d' autant plus que c' est la doctrine le plus communément enseignée dans les écoles de chirurgie. Cependant l'experience prouve le contraire; elle demontre que rarement la section de la cornée, dans ces circonstances, est suivie d' un bon succes, et que le plus souvent elle occasione des maux plus facheux que l'hypopion lui-même, malgre la modification suggérée par Richter, de ne pas vider tout d' un coup la matière

tière de l'hypopion, ni d' en solliciter l' issue par l' ouverture de la cornée, à l' aide des compressions repetées, ou des injections; mais de laisser sortir lentement, et d' elle-même, cette lymphe tenace. D' apres un nombre assez considerable d' observations sur ce sujet, il me paroit resulter que, quelque petite que soit l'ouverture pratiquée au bas de la cornée, pour donner issue à la matière de l'hypopion, elle reproduit le plus souvent l' ophthalmie grave aiguë, et qu' elle occasione un plus grand epanchement, qu' auparavant de lymphe concrescible dans les chambres de l' œil; et quand bien même encore, après la section de la cornée, on permettoit à la matière de l' hypopion de sortir d' elle même lentement et goutte à goutte, puisque elle est tenace, il lui faut plusieurs jours avant qu' elle soit entièrement evacuée. Pendant ce tems, la lymphe glutineuse maintient dilatées les levres de la plaie, les force à suppurer:—il en resulte un ulcère del a cornée, par lequel l' humeur aqueuse, située derrière la lymphe tenace et concrescible, s' écoule, et, après elle, on voit sortir au travers de l' ulcère de la cornée, un lambeau de l' iris, et quelquefois encore le crystallin vient s' y presenter.'—

Mr Ware concludes his first tract on ophthalmy with a few observations on pterygion and trichiasis.

By *psorophthalmy*, which is the subject of the next essay, is understood an acrimonious puriform discharge from the edges of the eyelids. The seat of the disease seems to be the sebaceous glands, and their ducts, which open on the inner edges of the eyelids. In consequence of inflammation and ulceration, the secreted fluid, instead of being moist and mild, and serving as a defence against the acrimony of the tears, is changed into a sharp, acrid, and adhesive humour, which causes a constant irritation of the eye and lids, ulcerates the inner edges of the latter, and, for want of proper attention, has often perpetuated the disorder for a great number of years.

The disease is often distressing, and does not yield to an general remedies, or to common treatment. Mr Ware's principal design in this tract is to recommend an application which he has found very successful, Unguent. Hydrar. Nitrat. of the last London Dispensatory. A little of the melted ointment must be rubbed into the edges of the affected eyelids once in twenty-four hours. Our experience confirms the character of this application. But we have more frequently used the unguent. hydrarg. nitrat. rub. and think it equally effectual.

The *purulent* eyes of new-born children is a disease of very formidable appearance, and, if neglected or improperly treated, actually becomes such. It much resembles the gonorrhæal ophthalmy, by the swelling of the eyelids, and the profuse puriform discharge from the whole surface of the adnata, and too often has terminated in the total destruction of the eye. There is is no method ſo effectual in checking the puriform diſcharge, and obviating the dangerous tendency of the diſeaſe, as the application of aſtringent lotions to the whole ſurface of the eye-balls. And the remedy particularly recommended by Mr Ware, from experience of its ſuperior uſefulneſs, is a ſolution of the ſulphate of copper, as preſented in the Aqua Camphorata of Bate's Diſpenſatory.

It is made as follows:

> ℞ Vitriol. Roman.
> Bol. Armen. á á ℥ iv.
> Camphor. ℥ j.

Fr. Pulvis, de quo projice ℥ j. in aquæ bullientis ℔ iv, Amove ab igne, et ſubſidant ſæces.

This is to be uſed in the proportion of two drachms to an ounce of water. The moſt effectual way of applying it is to inject it between the eyelids by means of a blunt conical-pointed ſyringe. This injection ſhould be frequently repeated; in bad caſes once or twice every hour; the ſtrength of the injection to be increaſed according to circumſtances. In this diſorder, where the ſwelling and inflammation are conſiderable, it is proper alſo to leech the temples, and apply bliſters. But our chief reliance is on the aſſiduous uſe of the injection. It becomes us to obſerve, that this remedy has been equally ſucceſsful in the hands of others; and that Scarpa, in treating of the cure of this diſeaſe, does little more than copy from Mr Ware, though without doing him the ſame juſtice, or making the ſame acknowledgment, which he has done in ſpeaking of the vinous tincture of opium.

The diſeaſe known by the name of *epiphora*, or watery eye, acknowledges a variety of cauſes, and, according to theſe, the appropriate treatment muſt neceſſarily be varied. The deſign of our author's eſſay on this ſubject is principally to exhibit the advantage to be obtained in certain caſes from the practice of Anel, of injecting through the puncta lachrymalia fluids into the lachrymal ſac, with the view of overcoming the obſtruction to the paſſage of the tears into the noſe, and of obviating the cauſes of that obſtruction. This obſtruction, which, if neglected, eventually terminates in fiſtula lachrymalis, may be produced by a thickening of the membrane lining the ſac, by the lodgment of inſpiſſated mucus, or by ſpaſm, or all together. In theſe caſes Mr Ware has experienced great benefit from injecting through the inferior punctum, by means of Anel's ſyringe, warm water, weak ſolutions of ſulphate zinc, warm or cold, according to circumſtances.

Mr

Mr Ware's method of treating the *fistula lachrymalis*,[a] we believe, is pretty generally known in this country. It consists in the insertion of a small silver style into the nasal duct, which is worn by the patient with little inconvenience, until the parts recover the power of carrying on their usual functions.

The style was first employed by Mr Ware to open and dilate the nasal duct, with the view of establishing a future passage for the tears after its removal. But he soon had the good fortune to observe, that its good effects were more immediate than he had expected. The watering of the eye almost wholly ceased as soon as the style was introduced, the tears passing freely into the nose. The neatness and simplicity of this practice are great recommendations, and the experience of Mr Ware of its utility has been confirmed by others who have given it a trial.

With regard to his observations on the *introduction of the male catheter*, it appears to us that he might save himself a great deal of trouble, by introducing the instrument, from the beginning, with its concave side towards the pubis.

When *hemorrhoidal tumours* have become highly distressing, and no relief can be obtained by the usual modes of treatment, recourse has been had to the knife or ligature for their complete removal, an operation painful, and not easily practicable, where the whole anus is beset with a mass of painfully inflamed piles. If these be accurately examined, it will commonly be found that the principal distress proceeds from one or two of the tumours more swelled and painful than the rest; and the intention of our author's observations is to show, that it is generally sufficient to remove the hard inflamed tumour which is the cause of the pain, and which is not unfrequently situated in the centre of the rest; all of which, he assures us, collapse and disappear after the excision of the principal one.

The method recommended is to secure the tumour with a common dissecting hook or forceps, and to snip it off, as close to its base as possible, with a sharp pair of curved scissars.

V.

Letters to Dr Rowley on his late Pamphlet, entitled, "Cow-Pox Inoculation no security against Infection." By Aculeus. 8vo. London. 1805.

Dr Rowley did not deserve a serious answer. His folly, not to use a harsher term, is exposed in these letters in a strain of indignant irony.

VI.

VI.

The Anatomy and Surgical Treatment of Inguinal and Congenital Hernia. By ASTLEY COOPER, F. R. S. &c. &c. Illuſtrated by Plates. London. 1804. Large folio. L. 2, 2s.

THIS work is already ſo well known that ſome of our readers may think it unneceſſary at this time to take notice of it; but the merits of the author, and the importance of the ſubject, induce us to give a ſhort analyſis, and to make a few curſory remarks on its contents.

The object of Mr Cooper, in the preſent volume, is to give the anatomical deſcription and ſurgical treatment of inguinal and congenital hernia, leaving the conſideration of femoral, and the other ſpecies, to a future publication.

There is no diſeaſe where minute anatomical diſſection has been more ſucceſsfully employed than in the pathology and treatment of hernia; for as this complaint ariſes more from an alteration in the relative ſituation of organs than from any morbid change of ſtructure, we muſt be well acquainted with the natural appearances in order to diſcriminate the effects of diſeaſe, or be able to point out the beſt means of affording relief.

Although Albinus ſeems to have been well acquainted with this part of anatomy, yet it is to Gimbernat, a celebrated Spaniſh ſurgeon, to whom we are indebted for the firſt accurate and detailed deſcription of the *abdominal*, and ſtill more particularly of the *crural* rings.

Mr Cooper, beſides availing himſelf of the deſcription theſe anatomiſts have given, advances a ſtep farther, and deſcribes ſome of the more minute parts of the anatomy of the abdominal ring with much preciſion and ingenuity. Neither Mr Cooper, however, nor, as far as we know, any other anatomiſt, has paid ſufficient attention to a deſcription of the bones of this part of the pelvis, when deſcribing the ſoft parts; for we have long believed that an accurate knowledge of them will lead to a ſimple deſcription, and give a clear notion of the ſoft parts with which they are connected. If we examine theſe bones, we find a ridge extending from the inferior part of the *venter* of the ilium, which forms the lateral parts of the brim of the pelvis, and the line of diviſion between the pelvis and abdomen, called *linea in-*

nominata; and there is alſo another line or ridge, which begins at the rough creſt or angle of the os pubis, and extends along the upper and inner edge of the bone to meet the former. The junction of the two ridges, in ſome ſubjects, is diſtinctly marked; but, in moſt bones, a ſmall portion of the edge is rounded at that part where the femoral veſſels paſs out of the pelvis. Although theſe two ridges have been deſcribed long ago by anatomiſts, yet they do not ſeem to have explained their uſe, or conſidered them in the deſcription of the ſoft parts. It will be found, however, that the pubic portion is intended for the inſertion of the inflected part of the ligament of Poupart, called Gimbernat's ligament, and the iliac portion for the attachment of the aponeuroſis of the iliac, pſoic, and abdominal muſcles. This knowledge of the bones, and of the different parts of them into which the aponeurotic and tendinous fibres are inſerted, enables us to form a clear and diſtinct notion of the relative ſituation of parts, and to be aware of the raſhneſs with which particular names have been given to continuations or parts of one faſcia, or of the ſame aponeurotic expanſion.

The oblique paſſage of the ſpermatic cord through the abdominal parietes was well known to and elegantly delineated by Albinus. Nevertheleſs, no author, except Mr Cooper, has conſidered it with that attention which it ſeems to merit. After having minutely deſcribed this beautiful piece of mechaniſm, he points out, with a good deal of ingenuity, the neceſſity of taking it into conſideration, in order to explain particular ſymptoms and varieties of inguinal hernia, to accompliſh the reduction of hernia, and alſo in the application of truſſes.

There is one part of the anatomy of which our author has not taken notice. It is the difference of the relative ſituation of the ligament of Poupart in the male and female. In Mr Cooper's deſcription no other difference is mentioned, than that the abdominal ring ſerves for the paſſage of the ſpermatic cord in the male, and of the round ligament in the female. Dr Monro jun. has obſerved a remarkable difference in the formation of theſe parts in the two ſexes, and he has deſcribed it accurately, and delineated it in his work on femoral hernia. It may be ſufficient here to mention, that this difference accounts very ſatisfactorily for the greater frequency of femoral hernia in the female than in the male, and for the rare occurrence of inguinal hernia in the female.

The next part of Mr Cooper's work treats of the pathology of hernia. He deſcribes the manner in which the ſac is formed, its ſize, mode of deſcent, coverings of faſcia, cellular ſubſtance, and, as he calls it, cremaſter muſcle. He alſo takes particular notice

notice of the situation of the spermatic cord, and mentions two varieties, in one of which, instead of the hernial sac passing on the outside of these vessels, it was found on their inner or pubic side. In the other instance, the vas deferens was found on the one side, and the rest of the cord on the other side of the sac.

The next chapter contains the diagnosis and the enumeration of those causes which most commonly produce hernia.

The subject of the fifth chapter is one of importance, and it is full of good practical information relative to the mode of action, application, and management of trusses.

"The object in applying a truss (says our author) is to close the mouth of the hernial sac, and destroy its communication with the abdomen; and this object can never be perfectly fulfilled by any truss which is applied in the usual manner upon the abdominal ring, and extending from it upon the os pubis. In this case the cure must be incomplete, because a considerable portion of the hernial sac remains uncompressed toward the abdomen, which portion is that situated between the abdominal ring and the opening of the sac into the cavity of the belly." He adds, "The proper method of completely obliterating the mouth of the hernial sac is to apply the truss, not upon the abdominal ring, but upon the part at which the spermatic cord, and with it the hernia, first quit the abdomen; for in this way only can a descent of the hernia be prevented entirely, and a cure by pressure, if practicable, can be performed." "Therefore, when a hernia has been returned into the abdomen by the surgeon, he should lay his fingers obliquely above and without the ring, and direct his patient to cough, and the furtheit part from the ring towards the spine of the ilium, where the hernial sac is felt to protrude, is the point which should be noted for the application of the pad of the truss, and the instrument made accordingly."

These remarks are no less ingenious than important. There are two circumstances, however, which appear to us to be of some moment, although they have not been taken notice of by our author. They regard the strength of the spring, and the form and size of the pad. It will be found that a person who has worn a truss for many years is not able to give up using it, chiefly on account of the strength of the abdominal muscles being diminished at that part where the pad rests. The pressure of the pad seems to produce an absorption of the abdominal parietes. As this effect will always be in proportion to the degree of pressure or strength of the spring, it is of importance never to employ in any case a spring stronger than what is necessary to keep up the bowels; and it is useful for a person labouring under hernia to have two trusses of different strengths, one for ordinary purposes, and the other when riding, or when

 taking

taking any violent exercife. Our author advifes that the pad be made of a conical form, the apex of which fhould reft on the internal ring or mouth of the fac. However ufeful this may be as a general rule, it ought to be known that there are many exceptions; and, with due deference to Mr Cooper's opinion, we beg leave to mention, that we have found fuch a variety, not only in the fize of the rupture, but alfo in the fituation and fize of the opening through which it paffes, that we apprehend it will be neceffary to vary the form and bulk of the pad according to every individual cafe. If the pad is too large and flat, it will prevent the bowels from paffing through the external ring, but it will allow them to pafs through the internal ring, and enter the inguinal canal. On the other hand, if the pad is fo fmall as to prefs into the mouth of the fac, and plug it up, there is no longer any chance of a permanent cure. The bowels may be prevented from entering the fac, but the pad will act as a dilator or bougie, keep the mouth of the fac continually open, and even increafe its diameter. It therefore appears to us, that, in every cafe of reducible hernia, a pad ought to be made according to the fize and fituation of the ring; that it be of fuch bulk and form as to make a preffure on the *internal* abdominal ring, along the *inguinal* canal, and on the *external* ring.

IRREDUCIBLE HERNIA.

"The following are the caufes which feem to bring the difeafe into this ftate.

1. When the protruded parts are fuffered to remain long down, they increafe fo much in fize as to be incapable of reduction.

2. When membranous bands form acrofs the fac, entangle its contents, and prevent its free motion.

3. When the protruded parts become clofely united by an adhefion to the fide of the fac fufficiently firm to render them immoveable."

The moft efficacious means recommended by our author to accomplifh the reduction of a hernia in this ftate, is to wear a bag trufs of fuch a form as to keep a fteady and uniform preffure on the fcrotum. The preffure produces a gradual abforption of the adipofe matter of the protruded bowels, and thus, after fome days confinement, the tumour becomes very much diminifhed, and at laft may be returned. The application of ice occafionally procures the return of a hernia which appears irreducible. Mr Cooper thinks that the good effects of this remedy are owing to its producing a contraction of the fcrotum, which performs the office of a ftrong and permanent compreffion of the tumour, and he relates two cafes where this practice proved fuccefsful.

OF

OF STRANGULATED HERNIA.

"If the tumour be examined after death, a quantity of clear ſerum will firſt be found under the ſkin. The hernial ſac contains a portion of bloody ſerum of a coffee colour. The inteſtine is of a chocolate brown, with here and there a black ſpot, which eaſily breaks down on being touched with the finger. A coat of the coagulable lymph, of the ſame colour as the inteſtine, may be peeled from its ſurface, and adheſions of no great ſtrength are found to extend from the inteſtine to the ſac. At the particular part where the inteſtine is ſtrangulated by the conſtricting membrane, it is either ulcerated through, or readily pulls aſunder under ſlight preſſure. If the inflammation has been very extenſive, there is a quantity of air in the ſurrounding cellular membrane."

"On examination after death, in ſtrangulated omental hernia, the omentum is found ſcarcely changed from its natural appearance; its colour is a little, and but a little, darker than uſual. I found it in ſome caſes, even during the operation, extremely offenſive to the ſmell; there is ſcarcely any fluid in the ſac. Though the cavity of the abdomen is inflamed, and the inteſtines ſlightly adhering to each other, they never appear to have ſuffered ſo much as by inteſtinal hernia." In old and large herniæ, Mr Cooper believes that the ſtrangulation is formed moſt frequently by the external abdominal ring; but, in other caſes, it is more commonly ſeated at the internal ring, the place where the ſpermatic veſſels quit the abdomen. "So if the ſurgeon, during the operations for hernia, examines accurately into the ſeat of the ſtrangulation, he will find, except in large herniæ, cutting through the ring is inſufficient to relieve the protruded parts, but he muſt proceed with his knife farther up towards the ſpinous proceſs of the ilium, before he can return the ſwelling."

"Moreover, though the abdominal ring be dilated with freedom, the hernia will, in many caſes, ſtill retain its colour of ſtrangulation, and remain irreducible, as before; but if the ſac be traced upwards with the knife, about one inch and a half, midway between the ilium and pubis, the ſtricture will there be found; and, when this is divided, the inteſtine recovers its colour, and can be readily returned."

TREATMENT OF STRANGULATED HERNIA.

The firſt object of our attention, in order to accompliſh the reduction of a ſtrangulated hernia, ought to be the poſition of the body of the patient. The celebrated Winſlow, the firſt anatomiſt who explained many of the phenomena of diſeaſe

 from

from a previous knowledge of the action of the mufcles, conceived it to be of importance that the body of the patient be placed in an inclined plane, and that the thighs be bent towards the trunk of the body. Our author advifes the fame practice, and remarks that fuch a pofture, by relaxing the fafcia of the thigh, relaxes alfo the aperture through which the hernia paffes. There is no doubt but every degree of tightening or relaxation of the femoral fafcia will be accompanied by a correfponding change in the abdominal ring; but the motion of flexion, while it relaxes the fafcia, relaxes at the fame time the abdominal internal iliac and pfoi mufcles, and it is the change produced by the relaxation of thefe mufcles which facilitates, and ought to be kept in view in the reduction of hernia. To be convinced of the truth of this obfervation, it is only neceffary to obferve in the dead body, when in a horizontal pofture, the fize of the crural ring. By introducing into it the fore-finger, a tight cord is readily felt at the upper part; when the thigh is bent upwards and inwards, the cord is relaxed, and the opening is enlarged.

The preffure which is employed on the tumour by the hands of the furgeon fhould always be directed upwards and outwards along the courfe of the canal of the cord, and our author advifes it to be continued from a quarter to half an hour; befides the mechanical means, he recommends tobacco glifters and cold as the moft fuccefsful in diminifhing the increafed action and bulk of the parts. Cold applications have been approved of by the moft celebrated furgeons, and they have been particularly recommended by Mr B. Bell in the form of ice: when ice cannot be procured, our author ufes a mixture of equal parts of nitre and fal-ammonia. To one pound of water in a bladder ten ounces of the mixed falts are added, the bladder tied up, and then laid over the tumour. "If, after four hours, the fymptoms become mitigated, and the tumour leffens, this remedy may be perfevered in for fome time longer; but if they continue with unabated violence, and the tumour refift every attempt to reduction, no farther trial fhould be made of the application."

OPERATION.

There is not a more difficult point in furgery, or one which requires more decifion, than to determine the exact period when recourfe muft be had to the operation. From the dreadful confequences of delaying it till the protruded parts mortify, fome eminent furgeons have recommended its early performance, whilft others, from the feverity and rifk which always attend it, advife it to be delayed till every means have failed of procuring a reduction.

Thofe

Those who urge the early performance of the operation (more particularly Dessault) have founded their opinion on the effects of a similar operation, when there is no hernia, or when the hernia is recent; for, in such cases, no serious consequences are to be apprehended, or any symptoms likely to occur more violent than what takes place after the common operation of hydrocele by incision; on the other hand, many cases have occurred, where, after repeated trials had been made to accomplish a reduction, and the operation about to be performed, the bowel has been suddenly and unexpectedly reduced.

The symptoms which ought to guide us in having recourse to the operation arise from an attack of inflammation in that part of the intestine contained in the hernial sac, and from its spreading into the abdominal cavity. It is in proportion to their violence, and after every fair and probable means has been employed, that we ought to urge the performance of the operation. Mr Cooper considers pain on pressing the belly, and tension, as the symptoms which point out its immediate necessity. He adds, page 27, " Indeed, there is scarcely any period of the symptoms which should forbid the operation; for even if mortification has actually begun, the operation may be the means of saving life, by promoting the ready separation of gangrenous parts."

Mr Cooper has explained at great length the different steps of the operation. He directs the incision to be made from the upper part of the abdominal ring to the bottom of the hernial sac. We are warned, however, by Camper against making this extent of incision downwards, for it sometimes happens that the spermatic vessels pass on the anterior part of the sac, and are very apt to be divided.

The sac is to be opened at its inferior part by pinching it up with a pair of forceps, and cutting the elevated portion horizontally with a scalpel.

We witnessed, in one case, a surgeon very much perplexed when he came to this step of the operation. The sac had a blue transparent colour, and looked very like a piece of strangulated intestine; the surgeon, for some time, conceived that it actually was so, and at last opened it with the utmost terror, when, to his surprise, he found it to be a thin hernial sac, much distended with water. We have seen the same puzzling appearance in the operation for hydrocele by incision, and it is one we may expect to find when either the hernial sac or tunica vaginalis is thin.

In order to divide the stricture, " the surgeon passes his finger into the sac as far as the stricture, and then conveys a probe-pointed bistoury on the fore part of the sac, and, insinuating it within the ring, cuts through it in a direction upwards, opposite to the middle of the sac."

Mr Cooper thinks there is an advantage from not dividing the *hernial ſac* in dilating the ring, as it takes away all danger from wounding the inteſtine; he alſo makes ſome uſeful remarks on caſes where there was more than one ſtricture.

OF MORTIFICATION OF THE BOWELS.

The next chapter contains many uſeful practical obſervations on the mortification of the bowels, and on the artificial anus; alſo ſome very intereſting and ingenious experiments of Mr Thomſon of Edinburgh, relative to the mode of tying two portions of divided inteſtine.

It appears from Mr Thomſon's experiments, that if the inteſtine of an animal be divided tranſverſely, reunited by ligatures, and returned into the abdomen, the animal ſuffers no inconvenience, and the ligatures are diſcharged at the anus.

"However (ſays Mr Cooper), as the protruded parts in hernia are ſo much inflamed as to endanger a ſpeedy ſeparation of the ligatures, and as it appears from my experiments (page 35.) that the animal did not ſuffer from the ligature hanging from the abdomen, I ſhould ſtill prefer performing the operation of uniting the divided inteſtine in ſuch a manner as to give an opportunity of extracting the ligatures, if any inconveniences aroſe from their application."

Since Mr Cooper's work appeared, an eſſay has been publiſhed at Philadelphia by Mr Smith, which contains a ſeries of ingenious experiments on the wounds of inteſtines. The concluſions he has drawn we ſhall quote in his own words.

"It appears from the reſult of my experiments on dogs, that not only the inteſtine may be returned into the cavity of the abdomen, but that the ligatures may be cut off and returned with the inteſtine, as was obſerved by Mr Thomſon of Edinburgh, and that we need not be under any apprehenſion of their being diſcharged into the cavity; for, by ſome proceſs of the animal economy of which we are ignorant, the ligatures have, in every inſtance, either been diſcharged with the fæces, or been found looſely attached to the *internal* coat of the inteſtine.

"It has been ſaid by Meſſ. Cooper and Thomſon, that there is a curious difference in the facility with which a longitudinal and tranſverſe wound unites. But, in all the experiments which I have made, it was found that, with care, the *longitudinal* united as kindly as the tranſverſe, only requiring a little more attention to the diet of the animal, which ſhould be very ſparing and liquid, until the wound has had time to heal. It certainly requires

requires more pains to close a longitudinal wound completely than one which is transverse. The longitudinal incision always occasions a diminution in the diameter of the intestinal canal, thereby producing dangerous obstructions. If it be of any considerable extent, probably the surgeon would be justified in cutting out the wounded portion, and treating it as a transverse division. This may be done without much endangering the life of the animal, as appears by two experiments, where three inches of the intestine were removed *."

Mr Cooper next proceeds to give some account of the mode of dressing, and after treatment of the patient. He particularly takes notice of the impropriety of giving strong purges, if an evacuation can be procured by more gentle means. He enjoins the patient to be kept in a horizontal posture till the cure is complete, and shows the necessity of wearing a truss during the rest of his life.

The object of some writers to produce a radical cure by tying the mouth of the sac, Mr C. considers as ineffectual and dangerous. Although the opening of the peritoneum is shut up by such an operation, the dilatation of the abdominal ring must ever remain open.

OF LARGE HERNIA.

Under this head our author records two important cases of large hernia, in one of which the bowels were reduced, after dividing the stricture, without opening the sac; in the other the sac was opened. The first patient recovered, the second died.

These cases, and the conclusions which our ingenious author has drawn from them, present to practical surgeons a point worthy of their mature consideration, Whether ought we, in general, to open the hernial sac? This mode of operation was first proposed by Dr Monro sen. and several cases are related in the appendix to his work on the bursæ mucosæ, where it was performed most successfully.

OF SMALL HERNIA.

Our author remarks, that it is by no means unfrequent to meet with cases of hernia where the hernial sac is so small as not to extend through the abdominal ring; and as in such there is little appearance of external tumour, the disease is very apt to

* Vide an Inaugural Essay on wounds of the intestines for the degree of doctor of medicine, submitted to the examination of the Rev. J. Andrews, D. D. Provost (pro tempore), the Trustees and Medical Professors of the University of Pennsylvania, June 1805. By Thomas Smith, of the island of St Croix.

to be overlooked by the patient and ſurgeon, and ſome other cauſe aſſigned for the ſeries of ſymptoms. The manner of operating in this form of the diſeaſe differs from that in the common ſcrotal hernia: the inciſion is to be made parallel to the direction of the ſpermatic cord, and the ſtricture will be found at the internal ring.

OF INGUINAL HERNIA ON THE INNER SIDE OF THE EPIGASTRIC ARTERY.

This variety of hernia, ſays Mr C. has now very often fallen under obſervation, and has been for more than 25 years deſcribed in the lectures delivered at St Thomas's and Guy's Hoſpitals.

The following note, which is tranſlated from Rougemont, the author of the French tranſlation of Richter's treatiſe on hernia, will alſo ſhow that this form of the diſeaſe has not only been *long* known and *well* underſtood on the continent, but the ſame mode of operation as Mr Cooper mentions has been adopted.

"After all theſe conſiderations, I conclude with Mr Deſſault, that the epigaſtric artery in inguinal hernia is commonly placed near the *internal* angle of the ring, and rarely towards the *external*. The caſes where that artery is placed at the external angle of the ring in inguinal hernia are very rare, and they do not happen unleſs when the viſcera eſcape on the inner part of the ring, and then the cord is placed to one ſide, and a little behind the ſac. I have had occaſion, two years ago, to obſerve this diſtribution on a dead body; I preſerved the preparation for ſeveral months, and ſhowed it to ſeveral profeſſional men."

Afterwards he adds,

"I believe, after what has been ſaid, that we may be allowed to conclude that we run leſs riſk of wounding the epigaſtric artery in cutting upwards and outwards, than in cutting upwards and inwards; that, in order to know exactly the ſituation of that artery, we ought to become acquainted with the relative ſituation of the ſpermatic cord and hernial ſac; and, ſuppoſing that this is impoſſible, *we ought to make the inciſion directly upwards, through the middle of the ſuperior edge of the ring.*"

OF CONGENITAL HERNIA.

The author, under this head, has nothing particularly intereſting to communicate, except a caſe deſcribed by Mr Foſter, where, on diſſecting carefully through the tunica vaginalis of the cord near the ring, a fluid eſcaped. "I then (ſays Mr F.) continued the inciſion to the bottom of the ſcrotum through the tunica vaginalis of the cord, and the tunica vaginalis teſtis, which I found to be one cavity, the edges of which being turned back on each ſide expoſed a hernial ſac pendent from the ring, and deſcending towards the teſticle." Mr Cooper adds, "The idea I have formed of this caſe is, that the tunica vaginalis, after the deſcent

descent of the testis, became closed opposite to the abdominal ring, but remained open above and below it. That the intestines descended into the upper part, and elongated both the adhesion and tunica vaginalis, so as to form it into a bag, which descended into the tunica vaginalis below the adhesion, and becoming wide at its neck, though narrow at its fundus, it received a portion of intestine, which was too large either to be returned into the abdomen, or to retain its functions, whilst it continued in the sac."

The work is embellished with eleven plates, illustrative of the anatomy and pathology of hernia. These and the letter-press are in very large folio, and although this size adds to the splendour of the book, it renders it so importable, and so teazing and difficult to read, that we cannot help thinking, that if the same materials had been printed in a different form, and sold at a more moderate price, it would have been more generally useful, and more within the reach of the great body of readers.

As drawings, we cannot help regretting that, situated as Mr Cooper is in the focus of the arts, he had not been fortunate enough in employing a more able draughtsman. To us they appear to be executed with great stiffness, formality, and labour; they seem not as they were drawings from the subject, but as copied from heavy brass casts.

When we compare them with Camper's drawings on the same subject, our English artist is completely eclipsed; Camper, with all the spirit and power of a master, expresses, with a single well-chosen line, what Kirtland tries to do by a hundred.

As engravings, they are well executed, but they are loaded and heavy with much unnecessary labour and superfluous work. They are far from being the *chef-d'ouvres* of Heath, and seem to be indebted to him for nothing but his name.

These remarks, however, apply only to the plates as works of art; with regard to their anatomical accuracy, we believe them to be true representations, and certainly they will ever be considered as a useful addition to surgical anatomy.

From this outline we have given of Mr Cooper's work, we hope our readers will be enabled to form a general idea of its contents, and to appreciate its merits. The attentive practitioner will, we venture to say, find in it much useful practical information; and the opinions and scattered observations of former authors, and of illustrious teachers, are so well arranged and so judiciously collected, as sufficiently to recommend the work to the careful perusal of every description of medical men.

PART

PART III.

MEDICAL INTELLIGENCE.

ASSOCIATION FOR MEDICAL REFORM.

Several meetings of medical men having been lately held at Sir Joſeph Banks' for the purpoſe of reforming the profeſſion, the following letter has been drawn up by Dr Harriſon, with the view of collecting a more correct knowledge of the extent of the abuſes which prevail, and of the opinions of practitioners reſpecting the beſt means of correcting them, previous to an application to Parliament.

Soho Square, *4th March*, 1806.

(CIRCULAR.)

I am requeſted, by an aſſociation of medical men, who have held ſeveral meetings at the houſe of the Preſident of the Royal Society, for the better regulation of the practice of phyſic, and to whom Government has been pleaſed to grant free poſtage for this letter, and the anſwer you may be pleaſed to return to it, to beg the favour of your ſentiments, and thoſe of ſuch other gentlemen, in and out of the profeſſion, as you may have the goodneſs to conſult, by holding meetings of the faculty or otherwiſe, reſpecting the propriety of an application to Parliament to eſtabliſh the practice of phyſic in the hands of qualified perſons. It may not be improper to add, that it is not intended that the regular faculty now exiſting, of any denomination whatever, ſhould be ſubjected to the meaſures in contemplation. They are to be confined entirely to ſuch perſons as ſhall hereafter preſent themſelves for admiſſion. It is greatly to be lamented that the practice of medicine, in many parts of the kingdom, is now engroſſed by phyſicians and ſurgeons without diplomas, accoucheurs without education, and apothecaries and druggiſts who never ſerved any apprenticeſhip; while regular and able practitioners are diſpoſſeſſed of the ſtations which they ought to hold in ſociety, and are deprived of the emoluments due to the expenſe of their education.

To prevent a continuance of the manifeſt abuſe of public confidence, and to increaſe the reſpectability as well as the uſefulneſs of the faculty, are the leading conſiderations of the gentlemen who have met on this ſubject. They are deſirous, in the commencement of their undertaking, to communicate with, and to obtain the cooperation of reſpectable practitioners in all parts of the kingdom. I therefore beg leave to ſolicit your aſſiſtance in promoting a meaſure which

which is eminently calculated to benefit the community at large, as well as to improve the condition of medical men.

The general principle only can now be proposed; its execution must be the result of much deliberation. It is proper, however, to acquaint you with two things; *1st*, That the scheme now under consideration does not interfere with any of the rights or privileges of the Colleges of Physicians and Surgeons. *2dly*, That these learned bodies do not possess powers for regulating the practice beyond the distance of seven miles from London, whatever may be their good dispositions for the benefit of society at large; consequently there exists no legal control over any person, however illiterate and ignorant, who ventures to assume the medical profession beyond these limits.

In order to facilitate the communication of the necessary information, I have taken the liberty of submitting to your judgment, and of requesting answers to the queries subjoined. The arrangement of free postage having been unavoidably delayed, a very early return to this letter is earnestly requested, to expedite the attainment of the desired object in the present session of Parliament.

I have the honour to be

Your faithful and very obedient, humble servant,

EDW. HARRISON.

*** *Please to address your answers to Dr Harrison, Horncastle, Lincolnshire—under cover to the Right Honourable Nicholas Vansittart, Treasury, London.*

First Query. Are you acquainted with any persons in your district, who practise physic, and are at the same time known to be so deficient in medical science and literature, that they may be considered incompetent to the responsibility they take upon themselves?

2dly, What may be, in your opinion, the proportion of such incompetent persons, under the heads of physicians, surgeons, apothecaries, druggists, and practitioners in midwifery, compared to the number of those whose education and talents render them deserving of the confidence of their patients?

3dly, In particular, what may be the proportion of persons usually distinguished by the appellation of quacks or empirics?

4thly, Do you find that the chymists and druggists, and other venders of drugs, are constantly supplied with medicines of such qualities, and with preparations in such a state, as a due regard for the public security obliges you to require? And do any of those persons interfere with the practice of physic or surgery?

5thly, What alterations appear to be wanted in your circuit to render the practice of physic most useful to the community?

N. B. It is by no means wished that the name of any incompetent person should be mentioned in the answers to these queries.

ROYAL

ROYAL JENNERIAN SOCIETY, FOR THE EXTERMINATION OF THE SMALL-POX.

At a Special Meeting of the Board of Directors, held at the Central House of the Society, No. 14. Salisbury Square, November 25. 1805. The Report of the Medical Council on the subject of Vaccine Inoculation having been laid before the Board,

RESOLVED,—That the same be immediately printed under the direction of the Medical Council, and that they be requested to subjoin their individual signatures to the Report for publication.

(Extracted from the Minutes,)

CHARLES MURRAY, *Secretary.*

REPORT.

THE Medical Council of the Royal Jennerian Society, having been informed that various cases had occurred which excited prejudices against vaccine inoculation, and tended to check the progress of that important discovery in this kingdom, appointed a Committee of twenty-five of their members to inquire, not only into the nature and truth of such cases, but also into the evidence respecting instances of small-pox alleged to have occurred twice in the same person.

In consequence of this reference, the Committee made diligent inquiry into the history of a number of cases in which it was supposed that vaccination had failed to prevent the small-pox, and also of such cases of small-pox as were stated to have happened subsequently to the natural or inoculated small-pox.

In the course of their examination the Committee learned that opinions and assertions had been advanced and circulated, which charged the cow-pock with rendering patients liable to particular diseases, frightful in their appearance, and hitherto unknown; and judging such opinions to be connected with the question as to the efficacy of the practice, they thought it incumbent upon them to examine also into the validity of these injurious statements respecting vaccination.

After a very minute investigation of these subjects, the result of their inquiries has been submitted to the Medical Council; and from the report of the Committee it appears,

I. That most of the cases which have been urged in proof of the inefficacy of vaccination, and which have been the subjects of public attention and conversation, are either wholly unfounded or grossly misrepresented.

II. That other cases, brought forward as instances of the failure of vaccination to prevent the small-pox, are now allowed, by the very persons who first related them, to have been erroneously stated.

III. That the statements of the greater part of those cases have been already carefully investigated, ably discussed, and fully refuted, by different writers on the subject.

IV.

IV. That, notwithstanding the most incontestable proofs of such misrepresentations, a few medical men have persisted in repeatedly bringing the same unfounded and refuted reports and misrepresentations before the public; thus perversely and disingenuously labouring to excite prejudices against vaccination.

V. That in some printed accounts adverse to vaccination, in which the writers had no authenticated facts to support the opinions they advanced, nor any reasonable arguments to maintain them, the subject has been treated with indecent and disgusting levity; as if the good or evil of society were fit objects for sarcasm and ridicule.

VI. That when the practice of vaccination was first introduced and recommended by Dr Jenner, many persons who had never seen the effects of the vaccine fluid on the human system, who were almost wholly unacquainted with the history of vaccination, the characteristic marks of the genuine vesicle, and the cautions necessary to be observed in the management of it, and were therefore incompetent to decide whether patients were properly vaccinated or not, nevertheless ventured to inoculate for the cow-pock.

VII. That many persons have been declared duly vaccinated, when the operation was performed in a very negligent and unskilful manner, and when the inoculator did not afterwards see the patients, and therefore could not ascertain whether infection had taken place or not; and that to this cause are certainly to be attributed many of the cases adduced in proof of the inefficacy of cow-pock.

VIII. That some cases have been brought before the Committee on which they could form no decisive opinion, from the want of necessary information as to the regularity of the preceding vaccination, or the reality of the subsequent appearance of the small-pox.

IX. That it is admitted by the Committee, that a few cases have been brought before them of persons having the small-pox, who had apparently passed through the cow-pock in a regular way.

X. That cases, supported by evidence equally strong, have been also brought before them of persons who, after having once regularly passed through the small-pox, either by inoculation or natural infection, have had that disease a second time.

XI. That in many cases, in which the small-pox has occurred a second time after inoculation or the natural disease, such recurrence has been particularly severe, and often fatal; whereas, when it has appeared after vaccination, the disease has generally been so mild, as to lose some of its characteristic marks, and, in many instances, to render its existence doubtful.

XII. That it is a fact well ascertained, that, in some particular states of certain constitutions, whether vaccine or variolous matter be employed, a local disease only will be excited by inoculation, the constitution remaining unaffected; yet that matter taken from such local vaccine or variolous pustule is capable of producing a general and perfect disease.

XIII. That if a person bearing the strongest and most indubitable marks of having had the small-pox be repeatedly inoculated for that

that diſeaſe, a puſtule may be produced, the matter of which will communicate the diſeaſe to thoſe who have not been previouſly infected.

XIV. That, although it is difficult to determine preciſely the number of exceptions to the practice, the Medical Council are fully convinced that the failure of vaccination, as a preventive of the ſmall-pox, is a very rare occurrence.

XV. That of the immenſe number who have been vaccinated in the army and navy, in different parts of the United Kingdom, and in every quarter of the globe, ſcarcely any inſtances of ſuch failure have been reported to the Committee, but thoſe which are ſaid to have occurred in the metropolis, or its vicinity.

XVI. That the Medical Council are fully aſſured, that in very many places, in which the ſmall-pox raged with great violence, the diſeaſe has been ſpeedily and effectually arreſted in its progreſs, and in ſome populous cities almoſt wholly exterminated, by the practice of vaccination.

XVII. That the practice of inoculation for the ſmall-pox, on its firſt introduction into this country, was oppoſed and very much retarded in conſequence of miſrepreſentations and arguments drawn from aſſumed facts, and of miſcarriages ariſing from the want of correct information, ſimilar to thoſe now brought forward againſt vaccination, ſo that nearly fifty years elapſed before ſmall-pox inoculation was fully eſtabliſhed.

XVIII. That, by a reference to the bills of mortality, it will appear that, to the unfortunate neglect of vaccination, and to the prejudices raiſed againſt it, we may, in a great meaſure, attribute the loſs of nearly two thouſand lives by the ſmall-pox, in this metropolis alone, within the preſent year.

XIX. That the few inſtances of failure, either in the inoculation of the cow-pock or of the ſmall-pox, ought not to be conſidered as objections to either practice, but merely as deviations from the ordinary courſe of nature.

XX. That, from all the facts which they have been able to collect, it appears to the Medical Council that the cow-pock is generally mild and harmleſs in its effects; and no inſtance has come to their knowledge in which there was reaſon to admit that vaccine inoculation had of itſelf produced any new or dangerous diſeaſe, as has been ignorantly and unwarrantably aſſerted; but that the few caſes which have been alleged againſt this opinion may be fairly attributed to other cauſes.

XXI. That, if a compariſon be made between the effects of vaccination and thoſe of inoculation for the ſmall-pox, it would be neceſſary to take into account the greater number of perſons who have been vaccinated within a given time; it being probable, that within the laſt ſeven years, nearly as many perſons have been inoculated for the cow-pock as were ever inoculated for the ſmall-pox, ſince the practice was introduced into this kingdom.

XXII.

XXII. That many well-known cutaneous diseases, and some scrofulous complaints, have been represented as the effects of vaccine inoculation, when, in fact, they originated from other causes, and in many instances occurred long after vaccination, but that such diseases are infinitely less frequent after vaccination than after either the natural or inoculated small-pox.

Having stated these facts, and made these observations, the Medical Council cannot conclude their report upon a subject highly important and interesting to all classes of the community, without making this solemn declaration,

That, in their opinion, founded on their own individual experience, and the information which they have been able to collect from that of others, mankind have already derived great and incalculable benefit from the discovery of vaccination; and that it is their full belief, that the sanguine expectations of advantage and security, which have been formed from the inoculation of the cow-pock, will be ultimately and completely fulfilled.

Edwd. Jenner, M.D. President.
J. C. Lettsom, M.D. V. P.
John Ring, V. P.
Joseph Adams, M.D.
John Addington
C. R. Aikin
Wm Babington, M.D.
M. Baillie, M.D.
W. Blair
Gil. Blane, M. D.
Isaac Buxton, M. D.
Wm Chamberlaine
John Clarke, M. D.
Astley Cooper
Wm. Daniel Cordell
Richard Croft, M.D.
Tho. Denman, M.D.
John Dimsdale
Henry Field
Edward Ford
Joseph Fox
Will. M. Fraser, M.D.
William Gaitskell
Will. Hamilton, M. D.
John Hingeston
Everard Home
Robert Hooper, M.D.
Joseph Hurlock
John Jones
Tho. Key
Francis Knight
E. Leese
L. Leese
William Lewis
William Lister, M.D.
Alex. Marcet, M.D.
Joseph Hart Myers, M. D.
James Parkinson
Tho. Paytherus
John Pearson
George Rees, M.D.
John Gibbs Ridout
J. Squire, M.D.
James Upton
J. Christian Wachsell
Thomas Walshman, M. D.
Robert Willan, M.D.
Allen Williams
James Wilson
J. Yelloly, M. D.

John Walker, *Secretary to the Council.*

Report of the Surgeons of the Vaccine Institution at the Public Dispensary of Edinburgh for 1805.

The Surgeons of the Vaccine Institution at the Public Dispensary of Edinburgh have much pleasure in reporting to the Managers that the inoculation for the cow-pock goes on with uninterrupted success.

Since the last general meeting they have inoculated 1658, being 221 more than were inoculated during the former year, and making in all 5371 since the commencement of the institution in February 1801.

In consequence of some recent publications against vaccination, particularly asserting that it operates as a preventive of small-pox only for four years, and that it produces new and dangerous diseases, the Surgeons have lately examined personally a great number of those children who were inoculated at this institution in the beginning of the year 1801, and have found that many of them have, within these three months, been freely exposed to the contagion of the natural small-pox in several quarters of the city, where this loathsome disease has unfortunately been very prevalent, without having been infected; and they beg leave particularly to notice, that they have not found one single instance, in which obstinate eruptions, or any new and dangerous diseases, have been produced in consequence of the introduction among mankind of this mild preventive of the small-pox.

Wm. Farquharson.
James Bryce.
Alex. Gillespie.
J. Abercrombie.

Account of Diseases treated at the Public Dispensary, Carey-Street, from 30th November 1805, to 28th February 1806.

CHRONIC DISEASES.

	No. of Cases.		No. of Cases.
Cephalæa	15	Chlorosis	1
Vertigo	2	Hysteria	8
Catarrhus Chronicus	67	Hypochondriasis	1
Asthma and Dyspnœa	16	Epilepsia	3
Hœmoptysis and Phthisis	20	Paralysis	4
Asthenia	22	Amaurosis	1
Dyspepsia	29	Rheumatismus Chronicus	34
Icterus	2	Lumbago	5
Constipatio	3	Pleurodyne	2
Hæmorrhois	5	Dysphagia	1
Tabes Mesenterica	7	Blenorrhœa	1
Vermes	6	Ascites	2
Enterodynia	9	Anasarca	7
Diarrhœa	12	Rachitis	1
Nephralgia	2	Prolapsus Uteri	1
Dysuria	7	Prurigo	3
Ischuria	2	Scrophula	3
Hæmaturia	1	Impetigo	6
Menorrhagia	4	Purpura	1
Leucorrhœa	4	Scabies	12
Amenorrhœa	11		

ACUTE

ACUTE DISEASES.

	No. of Cases.		No. of Cases.
Typhus	1	Variola conferta	1
Ephemera	3	Pertuſſis	6
Quotidiana	1	Rheumatiſmus	11
Cynanche tonſillaris	9	Podagra	2
——— parotidæa	1	Arthritis rheumatica *	10
Hemicrania	2	Dyſenteria	10
Hydrocephalus	2	Peritonitis puerperarum	1
Epiſtaxis	1	Inflammatio pudendi	1
Catarrhus	73	Febris poſt Partum	1
Pneumonia	10	Eryſipelas	2
Peripneumonia notha	8	Febris Infantum	3

The ſeaſon has been, on the whole, extremely mild, and the rains much more frequent than is uſual at this ſeaſon of the year. The firſt ten days of December were moderate in temperature, with the wind from S. W. to N. W.; a froſt of ſix or ſeven days enſued; and the remainder of the month was wet, with ſome gales from the S. W. This weather continued to the end of January, with the exception of the 10th and 11th, on which a ſlight froſt and a heavy hail-ſtorm occurred. February was uſhered in by a few days of moderate froſt; but, ſince the firſt week, the temperature of the air has been mild, with occaſional ſhowers and light gales of wind.

The metropolis ſtill continues, in an extraordinary degree, free from epidemic and contagious diſeaſes. One caſe of typhous fever, and one caſe of confluent ſmall-pox, both of which occurred in December, are the only inſtances of contagious diſeaſe which have fallen under our notice, with the exception of a few caſes of hooping-cough among children. The prevalence of the ſmall-pox has diminiſhed greatly ſince our laſt report, and has been conſiderably leſs fatal.

The catarrhal complaints have been, as uſual, numerous; and aſthmatics have ſuffered very ſeverely. In the former part of the period comprehended by this report, the inſtances of pneumonia continued to be connected with ſymptoms of great debility, and in ſeveral caſes proved fatal from effuſion and conſequent ſuffocation. But, during the preſent month, caſes of peripneumonia notha have been leſs frequent.

The moſt common form of the ſtomach complaints which appear at the Diſpenſary is the gaſtrodynia, or ſtomach-colic. This is a ſevere burning or ſtabbing pain about the region of the ſtomach, generally returning at intervals, but frequently, without any complete intermiſſion; and is accompanied with a loathing of food, occaſionally with vomiting, and often with that peculiar diſcharge of a clear watery fluid from the ſtomach which has been conſidered by Dr Cullen as a diſtinct genus of diſeaſe, under the title of pyroſis, or water-braſh. There is generally alſo a tendency to conſtipation.

2 In

* Sauvages Noſol. Chap. VII. Ord. I. Spec. 2.

In one of the instances, in which this pain was accompanied with extreme irritability of stomach, which rejected almost every thing for several days, and for many weeks bore very little, a numbness and debility of the fingers, first of one hand, and afterwards of the other, resembling the partial paralysis from lead, took place; this gradually increased, till the whole of both arms became absolutely paralytic, accompanied with great pains in the limbs and back. I must make my acknowledgments to Dr Hamilton * for the relief which I have been able to afford this patient. The bowels were not greatly constipated; the stools, however, were black, offensive, and of unhealthy consistence; and by frequent exhibitions of doses of about gr. iii. of calomel alone (for she bore this when every other medicine was rejected), the stomach was gradually brought to considerable strength, the pains have ceased, and the elbows and wrists have greatly recovered their motion; the fingers, however, remain considerably paralyzed. Whenever she neglected her bowels for two or three days, the irritability of stomach threatened to return, her pains increased, and her limbs became obviously more useless. It may be observed, that she has had electric sparks and slight shocks passed through the arms repeatedly of late, but without the smallest effect on the paralysis. The patient is a weak and delicate married woman, who has long laboured under considerable anxiety of mind. Her complexion is sallow, and her pulse generally small and frequent.

I have adopted the term *arthritis rheumatica* from Sauvages, to express a modification of rheumatism, which is not accurately expressed by the terms acute or chronic rheumatism; it is, in common language, called rheumatic gout. It is more properly an acute but partial attack of rheumatism, marked by a swelling, pain, and tension of the soft parts surrounding one or more of the larger joints, accompanied with a bright and shining redness of the skin, as in gout; not however, like the latter disease, occurring periodically, or connected with disorders of the digestive organs, or terminating by the deposition of concretions of urate of soda. I mention it more particularly with a view to the remedy which I have successfully employed; I mean the external application of *cold water*. This expedient has been lately adopted, in every instance which has come under my care, invariably with temporary relief, generally with speedy and permanent benefit, and never with any appearance of untoward consequences. A lotion of water and vinegar, or of equal portions of water and aqua ammoniæ acetatæ, has generally been used. This modification of local inflammation, being unconnected with the stomach, seemed to be without any probable danger of *retrogression*, and the event has hitherto accorded with this anticipation.

T. B.

28th February 1806.

TO

* The author of a late, excellent, and truly philosophical treatise "on the use of purgative medicines," which has contributed to throw much new light on some obscure diseases.

TO THE EDITORS OF THE MEDICAL AND SURGICAL JOURNAL.

GENTLEMEN,

The following statement of the number of patients admitted under the care of the Physicians and Surgeons of the Liverpool General Dispensary in the year 1805, and also of the diseases under which they have laboured, will, I hope, be acceptable to you. I will vouch for the statement being a correct one, having had a principal share in the investigation of the numbers, and in the arrangement of the diseases, myself. Should you think the list worth inserting in your next Number, have the goodness to give it a place therein.

Yours very respectfully,

JA. DAWSON.

Mount Pleasant,
Feb. 25. 1806.

List of Diseases in 1805.

Febres continuæ	795	Catarrhus	94
—— Intermittentes	35	Dysenteria	178
Inflammatio	91	Diarrhœa et Cholera	388
Ophthalmia	415	Apoplexia	12
Gangrena et Sphacelus	10	Paralysis	400
Cephalalgia et Vertigo	145	Hemiplegia	16
Cynanche tonsillaris	200	Hemicrania	26
Cynanche maligna	8	Paraplegia	5
Cynanche trachealis	15	Syncope	5
Pneumonia	67	Dyspepsia	328
Rheumatismus	656	Chlorosis	8
Variola	141	Vomitus	27
Varricella	12	Gastritis	4
Vaccinatio	1723	Enteritis	6
Rubeola	19	Hepatitis	4
Scarlatina	80	Nephritis	22
—— Anginosa	68	Peritonitis	3
Erysipelas	57	Hypochondriasis	21
Urticaria	9	Amenorrhœa	200
Aphthæ	110	Spasmi	16
Epistaxis	35	Convulsio	71
Hæmoptysis	76	Tetanus	10
Hæmatemesis	20	Chorea Sancti Viti	20
Phthisis	255	Epilepsia	57
Hæmorrhois	70	Palpitatio	65
Menorrhagia	97	Asthma	174
Leucorrhœa	63	Tussis et Dyspnœa	692
Blenorrhœa	14	Tussis convulsiva	125
Hæmaturia	18	Colica	100
Abortio	53	—— Pictonum	20

Diabetes

Diabetes	20	Schirrus & Cancer	28
Hyſteria	151	Polypus Naſi	12
Melancholia	2	Hernia	85
Inſania	8	——— incarcerata	5
Debilitas	226	Prolapſus Uteri	55
Maraſmus	6	Prolapſus Ani	38
Tabes Meſenterica	4	Luxatio et Diſtentio	85
Hydrops et Anaſarca	233	Amputatio	9
Aſcites	40	Vulnus, Contuſio, et Fractura	453
Hydrochephalus	9	Abſceſſus, Ulcus, et Uſtio	378
Congeſtio Capitis	10	Curvatura Spinæ	9
Hydrothorax	10	Tumor & Induratio	138
Hydrocele	6	Fiſtulæ	4
Rachitis	18	Herpes	30
Scrophula	145	Tinea Capitis	55
Syphilis et Gonorrhœa	799	Pſora	835
Scorbutus	21	Caries	10
Icterus	40	Hydrarthus	10
Amauroſis	16	Calculus Veſicæ	28
Dyſecœa	4	Vermes	246
Eneureſis	24	Dentitio	18
Obſtipatio	280		
Nephralgia	60		13,138
Aneuriſmus	3		

A Notice on the Preſence of the Phoſphat of Magneſia in Bones. Communicated by Mr Fourcroy to the Annales du Muſée d'Hiſtoire Naturelle, 36th Cahier.

The diſcovery of a new earthy phoſphat in the bones of animals is an intereſting fact in the hiſtory of phyſical ſcience. It was effected two years ago by Mr Vauquelin and myſelf, during the courſe of experiments which we were making on animal concretions, and of which we have frequently preſented the reſults to the public.

We had already diſcovered, *1ſt*, The preſence of the ammoniaco-magneſian phoſphat among the conſtituent principles of the urinary calculi in the human ſubject, and of the inteſtinal concretions in other animals; *2d*, That the phoſphat of magneſia exiſts in the urine of man, and is there characterized by the property of forming a triple cryſtallized ſalt, when urine gives out ammonia from its ſpontaneous decompoſition. It became, therefore, important to aſcertain whether that magneſian ſalt, formerly unknown in animal ſubſtances, might not likewiſe be preſent in ſome organs. Bones, which bear the greateſt analogy in their compoſition to urinary concretions, offered themſelves firſt to our inveſtigation; and although their analyſis appeared to have been already carried to a great degree of perfection, the new ſet of experiments to which they have been ſubjected has ſhown in them another conſtituent ſalt, by proceſſes, indeed, more complicated than thoſe which had been hitherto employed in that ſpecies of analyſis.

In

In order to discover the phosphat of magnesia in bones, well calcined and pulverized bones are treated with an equal weight of sulphuric acid; the mixture is allowed to stand for five or six days, is then diluted, first with ten times, and afterwards with five times its weight of water, filtrated each time and strained; ammonia is added in excess to the liquor, which, instead of phosphoric acid only, as was formerly supposed, contains phosphat of lime, and phosphat of magnesia, both held in solution by phosphoric acid, and in proportion as that excess of acid is saturated with the volatile alkali, a mixture of calcareous and ammoniaco-magnesian phosphat falls to the bottom. That precipitate is washed with some cold distilled water, and treated with some caustic potash, till the ebullition disengages no more ammonia. The ammoniaco-magnesian phosphat is decomposed by that process; the ammonia is volatilized, the acid unites with the potash, and the salt thus formed remains in a state of solution: magnesia is deposited at the bottom, and mixed there with calcareous phosphat. The liquor is then decanted, the precipitate washed, and boiling distilled vinegar is poured upon it, which dissolves the magnesia without attacking the phosphat of lime. The acetat of magnesia is then decomposed by carbonat of soda; the carbonat of magnesia resulting from that decomposition is dried, its weight determined; and, upon adding to it sulphuric acid, sulphat of magnesia is formed, under which form the presence of that earth is more easily determined.

In repeating the above process several successive times, in order to ascertain the reality of the presence of the magnesian phosphat in the bones of animals, or to determine its relative quantity, we have observed that the acetic acid always dissolved some lime along with the magnesia, while that lime could only come from the decomposition of a small part of the calcareous phosphat by the potash. Thus, notwithstanding our present laws of chemical affinities, it seems to be an ascertained fact, that potash may disengage lime from phosphoric acid, though in very small quantity, and that only when the quantity of the potash employed bears a large proportion to that of the phosphoric salt, whereas lime takes entirely and completely the phosphoric acid from the potash. We have here an instance of the influence of masses pointed out by Mr Berthollet, to explain apparent anomalies in the play of elective attractions.

Calcined ox bones contain about 1-40th of phosphat of magnesia.

The bones of the horse and sheep 1-36th.

Those of the chicken and hare very nearly 1-40th.

We have never been able to extract it in any considerable quantity from human bones.

The bones of the ox, which have been most frequently the subject of our analytical researches, appear to us to have the following constituent parts.

Gelatin, (solid)	-	51
Phosphat of lime	-	37.7
Carbonat of lime	-	10
Phosphat of magnesia		1.3

The

The presence of the phosphat of magnesia in various parts of animals manifestly derives its origin from the food which they use. We have found that salt in barley, wheat, oats, &c.; it exists in the *cerealia* in the proportion of 1.5·100 of their weight, that is to say, in a proportion nearly double that of the calcareous phosphat which they contain. There is undoubtedly some connexion between that fact, and that of the existence of those intestinal concretions in animals which are composed of the ammoniaco-magnesian phosphat.

It is not very difficult to explain how it happens that bones in the human subject contain no magnesian phosphat, although that salt exists in larger quantity than the calcareous phosphat in wheat flour. It is probably carried away by the urine, where we have found it, while it is not discoverable in that excrementitious fluid in animals in which the skin or the intestines are the natural emunctories for that neutral salt.

Without laying too much stress on the influence of those chemical discoveries which result from the analysis of natural bodies, in illustrating the animals of economy, we can no longer overlook or neglect their more immediate applications. We may even confidentially expect that their sober multiplication will slowly promote and improve the science of physiology.

Dr Henderson is preparing for the press a translation of Cabanis' work, reviewed in the present Number.

TO CORRESPONDENTS.

We have received communications from Professor Rosenmuller, Leipsick, Mr Roberts, and from one of the surgeons of the Newcastle Dispensary; and the Memoirs of the Medical Society, vol. vi. Dr Buchan on sea-bathing, and Dr Lambe on spring-water, have been sent for analysis. The suggestions of Medicus and Tyro are under consideration; and the reviews of Dr Stock on cold, Dr Bourne on consumption, Fabbroni on the genus cinchona, and Dr Hunter on the diseases of Lascars, have been postponed for want of room.

ERRATA.

Vol. ii. p. 29. line 19. for *idiosynery*, read *idiosyncrasy*.
—— p. 139. 3 l. from bottom, for *us*, read *as*.
—— p. 143. l. 14. for *agitating*, read *agitations of*
—— p. 105. l. 22. for *master*, read *member*.

It is with much regret that we must call the attention of our readers to a most unlucky misprint in the sketch of the life of Dr Currie. It is there stated, page 47. line 2. from the bottom, that that illustrious character *had a* bad *memory for his friends, but not for his enemies.* By an inexcusable typographical interpolation, the biographer is thus made to record a censure on the memory of his deceased friend, when he intended a panegyric. We, therefore, request our readers to correct this important error, by deleting the injurious epithet.

*** Communications may be addressed to Mess.* Constable & Co. *Booksellers, Edinburgh*, Longman, Hurst, Rees, & Orme, *London; or* Gilbert & Hodges, *Dublin.*

No. VII *will be Published on Tuesday, July* 1. 1806.

THE

EDINBURGH
MEDICAL & SURGICAL JOURNAL.

JULY 1. 1806.

PART I.

ORIGINAL COMMUNICATIONS.

I.

Observations on the Structure of the Parts concerned in Crural Hernia. By ALLAN BURNS, Member of the Royal College of Surgeons in London, and Lecturer on Anatomy and Surgery in Glasgow.

HERNIA is a disease extremely frequent in its occurrence, always dangerous while it continues, and in its issue often fatal. Sometimes it is remediable without the performance of a surgical operation; at other times it is absolutely necessary to have recourse to the knife. Now, to enable the surgeon to act most advantageously on the prolapsed parts, in order to reduce them without cutting, or to operate with most ease to himself, and safety to his patient, he must obtain a thorough knowledge of the structure of the parts situated in the vicinity of the disease. In crural hernia, a correct acquaintance with the anatomy of the parts at the upper part of the thigh is of the highest value to the surgeon; for, not possessed of this information, he is extremely apt unintentionally to increase the obstacles to reduction, or, in operating, to injure parts he ought not to have touched; but, acquainted with the parts concerned, he knows how to obviate, in so far as can be done by art, the mechanical agents which resist the replacing of the gut, and he is made acquainted likewise with the safest and most advisable mode of operating.

Previous to the year 1768, little was known to anatomiſts with regard to the ſtructure, connexions, and relative ſituation of Poupart's ligament. It had till then been generally deſcribed as a diſtinct ligamentous production attached to the lower margin of the oblique muſcles, and extended from the ſpine of the ilium to the creſt of the pubes, poſſeſſed of but ſlight attachment by means of cellular membrane, to the parts in the vicinity. It was about this time that Mr Gimbernat, a Spaniſh ſurgeon, diſcovered two eſſential points reſpecting the formation of the crural arch. He found a ſeptum extended from the lower margin of the ligament, to be implanted into the brim of the pelvis, and he diſcovered ariſing from the inferior fifth of the arch, a membranous production, which is inſerted all along the linea pectinea. This duplicature may either be ſaid to ariſe from the femoral arch, or it may be deſcribed as taking its origin from an aponeuroſis to be afterwards deſcribed. In itſelf, it is triangular in ſhape, the apex looking to the ſymphyſis of the pubes, the one ſide fixed to the crural arch beneath the inguinal canal; the other attached to the pubes, and the creſcent ſhaped baſe turned toward the iliac vein. Theſe two proceſſes, diſcovered by Gimbernat, tend to bind down the arch, to retain it firmly in its ſituation, and, beſides, to divide it into two unequal portions. To the outer and largeſt diviſion he gave no name; to the inner, or the one neareſt the pubes, he gave the name of crural ring; and through this aperture, in which the iliac vein and a ſet of lymphatics are lodged, the herniary contents invariably protrude in femoral hernia.

After Mr Gimbernat, ſucceeding anatomiſts have, by their reſearches, continued to extend our acquaintance with the ſtructure of theſe parts; but ſtill from ſome diſſections made by my brother and myſelf during the ſummer of 1802, we have been led to ſuppoſe that ſome peculiarities had at that time remained unnoticed and undeſcribed, more eſpecially with regard to the ſtructure and connexion of the faſcia of the thigh; and it is theſe that I now chiefly intend to deſcribe.

By diſſecting away the peritoneum and adipoſe matter, we find that all the inner ſurface of the pelvis is lined with a pretty firm and denſe aponeuroſis, which completely covers the iliac and pſoac muſcles, and dips down into the cavity of the pelvis, covering the muſcles and ligaments there, as well as the bones. This aponeuroſis is ſeparable into at leaſt two layers; perhaps, by maceration, we may obſerve more. That portion of the aponeuroſis, which inverts the iliacus muſcle, is inſerted into the inner margin of the crural ligament, in the way which I am now to deſcribe. The aponeuroſis divides into two layers; one

one paſſes before the arteria circumflexa ilii, the other behind it; or, in other words, this veſſel inſinuates itſelf between the laminæ. The outer layer is inſerted into Poupart's ligament all the way from the ſpine of the ilium down to the point beneath which the femoral artery emerges from the abdomen; and, juſt at this ſpot, or rather a little nearer the ſpine of the ilium, a narrow production from the outer layer of the aponeuroſis runs forward, implanting itſelf into the crural arch beneath the ſulcus leading into the inguinal canal, and terminates in a pointed extremity directly over the entrance of the great vein. It turns upward along the internal ſurface of the abdominal muſcles, forming an internal faſcia. The inner lamina paſſes down behind the iliac veſſels, and incorporates itſelf with the aponeurotic expanſion covering the pſoas muſcle, is continued along the brim of the pelvis, dips down into the cavity of the pelvis, and expands over it, forming a general lining for the muſcles and bones; part alſo turns over the body of the pubes, or brim of the pelvis, and paſſes out on the thigh, forming a deep aponeuroſis behind the femoral veſſels, which may be traced expanding from the tendon of the pſoas and brim of the pelvis over the pectineus and triceps muſcles, and is ſeen afterwards uniting with the faſcia of the thigh. A little nearer the ſymphyſis of the pubes than the great vein, the outer layer of this aponeuroſis quits the bone, forming a duplicature, which riſes up to the inferior margin of the femoral ligament, and, having joined it, is continued with it all the way to its final implantation into the creſt of the pubes, forming thus a triangular membranous proceſs, whoſe apex is directed toward the ſymphyſis of the pubes; and the baſe, which is creſcent ſhaped, has the concavity directed toward the great vein. This duplicature has been deſcribed by Mr Gimbernat; and my friend Dr Monro junior, the preſent learned profeſſor of anatomy in Edinburgh, has aſcertained, by diſſection, that it is conſiderably broader in females than in males, which, by increaſing the diameter of the crural aperture, is, in his opinion, one reaſon why women are ſo much more ſubject to femoral hernia than men. And, in all thoſe caſes where we have had an opportunity of examining crural hernia, this ſeptum or duplicature has invariably been found to meaſure at leaſt one-third more, from its point of junction with the crural ligament, to its inſertion into the linea pectinea, than, in a healthy condition, it ought to have done. But whether this depth of the duplicature depended upon an original formation, or was the reſult of alterations induced by the protruded parts, is a queſtion not eaſily anſwered.

Next, it is to be remarked, that the aponeuroſis of the pſoas muſcle, as it extends along the bone, ſends up a duplicature or ſeptum between the great artery and vein, which is inſerted into the lower edge of Poupart's ligament, juſt beneath the termination of the point or narrow ſlip of the proceſs from the outer layer of the iliac aponeuroſis. It is alſo implanted into the under ſurface of the femoral faſcia, through the whole length of the thigh, accompanying the veſſels to that ſpot where they perforate the triceps tendon. This ſeptum ſeparates the artery from the vein, and divides the oval ſpace formed beneath the arch into two portions; the outer compartiment containing the tendon of the pſoas muſcle, the inner containing the great vein, and a ſet of lymphatic veſſels, with one or two ſmall glands, which fill up the vacant ſpace between the vein and the duplicature at the pubes. Theſe are the general contents of the crural foramen; ſometimes, however, the glands are wanting, and cellular matter ſupplies their place; and, more than once, I have obſerved this aperture almoſt cloſed up by a ligamentous expanſion ſtretched acroſs it. Indeed, no opening exiſted, if we except a ſmall perforation ſeated in the centre of this unnatural ſeptum.

Theſe different proceſſes, which are three in number, one at the iliac muſcle, one at the pubes, and a third between the great artery and vein, tend to bind down the crural arch more firmly, and to connect it better and more ſtrongly to the bone, and prevent its yielding ſo much as it would otherwiſe do; but this tenſion is ſtill more kept up by the faſcia of the thigh, which muſt next be examined: But, before doing ſo, I may mention, that ſometimes an unnatural aperture is found ſituated between the crural foramen and the lower margin of the inguinal canal, formed in the line of junction of Gimbernat's duplicature with the crural arch, and placed near to the creſcentic edge of the former. Now, when protruſion takes place through this vacuity, then a particular ſpecies of hernia is produced; for the tumour lies behind the ſpermatic cord, yet follows its courſe, partaking thus, in ſome reſpects, of the nature of both crural and inguinal hernia. It is not a frequent occurrence to find this foramen, yet, in two inſtances, I have met with it.

The faſcia conſiſts of two layers, the outer thin and cellular, the inner firmer, thicker, and more membranous. The outer layer deſcends from the aponeuroſis covering the external oblique muſcles, and is traced attached to the whole extent of the crural arch, and ſpreading down the thigh over all the veſſels and glands; but its ſtrength and thickneſs are inconſiderable, and it looks almoſt like firm, cellular ſubſtances, except in the fœtus, where it has a diſtinct fibrous appearance, and the ſtriæ run tranſverſe, which diſtinguiſhes this layer from the inner,

inner, in which they all tend from above downward. The inner lamina arifes only from the outer part of the arch, from that portion which extends from the ilium to the femoral vein; it keeps the ligament tenfe, and all the mufcles firm. Juft where this layer ceafes to arife from the arch, we find the fuperficial vein entering, and therefore this vein is not covered with the inner or principal layer of the fafcia, and, on diffecting away the vein, we fee ftill better the ftructure of thefe parts: we find that the fafcia ftops juft at the entrance of this vein, and, in many cafes, it terminates abruptly with a neat, firm margin, which is traced fome way down the thigh. The edge is lunated, and the concavity is directed toward the pubes, or fuperficial vein. This is the ufual appearance of the parts; fometimes, however, the ftructure is not quite fo diftinct, for occafionally a confiderable quantity of reticular cellular matter is placed about, and adheres to the crefcentic margin of the fafcia. Neverthelefs, in every inftance, this lunated edge may be difcovered, by paffing the finger from the abdomen through the crural ring, and preffing outward; and by diffection it may be clearly demonftrated in emaciated, anafarcous fubjects. It has been named by my brother the falciform procefs, or margin of the fafcia; and is highly worthy of notice, for, as we fhall afterwards fee, it performs an important part in femoral hernia, and a knowledge of its fituation and connexion elucidates fome points in the pathological hiftory of this difeafe. The top, then, of the pectineus, and long head of the triceps, is not covered by this fafcia; but, as I have already remarked, they are covered by a firm aponeurofis, into which we trace the invefting fheath of the pfoas. About an inch and a half below the creft of the pubes, the pectineal aponeurofis fends off a procefs or duplicature to be inferted into the under furface of the fafcia, at a very little diftance from the falciform procefs; and this duplicature divides the fuperficial vein and lymphatics, which enter with it completely from the large veffels lying beneath the fafcia; and over the edge of this procefs we, in general, find an oblong conglobat gland folded, one half ftretching beneath the aponeurofis; the other defcends above it, and thus between the two portions this duplicature is interpofed. On the outer fide of the duplicature we difcover the vena faphena lying in a hollow or channel, which is covered only by the fuperficial thin layer of fafcia, and which leads us up to the crural foramen of Gimbernat, fituated between the great vein and the crefcentic fold at the pubes; and, in femoral hernia, it is in this hollow, which may be called the vagina of the faphenic vein, that the gut is lodged. Whenever it comes out, it is feparated from the great veffels

 by

by the ſeptum, or proceſs which I have deſcribed as ariſing from the pectineal aponeuroſis, and it is bound down not only by the arch at the crural aperture, but alſo by the falciform proceſs, after it has got beyond the ring; and thus there is a double ſource of ſtrangulation, and the gut being tied down thus firmly, and alſo covered with the thin layer of the faſcia, has a hard feel, a flattened ſurface, and its ſac lies on the pectineus muſcle, and fills up completely the vagina of the ſuperficial vein, and the protruded parts are difficult of reduction. In inguinal hernia we can graſp the tumour in our hand, and entirely ſurround its baſe, which gives us a great command over its contents. But this advantage we are deprived of in crural hernia, for in it the tumour is flat, narrower above than below, and often doubled back upon itſelf, the one portion lying in the vagina of the vein, the other folded over the falciform proceſs of the faſcia, and the inverted edge of Gimbernat's duplicature; for the one is a continuation of the other; and, in femoral hernia, from the ſtructure of the parts, the upper horn of the creſcentic duplicature at the pubes is frequently protruded before the gut; a fact, if I am not miſinformed, which has been aſcertained by Mr John Thomſon, profeſſor of ſurgery in Edinburgh. This turning up of the tumour has been fully deſcribed by Dr Monro; and Mr Charles Bell aſſures us, that the receſſion depends upon a rupture of the faſcia. But this is a ſuppoſition to which we cannot aſſent; for it would in reality ſeem to depend upon the upper part of the tumour being confined by the vagina of the vein; while, on the other hand, the inferior part of it is allowed to expand from the deficiency of the faſcia, immediately after it has emerged from beneath the falciform margin. By this want, and by the pectineal aponeuroſis riſing up to join the femoral faſcia, the tumour is naturally elevated at this ſpot conſiderably above its original level; and this, it is evident, cannot be accompliſhed without giving the inferior part a tendency to incline upward from the leſs reſiſtance in that direction. From this tilting of the tumour, one of the ſtrongeſt proofs, independent of diſſection, of the exiſtence of a falciform proceſs may be drawn; as, without ſome conſtruction of this kind, this phenomenon never could take place; and the farther out and leſs perfect the falciform proceſs is, the more obſcure this elevation of the herniary tumour muſt of courſe be; and this, together with the inaccuracy of ſome examinations, is a ſufficient explanation of the fact, that the tilting is not invariably detected.

Further, with regard to the falciform proceſs, I have yet another remark to offer, and that is, to beware of attempting reduction by the taxis, without first considering and obviating, as far as it is possible to do so, the obstacles retarding the accomplishment of this end. We have already seen that the tumour in crural hernia is frequently doubled back upon itself, and this retroversion we have pointed out as one source of embarrassment to the surgeon. Now, I must mention, that, in certain positions of the limb, the falciform process exerts a more powerful action upon the gut than it does in others, and thereby renders what is difficult still more so. To overcome this difficulty, it behoves the surgeon to study well the situation and connexion of this process, as, by a knowledge of its locality, he will be led to an acquaintance with its action. By reason of the mode of junction with the femoral ligament, the falciform process, when the limb is extended, and at the same time separated, and the toes rolled outwards, comes to gird the gut more powerfully than when the member is in an opposite direction. For, by abduction, extension, and rotation outwards, we endeavour to elongate the falciform process, which is, in femoral hernia, stretched over an arched surface formed by the upper segment of the sac; and this elongation, it is clear, can only be accomplished in one of two ways, either by removing to a greater distance from each other the individual fibres composing the process, or otherwise, by making the margin of the process sink into the tumour, whereby it will approach nearer to the straight line. And the latter is the most obvious mode; for we well know that fascia is not over and above extensive, and that, of consequence, while a less force will be sufficient to press it into the tumour, a greater one will not be employed to operate upon the process itself. Now, mark the effects of this action of the falciform process upon the gut: The tumour is divided into two portions, and the part immediately subjected to the pressure of the process is firmly and immoveably tied down, and, of course, resists every endeavour of the surgeon to replace it. He acts, as it were, upon a sand-glass; his endeavours are exerted to overcome a power to which he has unknowingly added potency. The contraction of the ring does not act more powerfully in preventing the restoration of the displaced parts, than does this other cause of strangulation, which it is, in a great measure, in our power to overcome, not, indeed, by force, but rather by the employment of artifice. Let us, therefore, before undertaking to reduce the parts by taxis, obviate, in as far as we can, all those obstacles which have a tendency to foil our wishes, and then we may, with a greater prospect of success, proceed to restore the gut.

From what has been already said, it will be evident, that after having premised the usual auxiliaries of this operation, such

ſuch as the warm bath, blood-letting, and the other depreſſing agents, the poſition of the limb next merits our regard; and on this head a very few words will ſerve to convey all the requiſite information. A ſhort ſentence will contain all the directions we have to give. Extend the leg, bend the hip joint, roll the toes inwards, and rather croſs the affected thigh over the other; and theſe done, we have, to the utmoſt of our ability, removed all the obviable mechanical obſtruction to the reſtoration of the gut into the ventral cavity. But how often this fails, is beſt known to thoſe engaged in actual practice. After the taxis has proved ineffectual, we have yet another reſource left, by the performance of a ſurgical operation, which never fails, if we wiſh it to permit of a return of the diſplaced parts, although even it often proves unſucceſsful in reſtoring the health.

To relieve the ſtrangulation, it has been propoſed to cut the ligament or arch, giving the inciſion various degrees of obliquity; but the objections to theſe are ſolid and well known. To avoid theſe, Mr Gimbernat propoſes to cut only the duplicature at the pubes: "Sed incidit in Scyllam, dum cupit vitare Charybdin;" for, in rare inſtances, the epigaſtric artery, as it comes off from the iliac, makes a ſweep inward, and lies on the duplicature, and the hernia comes down within the concavity or ſweep of the veſſel, and preſſes it on the very ſpot cut by Gimbernat; and whenever this is the caſe, which, it muſt be confeſſed, is not often, we ſhall divide not only the artery, but alſo the vas deferens, which always turns over the loop formed by the veſſel. But, even granting that the epigaſtric is in every inſtance ſafe, ſtill it is to be remarked, that the epigaſtric and obturator arteries, in many caſes, ariſe by a common trunk, and that the latter, after ſeparating from the former, often attaches itſelf to the creſcentic duplicature at the pubes, ſometimes by cellular membrane, ſometimes by ligamentous fibres, and not rarely by an intricate plexus of ſmall veins. Now, whenever this happens, the veſſel is, by the deſcent of the gut, brought into contact with the lunated edge of the production at the pubes, and muſt inevitably, in Gimbernat's mode of operating, come to be injured. It is equal in ſize to the epigaſtric, and it muſt be equally dangerous to divide either of theſe veſſels. It may be ſaid that this diſtribution is rare. I ſhall only reply, that we have, in the courſe of our obſervation, met with above thirty examples of it, and, in ſeveral of the ſubjects, it aroſe by a ſimilar origin on both ſides. In ſome rare caſes, even where the artery does come off along with the epigaſtric, it may ſtill be ſafe; but this is only when it is very

EDINBURGH MEDICAL & SURGICAL JOURNAL

Nº VII page 273.

Internal View
of the parts concerned in
CRURAL HERNIA

Fig. 1.

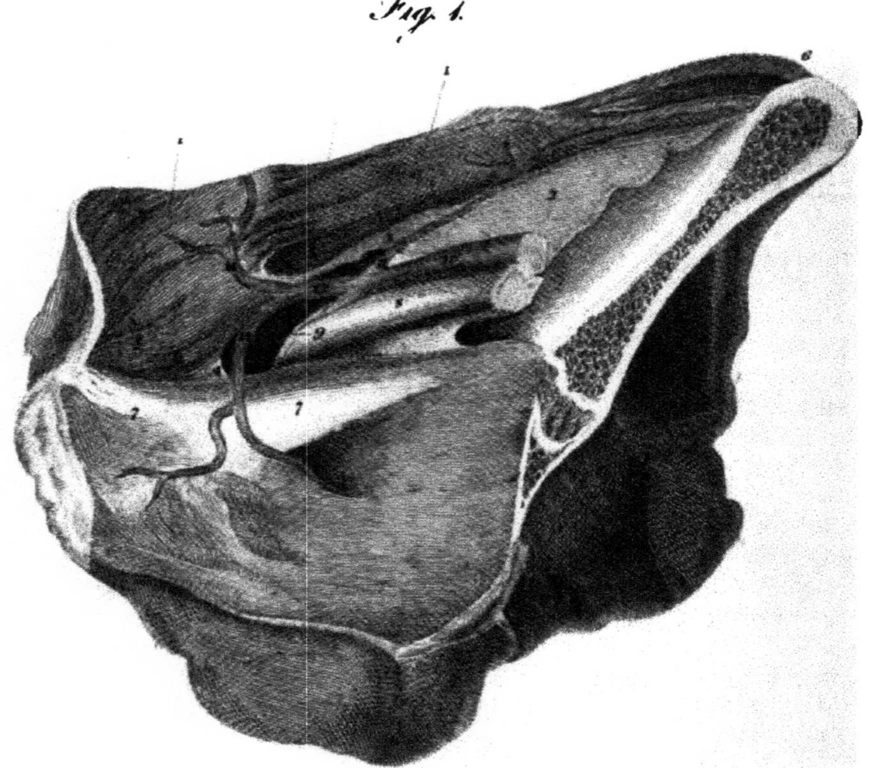

Published by A Constable & Cº — July 1806

J. T. Wedgwood, sculp.

very ſhort, and applied cloſe to the great vein, inſtead of the proceſs at the pubes.

There is, however, I imagine, in moſt herniæ, very little cutting neceſſary with a view to dilatation; for when the ſac is opened, and the inteſtine expoſed, we can act upon it for reduction with great advantage; but, when this is not practicable, we may have, only in femoral hernia, to divide the falciform proceſs of the faſcia with a pair of blunt-pointed ſciſſars, and this not only takes off one direct cauſe of ſtrangulation, but it is ſtill more uſeful by ſlacking the arch, and allowing it to yield at the crural ring; then if we open the ſac, and try to introduce the finger upward and outward, we can eaſily feel the tightening made by the margin of this proceſs. I have even felt it where the parts were completely gangrenous; and, after cutting it, and pulling out a little more of the gut, to make it change its poſition at the ring, and to deſtroy any adheſion which may exiſt, we may with eaſe return it.

To illuſtrate the deſcription, I have added two views, taken from a preparation made during the ſummer of 1802.

Explanation of Plate I. which is an internal view of the parts concerned in crural hernia.

1. The abdominal muſcles dried in ſitu. 2. The iliac aponeuroſis. From beneath it the fibres of the muſcle are cut away, ſo as to expoſe the coſta of the ilium. The poſterior part of the ala ilii is cut away. 3. The peak of the outer layer of the iliac aponeuroſis, ſhowing its implantation into the crural arch juſt over the exit of the great artery. 4. The duplicature at the pubes, diſcovered by Gimbernat. In this view, the ſeptum dividing the ſpace beneath the arch into two compartiments cannot be expreſſed. 5. The internal orifice of the inguinal canal. 6. The anterior ſuperior ſpine of the ilium. 7. The body of the pubes. 8. The external iliac vein. 9. The vacant ſpace between the vein and the duplicature at the pubes, named by Gimbernat the crural foramen, and through which the gut protrudes in femoral hernia. 10. The iliac artery. 11. The arteria circumflexa ilii, winding round the curve of the ilium between the two layers of the iliac aponeuroſis. 12. The common trunk of the epigaſtric and obturator arteries. 13. The obturator veſſel. This preparation illuſtrates the ſweep it makes in its courſe to the thyroid foramen, and exhibits the proximity of its coats to the creſcentic fold at the pubes. In a ſimilar diſtribution of this veſſel, the gut muſt, in crural hernia, invariably deſcend within the loop of the artery, preſſing it upon the lunated margin of the duplicature, or upon the very ſpot divided by Gimbernat. 14. The epigaſtric artery.

Fig.

Fig. II. explains the ſtructure of the parts at the top of the thigh.

(A) the ſpine of the ilium. (B) The tubercle of the pubes. (C) The abdominal muſcles. (D) The crural arch. (E) The external or inferior orifice of the inguinal canal. (F) The anterior fillet of the ſpermatic canal, ſeen terminating in the creſt of the pubes. (G) The poſterior faſciculus, ſhowing its twofold inſertion. The one diviſion implanted into the tubercle of the pubes, juſt behind the former, the other band comes along the triceps and gracilis muſcles, to reach, in ſome ſubjects, even to the gluteus tendon to which it is attached. (H) The inner layer of the femoral faſcia, or the faſcia vera. It is obſerved to take its riſe from the ſuperior and middle parts of the crural arch. (I) The falciform proceſs of the faſcia vera, ſeated juſt over the head of the pectineus muſcle, and in this ſubject peculiarly diſtinct, more ſo than in general. It is a continuation of Gimbernat's duplicature, which turns outwards, and its diviſion relaxes the crural arch as much as does the cutting of the creſcentic fold at the pubes. (K) The vena ſaphena, dipping in beneath the falciform proceſs to join the femoral vein. (L) The pſoas aponeuroſis emerging from the pelvis by the foramen crurale, and covering the heads of the triceps and pectineus muſcles, then ariſing at (M) from theſe muſcles, paſſing acroſs between the ſaphenic and femoral veins, and finally uniting itſelf to the faſcia vera. (N) The femoral artery ſeen through the dry and tranſparent faſcia. (O) A ſmall foramen in the faſcia, through which we traced a ſet of lymphatics paſſing in their way to the abdomen.

Glaſgow, 17th April, 1806.

II.

Obſervations on the State of the Venereal Diſeaſe in the South Sea Iſlands. By JOHN WILSON, Surgeon to his Majeſty's Ship Porpoiſe.

HIS Majeſty's ſhip Porpoiſe arrived for the firſt time at Otaheite from Port Jackſon in June 1801, and an inquiry reſpecting the diſeaſes of the iſland, but more particularly thoſe by which the

N° V [illegible] 274

External View

Fig. 2.

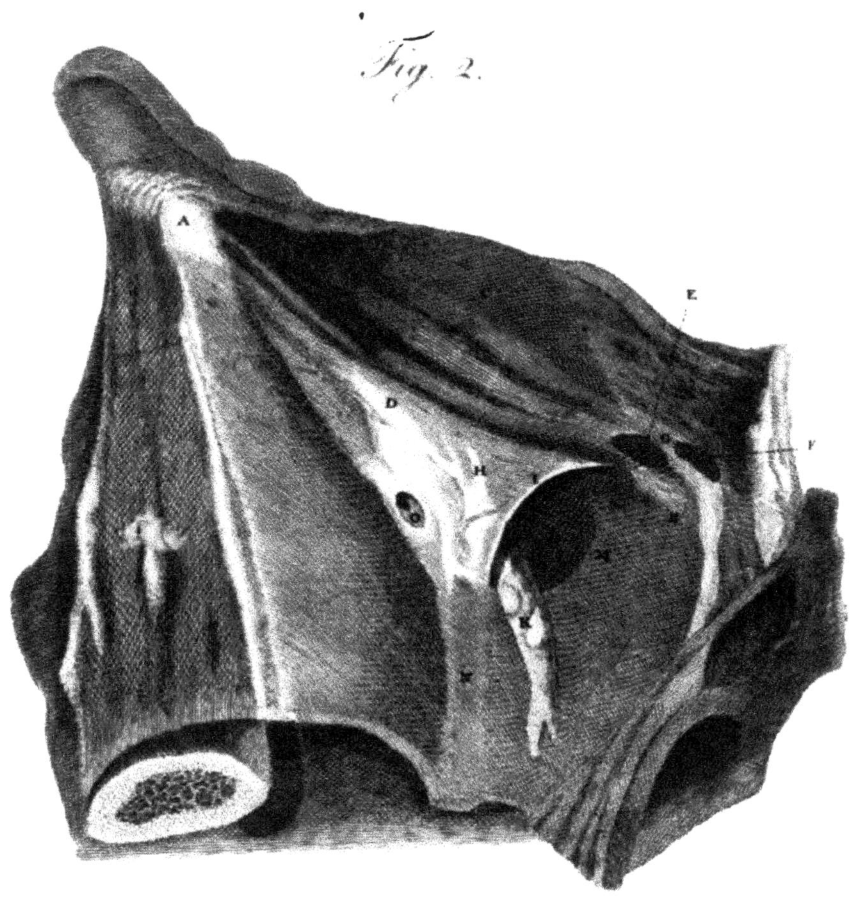

Published by A. Constable & C° — July 1806

I. T. [illegible]

the health of the ship's company might be affected, immediately became a part of my duty.

Having arrived at this island with a deep impression upon our minds of what we had read in voyages relative to the venereal disease, and its dreadful effects on the inhabitants, and as it was apprehended that its dissemination on board might eventually disable the ship from accomplishing the important service on which she was sent, this disease naturally claimed my first attention, in order that measures for preventing such a serious consequence might be recommended.

It also immediately occurred to me, that much useful information on this head might be obtained from the missionaries, who had been residents on the island for several years; and accordingly the first step taken towards ascertaining the most effectual preventive measures was to consult them.

From these gentlemen I received, without surprise, a farther confirmation of my ideas respecting the prevalency and fatality of lues venerea, to which, with good reason, we were fearful many of the ship's company would soon become victims, especially as it appeared, in a few days after our arrival, that an early application to the surgeon was almost the only practicable measure of precaution left us; restrictions being found not only to be inadmissible, but, from the necessary frequent intercourse of the ship's crew with the shore, to be unattended with the desired advantage.

Free admission into the ship was therefore given to the women soon after our arrival, and it may be easily imagined that the seamen did not fail to avail themselves of this indulgence; at the same time they were strictly enjoined to apply to me the moment any venereal symptom, however slight, made its appearance.

From this period it was expected that many venereal cases would occur; fortunately, however, our apprehensions were proved, by the result, to have been groundless; for after we had remained one month in Mattavai bay, during which time the connexions of the seamen with the native women were perfectly unrestrained, the venereal disease in no mode whatever appeared amongst them; and even in the remaining part of our visit, which was a space of nearly four weeks more, only three of them contracted gonorrhœa in a mild form, and were cured by injection alone in a few days.

The number of women, who were on board at different times during our stay in this voyage, amounted at least to two hundred, which was probably more than one fourth part of the whole of the young females at that time upon the island; and as these

theſe were certainly not the moſt chaſte part of the community, it muſt be from thence inferred, that gonorrhœa was at that period extremely uncommon amongſt them.

The total exemption of the inhabitants from lues venerea, and the unfrequency of gonorrhœa, both ſo irreconcileable with the accounts in voyages, and more eſpecially with the aſſertions of the miſſionaries, could not fail to excite ſurpriſe, and, at the ſame time, an attempt on my part to inveſtigate the merits of opinions ſo very repugnant to our experience; and the reſult of my inquiry proved, that the miſſionaries at leaſt had adopted erroneous opinions reſpecting the nature of the many tumours and ulcers which are to be met with among the inhabitants; for they did not heſitate to pronounce, that almoſt every tumour or ulcer, which came under their obſervation, had its origin in a venereal ſource.

Their miſtake originated partly from prejudice, and partly from being unqualified to diſcriminate; for they arrived at this iſland with as thorough a conviction of the prevalency of lues venerea amongſt the inhabitants as we did, and it cannot be ſuppoſed that any of them have much medical knowledge. At the ſame time it muſt be confeſſed, that the accounts of the natives often tended to confirm them in this error; for, from a kind of vain credulity, they believe, or rather pretend, that their iſland, before their intercourſe with ſtrangers, was free from moſt of the diſeaſes to which they are now ſubject; and thus lues venerea being, on all hands, allowed to be a foreign diſtemper, they of courſe moſt commonly aſcribe their ſores to that ſource.

I have now given an account of the venereal diſeaſe as it affected us in our firſt voyage, and it remains to be ſtated what came under obſervation in the ſecond.

In the interval between our departure from and arrival again at Otaheite in Auguſt 1802, the iſland was viſited at different periods by four ſmall veſſels from Port Jackſon, one of which, viz. the Norfolk colonial veſſel, was ſtranded in Mattavai bay, and her crew, to the amount of twenty-one, we found living on ſhore.

Soon after this our ſecond viſit, ſeveral of our ſhip's company were infected with gonorrhœa; and during two months continuance here, and one at the neighbouring iſland Eimeo, no leſs than thirty of them contracted it.

The ſymptoms were generally mild, and it often yielded to injection alone in three or four days. Only one caſe of ſwelled teſtes occurred, which took place four weeks after leaving the iſlands, and was the only one on board which was

not

not cured at that time. Several had alſo excoriations on the glans penis; but this ſymptom being always preceded by a diſcharge from the urethra, and obviouſly occaſioned by an inattention to cleanlineſs, no variation was obſerved in the treatment, and it always diſappeared on removing the cauſe.

The plan of cure adhered to was, to throw up an injection of zinc vitriolat. five or ſix times a-day, with occaſional laxatives; and if chordee was troubleſome, a grain or more of opium was adminiſtered at bed-time; but in no inſtance was any mercurial preparation uſed. The crew of the Norfolk were brought to Port Jackſon in the Porpoiſe, after having lived on ſhore eight or nine months; during which period none of them eſcaped the infection of gonorrhœa, yet no ſymptom of lues venerea had appeared amongſt them on our arrival in the colony, two months after leaving all the iſlands.

This great increaſe of gonorrhœa, ſince our former voyage, was no doubt occaſioned by the ſubſequent arrivals from Port Jackſon, but more particularly by the crew of the ſtranded veſſel, one of whom, it appeared, had arrived at the iſland with a virulent clap.

The intercourſe of theſe ſhips' companies, including our own, with the women, was carried to ſuch an extent, that I am well aſſured that, during their ſtay, they had connexion with nine-tenths of the whole of the young ones on the iſland.

This indelicate ſtatement is neceſſary, as it ſtrongly elucidates the ſubject on which I am writing, and ſupports inferences which are directly oppoſite to the generally received opinion reſpecting lues venerea, and its effects on the Otaheitians; and, in order to ſhow the authority on which that opinion has been founded, I have taken the liberty of giving the following extracts from Captain Cook's voyages. In the ſecond volume of the firſt voyage, he ſays, "Their commerce with us has entailed the venereal diſeaſe; and nothing is more certain than that, when we arrived, it had made moſt dreadful ravages in the iſland. One of our people contracted it five days after he went on ſhore." He ſays further, "That the natives ſaid it was brought by the veſſels which had been there about fifteen months before us, and that they diſtinguiſhed it by a name ſignifying rottenneſs, ſaying it cauſed the hair and nails to fall off, and the fleſh to rot from the bones; that it ſpread an univerſal terror among them, and that the ſick were abandoned to periſh alone." He obſerves in the ſame page, "We had ſome reaſon to hope that they had found a ſpecific remedy for it. During our ſtay we ſaw none on whom it had made a

great

great progress; and one who went from us infected returned after a short time in perfect health; and by this it appeared, either that the disease had cured itself, or that they were not unacquainted with the virtues of simples. If we could have learned their specific remedy for the venereal disease, if such they have, it would have been of great advantage to us; for when we left the island, it had been contracted by more than one half of the people on board."

SECOND VOYAGE, vol. i.

"The Otaheitians complained of a disease communicated to them by the people of this ship, which, they said, affected the head, throat, and stomach, and at length killed them. They seemed to dread it much, and were continually inquiring if we had it. This ship they distinguished by the name of *Pabai no Peppe*, just as they call the venereal disease *Apa no Pretane* (English disease), though they, to a man, say it was brought to the island by M. De Bougainville; but I have already observed that they thought M. De Bougainville came from Pretane, as well as every other ship that has touched at the isle. Were it not for this assertion of the natives, and none of Captain Wallis's people being affected with the venereal disease, either while they were at Otaheite, or after they left it, I should have concluded that, long before these islanders were visited by Europeans, this, or some disease which is near akin to it, had existed amongst them; for I have heard them speak of people dying of a disorder, which we interpreted to be the pox, before that period. But, be this as it will, it is now far less common amongst them than it was at the year 1769, when I first visited these isles. They say they can cure it, and so it fully appears; for, notwithstanding most of my people made pretty free with the women, very few of them were afterwards affected with the disease, and those who were had it in so slight a manner that it was easily removed; but amongst the natives, whenever it turns to a pox, they tell us it is incurable. Some of our people pretend to have seen some of them who had the last disorder in a high degree, but the surgeon, who made it his business to inquire, could never satisfy himself in this point. These people are, and were before Europeans visited them, very subject to scrofulous diseases, so that a seaman might easily mistake one disorder for another."

We are here only told by Captain Cook, in very general terms, that the venereal disease affected his ship's company, but unfortunately the symptoms are no where described. The marks of of the disease which were observed on the bodies of the natives are by no means conclusive, and their accounts of its effects do not correspond with the symptoms of lues venerea which usually occur with us.

The unequivocal symptoms of chancres and buboes about the pudenda do not appear to have been remarked; and indeed, as far as my observation went, I have reason to believe that an examination of the parts, which affords the most certain proof of the existence of venereal infection, was generally found to be impracticable; for although obscenity for the most part predominates in the dances and games of these people, yet, at any other time, as, for example, when they bathe, they are much more decorous in concealing, and infinitely more reluctant in exposing, these parts than Europeans. It must also be observed, that no dependence whatever should be placed on the accounts of the inhabitants, who, if they are to be credited, had few or no diseases amongst them before their intercourse with strangers; and they will, even at this time, name the particular English ships from which they pretend to have derived several of their complaints. But this is a topic which, above all others, they detest, and impart with no regard to truth whatever; for they apparently consider persons labouring under age or sickness in something of a criminal point of view, and under the immediate displeasure of some supernatural being.

Farther, Captain Cook's observing none in whom the disease had made great progress was certainly a contradiction to their assertions. Is it not more than probable that the native who went from the ship infected, and soon returned in good health, had nothing more than gonorrhœa? and also, that the mild disease, with which his own people were affected in the second voyage, was so likewise? The prevalency of scrofulous affections obviously appears to have led the captain into a mistake in the first voyage, and the doubts of his surgeon in the second, seem, in some degree, to have altered his opinion. That his concluding remark, that a seaman may easily mistake one disease for another, was well founded, will appear by the following extract from the same voyage.

Speaking of Rotterdam, or Anamocka, he says, "The people of this isle seem to be more affected with leprosy, or some scrofulous disorder, than any I have seen elsewhere. It breaks out on the face more than any other part of the body. I have seen several whose faces were ruined by it, and their noses quite gone. In one of my excursions, happening to peep into a house where one or more of them were, one only appeared at the door by which I must have entered, and which he began to stop by drawing

drawing several parts of a cord across it. But the intolerable stench which came from his putrid face was alone sufficient to keep me out, had the entrance been ever so wide. His nose was quite gone, and his whole face in one continued ulcer, so that the very sight of him was shocking. As our people had not all got clear of a certain disease they had contracted at the Society Isles, I took all possible care to prevent its being communicated to the natives, and, I have reason to believe, my endeavours succeeded."

It may be observed, that the Friendly Islands, of which this is one, had been visited by Europeans long before the Society Islands were discovered, by which they had certainly as great a chance of getting the venereal infection as the latter: yet if people wanting their noses had been observed at the Society Islands, it may be presumed that their complaints would have been ascribed to a very different source. What he says about leprosy will, as far as my observation goes, apply to all the South Sea Islands with which the Porpoise had any communication.

Mr Anderson, who was surgeon of the Resolution in Cook's third voyage, speaks in still more positive terms of the frequency of lues venerea at Otaheite, as appears by the following extract: "They only reckon five or six which might be called chronic or national disorders, amongst which are the dropsy and the fefai, or indolent swellings, before mentioned, as frequent at Tongataboo. But this was before the arrival of the Europeans; for we have added to this short catalogue a disease which abundantly supplies the place of all others, and is now almost universal. For this they seem to have no effectual remedy. The priests, indeed, give them a medley of simples, but they own it never cures them. And yet they allow that, in a few cases, nature, without the assistance of a physician, exterminates the poison of this fatal disease, and a perfect recovery is produced. They say, that if a man is infected with it, he will often communicate it to others in the same house, by feeding out of the same utensils, or handling them; and that, in this case, they frequently die, while he recovers, although we see no reason why this should happen."

But as this ingenious gentleman has neither informed us of the symptoms which appeared among the ship's company, nor described in what manner the disease showed itself on shore, it may be fairly presumed that he adopted the opinion of his captain, and confounded the most common disease, viz. scrofula, with lues venerea. And this opinion seems more probable, if it is considered, that at the period at which this gentleman wrote, gonorrhœa

gonorrhœa, which I ſuppoſe to have been the diſeaſe he ſaw on board, was generally conſidered as a modification of lues venerea, and excoriations on the glans, or ſymptomatic ſwellings in the groin, were invariably treated as chancres or buboes.

If lues venerea was at that time ſo common, how can its diſappearance be accounted for? As I preſume no fact can be better eſtabliſhed than that it did not exiſt, at leaſt in a mode capable of communicating the infection in the uſual manner, at the time of the Porpoiſe's viſits; ſince none of her crew, or the Norfolk's contracted it, after having ſuch unlimited connexion with the women, as has been already ſtated; and it would be highly abſurd to imagine, that if any of the latter had been infected, they would, on that account, have been inclined to any particular reſtriction. This opinion receives farther confirmation from the reſidence among the inhabitants, for ſeveral years, of many Engliſh ſeamen who deſerted from their ſhips. Some of theſe I have had an opportunity of ſeeing, who declared that they had frequently contracted gonorrhœa, which they ſpoke of as a complaint of a trifling nature, and which they obſerved generally went off ſpontaneouſly, or on uſing ſalt water and cocoa-nut milk as a purgative; yet none of them have ever had any ſymptom of lues, nor have they had an opportunity of taking any medicine whatever; and it may be ſuppoſed, that had this diſeaſe exiſted in the iſland, they muſt have contracted it, as the women were the principal attraction which induced them to deſert their ſhips.

It may be alſo advanced, from all the knowledge we have of lues venerea, that had it been imported by the firſt navigators, its extinction could not have been effected, even if the inhabitants were in poſſeſſion of a ſpecific remedy, of which I am well aſſured they are not; for, after a very careful inquiry, it appeared, that although they ſometimes uſe ſimples by way of medicine, ſuch as ſalt-water and cocoa-nut milk, as a purgative, they, like other uncivilized nations, have more faith in various ceremonies of a religious tendency; and, if we are permitted to judge from analogy, the effects of lues would certainly be more rapid and violent, in a country where chaſtity is not accounted a virtue, than in Europe.

The inhabitants whom I have obſerved affected with gonorrhœa chew great quantities of ſugar-cane, and ſometimes apply a poultice of the kernel of the cocoa-nut to the penis; the firſt of which is probably more advantageous than our preſcriptions of mucilaginous drinks, as it poſſeſſes all their virtues, with the addition of a laxative quality; and the latter muſt certainly have all the effect of an emollient poultice in chordee. By these means I have witnessed two or three very good cures.

Their manner of living, and strict attention to cleanliness, in which they excel us, are certainly very favourable in this complaint; therefore the symptoms are generally mild. And it may be here observed, that had the same number of our ship's company contracted gonorrhœa in a European port, they would have been affected with much severer symptoms; which is sufficiently accounted for by observing that they did not drink their allowance of spirits, and lived on what might be termed an antiphlogistic diet; that they generally applied to the surgeon the moment they found themselves infected, and were rigidly restricted from women while the disease continued. Indeed, the single case of swelled testis occurred in a person who did not observe those precautions.

One of the missionaries, who is a little acquainted with medicine, has had considerable practice among the natives in gonorrhœa, and had been in the habit of administering preparations of mercury for it. These he was persuaded to lay aside for the more simple plan of injection, and, before our departure, he was perfectly convinced of the propriety of this change; for, independent of its being unnecessary, they bathe with such a kind of religious punctuality, that mercury cannot be administered without incurring much danger.

The natives name gonorrhœa *O-pee*, and maintain that the British introduced it; and to the same source, as has been already observed, they attribute most of their diseases. But it must by no means be inferred from their relations that this was really the case; for although the crew of the Dolphin, which was the first European ship that paid them a visit, did not contract this complaint, yet this circumstance does not prove the disease to have been unknown to them anterior to the visit of that ship; especially if it is considered that, in the Porpoise's first voyage, only three of the crew were infected; and, if her stay had been limited to one month, they would have escaped it altogether.

I presume that it will always remain doubtful whether even this trifling complaint is one of their imported evils, although it appears to me to be more probable that it is not*; for the medical establishment of all the ships on discovery was carefully selected; and more than sufficient time for the cure of gonorrhœa must have elapsed between their leaving any port where they could contract it, and their arrival at these islands.

The

* Mr B. Bell, p. 35. vol. 1. says, that he has authority for saying that, in Cook's second voyage, gonorrhœa had not appeared among the Otaheitians.

1

The discovery of other islands in the same sea at some future period will throw light upon this subject, if due attention is paid to it: however, if I may be permitted to hazard an opinion, I think, that wherever man is found, gonorrhœa will be found also *.

From the foregoing statement it may be concluded, I hope, without incurring the censure of presuming too much, that, notwithstanding the melancholy accounts we read of the ravages of lues venerea at Otaheite, and even disputations about its first importers, this disease was not introduced there antecedent to the Porpoise's voyages †; and that Captain Cook and others met with gonorrhœa only, which they supposed sufficient to produce all the symptoms of pox; and also that it must be sufficiently obvious that the nature of these infections is different, as we found the one prevailing, yet in no instance met with the other.

However, although the first navigators are thus freed from having introduced this scourge of mankind, it is melancholy to reflect that its speedy importation was almost certain; for before we departed from these islands, a small vessel arrived from Port Jackson, on board of which there was a man affected with bubo and chancres; and it is probable that the efforts of the master to prevent him from disseminating the infection would prove unavailing.

Yet there remained a still more certain source of infection from two vessels which afterwards arrived from the Sandwich Islands, where, I have good authority for saying, the disease is very common ‡. And whenever it is imported, there can be little doubt of its making a rapid progress, notwithstanding the benevolent efforts of the missionaries; for, from the danger, and, indeed I fear, the impossibility of making the natives submit to a mercurial course, it will be a very difficult matter to cure any of them.

The great probability of their future intercourse with New South Wales becoming frequent, will also be a constant source

2 of

* Gonorrhœa has been observed in natives of New Holland, at a distance from the settlement sufficient to preclude the possibility of their having, either directly or indirectly, contracted the infection from the British.

† I am positive that in neither of our voyages did we carry to Otaheite venereal infection of any kind. One man complained of chancres in the second voyage, soon after leaving Port Jackson; and although he might have been cured on board, the possibility of his introducing the infection was considered as a matter of such a serious consequence, that he was not permitted to proceed on the voyage, but sent on shore at Norfolk Island.

‡ Mr Bass, surgeon R. N. the discoverer of the Streights in New Holland, which bear his name.

of infection, and bids fair to destroy the intentions of the mission; for from that settlement they have already received, and will continue to receive, deserters, whose baneful example and instructions will not fail to counteract the benefit which would otherwise accrue to these courteous islanders from its exertions.

III.

Remarks on the Depopulation of Otaheite and Eimeo, with an Account of some of the most common Diseases. By JOHN WILSON, Surgeon to his Majesty's Ship Porpoise.

ON comparing the present population of these islands with what existed at the time of Captain Cook's voyages, an interesting, but, at the same time, most deplorable picture presents itself. The reduction of the inhabitants is so incredibly great, that, were it not for the acknowledged accuracy of that great navigator in most particulars, we could with difficulty suppose him to have been in earnest, when he calculated the number on Otaheite at two hundred and four thousand, especially as it has been lately ascertained by the missionaries, by a mode almost amounting to the accuracy of actual enumeration, that the number of souls on the island does not amount to seven thousand. However, allowing the former to have exceeded by one half, there still remains a reduction of ninety-five thousand in about the space of thirty years; a mortality to which there is perhaps no parallel on record.

That the island was formerly infinitely more populous than at present is beyond a doubt, and perhaps the many well-constructed and extensive morais or places of worship, now seen in a ruinous condition, afford one of the best proofs of a former numerous population; and the assertions of the inhabitants, which deserve some credit in this instance, corroborate this conjecture; for they say, that, at no very late period, no land was unoccupied, as is the case at present, and that the population now will not bear comparison with what existed then.

The introduction of the venereal disease by Europeans has been hitherto invariably considered by voyagers as the most active cause of their declension; but from what has been already related respecting that disease, it is presumed no one will impute it to that source, especially as other causes are obvious, and are at present operating with a most fatal sway; the operation of some of which appears to me to have commenced about the time of the visits of Cook and others, and to have had a gradual increase of force ever since.

The diseases which have had the greatest share in the depopulation may be reduced to the following, viz. Fever, dysentery, phthisis pulmonalis, and scrofula. But by far the greatest proportion must be ascribed to the first, which the inhabitants name Hottute, and which, at the beginning, is most commonly of the intermittent kind, but, before its termination, which is almost universally fatal, it becomes a remittent. On the other hand, if the patient recovers, scrofula so commonly supervenes in the form of glandular swellings and distortions of the thorax and spine, that the natives hail these dreadful maladies as a very salutary kind of crisis *. Although many who were affected with this complaint in all its stages daily came under my observation, it was found to be impracticable, from their constitutional ficklenefs and levity, to persuade any one patient to remain stationary in a place where I could conveniently attend to the progress of the disease; consequently my knowledge respecting it must be very circumscribed. At the beginning the head and stomach are much affected, and the good effect of emetics in cutting it short was completely ascertained in the few cases for which I prescribed them; but it was also observed, that the disease often recurred in two or three weeks.

It was impossible to learn with certainty, whether it is esteemed contagious by the natives, as they differed as much in their accounts upon this head as in most other cases; however, the many deserted houses which are to be met with, the whole of whose inhabitants had fallen victims to it in a short space of time, afford a presumption that it is infectious †; at the same time, it should be observed, that they are much exposed to a very powerful cause of fever, from the many marshes that

3 are

* We do not read, in any voyages, that many cases of deformity were observed among these islanders; but it is now so common, that the most superficial observer would conclude them to be comparatively a deformed race.

† Although several affected with this fever were on board of our ship, and even slept there, yet none of the crew were attacked with it; and, among the missionaries, only one of their wives has had it. She recovered, and, I was informed, had taken considerable quantities of bark.

are to be found on these islands; and these spots, on account of their conveniency for the favourite habit of bathing, are generally preferred for erecting their houses. The usual custom of sleeping on the ground, and even in the open air, exposes them much to these miasmata, and perhaps the missionaries could not exercise their humanity in a more laudable manner than by teaching them to construct bedsteads, and impressing them with their utility*.

I do not know that they use any thing of a medicinal nature in this complaint, but they seem to be well acquainted with the beneficial effects of a change of air, for they frequently transport themselves to Tethevroa, and other islets, about eight leagues to the northward, from whence they generally return in good health and condition. Indeed, these isles are the Montpellier of Otaheite, to which not only invalids, but persons in good health, resort, particularly females, with the view of improving their complexion and general appearance. Their principal food there is fish.

Dysentery is to be ranked in the second class of their mortal diseases, and it is pretty frequent, and often fatal. While the Porpoise was at Eimeo, it raged with great violence, there being scarcely a house on the island in which there was not found one or more afflicted with it.

Phthisis pulmonalis, I believe, is more frequent, and proves sooner fatal than with us.

Rheumatism was frequently met with, and it is in this disease that the operation of taroomee, or squeezing the affected parts, is performed with advantage. Several cases of elephantiasis were observed, but it is by no means common.

Scrofulous tumours and ulcers appear to be much more common than in Britain, and this disorder, as with us, chiefly attacks people with delicate complexions, and those who, from this and some other external appearances, are supposed to be peculiarly predisposed to it. It generally makes its appearance before or about the age of puberty, and, I believe, almost universally attacks those whom the fever spares, which seems to leave the system in a state well adapted for its action. The glands about the neck are most commonly affected. However, it should be observed, that the most common dress of the natives covers only a small portion of their bodies, and consequently their sores, if they have any, are exposed; and this will lead a superficial observer to imagine, that they are afflicted with this disorder in an infinitely greater proportion than in European

* Bedsteads made by the missionaries were sometimes observed.

European countries, where the face and hands only are left uncovered.

These are, I think, their principal dangerous diseases; and although they very probably have many others to which humanity is subjected, they may likewise be unacquainted with some to which more refined nations are liable.

Epilepsy and, I think, hysteria are not uncommon, but confer a degree of sanctity on the proprietors of them, as they are supposed, during the fit, to be favoured with supernatural visions; and although it is not altogether connected with the present subject, an instance which came under my observation proves that they, in common with the ignorant part of more civilized nations, believe these and some other spasmodic diseases originate from the immediate impulse of a good or bad spirit. In one of my excursions I was introduced to a middle aged woman, who was said to be occasionally favoured with the gift of seeing into futurity; and a sick child happening to be in the same house, whose speedy dissolution appeared to me to be certain, she received the divine impulse, or, as the natives expressed it, the eatooa, or God entered her, for the purpose of predicting its fate.

She accordingly seated herself on the ground, and continued in a musing attitude for about a quarter of an hour, when she was violently seized with a violent hysteric paroxysm, during which three men held her down with difficulty. The fit lasted about ten minutes, and, when she recovered her senses, she gave a favourable prognostic. This, I had no doubt, was a real hysteric fit, brought on, perhaps, by the force of imagination, which is acknowledged to have great influence in this and some other analogous diseases. There are even some pretenders to this science who are generally believed to be impostors; but as what they utter during the fit has great weight in their most important national affairs, this supposition, perhaps, often arises from a collision of interests, and the many different interpretations which their incoherent rhapsodies will always admit of.

Some of the diseases which at present ravage these islands may, by some, be supposed to have been imported; but of this we can have no evidence; and probably all the elucidation the subject will admit of may be found in the analogy of many countries which have been long healthy and populous, suddenly becoming overwhelmed with disease and death, from some revolution in nature, which is likely always to remain a mystery.

Although disease must have had a very powerful influence on the depopulation, yet the greatest share is to be attributed to a custom which, although it has been practised as a system by others, perhaps more civilized people, is of a nature the most barbarous and cruel that ever disgraced the species. This is infant murder, which is carried to such an extent, that some of the best informed of the missionaries have asserted, that at least two-thirds of the whole of the births on the island are destroyed the moment they have seen the light *. Not only is the offspring of an unequal connexion with respect to rank, either on the male or female side, invariably destroyed, but young men and women who are every way equal, frequently agree to murder the innocent fruit of their pleasures †; and more females are destroyed than males.

They appear to have no idea of any criminality being attached to this deed, and many of the women who had born children, on being requested, did not scruple or appear abashed to tell us the number they had destroyed. The young king's wife, although not twenty years of age, has, I think, killed two, which, she pretended, were begot by some of her domestic attendants.

I have remarked, that at least two-thirds of the whole of the women on Otaheite are either middle aged or old, and that children are principally observed to be possessed by the former: for it is a very rare occurrence, indeed, to meet with a young woman rearing a child: likewise, that the whole of the females do not amount to above one-tenth part of the males; from which it may be inferred, that they do not often save their children until about or after their meridian, and that infant-murder has been of late years more frequent than at the time when those middle-aged and old women were born. The more frequent destruction of females sufficiently accounts for their disparity to the males. It is a mere question of course with the natives, on hearing the news of a birth, to ask whether it is preserved.

They have many absurd customs in their treatment of children, particularly females, which certainly render the rearing of them exceedingly troublesome; but there is nothing of a sacrificial nature in their destruction: for, although they do not suppose that they incur their displeasure by it, yet they do not pretend that it is acceptable to any of their divinities: and, indeed, although they have some notion of a future state, it does

* This custom has by some been considered to be peculiar to a class of people called Arreoyies; but, from the dissolute life they lead, they must have much less frequent occasion to practise it than the other inhabitants.

† They also induced abortion by pressure, but this is a painful operation, and is sometimes fatal.

not seem to have any influence whatever on their moral actions in this world.

I am of opinion that infant-murder is more frequently practised since their connexion with us, and that it will continue to increase in proportion to the number of ships which may for the future visit them, principally from the following considerations:

First, From all the information which I could procure, I believe their only inducement to this cruel deed, independent of inequality of rank, or being an Arreoyie, which are always insurmountable, and from the construction of their succession *, are love of pleasure and avarice; and these passions, but more particularly the latter, have gained much ground since their intercourse with us: indeed, I have often been struck with astonishment, when observing the eagerness with which they hoard European manufactures †. They are also as well aware as we are, that the charms of women who rear families sooner decay; and having experienced that female beauty is always a marketable article with their visitors, they have recourse to murder to preserve it.

Secondly, At the Society Islands, where the same manners and customs prevail, and which have been less frequently visited by Europeans, infant murder is not so often practised; consequently these islands are more populous, although they appear at present to labour under disease in the same degree as Otaheite. It must, therefore, be concluded, that the frequent visits of ships tend to decrease their numbers, not only by inducing a scarcity of food, but by striking at the very root of population ‡.

War, undoubtedly, must be supposed to have considerable influence on their declension. In that which occurred in the interval between our voyages, it was said that five or six hundred perished, but these were chiefly old men and women; and this was the only war of any consequence since the arrival of the missionaries. There is also reason to believe that it was more frequent formerly than of late years, as the Bounty's mutineers and other deserters strengthened the authority of the present reigning fa-

* The moment a son is born, he is considered as the head of his family, and the father sinks into his executor, until he is able to manage his affairs himself. The effects of this absurd custom must be sufficiently obvious.

† An old female chief favoured me with a sight of her treasure-chest; among other articles, it contained 46 axes and hatchets.

‡ The oftentimes superabundant quantities of provisions which the chiefs bring on board of ships, has induced voyagers to believe that a never-failing plenty reigns here; however, this is by no means the case, and, even in plentiful times, the common people do not often taste animal food.

mily to a degree never before enjoyed by any chief. Therefore, war cannot be admitted to have had much influence in the present deficiency of numbers.

The cuſtom of offering human ſacrifices we have no reaſon to believe to have been more frequent ſince their diſcovery. Probably the number offered will amount to twenty in a year, and, as they are always males, this cannot have a very powerful operation.

Polygamy may alſo have ſome effect; but as this cuſtom muſt be ſuppoſed always to have exiſted, it cannot be conſidered to have had contributed to preſent depopulation.

IV.

Report of the Phyſical and Mathematical Claſs of the Inſtitute, upon the Queſtion, Are thoſe Manufactures which emit a diſagreeable Smell prejudicial to Health?

[Read at the Sitting of the 26th Frimaire, year 13. by Meſſ. Guyton-Morveau and Chaptal *.]

THE Miniſter of the Interior has conſulted the Claſs upon a queſtion, the ſolution of which is of the greateſt importance to our manufacturers, Is the neighbourhood of certain manufactories prejudicial to health?

The ſolution of this problem muſt appear the more important, as, by the confidence naturally placed in the opinions of the Inſtitute, it may henceforth form the baſis of judicial deciſions when the fate of a manufactory and the health of the people are concerned.

This ſolution is the more urgent, and is become the more neceſſary, as the fate of the moſt uſeful eſtabliſhments, nay, even, the exiſtence of many arts, has hitherto depended on ſimple regulations of the police, and as ſome, driven to a diſtance from materials, from labour, or from a due conſumption, by prejudice, ignorance, or jealouſy, continue to ſtruggle with diſadvantage againſt the numberleſs obſtacles oppoſed to their proſperity. Hence we have ſucceſſively ſeen manufactures of acids, of ſal ammoniac, Pruſſian blue, beer, and leather, baniſhed from the precincts of cities, and hence theſe ſame eſtabliſhments are ſtill daily complained of by captious neighbours, or invidious rivals.

So

* See Annales de Chimie, vol. liv. p. 86.

So long as the fate of these manufactures is insecure; so long as a legislation, purely arbitrary, can interrupt, suspend, or fetter the efforts of the manufacturer; in a word, so long as a mere magistrate of police shall wield in his hands the prosperity or the ruin of a manufacturer, how can we suppose that he will have the imprudence to embark in enterprises of this nature? How can we hope to see the manufacturing industry established on so feeble a basis? This state of uncertainty, these perpetual animosities existing between the manufacturer and his neighbours, the eternal apprehensions he must entertain with regard to the fate of his establishment, confine and paralyse his efforts, and gradually impair his property and his spirit of enterprise.

It is then of material importance to the prosperity of the arts that limits should be fixed, which leave nothing to the caprice of the magistrate; which point out to the manufacturer that sphere within which he may, with freedom and security, exercise his industry, and guarantee to the neighbouring proprietor the sure enjoyment of his health, and produce of his estate. To solve this important problem, it appears to us indispensable to take a view of each of those arts against which the greatest objections have been started.

To this end, we shall divide them into two classes. The first will comprehend all those in whose operations gaseous effluvia, the consequence of putrefaction or fermentation, which may be accounted unpleasant to the smell, or noxious in their effect, escape into the atmosphere.

The second class will include all those where, by the action of fire, the artist developes and diffuses in vapours or in gas, various principles which are more or less disagreeable to breathe, and are reckoned more or less prejudicial to health.

In the former we may insert the steeping of flax and hemp; the manufacture of catgut; slaughter-houses; starch manufactories; tanneries; breweries, &c. In the latter, the distillation of acids, of wines, of animal matters; the art of gilding metals; preparations of lead, copper, mercury, &c.

The arts comprised in the first class, considered with regard to public health, deserve a most particular attention; because the fumes which are emitted by fermentation or putrefaction are really prejudicial to health in some cases, and under some particular circumstances. For example, the steeping of flax, which is practised in stagnant pools or pits, infects the air, and is fatal to fish. The diseases to which this gives rise are all known and described. Wise regulations, therefore, have ordained that this operation should be performed without the limits of cities,

at

at a certain diſtance from all dwellings, and in waters whoſe fiſh are of no importance to the inhabitants. Theſe regulations ſhould undoubtedly be maintained; but as the execution of them is attended with inconvenience, it is deſirable that the proceſs of M. Brâle, the ſuperiority of which is confirmed by the teſtimony of M. M. Monges, Berthollet, Teſſier, and Molard, ſhould ſoon be known and adopted.

Other operations, which are practiſed on vegetables, or certain products of vegetation, in order to obtain from them fermented liquors, as in breweries; to prepare colours, as in manufactories of turnſol, archil, and indigo; or to diveſt them of ſome of their principles, as in ſtarch manufactories, paper mills, &c. do not appear to us, by their nature, to furniſh any cauſe for ſolicitude on the part of the magiſtrate. At all events, the fumes which ariſe from theſe fermenting matters can be dangerous only in the immediate vicinity of the veſſels and apparatus which contain them; they ceaſe to be ſo the moment they are combined with the external air; therefore a little prudence only is neceſſary to avoid danger. Moreover, this cannot affect the inhabitants of neighbouring dwellings; it concerns and can injure only thoſe employed about the works; ſo that a law, which ſhould order the removal of theſe works without the cities, and to a diſtance from all habitations, would be, on the part of government, an act at once oppreſſive and unjuſt, in oppoſition to the progreſs of the arts, and not at all likely to remedy the evil ſuppoſed to be produced.

Some preparations which are extracted from animal bodies often require the putrefaction of theſe ſame bodies, as in thoſe connected with the making of catgut; but more frequently the animal ſubſtances employed in manufactures are liable to putrefaction, by remaining too long in the manufactory, or by reaſon of too hot a temperature. This is particularly exemplified in the dying of red cotton, where much blood is uſed. The infection which this corrupted matter exhales is far diffuſed, and forms in the neighbourhood an atmoſphere very diſagreeable to breathe. It would be well, therefore, to cauſe the materials to be frequently renewed, in order to prevent their corruption, and to keep the place clean, ſo that none of the refuſe of the animal ſubſtances employed ſhould be ſuffered to remain too long, and thereby putrefy.

In this laſt reſpect, ſlaughter-houſes are attended with ſome inconvenience; but this is by no means of ſo ſerious a nature as to demand their baniſhment without the limits of cities, and their being collected in one place, as ſpeculators are daily ſuggeſting to government. A little attention on the part of the magiſtrate,

that

that butchers do not throw out the blood and certain offals of the animals which they kill, is sufficient to obviate any disgusting and unhealthy effects arising from slaughter-houses.

The manufacture of *poudrette* is now establishing itself in all the great cities of France; and the operation by which night soil is reduced to a state of powder necessarily diffuses for a long time a most disagreeable smell. Establishments of this kind ought therefore to be formed in airy situations, and far from any dwelling, not that we regard the gaseous exhalation from them as prejudicial to health, but we cannot deny that it is inconvenient, tainted, disagreeable, and difficult to breathe. On this account, therefore, these ought to be removed to a distance from the habitation of man.

There is one very important observation to be made on the spontaneous decomposition of animal substances, which is, that the emanations from them appear to be the less dangerous, in proportion as the matters undergoing putrefaction are less humid. In this latter case, a considerable quantity of carbonate of ammonia escapes, which imparts its predominant character to the other matters volatilized, and corrects the bad effect of those which would otherwise be deleterious. Thus, the decomposition of stercoraceous matter, and of the refuse of the cocons of the silk-worm, in the open air, and in situations the position and inclination of which permit the escape of the liquids, evolve an enormous quantity of carbonate of ammonia, which counteracts the poisonous quality of certain other vapours, whilst these same substances, decomposed in water, or very wet, emit sweetish and nauseous fumes, the respiration of which is extremely dangerous.

The numerous arts in which the manufacturer produces and diffuses into the air in the course of his operations, and by the aid of fire, vapours more or less disagreeable to breathe, constitute the second class which we are to examine. These, more interesting than the former, and much more intimately connected with the prosperity of national industry, are still oftener objects of reference to the decision of the magistrate; and on this account, they appear to us deserving of more particular attention.

We shall begin our examination with the making of acids.

The acids, against the preparation of which the neighbours of a manufactory may complain, are, the sulphuric, nitrous, muriatic, and acetic. The sulphuric is obtained by the burning of a combination of sulphur and saltpetre. It is very difficult, in this operation to prevent a more or less observable smell of sulphureous

ſulphureous acid from being diffuſed around the apparatus in which the combuſtion is going forward; but, in works ably contrived, this ſmell is ſcarcely ſenſible in the manufactory itſelf; the workmen daily breathe it with impunity, and any complaint on the part of the neighbours muſt be unfounded. When the art of making ſulphuric acid was introduced into France, the popular voice was loud in oppoſition to the firſt eſtabliſhments: the ſmell from the matches uſed in our houſes contributed not a little to exaggerate the effect ſuppoſed neceſſarily to follow the rapid burning of ſome hundred pounds weight of ſulphur. The opinion at the preſent day is ſo completely reverſed, that we ſee many of theſe manufactures flouriſhing in peace and quietneſs in the midſt of our cities.

The diſtillation of aquafortis, and of ſpirit of ſalt (nitrous and muriatic acids), is not more dangerous than the making of ſulphuric acid. All the proceſs is conducted in veſſels of earthen ware or glaſs, and the chief concern of the manufacturer is undoubtedly to diminiſh the loſs or volatilization as much as poſſible. Neverthelеſs, whatever attention be given to the proceſs, the air which is breathed in the manufactory is always impregnated with the peculiar ſmell of each acid, notwithſtanding which the reſpiration there is free and ſafe, the people daily employed there are not at all incommoded by it, and any complaint from neighbours would be unjuſt.

Since the manufactories of white lead, verdegris, and ſugar of lead, have become ſo numerous in France, vinegar has come into more general uſe. In diſtilling this acid, to render it more fit for ſome of theſe uſes, a very ſtrong ſmell of vinegar ſpreads itſelf, which is not dangerous; but when a ſolution of lead in this acid is evaporated, the vapours aſſume a ſweetiſh character, and produce upon thoſe who are in the habit of breathing them all the effects peculiar to the vapours of lead itſelf. Happily theſe effects are confined to the men who work in the building, and cannot injure thoſe who reſide in the neighbourhood.

Preparations of mercury and lead, thoſe of copper, antimony, and arſenic, the proceſs of gilding metals, are all ſomewhat dangerous to thoſe who inhabit and aſſiſt in the works; but the effects are confined within the encloſure of the manufactories, and are dangerous only to thoſe concerned in them.

It is an object deſerving of the attention of chemiſts to inveſtigate the means of preventing theſe unpleaſant effects. Already much inconvenience has been obviated by the help of chimnies which convey the vapours out of the reach of reſpiration. At preſent, all the attention of adminiſtration ought to

be

be confined to directing ſcience towards the improvements of which theſe proceſſes are ſuſceptible with regard to health.

The making of Pruſſian blue, the extraction of carbonate of ammonia by the diſtillation of animal bodies, in the new works of ſal ammoniac, produce a great quantity of fœtid vapours. In truth, theſe exhalations are not dangerous to health; but, in theſe times, to be reckoned a good neighbour, it is not enough not to be dangerous, we muſt alſo not be diſagreeable. The projectors of theſe eſtabliſhments, when about to fix upon a ſituation, ought to prefer one at a diſtance from any dwelling; but when the eſtabliſhment is already formed, we ſhould be careful of adviſing the magiſtrate to order its removal. In this caſe, it will ſuffice to require of the proprietor that he ſhall carry his chimnies to ſuch a height as to diſſipate in the air the diſagreeable vapours produced by his operations. This plan is particularly well calculated for the making of Pruſſian blue; by putting it into execution, one of ourſelves has been the means of preſerving in the centre of Paris one of the moſt important manufactories of this kind, againſt which the neighbours had already combined.

In the report which we ſubmit to the Claſs, we have thought it our duty to confine ourſelves to the chief manufactories, againſt which violent complaints have been preferred at various times and places; and, after what has been ſaid, it is apparent that the neighbourhood of a few only is prejudicial to health.

Hence, we cannot too ſeriouſly adviſe the magiſtrates intruſted with the care of the public health and ſafety to diſmiſs thoſe ill-grounded complaints, which too often are directed againſt eſtabliſhments, daily threatening the proſperity of the honeſt manufacturer, retarding the progreſs of induſtry, and compromiſing the fate of the arts themſelves. The magiſtrate ſhould be on his guard againſt the inſinuations of a jealous and troubleſome neighbour; he ſhould carefully diſtinguiſh between what is only inconvenient or diſagreeable, and what is really noxious or dangerous; he ſhould recollect that the uſe of pit-coal was, for a long time, aboliſhed, under the frivolous pretext of its being unwholeſome; he ſhould, in a word, be fully ſenſible, that, by liſtening to complaints of this nature, not only the eſtabliſhment of many uſeful arts in France might in time be prevented, but that it might be the means of inſenſibly baniſhing from cities, farriers, carpenters, joiners, braziers, coopers, founders, weavers, and all thoſe whoſe profeſſion is more or leſs inconvenient to the neighbour. For certainly theſe trades are more diſagreeable to the neighbourhood than the manufactories above

above mentioned, and the only advantage they enjoy over them is their antiquity. Their right of toleration has been eſtabliſhed by time and neceſſity, and we make no doubt, but when our manufactories become older and better known, they will peaceably enjoy the ſame advantage in ſociety. In the mean time, we think the Claſs ought to profit by this circumſtance, to place them under the ſpecial protection of government, and declare that manufactories of acids, ſal ammoniac, Pruſſian blue, ſugar of lead, white lead, and of ſtarch, ſlaughter-houſes, breweries, and tan-pits, are not prejudicial to the health of the neighbourhood, when well conducted.

We cannot ſay ſo much for the ſteeping of hemp, catgut manufactories, lay-ſtalls, and all thoſe eſtabliſhments where great quantities of animal or vegetable matter are expoſed to humid putrefaction; for, beſides the diſagreeable ſmell that exhales from theſe, vapours are emitted which are more or leſs hurtful.

We ſhould add, that although the manufactures of which we have been ſpeaking, and which we have conſidered as not being hurtful to health by their vicinity, ſhould not be removed, yet adminiſtration ſhould be deſired to exerciſe over them the moſt active watchfulneſs, and conſult perſons capable of preſcribing to the proprietors the moſt proper meaſures for preventing the ſmoke and ſmell from being diffuſed in the neighbourhood. This end may be attained by improving the proceſſes, by elevating the outer walls, ſo as to prevent the vapours from being diffuſed in the neighbourhood; by improving the chimnies, which might be ſo conſtructed that the ſmoke itſelf be burnt in the fire-place, or condenſed; by keeping the premiſes very clean, ſo that there ſhall be no putrefaction in them; and by conveying off into deep pits all the remains ſuſceptible of fermentation, ſo as not to become in the leaſt inconvenient to neighbours.

We muſt again obſerve, that when new eſtabliſhments are about to be formed for making Pruſſian blue, ſal ammoniac, leather, ſtarch, and all thoſe manufactories in general which emit vapours offenſive to the neighbours, or which are in frequent danger of fire or exploſions, it would be at once wiſe, juſt, and prudent, to declare that theſe eſtabliſhments cannot be formed within the limits of cities, and near habitations, without ſpecial authority; and that where the founders of them do not comply with this indiſpenſable condition, the removal of ſuch eſtabliſhments may be ordered without indemnity.

The reſult, then, of our report is, 1*ſt*, That eſtabliſhments for the making of catgut, dunghills, ſteeping of hemp, and, in general,

general, all those in which a great mass of animal or vegetable matter is heaped up to rot or putrefy, are prejudicial to health, and that they ought to be carried on at a distance from cities, and every other habitation. *2dly*, That buildings from which disagreeable smells are emitted by the action of fire, as in the making of acids, of Prussian blue, and sal ammoniac, form a dangerous neighbourhood only from want of due precaution; and that the care of administration ought to center in an enlightened and active superintendence, having for its objects the perfection of the processes employed, the management of the fire, and the maintenance of cleanliness. *3dly*, That it would become a good and wise administration to enact regulations for prohibiting in future, without previous authority, the establishment of manufactories in towns, or near dwelling-houses, the vicinity of which is necessarily dangerous or inconvenient. In this class may be comprehended the manufactories of *poudrette*, tan-pits, starch-manufactories, founderies, melting-houses for tallow, slaughter-houses, rag-warehouses, manufactories of Prussian blue, varnish, glue, sal ammoniac, potteries, &c.

Such are the conclusions we have the honour to submit to the Class.

These conclusions have been approved of by the Institute, and transmitted to Government, with an invitation to adopt them as the basis of its decisions.

OBSERVATIONS BY THE EDITORS.

The preceding report we consider as particularly interesting, not only on account of its containing the principles upon which the law of nuisances is to be executed in one of the most enlightened nations of the world, but also as affording us an opportunity of calling the attention of the medical men of this country to so important a subject.

Although, in this great manufacturing kingdom, numberless decisions connected with it have been given, the principles by which they ought to be regulated have never been scientifically developed, nor have they, so far as we know, been ever collected or arranged. Hence they are, in general, arbitrary, often contradictory, and sometimes unjust. What on one occasion has been proscribed as a nuisance, on another has been declared to be a matter of indifference, and, on a third, has been cherished as salutary. But so long as this uncertainty continues, so long as as juries and judges are not in poſſeſſion of general principles to guide them in their determinations, innocent eſtabliſhments muſt run the riſk of being ſuſpended on groundleſs fears, or pernicious ſpeculations tolerated until they have committed irreparable injury.

Although it is rather the buſineſs of the lawyer to collect deciſions, yet this ſubject is ſo cloſely connected with the prevention of diſeaſe, and queſtions concerning it often, as indeed they always ſhould be, referred to medical men for their opinions, that we do not think that a few pages of our Journal could be better employed than in recording, from time to time, thoſe important caſes on which our correſpondents may have been conſulted. In this way, we are not without hopes that our Numbers may render an eſſential ſervice to the adminiſtration of juſtice, by collecting materials for a ſcientifical elucidation of this branch of medical police.

Blackſtone defines a nuiſance to be "any thing which worketh hurt, inconvenience, or damage." Nuiſances, therefore, may affect either inanimate matter or living animals. The former claſs of nuiſances ſeldom comes within the ſphere of the phyſician, the latter is intimately connected with the exerciſe of his profeſſion. It may, again, be ſubdivided into thoſe nuiſances which merely excite unpleaſant ſenſations, and thoſe which are injurious to health. To the former variety belong diſagreeable ſights, ſounds, and ſmells, when they do not impair or endanger health. Any perſon, who fixes his abode near a nuiſance of this deſcription, has only himſelf to blame, and it cannot be removed until its poſſeſſor be indemnified for the injury he may thereby ſuſtain. But a ſpeculator has no right, with a view to his own advantage, to erect any eſtabliſhment which ſhall diminiſh the value of the neighbouring property, or render unpleaſant an abode which was formerly otherwiſe. In every caſe the offender may juſtly be obliged to uſe every precaution to leſſen, as much as poſſible, the nuiſance complained of; but in this country, whoſe proſperity ſo much depends on its manufactures, the ſpirit of enterpriſe muſt not be checked on capricious or arbitrary objections.

The ſecond claſs is of infinitely greater importance, and the nuiſances included under it not being, like the former, direct objects of our ſenſes, are more obſcure, and give riſe to greater contrariety of opinion. In general, however, they act either by rendering the atmoſphere unwholeſome to breathe, or by contaminating public waters, ſo that they become unfit for the uſe of man and domeſtic animals, or poiſonous to the fiſh contained in them. The atmoſphere may be rendered unwholesome by being deprived of its oxygen, or by being loaded with deleterious vapours.

The first effect can only take place in very confined situations, and can scarcely ever become a public nuisance. If, however, in any case it should be suspected, it admits of positive determination by eudiometrical experiments.

It is to the second head of this division that the report of the French Institute is chiefly confined, which, upon the whole, is the result of much scientifical and political information, but, in some instances, seems rather too despotically and rashly to sacrifice the rights of the people to the appearances of national prosperity. Indeed, previous to experience, it is no easy matter to determine what vapours are capable of rendering the atmosphere unwholesome, for, to the question of the French Minister of the Interior, we have no hesitation in giving a decided negative. A disagreeable smell is by no means a certain criterion of an unwholesome atmosphere. And, on the other hand, the air is often pestilential, when, to our senses, it seems uncontaminated, and unfortunately eudiometry is not yet capable of elucidating this important question; we must therefore almost entirely content ourselves with the information derived from analogy and experience. The principal causes, however, which render the atmosphere unwholesome, are either the volatilization of poisonous metals by fire, or the decomposition of organic matters, especially by humid putrefaction. The danger from the first of these sources may fortunately be almost entirely obviated, by connecting with the works proper chimnies, and other condensing apparatus, and any deficiency in this respect is, on no account, to be tolerated.

But, of all these sources of disease, that which requires the most active vigilance of the police is the contamination of the air by putrefying animal or vegetable matters, because it is the most common, least suspected, and most dangerous. Were a single death to be traced to arsenical vapours from a smelting-house, the establishment would be instantly suspended; whereas we could point out shambles which have been a source of disease and death year after year. It is dreadful to think that we should have to record a fact, a crime, of such enormity. For is it not a crime of the most atrocious nature to bring the lives of a whole neighbourhood, nay, of a whole district, into danger, from indolence or avarice? A slaughter-house, when the offals are regularly removed, is no nuisance; but when the filth and blood are collected in heaps to putrefy, it is pestilence itself. Surely such an abuse is tolerated in this civilized country, in these enlightened times, only because it is unknown to those who would put a stop to it, from being confined to the neighbourhood of the very lowest class, who are ignorant of their rights, or do not complain. But, though the poor are indeed the immediate sufferers, the rich are eventually in danger; for instances are not wanting of pestilences, engendered under such circumstances, depopulating whole cities. Let, then, all such trades, not in themselves dangerous, but becoming so from indolence or avarice, be exercised under the most jealous and unremitting superintendence. Let the punishment attending the breach of such regulations as may be thought necessary be exemplary and severe. The welfare of the community is interested. To prevent the introduction of foreign contagion, our whole commerce is subjected to restraints, which are often unnecessary, sometimes oppressive. But the danger from home-bred pestilence is at least as great, and ought to be counteracted by measures equally prompt and energetic.

The degree to which water is contaminated by any cause is more easily estimated by direct experiment and observation. When the fish are poisoned, it is certainly unfit for the use of man, but, even when they continue to live, it may be sometimes rendered disgustful and injurious; a nuisance which ought not to be permitted, if a town, or even a hamlet, depend upon it for an article of such prime necessity.

—— Cunctis fluat unda salubris
Quæ levet arentem, si cupis, apta sitim.

V.

History of the Guinea Worm, and the Method of Cure employed by the Hindoos.

THE account of the dracunculus, or Guinea worm (Gordius Medinensis), contained in the following correspondence is highly interesting. Mr Dubois is a respectable and learned missionary, who joins a talent for minute observation to a perfect knowledge of the languages of the East. The answer from Dr Anderson renders the history of this singular disease more complete, and the notes have been added, with the view of explaining some particular expressions, by an intelligent physician, Dr Griffiths, who has practised some time in India, and by Dr De Carro of Vienna, to whom we are obliged for forwarding this communication.—*Editors*,

LETTER

Letter to Dr James Anderson, Physician-General at Fort St George.

Dear Sir,

The principal motive of this application is to communicate to you two popular remedies, whose efficacy I have witnessed in a great number of cases, against two disorders prevailing in this and many other districts. I mean the disease known to Europeans under the name of *Guinea worm*, to Hindoos under that of *Naramboo* or *Nurapoochalandy*, and the pain occasioned by the sting of scorpions. These two simple, and, as I suppose, inoffensive remedies were communicated to me by the same person, a native doctor, who administered them in this district with much success to a great number of persons, who almost daily called upon him for relief. As that person was under obligations to me, I prevailed upon him to communicate them; and as he exacted no promise of secrecy, I hope I shall not be accused of a breach of confidence by making them public. Since I became acquainted with these remedies, I have had many opportunities of trying their efficacy. I chiefly administered that which is used against the Guinea worm, and almost always with success. I say *almost always*, because, in two or three cases, it failed of producing its effect; the person who took it a first time, refusing to take it again, which is often necessary when the disease is inveterate. However obstinate it may be, the remedy, being taken a second time, will carry it off, by forcing the worm to come out, if it be already formed, or by preventing its formation, if taken at an early stage of the disease. The remedy used against the sting of scorpions, I have yet had but few opportunities of trying, having only administered it in three cases, where it proved so successful, that given in two of them, when the pain was insupportable, about an hour after their being stung, within half an hour after being taken, the pain was considerably abated, and in an hour ceased altogether. It is well known how painful and burdensome the Guinea worm is to persons who are subject to it; for, besides the smart pains it ordinarily produces, it obliges them to sustain a great loss of time, as it attacks chiefly the legs, rendering them incapable of all movement for many months. I have known poor fellows deprived, in this way, of all power to procure for themselves and their needy family a scanty subsistence, being incapable of any labour for six months, and sometimes more; one worm having no sooner come out than another made its appearance. It is not rare to see persons from whose legs six or seven of those worms, and sometimes more, come out in succession, after occasioning great pain, for many months. When this disorder (which prevails all over this district, as well as many others in the Carnatic and Madura, to within the diſtance of one or two days journey from the ſea-coaſt) breaks out, it is ſometimes epidemic, ſo that I have often ſeen villages in which more than half the inhabitants were affected by it at the ſame time. Although it appears at every ſeaſon of the year, yet it more generally breaks out in the months of December, January, and February: it is then that it becomes general in many cantons; at other times of the year there are fewer perſons viſited by it. The ſymptoms which announce this diſeaſe are almoſt always the ſame; an uneaſineſs is experienced during ſome days, which is by intervals accompanied by headach, pain in the ſtomach, and nauſea. One or two days before the pain is fixed in the part through which the worm is to make its paſſage, an eruption of ſmall pimples, accompanied with a very unpleaſant itching, takes place over the whole body: this itching becomes more violent in the place where the worm is to paſs, until the pain is fixed in it, when the part ſwells; ſometimes to a great extent, with conſiderable inflammation, which is ſoon followed by ſuppuration. In this caſe, the worm often comes out with the pus, or makes its appearance when the ſuppuration is at an end: ſometimes the place where it is lodged puffs up in the form of a bladder, filled with a limpid matter, and ſometimes only a hardneſs is produced, without any conſiderable inflammation taking place. The period for the worm to come out is not determined within the firſt eight or ten days of the diſeaſe: in many caſes, two or three months elapſe before it makes its appearance, and, during the whole of that time, the limb will continue in a ſtate of ſwelling, inflammation, and ſuppuration. Sometimes it will come out all at once, being gently aſſiſted; and, in this caſe, it is often in a living ſtate. I have many times ſeen theſe inſects extracted from the leg continue to live and move for many minutes; however, for the moſt part, the worm comes out by little and little, about an inch being extracted every day: care muſt then be taken to roll it round a ſtraw, or ſome other ſubſtance, to prevent its returning again. If it be drawn rudely, it is liable to break, as often happens, and, in theſe caſes, the part which remains, will again occaſion ſwelling and inflammation, attended with ſmart pain, which will be again followed by ſuppuration, and the diſorder will prove tedious and obſtinate. However ſevere the diſorder, it is never, or very ſeldom, followed by mortification; nevertheleſs, it is not uncommon to ſee caſes in which ſome of the principal nerves have been ſo much injured by it, as to produce lameneſs, or ſome deformity of the legs.

These worms are of different sizes; I have seen some more than a cubit in length, although they are commonly shorter; but, in general, their size and form may be compared to the treble string of a violin. The places in which they make their appearance are the extremities, chiefly the legs: sometimes they appear on the arms. I have been assured in many places by natives, that they were sometimes observed in the other extremities, such as the nose, ears, eye lids, &c.; but I have never seen them myself, excepting in the legs and arms. I feel myself no ways qualified to undertake a discussion on the origin and causes of this singular disease. The natives, accustomed to attribute most of their disorders to the offensive quality of bad water, are generally of opinion that this also proceeds from that source, pretending that these worms are generated in it, and swallowed in a living state, and that they continue to grow in the human body, until they have found a passage to come out. It would be difficult in following this notion, to explain how these insects may pass through deglutition, digestion, &c. in a state of life. On the other hand, admitting that water has no share in their formation, it will not be easy to explain how the inhabitants of a village, who drink water from one well, are attacked by the disease; whilst the inhabitants at the distance only of half a mile, who drink water from another well, are not exposed to it: or how it happens that those living on the shores of the Cavary, and other rivers, who constantly drink their limpid waters, are never visited by it: whilst those who live at the distance of one mile on both sides, and are obliged to drink the saltish water of wells, are all, or the most part, yearly exposed to it The climate may perhaps also be allowed to contribute to the prevalence of the disease, as I am informed it is very seldom observed amongst people living near the sea. I never saw it in any part of the Mysore, and its very name is not known above the Ghauts; whilst it prevails generally over the Carnatic, and other districts below the Ghauts, the vicinity of rivers excepted, as I have already observed But whatever may be the cause and origin of the disease, it will be enough for me if the remedy I propose proves a specific for its cure; and I will now relate an instance which, independently of experience, would prove its efficacy. A long time before I was acquainted with this remedy, conversing with the natives on the disease, it was many times remarked that Bramins were never or very rarely affected with it, although living in villages where the other inhabitants were constantly visited by it every year; but I never paid any attention to such a remark, considering it as one of those idle assertions so common amongst the natives, for

which

which no apparent cauſe can be alleged, excepting in this caſe, to attribute that exemption as a privilege excluſively attached to the ſacred character of that order of men. Reflecting, however, on that remark, after being acquainted with the remedy, I was led to ſuppoſe that this exemption of the Bramins from the diſeaſe muſt be attributed to the conſtant and daily uſe which they make of the *aſſafœtida*, or *peroongabyam*, as one of the principal ingredients in their food, which is alſo the principal ingredient in the remedy. That uſed againſt the ſting of ſcorpions may likewiſe be applied with equal ſucceſs, for the ſting of winged inſects, agreeably to the encloſed receipt. The ſhrub whoſe root proves a ſpecific in this caſe, is called by the natives *kaletchy-cheddy*. Not being acquainted with the name given to it by European botaniſts, I encloſe two of its fruit, called *kaletchy-kabye*, that you may by them know the ſhrub which produces them. It is to be found in every hedge, but as there are different kinds, only thoſe which produce white fruit, like thoſe I ſend you, muſt be choſen, the root of the other kinds not poſſeſſing the ſame virtue.

I have the honour to be, &c. &c. &c.

(Signed) Dubois, *Miſſionary*.

Sattimungalum, March 23. 1805.

REMEDY AGAINST THE STING OF SCORPIONS.

Take, at the time of the new moon, the root of the ſhrub called, in Malabar, *kaletchy-cheddy*, of the kind producing white fruit*: Cut it into pieces three or four inches in length, and let them dry in the ſhade. When any perſon has been ſtung by ſcorpions, cut a bit of that root as big as an ordinary bean: let the patient put it into his mouth, and, preſſing it gently between his teeth, let him ſwallow his ſpittle, taking a freſh bit of the root every 12 minutes. At the ſame time, a ſmall quantity of the root being reduced to a fine powder, pour on it three or four drops of water; let it be worked into the conſiſtence of a ſoft paſte, and applied to the wound.

REMEDY AGAINST THE GUINEA WORM.

1. Take of genuine *aſſafœtida*, called by the Tamuls *peroongabyam*, ſeven gold fanams weight. 2. The fruit well known in all the Indian gardens, called by the Tamuls *katri-*

1 *kabe*,

* This diſtinction of the miſſionary appears very vague to the Profeſſors Jacquin, as the ſeeds of every guilandina, of which five ſpecies are known, are all white.

kabe, and by the Portuguese *beringelle* *. 3. Oil of sesamum, called by the Tamuls *natta-yennie*, a quantity in which the katrikahe, or beringelle, may be fried. Bruise the assafœtida, and having divided with a knife the beringelle into three equal parts, leaving them only united by the stalk, insert a third part of the assafœtida into each of the parts; afterwards sew them together with a thread, and fry the beringelle over the fire, in any convenient vessel, with the oil. Give one part to the patient on his going to bed, another in the morning, and the last on the evening of the next day; and rub with the oil, in which the ingredients were fried, that part of the limb where the worm is lodged, three times a-day for three days.

Extract of a Letter, dated Fort St George, March 29. 1805, *from Dr Anderson to the Rev. Mr Dubois.*

The Kaletchy which you have recommended as a remedy for the sting of insects, is of the order *Lomentacea*, and genus *Guilandina* of Linnæus, of which botanists have distinguished two species, the bonduc and the bonducella, without any remark on the colour of the seeds; but those of a light-brown colour I have seen given with advantage by a Bengal lady here, on her passage to Europe, to her own child, labouring under an intermitting fever, in preference to Jesuit's bark. The reason you have supposed for the Bramins not being so much subject to the Guinea worm as the other inhabitants of the country, leads to a very natural conclusion, on which I shall only remark, that having observed a similar difference between the liability of our officers and privates, having had sometimes thirty of the latter, without any of the former, at a time under my care for this disease, and, unable to find any such difference in the diet to warrant the conclusion which you have made, I was led to think that the privates contracted the disease by sleeping upon earthen pyales †, as practised at that time, which has since been greatly remedied by the introduction of wooden benches into the barracks and guard-rooms of the men. It is well known that the

* According to Dr Griffith, the *Beringelle* of the Portuguese, called by the English in India *Brinjaul*, is the fruit of the *Solanum Melongena Linn.* This fruit, which is well known, and often eaten on the continent of Europe, particularly in Italy and in the south of France, under the name *Aubergine*, is of an insipid taste. The manner in which it is commonly fried seems to constitute its sole merit as a comestible; and it is indeed difficult to suppose that it possesses any anthelmintic power. It must, therefore, be considered rather as a vehicle for the assafœtida than a necessary ingredient in the remedy.

† Pyales are those mounds of earth formed like ordinary benches, upon which the natives of India are accustomed to sleep before their houses. They are usually defended from the sun by a thatch of Palmyra leaves.

the ichneumon fly lodges its eggs in the silk-worm, as a proper nidus for their future subsistence, and we daily find flies in the very kernels of fruits that have been deposited when ova, without leaving any external mark; nor can we cavil with the idea of an entrance by the chylopoetic organs, when we see worms in the eyes of horses *, and in the livers of sheep. I have been inclined to think that the Guinea worm was introduced into the human body after the manner of many other insects, in providing for their offspring, or that, in the state of ova, they might have been taken up from the moist earth through the absorbents of the skin. Let this be as it will, it is our business to get rid of them as easily as possible; and there cannot be a doubt that an additional remedy is always a consolation to the afflicted, and the well-known *assafœtida* being in the hands of every one, its agency on animal sensibility will frequently be had recourse to, as well for prevention as cure. In my own practice, I have found nothing so beneficial as poultices of the Cattale of the Tamuls, (*aloe-littoralis* †) which I likewise learned from a native of India The saponaceous quality which it seems to possess, by softening the integuments in high degrees of inflammation, checked the tendency to gangrene and mortification in many instances, as well as admitted a more free exit to the worm, which I have seen in the breasts of men, as well as in all the lower extremities. When you consider that insects sometimes come as blights over countries where they never appeared before, you will find it difficult to establish the local situation of some species such as this perhaps, known by the name of the Guinea worm, as our ships only frequent the mouths of rivers in Africa, from whence the first notice of them has come. Rajamundry, which is on the bank of the Godavery, the largest river on the coast, is, to my knowledge, very subject to them, and it is notorious that they prevail at Trichinopoly, which lies upon the river Cavary: nor are we without evidence of their existence at Bombay, which is altogether a maritime place; and, indeed, your notice of wells of saltish water, where they are most frequent with you, renders it in some

* This disease, '*a worm in the eye of a horse*,' is, I believe, unknown in Europe, but is common in India, and is cured by the native farriers by an operation similar to the extraction of the cataract. The insect is seen floating in the humour of the eye; the horse appears to suffer great uneasiness, and a constant weeping takes place. For further particulars, application might be made to the surgeons attached to the regiments of native cavalry on the Madras establishment.

† This species of aloë is quite unknown to the celebrated botanists of Vienna, M. M. Jacquin.

some degree probable that vitriolic and marine salts, which are found both in wells and in the sea, are not unfavourable to their propagation, although I have seen them where nothing but the purest rock water was made use of.

VI.

Case of Sphacelated Hernia, with Observations.

By George Kellie, M. D. Fellow of the Royal College of Surgeons, Edinburgh.

The usual termination, and indeed the natural crisis, of strangulated hernia, when neglected, is gangrene of the intercepted parts, generally followed by the death of the unfortunate sufferer. Sometimes, indeed, after the separation of the sphacelated gut, an uncomfortable existence is preserved by the formation of what has been called an artificial anus. Uncertain, however, as this event must be, the process of nature, in effecting it, is so clear and intelligible, as to enable the practitioner to anticipate and assist her efforts, or, aiming at a higher advantage, to restore the continuity of the intestinal tube, and the natural course of the faeces towards the rectum, by a proper apposition of the ends of the divided gut. And the success which crowned the operation of Ramdhor, and the result of experiments made on brutes, encourage the trial of the latter method in those cases which admit the attempt.

Every book on the subject speaks of this accident of an artificial anus. But there is yet a more fortunate, though perhaps a rarer, natural crisis of sphacelated hernia, where, although the hernial tumour and its contents are affected with gangrene, and the fæces make their appearance through the sphacelated gut, the continuity of the intestinal canal is yet preserved, and the natural course of the bowels restored, without the interference of art, and when not a hope had been indulged of so happy an occurrence. Many such cases, however, are to be found in the records of surgery. The circumstances under which this has happened would appear to be these.

1*st*, The most simple case is when a portion of the circumference only of the intestine has been exposed to stricture, and suffered sphacelation. When the whole diameter of the gut has not been acted on by the stricture, and the gangrene is confined

confined to the small part of the circumference intercepted, then, though feculent matter may be for a time discharged by the opening, part also may pass on and be discharged per anum; and the continuity of the gut having never been altogether destroyed, on the cicatrizing of the wound, the natural course of the bowels will be restored. Several cases of this description are related by M. Louis, in an excellent memoire "Sur la Cure des Hernies avec Gangrene *."

2. The caput coli may be displaced, and, descending through the ring, form the herniary tumour. Becoming strangulated, with the usual symptoms, mortification may ensue, the cœcum be thrown off, and the fæces discharged by the wound, which may afterwards close without any interruption of the natural passages.

3. In like manner, a favourable termination of sphacelated hernia may be expected, when the part destroyed has not been any portion of the regular intestine, but a preternatural appendix, cul de sac, or diverticulum, as such a process of the intestine has been variously called. These diverticula have been frequently observed, either as lusus naturæ, or as the products of disease †. According to the observations of Ruysh and Morgagni, they occur most commonly in the ileum, though they have also been found in other portions of the intestine. Such a cul de sac has been the only part protruded and strangulated in some cases of hernia which have terminated fatally ‡.

Whether a small portion only of the diameter of the intestine has been intercepted, and pinched as the French surgeons describe it, or the caput cœcum, or a preternatural diverticulum,

* Memoires de l'Academie Royale de Chirurgie.

† Esse autem interdum præter naturalem illam (apophysin cœci intestini) alias aliquas appendices quas et diverticula vocant, herniæque sacculum subire, certum est, sive illæ sensim præter naturam producantur, sive a prima origine quibusdam corporibus sint datæ.

Morgagni, Epist. xxxiv. 16.

‡ A full account is given of a case of this kind by Morgagni. The following is the description of the diverticulum, as observed on dissection after the death of the patient. "Erat ejus cavitatis qua sensim ab intestino incipiebat, major axis trium circiter digitorum secundum intestini longitudinem; minor axis multo brevior, quippe per anteriorem intestini faciem digituli intervallo a mesenterii insertione ad inferiorem faciem se extendens. Illis ex initiis paulatim cavitas magis magisque; ut semiovalis requirit figura, se contrahebat, donec ad pollicis profunditatem in medio descenderet. Hanc igitur sive cavitatem malis, sive diverticulum appellare, hernia solam intercipiebat, non reliquum intestini tubum, simulque cum omenti extrema parte concludebat."

Lib. III. Epist. xxxiv. 18.

verticulum or cul de ſac has been ſtrangulated and thrown off by ſphacelation, we underſtand how the cure may be ſo fortunately completed by nature, and the fæces, though at firſt diſcharged by the wound, reſume their natural courſe; for the continuity of the inteſtinal canal has not been deſtroyed, and has ſcarcely been interrupted.

4. If, however, the whole circumference of the gut be ſtrangulated, if a complete link of inteſtine be intercepted and deſtroyed by gangrene, we could not, without the interference of art, expect any more favourable termination than the formation of an artificial anus.

Even in ſuch caſes, however, the ſurgeon has been ſurpriſed by a happier criſis. After the loſs of ſeveral inches of gut, including the whole circumference of the ſeparated portion, the artificial anus has cloſed, and, as unexpectedly, the fæces have afterwards continued to paſs by the natural outlet. M. Pipelet, aſſiſted by M. Guerin, had the good fortune to treat a caſe of this kind. The eleventh day from the operation, the ſphacelated inteſtine ſeparated from under the crural arch; it was five inches in length. From that moment the fæces, which had hitherto partly eſcaped from an opening in the gut, and had partly paſſed by the anus, were only paſſed by the wound. The wound gradually contracted, and, at the end of four months, the fæces were ſtill entirely diſcharged by the artificial anus. No more favourable termination was or could be expected. In conſequence, however, of ſome indiſcretion committed by the patient, ſhe was attacked with diſorder of the bowels and fever, for which M. Pipelet preſcribed a laxative, when, to his great aſtoniſhment, the fæces, which had ſo long paſſed entirely by the wound, were diſcharged in the natural way by the anus. In twelve or fifteen days more, the wound was completely cicatrized, the natural function was fully reſtored, and the woman enjoyed good health for ſixteen years after. The proceſs by which nature alone accompliſhed this fortunate cure cannot be better explained than in the words of M. Louis. "Si les deux portions ſaines de l'inteſtin contractent dans leur adoſſement au-deſſus de l'anneau une adherence mutuelle; il eſt clair qu' apres la ſeparation de l'anſe pendante au dehors, ces portions réunies formeront un canal continu, qui ne ſera ouvert que dans la partie anterieure, c'eſt-à dire, dans la partie qui regarde l'anneau; et ſi les bords de cette ouverture ſont adherens de chaque coté à la circonférence de l' anneau, celuici en ſe reſſerrant, en fera neceſſairement la reunion parfaite." "Ces cas," he adds, "ſe preſentent quelquefois pour le bonheur des malades *."

The

* Memoires de l' Academie Royale de Chirurgie.

The general rule for the surgeon, however, must always be to guard against so formidable an accident as sphacelation of the protruded gut, by a seasonable division of the stricture, when the hernia is otherwise irreducible. But those rarer examples of fortunate escapes, after mortification of the herniary contents, do not the less deserve to be recorded. They teach us not to withdraw our efforts through despair, even in the worst cases, and point out to us the resources of nature as rules for the interference of art.

Elizabeth Craig, æt. 60, a corpulent woman, of a loose habit of body, showed me, when called to her assistance on the 12th February 1804, the largest crural hernia I had ever seen. It measured nine inches across, and was nearly as prominent as broad. Its figure was equal and round. It was tilted upwards on the right side of the abdomen; and so yielding and relaxed was this poor woman's skin, that, grasping the tumour with both hands, the fingers could be pressed beneath it all round, and distinctly perceive, like a large cord, the narrow neck of the hernia passing under the crural arch. The tumour was hard, and inelastic to the feel; handling it occasioned no pain; the skin was no way discoloured.

For years past she has been subject to this descent, but the tumour never before attained its present size, and was easily reduced. It had now been down 14 days. For ten days she has passed nothing by stool. She is still obstinately constipated. She complains of constant pain in the epigastric region; she calls it a tearing pain, which, increasing by paroxysms, brings on sickness, erructations, and occasional vomiting. Neither food nor drink have been retained by her stomach these three last days. Her tongue is red and parched. Pulse 100, small, but not very hard. Face flushed, and skin hot. The hernia is irreducible. She was blooded; several injections were given; and purgative and occasional anodynes were prescribed during this and the following day, but in vain; nothing was retained by the stomach, and the injections were ineffectual.

Feb. 14*th*. I had an opportunity of consulting with my friend Mr John Thomson, whose humanity and professional curiosity led him to visit the poor woman at my request.

The great bulk of the herniary tumour we concluded to be omental. The operation was proposed, but resisted by herself and friends. She had given herself up, and wished to resign herself to her fate.

15*th*. Her stomach received and retained one drachm of aloetic pill, and eight grains of calomel, yesterday prescribed to be taken in divided doses. She has since had very severe griping

ping pains about the umbilicus, occasional but ineffectual calls to stool; and, on such an attempt this evening, she was seized with stercoraceous vomiting in my presence. To have a draught with 50 drops of laudanum.

16th. Slept a few hours. Vomited once only; but has retained a cup of tea, which she took for breakfast this morning. The tumour appears less bulky, though as firm and irreducible as ever. This evening she passed a great deal of wind, and even some feculent lumps by stool. Pulv. Jalap. comp. ℈ss. 3tia. q. q. hora.

17th. Several liquid stools, with scybalæ, this morning. The tumour is diminishing very sensibly in bulk. No vomiting or pain since yesterday. Tongue white, and furred in the middle. Pulse 60. To have a laxative in the morning, and anodyne at night.

21st. Has every day convalesced. The tumour has been gradually diminishing, and what remained was this day quite reduced.

23d. Continues well. Belly and functions natural. She is going about her house as usual.

This woman, however, was again to alarm me by her danger, and surprise me by her escape.

On the 28th April I was requested to visit Mrs Craig, as she was again ill. She had been negligent of her bowels, and, while stooping yesterday at her washing-tub, the hernia again protruded. She has had a restless night. The tumour is not larger than the clenched fist. She complains of nausea and cholic pains. A laxative injection was ordered.

29th. The size of the tumour not larger, but it is so painful, that it can hardly be allowed to be examined, and the skin is discoloured. No stool. Constant vomiting since morning. Pulse 120. Tongue foul. To be blooded; a purgative clyster to be given and repeated. An anodyne draught at bed-time. Cold solution of acetite of lead to be applied to the tumour.

30th. Vomiting continues. No evacuation by stool. Complains greatly of the pain of the tumour. The skin is red. Mr Charles Anderson was requested to visit her along with me. She refuses to submit to the operation, which now appears the only hope. Two grains of calomel to be taken every hour. The anodyne to be repeated at bed-time. The cold applications to be continued.

May 1st. A restless night, with delirium. Vomiting continues. The tumour is more prominent and more discoloured, of a dark shining red; two small erysipelatous vesicles on its surface.

ſurface. Calomel to be omitted. Fomentations to the tumour, and anodyne at bed-time.

2d. Complains dreadfully of burning pain in the tumour. It feels ſofter; there is a perceptible fluctuation under the ſkin, which is prominent in the centre of the ſwelling, and pointing like an abſceſs. Has not vomited ſince laſt night. Wind paſſed by the anus, but no fæces. Pulſe 120. To take an ounce of caſtor oil.

3d. Diſturbed and reſtleſs night. No ſtool. Stomach rejected the oil, but ſhe has not ſince vomited. Her chief complaint is of the inſufferable pain, heat, and tenſion of the tumour. The ſkin is now very thin, of a gloſſy red, and ſeems ready to give way. She is urgent that ſomething may now be done to relieve her ſufferings, and, with little other view than to immediate eaſe, it was agreed to lay open the tumour. A ſmall opening was accordingly made (Mr Anderſon being preſent), through which there was immediately diſcharged, with great impetuoſity, mixed with a little pus, an abundance of fluid fœcal matter, which more than filled a half-pint baſon. The tumour ſubſided, and the poor woman expreſſed a grateful ſatisfaction, in which we were far from ſympathizing. An emollient poultice was applied. An anodyne draught in the evening.

4th. Has ſlept well, and continues eaſy. Pulſe 100. Tongue foul. She has not vomited. The belly is neither tenſe nor painful. There is a purulent diſcharge, and ſeveral ſmall feculent lumps on the poultice. The tumour has greatly ſubſided. It has a looſe and knotty feel. The ſkin is better coloured. Poultices to be continued.

5th. Yeſterday ſhe went to ſtool, and has again this morning had two natural evacuations per anum. Feculent matter is alſo diſcharged by the wound. A long portion of a ſoft, white ſlough, protruding from the wound, was eaſily withdrawn. It is about three inches long, but its organization ſo deſtroyed as to afford no diſtinct marks of its origin.

6th. A good night. Continues in every reſpect better. Pulſe 90. Frequent looſe ſtools, in the natural way. A very ſmall portion of thin feculent matter on the poultice, with ſmall membranous ſloughs.

7th. The herniary contents have returned within the abdomen; for the tumour has entirely ſunk. Belly open; functions natural. Diſcharge from the wound ſimply purulent.

8th. Purulent diſcharge continues. A long ſlough protruded, and was removed.

11*th.*

11th. Wound looking well. Discharge diminishing. Belly natural.

14th. Wound contracting daily.

20th. The wound is now cicatrized. She continues free from all complaint; only, when in the erect posture, the hernial tumour reappears of considerable size. It is easily returned when in bed; and a very careful examination of it, at different times, has convinced me that it is entirely intestinal. I have this day, May 20. 1806, examined it once more. It is large, elastic, and easily returned, with a gurgling noise, and again descends when the pressure is removed. She has tried a truss, but was obliged to lay it aside, on account, as she says, of the cholic pains which it always brings on.

I cannot pretend to offer any particular explanation of this case. It is probable that a very small breach only had been made in the intestine, through which the fæces had passed into the hernial sac.

Leith, May 20. 1806.

We add the following very interesting Case of Sphacelated Hernia, communicated, at the request of the Editors, by the Physician who attended the Patient:

On Wednesday the the 18th December last, I was called in haste to see a man from the country, said to be dying. He was a stout, hale-looking man, of between 40 and 50 years of age, not, by his own account, subject to any complaint, except habitual costiveness, and occasional flatulency in his stomach, which he imputed to dram-drinking.

The day before (Tuesday), while on the road from Haddington to town, he had been taken ill with fits of severe pain in his bowels, and he had had a good deal of vomiting and retching. Nothing would stay on his stomach, and several purgative medicines had been given him, but without effect. When I saw him, he also complained of a severe pain frequently seizing him in the left groin, and shooting up that side of the abdomen. I immediately suspected the cause of the patient's distress, and, on examination, discovered a large hernial tumour, extending into the scrotum of the left side. This, however, he seemed to make no account of, as he has had it for about eighteen years, and it had never given him any uneasiness, except

slight

ſlight pains in the part and in the belly when he caught cold. The pulſe was rather frequent, the tongue a little clammy, but the ſkin was cool.

With ſome difficulty I ſucceeded in reducing the tumour, and its reduction was accompanied by a gurgling noiſe. A proper truſs was afterwards applied, and on Saturday he left town quite recovered.

On the 30th, however, I was informed that he was confined to the houſe from a ſwelling in his right groin, which had become ſo painful, that he could not extend the thigh, and that the ſurgeon in the country had directed the application of a poultice to it. This did not excite in me any great apprehenſion, although, on one occaſion, as I was examining the *left* ſcrotal hernia, I had been ſtruck with the appearance of a ſmall ſwelling in the *right ſide*, which ſeemed hard, knotty, and ſlightly moveable. It originated two years before from a blow on the part, and had never been productive of any uneaſineſs. At the time, I conſidered it as an indolent enlarged gland, and am ſtill perſuaded, although it perhaps did not meet with the attention it deſerved, that at that period no hernia exiſted in the right ſide, as, after the reduction of the left hernia, all the ſymptoms ceaſed. In the afternoon, however, of the following day, I received a meſſage to viſit him immediately, as the ſwelling had mortified, and the greateſt danger was dreaded.

When I ſaw him, his looks did not indicate much diſtreſs; his pulſe was by no means bad; he was in good ſpirits, took his food with appetite, and had enjoyed a good night's reſt. He was perfectly free from pain in the abdomen, and felt but little in the affected groin. He confirmed to the fulleſt extent the account which had been given me of his having been entirely free from retching or vomiting, and of his having daily had natural and eaſy motion of his bowels.

After this account, my ſurpriſe and diſappointment will not ſeem ſtrange, when I ſaw the appearances the affected parts exhibited. The ſkin and cellular ſubſtance of the groin, to the extent of about two inches and a half in length, and one in breadth, had ſloughed off, and the ſurrounding ſkin was inflamed, and rather of a livid hue. The greater part of that portion of the peritoneum which had formed the herniary ſac was quite deſtroyed, leaving only a kind of cobweb fringe attached to the edges of the wound, and expoſing a portion of inteſtine. This, in ſize and ſhape, reſembled the half of a hen's egg divided in the direction of its longeſt axis. It was ſituated higher up than the ſeat of femoral hernia, and more towards the ſpine of the os

ileum

ileum, than the feat of common inguinal hernia, appearing to me to be exactly in the fituation of the internal ring. This tumor of the inteftine had a pretty natural appearance, that is to fay, it was whitifh, and bore little mark of inflammation; but, upon preffing it, air-bubbles iffued from feveral points of it. A confiderable quantity of a thin brownifh fluid, of a very offenfive foetor, flowed from it, and fmall quantities of foeculent matter could alfo be preffed out. After the preffure, it remained flaccid, and the upper fide of it at leaft was in firm adhefion to the contiguous parts of the abdominal parietes. So far as I judged prudent to examine, there was little ftricture upon the gut, infomuch that had there not exifted an adhefion, the inteftine could, in my opinion, have been replaced into the abdomen.

Notwithftanding that the pulfe and vires vitæ in general were much improved to what they had been for fome days before, yet our prognofis was very unfavourable. We had, indeed, the hope that the patient might efcape with the inconvenience of an artificial anus, but we were rather difpofed to dread the worft. We did not fee that any furgical operation could be of ufe, as nature had fulfilled the only rational indication in view, viz. fecuring the gut to the internal wound, fo that the difeafed gut might not flip into the abdomen, and a paffage be fecured through the external wound for the fæces. If the cafe fhould terminate in this way, we alfo hoped that in time the patient might obtain a complete cure, particularly as we concluded that the whole caliber of the inteftine was not affected, fince he all along had enjoyed natural and eafy paffage of his bowels. A carrot poultice, with fome yeaft, was applied to the part, and a liberal exhibition of bark and wine was ordered.

I returned to town, and received the following account of the ftate of our patient, on the 7th January, from the furgeon attending him.

"Dear Sir,—I have delayed giving you an account of the interefting cafe at Linton, until I vifited the patient yefterday.

"I am happy to fay I found him in better fpirits, with a better countenance and better pulfe than the day on which you vifited him. The gut in the fame ftate as you obferved it, the fphacelation going on, and more evident marks of decay.

"The external wound or fore has now fine granulations, a good difcharge and healthy appearance, and the offenfive fmell is corrected.

"But what appears moft fingular in the cafe is the regular, eafy, and natural ftools which daily take place.

"The pulfe is firmer, at 68, and his appetite good.

 He

He is going on in the same plan, bark, wine, an opiate in the evening, and the antiseptic poultices."

Upon the receipt of this letter, considering that the gut was much decayed, that the fæces did not force their way through the wound, but had a free and easy discharge per anum, it occurred to me, that this diseased gut must be the anterior part of the cœcum, or caput coli. For although, from the contiguity of the ileum to the groin, and from the length of the mesentery allowing it to move very freely within the abdomen on the one hand, and from the close, strong, and ligamentous attachment of the cœcum and right side of the colon to the kidney, on the other, one should naturally suppose the ileum to be most frequently the subject of hernia; yet experience does not confirm this. Mr Pott, on this subject, has the following passage in his Treatise on Ruptures: "That the descent, or more properly protrusion, of a part of the cœcum and colon is rare, is not true, for it happens very frequently. Perhaps it would not bear to be established as a general rule; but from what has fallen within my observation, in frequently performing the operation for a strangulated rupture, it has appeared to me, that the greater number of those in whom it has been necessary (all attempts to reduce the parts by the hand having proved fruitless) has consisted of the cœcum, with its appendicula, and a portion of the colon."

In the course of a few days I received the following very satisfactory confirmation of my opinion.

"13*th January*, 1806.

"Dear Sir—Agreeably to my promise and your desire, I sit down with much pleasure to give you an account of our patient, who, I am happy to say, has most completely deceived the doctors, and every one who visited him.

"On the 7th of January the sphacelated portion, which formed the hernia, separated and came off with the poultice, and it was fortunately preserved in water.

"Upon examination, on the 8th, it appeared to consist entirely of the blind sac of the colon or cœcum, which satisfactorily explains the regular, easy, and natural stools which of late had daily taken place. The external sore was clean; healthy granulations appeared, and there was a rich discharge of pus, free from fœculent matter and smell. Having a desire to empty his bowels on this day, whilst I was with him, upon inspection, I found it easy, and in every respect natural. The pulse 64, and feeble; appetite and spirits better.

"From

" From every consideration of what has taken place in this case, I entertain a hope that adhesion of the remaining part was going on even at the time you visited him, and is now completed internally.

" Dressed with charpee compress and gentle pressure by bandages. Continued the bark, wine, and opiate, with nourishing diet.

" From the 8th to this day, the external sore has been healing rapidly, and, to a wish, his appetite and spirits improving, with a gradual return of strength; though, I must confess, this does not evidently appear in the pulse, which I found this day still low and feeble, about 60; which induces me to go on with the bark and wine, and nourishing diet, for some time longer.

" I would have informed you of the result ere this, but was inclined to delay; for, candidly speaking, I must confess I did not expect so favourable a termination.

" I remain," &c.

The foregoing case is uncommon, and, so far as my surgical knowledge extends, is, in many respects, new. It has terminated, beyond expectation, most fortunately for the patient, although professional curiosity would have been satisfied with the internal inspection of the parts. If the surgeon be right in his conjecture, which, in my opinion, he is, that there is a complete adhesion of the remaining part of the cœcum internally, it will resemble one of those rare varieties of hernia, where the opposite sides of the intestine, just above the protruded portion, adhere, while the part has no communication with the intestinal canal, and forms a cul de sac. The present case would form one of the most favourable of these varieties, since the cœcum having formed the cul de sac, no narrowness or tightness will remain at the affected part of the alimentary canal.

Mr Pott relates a very wonderful case of hernia, where about three inches of protruded ileum became completely sphacelated. The part cast off, and the patient discharged the fæces for some time through the wound; but, in about the space of a month, that entirely ceased, the wound healed, the fæces were discharged naturally and regularly per anum, and the patient continued afterwards well. I may be allowed to make the same remark in my case that Mr Pott has made in his, viz. That, had the usual surgical operation been here performed, or, to speak plainly, had the sphacelated portion of gut been prematurely removed, and the intestine stitched to the external wound, although the patient might have escaped with life, yet, in all

 probability,

probability, he might have been subject to the inconveniency of an artificial anus.

I have only to add, that the patient is now perfectly recovered, feels no inconvenience whatever, and is following his usual occupation of life, which is rather a laborious one.

Edinburgh, 9th May, 1806.

VIII.

Case of Tumour in the Tongue, cured by Calomel and Cicuta. By one of the Surgeons of the Sunderland Dispensary.

EMMA HAZARD, a married woman, in the 55th year of her age, applied for relief to the Sunderland Dispensary, in consequence of a hard tumour, seemingly of a schirrous disposition, occupying the middle and fore part of the tongue, but extending farther back on its under than upper surface. She had been troubled with it for more than three years, during the latter part of which period it became so uneasy and painful, as to induce her to apply for medical assistance on September 9. 1805. The tumour, from its bulk, and being situated in the middle of the tongue, equally between its upper and under surface, not admitting of excision, she was desired by a respectable surgeon, under whose care she had been placed as a patient of the Dispensary, to employ the cicuta, which she continued to take in the form of a pill, to the extent of a drachm daily, till the 23d of November, but without effect. A consultation of the surgeons of the Dispensary, of whom I am one, being at this time called, and it appearing manifest that, so far from getting better under the above-mentioned treatment, she daily became worse, it was agreed, at my suggestion, to combine with the cicuta half a grain of calomel daily, which was afterwards increased to a whole grain. Being made to observe this plan for some time, she appeared to derive manifest advantage from it, excepting that, on the 16th of December, her bowels became affected; which inconvenience, however, was speedily remedied, by having recourse to opium. This plan being observed, on the 23d of the same month the tumour became much less painful and indurated, and some small ulcers which

surrounded

furrounded it were obferved to heal up. It being ftill perfifted in, fhe continued to mend daily. On the 30th of January her tongue was almoft well, and, on February the 3d, fhe was difmiffed completely cured.

I fhall refrain from making a fingle remark upon the cafe I have detailed, contenting myfelf with confidering it as an ufeful addition to our prefent ftock of medical facts, from which future advantage may be derived to the practice; and, as fuch, I feel defirous of its being announced to the public through the medium of the Edinburgh Medical and Surgical Journal.

It may be neceffary to obferve, that the woman has remained in perfect good health ever fince the time of her difmiffal from the Difpenfary.

Sunderland, March 7. 1806.

IX.

Cafe of Tic Douloureufe. By George Kitson, Member of the Royal College of Surgeons, London.

Thomas Andrews, aged 29, was attacked with pain over the orbit of the left eye in the morning of Feb. 8, 1806, which continued till about three in the afternoon, when it ceafed, and did not return till the next morning; it ceafed again in the evening, and returned moft violently on the 10th, when I was defired to fee him. I found him affected with univerfal fpafm; his pulfe weak, tremulous, and irregular; his eyebrows drawn down, and the eyelids conftantly clofed. The fpafms would relax for a fhort time, and return with violence. He was perfectly fenfible, and complained of great pain over the orbit of the left eye, immediately in the fituation of the frontal nerve. He faid he could cover the part with the point of his finger, but that the pain extended into the orbit, and over the forehead. The part was not fwelled, nor was the fkin inflamed. The pain was increafed on preffure, which would inftantly bring on the fpafms. It was with difficulty he could be prevailed on to open his eyes. I gave him fome wine, and other ftimuli, with little advantage. The pains and fpafms increafed, and the man ftill perfifting that it proceeded folely from the fpot over the orbit, and that he was free from pain in every other part, I determined to divide the frontal nerve, and made an incifion about half an inch in

 length

length directly above the eyebrow down to the bone; the supra-orbitary artery was divided, but not more than two ounces of blood were lost. The operation gave him great pain, and brought on a violent attack of spasm. In a few minutes he said he was free from pain, and the spasms ceased. I brought the divided skin together by sticking-plaster, and directed a mixture composed, of comp. sp. of vitriolic æther, lavender, and camphorated mixture, to be given occasionally in the evening. I found he had had some sleep, that he was quite free from pain, and considered himself well. Pulse 102, irregular.

Feb. 11th. He has had no return of the pain or spasms; slept well, and was down stairs this morning. He says he is as well as before this attack. Pulse quick, small, and irregular. Ordered to take two table-spoonfuls of the cordial mixture three or four times a-day.

Feb. 12th. He is in his usual state of health. Pulse irregular. Ordered to discontinue medicine, and live chiefly on animal food.

March 13th. The wound united by the first intention. That part of the skin of the forehead, to which the divided nerve is distributed, is still deprived of sensation. He has had no return of the pain; but should it return with the sensation of the part (as has been the case in some instances), I will inform you of it. The irregularity of the pulse proceeds, I have reason to believe, from a disease of the heart, with which he has been affected some time.

Bath, 13th March, 1806.

X.

Account of Dr Gall's Discoveries regarding the Structure of the Brain. By T. C. Rosenmuller, Professor of Anatomy at Leipsic.

From careful observations and examinations of the brain and skull, in men and animals of every class, continued for a long series of years, Dr Gall of Vienna has been convinced that peculiar nerves are appropriated to each of the functions of the mind, as they are to the different senses. When, in any individual, there is a greater disposition to or perfection in in any mental faculty than in the others, the nervous apparatus belonging to it is distinguished by a greater prominency on the convolutions which are observed on the surface of the brain; and this prominency of the brain, or nervous mass, produces on the corresponding part of the skull a gentle rising, or eminence, which is to be seen or felt on the outside.

Many authors have occupied themselves in describing minutely the situations in which, according to Dr Gall's numerous observations and experience, the organs for several functions of the mind are expressed by eminences on the skull. But I am disposed to consider, as of infinitely greater importance, Dr Gall's examination of the brain, which I shall endeavour to communicate as concisely as possible, abstracted from all the results deduced from it. On account of its importance, I shall also confine myself to that part of his inquiries which relates to the human brain; for although, in reality, he was led by a comparison of the brain of animals to his opinions concerning the human brain, it would be too tedious to enumerate, on this occasion, these comparisons, and they will be very circumstantially detailed by Dr Gall himself in a complete treatise which he is preparing on the subject.

According to Gall's investigation, the whole of the medullary substance of the cerebrum and cerebellum consists of nervous fibres, and the whole of the cortical substance of ganglions, by means of which the nervous fibres are nourished, strengthened, and more intimately connected.

The nerves which constitute the essential part of the cerebrum and cerebellum, as well as of the spinal marrow, are, like the blood-vessels, of two kinds; the excurrent or diverging, and the recurrent or converging, which all arise from the spinal marrow, or terminate in it.

The excurrent nerves pass through various ganglions; but a ganglion, according to Gall, consists in an enlargement, in which the nervous filaments separate from each other, and each filament is surrounded with a softer, gelatinous, dirty reddish mass, of a glandular nature, which serves, perhaps, for the nourishment of the nerve, and contains its accompanying blood-vessels. On passing out of such a ganglion, the convolution of nervous filaments is always larger than on entering it. The darker and softer substance, which constitutes the essential part of a ganglion, spreads itself not only over the whole surface of the cerebrum and cerebellum, but is also found in the corpora striata, the thalami nervorum opticorum, the tuber cinereum, between the nervous filaments of the spinal marrow, in the

pons

pons varolii, corpora olivaria, and in all the ganglions unconnected with the brain.

The recurrent nerves, from both hemispheres of the cerebrum and cerebellum, meet at certain places, and form mutual connexions or commissures. Thus, the corpus callosum is the commissure of the cerebrum, and the pons of the cerebellum.

The spinal marrow consists, like the brain itself, of two symmetrical halves, and each half is formed of from eight to twelve distinct bundles of nerves, but contiguous and parallel.

Each of the eight pairs of nervous bundles, which Gall has hitherto ascertained in the spinal marrow, contains the materials of a determined nervous apparatus. Beneath the corpora pyramidalia, the bundles, which were originally parallel, cross each other, so that the nerves of the left half go to the right side, and those of the right half to the left. This decussation may be distinctly observed, if we gently separate the halves of the spinal marrow with the handle of the scalpel, after having removed the pia mater.

The bundles of both sides now ascend thickened, forming the corpora pyramidalia and corpora restiformia (the crura pedunculi, or processus cerebelli ad medullam oblongatam), from the former of which the cerebrum, and from the latter the cerebellum, receives its nerves.

From the corpora pyramidalia, the nervous bundles pass into the pedunculi cerebri, by penetrating through the pons varolii. When the pia mater is removed, we immediately perceive distinctly the transverse fibres of the commissure, which conceal the excurrent nerves of the cerebrum; but the course of the latter is also distinctly seen, when an incision is made into the pons varolii, in the direction of the pedunculi cerebri, towards the corpora pyramidalia, and, by separating the edges of the cut, the transverse nerves of the commissure are scraped off, with the handle of the knife, from the longitudinal nerves of the pedunculi cerebri, which are interwoven with the former like the threads of linen.

The pedunculi cerebri, or the continuation of the corpora pyramidalia, now proceed in an excentric direction of the nervous filaments through a ganglion, viz. through the corpora striata and thalami nervorum opticorum as they are called, but which, in reality, have no connexion with the optic nerves.

If a portion of the posterior lobe of the brain be cut off horizontally from the fossa sylvii backwards, there appears a central lobe of the brain, bounded by a deep groove, which Gall denominates the *insula*. This insula conceals the corpus striatum. By gradually scraping off the substance of this ganglion

glion with the handle of the knife, from within and behind, forwards and outwards, the nervous filaments of the pedunculi cerebri, which proceed through it in their excentric direction, soon become visible. After they leave this ganglion, they again acquire a greater extension, as they continue their course toward the cortical substance of the brain, where they terminate. But this superficial ganglion, in addition to the nerves immediately terminating in it, consists of a large, flat, membranous expansion, which could not be contained within the skull, if it were not folded up like a napkin. In the morbid state of the brain, when water is accumulated in the ventricles, this folded membrane, along with the bones of the skull, gradually becomes so expanded, that the folds or convolutions entirely disappear*, and the nervous fibres, which previously were folded up, are now extended. But they can also be extended, when the circumference of the brain is unfolded into its membranous form, by introducing the finger moistened with water into a lateral ventricle, and gently stroking towards the convolutions, until they disappear.

From this superficial ganglion the recurrent nerves commence, either by originating in the cortical substance, or by the excurrent nerves taking an opposite direction at this place. The recurrent nerves are distinguished from the excurrent by their greater softness, as well as by their opposite course; for they proceed from both sides towards the corpus callosum, and become there blended with each other in their commissure, so that they lie in contiguous transverse bundles, which always grow thicker towards the middle, as more nervous fibres are added. At last they return to the pedunculi cerebri and spinal marrow, from which the nerves of the brain took their rise.

To the cerebellum nervous filaments proceed through the corpora restiformia from the spinal marrow, running upwards and outwards, as they form a part of the pedunculi cerebelli, and then pass through a particular ganglion, the corpus ciliare, or rhomboideum. From this ganglion they again proceed thickened, and terminate in the superficial ganglion, (the cortical substance). From this the recurrent nerves now also take their rise, and, as a broad trunk, pass by the corpus ciliare, unite from the opposite sides in their commissure, the pons varolii, and

* We lately examined a case of hydrocephalus internus, in which this observation was remarkably exemplified. The brain resembled a bladder filled with water, and although its parietes were thin, this was owing to expansion, not to absorption, for it did not weigh less than a healthy brain would do.—*Editors.*

and return, as a part of the pedunculi cerebelli, to the spinal marrow.

In regard to the nerves proceeding from the brain to the organs of sense, there is also some peculiarity of arrangement.

The olfactory nerve arises from its bundle in the spinal marrow, ascends towards the testis as its ganglion, spreads from this as a broad fibrous band outwards upon the pedunculi cerebri; winds around the under and outward part of the corpus striatum in the same manner as the optic nerve, and can, like it, be peeled off the corpus striatum. The trunk again expands beneath the anterior lobe of the brain into a ganglion, from which the single fibres are distributed upon the Schneiderian membrane.

The second pair arises from the spinal marrow, ascends towards the nates as its ganglion, and, on quitting them, winds around the pedunculi cerebri, from behind and without, forwards and inwards, near and behind what are called the thalami nervorum opticorum, but without intermixing with them, so that where it first touches the pedunculi cerebri, it receives fibres from them, but, afterwards partly decussating, unites from the opposite sides, and is, in some degree, connected with the olfactory nerves by means of the fundus ventriculi tertii, or tuber cinereum.

The third pair is also to be found as a bundle in the spinal marrow, is thickened in the corpus olivare as its ganglion, penetrates through the black mass of the pons varolii, in which some fibres separate, and, on leaving it, again unite to form that bundle called the third pair.

The white nervous filaments lying in the fourth ventricle have no connexion with the portio mollis of the seventh pair. They proceed from the inner layer of the spinal marrow into the fourth ventricle, and supply with nerves the nearest convolutions of the cerebellum. In many animals which hear acutely, they are entirely wanting.

THE

THE INQUIRER, Nº VI.

On Herpes.

THE diſeaſes of the ſkin, though numerous and important, have been much overlooked. We have only to conſult the writings of phyſicians to be convinced how neceſſary it has become to determine with preciſion the genera of cutaneous diſeaſes *. The term *herpes* has, in particular, been greatly abuſed; it has, indeed, been ſo variouſly applied by different authors, both ancient and modern, that it has now become not a little difficult to ſeize the true character of thoſe affections which ſhould be claſſed together under that title.

Herpes ſeems to have been originally employed by the Greek phyſicians to expreſs any ſuperficial ſpreading eruption. It is not uſed by Celſus to denote any particular diſeaſe; but, under the genera papulæ and ignis ſacer, he deſcribes thoſe cutaneous diſorders which later phyſicians have comprehended under the term herpes.

Galen admitted three ſpecies of theſe diſeaſe, ἑρπης κεγχριας, εσθιομενος, and φλυκταινωδης; a diviſion which has deſcended to us by the names of herpes *miliaris*, *erodens*, and *phagædenicus*; the firſt from its form and appearance, the ſecond from its malignity and rapid courſe, and the third from its deep ulceration.

There are three orders, however, of cutaneous diſeaſes, which it is highly neceſſary to diſtinguiſh; the papulous eruptions which, without any diſcharge, terminate in ſcurf; thoſe eruptions which, though not prone to ſuppuration, diſcharge a ſerous fluid, and terminate in ſcurf or ſcales; and the puſtulous eruptions, which ſuppurate, and terminate in cruſts or ſcabs, covering ulcerated ſurfaces. The genera lichen, herpes, and impetigo, are examples of theſe different appearances. Lorry, however, one of the beſt modern writers on the diſeaſes of the ſkin, confounds both lichen and impetigo with herpes. And the herpes farinoſus of Sauvage ſhould, in the opinion of Willan, be referred to the genus lichen. The term herpes ſhould therefore be confined to thoſe cluſters of minute puſtules which do not end in ſuppuration, but diſcharge a ſerous lymph †, and

* There is reaſon to hope that this will ſoon be accompliſhed by the labours of Dr Willan.

† "It neither matters nor comes to digeſtion, but, being rubbed, will ſometimes gleet a thin ſharp water."—*Turner*.

"Non raro exudant humorem tenuem et acrem, ſed non ſuppurantur nec reſolvuntur."—*Sauvage*.

and terminate in ſcurf, ſometimes in cruſts. It will thus be ſeparated from the ſimple papulous eruptions on the one hand *, and from puſtular ulcerating affections on the other †.

DEFINITION.

It is difficult to fix the character of this diſeaſe in the terms of a definition. That given by Dr Cullen is too general, and might be applied with equal propriety to other diſeaſes of the ſkin.

"Phlyctenæ vel ulcuſcula plurima, gregalia, ſerpentia, dyſepulenta." The words phlyctenæ ‡ and ulcuſcula convey but an imperfect idea of the herpetic puſtules.

The definition of Sagar applies more ſtrictly to the ſtrophuli and lichenes than to herpes. "Papularum prurientium corymbus in ſquamas furfuraceas fatiſcentium."

Thoſe of Linnæus and of Vogel are rather more accurate. The former defines *herpes* "Puſtulæ eſcharoticæ baſi communi eryſipelacea;" and the latter, "Papula ardens cutem ſerpentibus minimis puſtulis erodens." The definition given by Sauvage, which we ſhall adopt for the preſent, differs little from that of Vogel. "Herpes eſt papularum congeries, ſeu efflореſcentia ex tumoribus exiguis, rubris, aggregatis, pruriginoſis, in ſquamas furfuraceas, raro cruſtaceas abeuntibus ‖."

The accuracy of this definition, however, depends much on the idea underſtood by the term papula, which is explained by Sauvage as differing from the puſtule, "Ex eo quod non ſuppurantur (papulæ), ſed quid humidi apice rejiciunt, dein abeunt in ſquamas furfuraceas §."

HISTORY.

Herpes commonly makes its firſt appearance by an eruption of a number of red elevated papulæ, diſpoſed ſo as to form a ſmall circular areola, a little raiſed above the ſurface, rough to the touch, and ſurrounded with ſome degree of erythema. The areola ſpreads

* Willan deſcribes as genera of papulæ, the ſtrophulus, lichen, and prurigo.

† Scabies, impetigo, ſerpigo, &c.

‡ "Veſſels with a dark red and livid-coloured baſe are uſually denominated Phlyctenæ."—*Willan.*

‖ Noſolog. Methodic. Sauvageſii.

§ This is ſomewhat different from the papula of Willan, "a very ſmall and acuminated elevation of the cuticle, with an inflamed baſe, not containing a fluid, not tending to ſuppuration."—*Willan on Cutaneous Diseases.* We ſhall continue to uſe the term papula in the ſenſe of Sauvage.

spreads more or less rapidly in every direction, by the eruption of new papulæ, and the extension of the erythematic circle. The parts are affected with a troublesome itching, burning heat, and tingling pain. If the papulæ are scratched or rubbed, they discharge a serous fluid, which oozes out from their ruptured apices. This, however, far from relieving, seems rather to increase the itching, which often becomes intolerable. While the first formed eruptions discharge themselves, dry up, and fall off in scurf, a new crop succeeds; on leaving the originally affected parts, the disease spreads over the neighbouring surface. Thus, by the evanescence of one set of pustules, the succession of others, and the spreading erythema, the disease continues often for a long time. But, in slighter cases, the papulæ gradually shrink, or, after discharging a little serous lymph, dry up, leaving the skin discoloured and rough, covered with a furfuraceous scurf, and sometimes with crusts.

Different parts of the body are frequently at the same time affected. The heat and itching which accompany these eruptions are commonly aggravated towards evening, and often prevent the patient sleeping at night; the irritation is also increased by external heat, and after taking food, or swallowing warm and stimulating drinks.

The functions are commonly natural, and the general health seldom suffers, unless in more violent cases, where the irritation may give occasion to some degree of symptomatic fever.

Every part of the skin is occasionally subject to herpes, but the thighs, arms, back, and face, are more frequently affected.

It is generally in spring or summer that herpetic eruptions make their first appearance, and it is not uncommon for the disease to disappear altogether during the colder months, and to return again with the spring.

The system is said to have been relieved from many chronic ailments by the eruption of herpes, and dangerous symptoms are proclaimed to have arisen from its sudden repulsion.

CAUSES.

Predisposition.—There would seem to be, in some individuals, a particular predisposition to this cutaneous affection. Some families are more liable to it than others, and women more than men.

There are two periods of life, Professor Lorry observes, more especially subject to herpes; that which immediately succeeds the complete growth of the body, and, again, about the first decline of the system. "Certè sunt duæ vitæ periodi in quibus maximè emicant herpetes. Prima est periodus illa, in quâ corpus incrementi apicem pervenit, jamque ſuperflua exundant. Altera eſt ubi menſtrua ceſſante in fœminis vacuatione, organis verò ſimul perſpiratoriis in utroque ſexu minus liberis, appelens ad cutem reſiſtat lympha *."

Occaſional Cauſes.—Among theſe we may number, 1. External irritation. Thus, Sauvage informs us that the prieſts of his time were often affected with what he terms *herpes collaris*, "propter acrem tincturam quâ lineum ipſorum collare inficitur †." There is another example better known, the *herpes periſcelis*, la jarretière of the French, "qui poplitem, ubi zona vinciri ſolet, infeſtat †."

2. In ſome individuals, particular ſubſtances received into the ſtomach, as ſome kinds of fiſh, muſcles, bitter almonds, &c. give occaſion to cutaneous eruptions ‡; but it is doubtful if herpes is ever produced in this way. Errors in diet, however, and more eſpecially habitual exceſſes in eating and drinking, may be admitted as cauſes of this diſeaſe ||.

3. Herpes is not unfrequently the immediate conſequence of the body being overheated by violent exerciſe. This cauſe is indeed allowed by almoſt every writer. I have at this time a patient under my care with very extenſive herpetic eruptions on the arms and thighs, in whom the diſeaſe firſt appeared a few hours after returning home much heated and fatigued with more than uſual exerciſe.

A ſimilar caſe is mentioned by Turner: "A ſervant-maid, of a fine ſkin and clear complexion, being red haired, was, after walking in the heat of the day from her maſter's country-houſe to London, ſeized with a burning heat and tingling in her thigh, in which diſcovering a cluſter of pimples in the ſkin, ſhe acquainted her miſtreſs with her fears of the ſmall-pox, which, ſhe ſaid, were very thick in one of her thighs §."

4. Herpetic eruptions ſometimes occur in caſes of ſyphilis, and hence ſyſtematic writers have mentioned a herpes ſyphiliticus, or venereus ¶. The propriety of admitting this ſpecies is, however, queſtionable. There is greater reaſon, perhaps, to attribute ſome caſes of herpes to the mercurial irritation; at leaſt eruptions of this diſeaſe are not uncommon after courſes of mercury.

5.

* Lorry de Morbis Cutaneis, p. 313.

† Sauvag. Noſolog. Methodic.

‡ See Van Swieten Commentar. in Aphoriſmos. Dr Gregory's Lectures, &c. &c.

|| An example may be found in Turner. See alſo Lorry de Morbis Cutaneis.

§ Treatiſe of Diſeaſes incident to the Skin.—*Turner.*

¶ Sauvage Aſtrua.

5. It is asserted by many authors that herpes may be propagated by infection, or casual inoculation, from contiguous intercourse with an affected person *. But the same has been said of almost every cutaneous eruption. For my own part, though I have often seen this disease, I have never known it communicated from one person to another. Negative experiments are certainly not very decisive; but I have attempted to inoculate myself with the serous fluid which oozed from the herpetic papulæ of the patient already mentioned. I introduced the matter in the usual way, under the cuticle of my arm, but without effect.

Lastly, Various other circumstances affecting the general health of the system, such as, suppression of the catamenia, grief, and other debilitating passions, have been assigned as causes of this cutaneous disease †. On these, however, I have no remarks to offer.

DIAGNOSIS.

There is no danger of confounding herpes with any of the exanthemata or impetigenes of Dr Cullen; and the papulous eruptions and itching readily distinguish it from erythema.

Herpes, however, has more resemblance to the lichenes, and other papulous diseases of the skin. But the papulæ of herpes are larger, more distinct, and more elevated than those of lichen; they have more the appearance of pustules; the former contain a fluid, the latter are dry. The eruptions of herpes are more confined, crowded together into distinct and commonly regularly circumscribed forms, the lichens are more diffused and irregular; herpes frequently terminates in crusts, the lichenes in scurf; lichen is commonly preceded by some disorder of the system †, herpes very seldom.

PROGNOSIS.

Herpes is not a disease of any danger, but one of very uncertain duration, sometimes passing away in a few days, sometimes continuing with great obstinacy for a long while.

Solitary

* "In contagio consistit, quod negare pariter medicis expertis impossibile est. Vidi in uno decubitur contractos herpetes, nec facile sanabiles, idque non una vice."—*Lorry de Morb. Cut.* p. 312.

"Per contagium adhuc herpes communicatur, uti osculando, si herpes in facie sit, vel concubando."—*Tractat. duo Patholog. Medico Monspel.* tom. ii. p. 273.

† Willan on Cutaneous Diseases.

Solitary eruptions are more evaneſcent; when different parts of the body are at the ſame time affected, the cure is always more difficult. An extending erythema, with interſperſed papulæ, generally marks an obſtinate diſeaſe.

CURE.

Cutaneous diſorders, in general, ſeem to have afforded ample ſcope to the ſpeculations of the humoral pathologiſts. In theſe complaints, they were at no loſs to demonſtrate the already concocted humours which had vitiated the circulating maſs, and which, by an effort of nature, were thus ſeparated, expelled, and depoſited on the ſurface of the body. Lorry, for example, the very learned author of an excellent work, *de Morbis Cutaneis*, gravely enumerates no leſs than ten different kinds of acrimony generated within the body, and giving riſe to diſeaſes of the ſkin, acrimonies of the bile, of the lymph, of the ſerum, of the mucus, of the milk, and of the fat; a ſcrofulous, venereal, variolous, and morbillous acrimony *. To one or other of theſe fancied acrimonies, it was uſual to refer the different diſorders of the ſkin.

According to Galen, and ſeveral of the Greek phyſicians, vitiated bile was the cauſe of herpes; while Avicenna, it ſeems, blamed, with Hippocrates, an incraſſated pituita. Lorry himſelf finds ſeemingly much difficulty in determining to which of the humours herpes ſhould be referred. He frequently ſpeaks of an herpetic virus wandering over the body, and producing various chronic diſeaſes, till at length it arrives at the ſkin, and relieves the ſyſtem from all its ills. He appears, however, upon the whole, to conſider the lymph as the peccant humour. "In herpetibus etiam non ſerum, non bilis per ſe, quanquam aliter ſenſerunt antiqui preceptores noſtri, luem accipiunt, ſed mucor ille qui proprié lympham conſtituit †."

The practice which has prevailed in the treatment of herpes was the natural offspring of ſuch notions of the diſeaſe.

The cure was always begun by blood-letting and purging; then the patient was bathed, and put on a courſe of diluent ſoups and ptiſans, blooded and purged again, while a variety of alterants were preſcribed with the view of diluting, correcting, and expelling the morbific humour. At length, with the greateſt caution, they ventured on topical applications, which were often inſignificant; for they were fearful leſt, by repelling the humour into the blood, it might fix on ſome important organ, and produce a more dangerous diſeaſe.

* De Morbis Cutaneis, Introduct. p. 51, 48.

† Tractat. de Morbis Cutaneis, p. 304.

Those, however, whose fears were not alarmed by visionary speculations, employed, at all times, external applications with a happy freedom; for their practice was successful, nor did they experience those complicated evils which the theory of the humoral pathologists led them to expect, and which their practice sometimes perhaps gave rise to.

Celsus trusted much to external remedies; he ordered the parts affected to be fomented with wine, and recommended several healing applications *. Ambrose Parée, after some general evacuations, at times, no doubt, necessary, prescribed astringent ointments, with the powder of oak-galls and alum †. And Turner, who, not much addicted to theory, generally details the result of his own successful practice in the simple language of truth, recommends topical applications of a similar naure, solutions of alum, and of white vitriol, and astringent ointments, containing often the submuriate of mercury ‡. The vulgar, too, no way suspicious of danger, and experiencing none, often put a stop to the progress of herpes by the simple application of ink.

Let us then banish those lurking fears to which a fanciful pathology has given birth, and at once attempt the cure of a very troublesome and often distressing disease.

After all, we shall soon find how little it is in our power to repel or to cure these eruptions. In the beginning, indeed, this may be frequently accomplished; but when the disease has extended, when larger portions of the skin have assumed a morbid action, so soon as we think we have repelled one set of eruptions, another succeeds, or the disease will radiate, as it were, from the original focus in every direction. When the erythema is extending, we shall be convinced that there is no danger of this repulsion, that no application merits the name of repellent; for if the powerful astringents are now employed, so far from repressing, they will rather seem to accelerate the progress of the disorder §.

Our applications, therefore, must be varied, and suited to the different appearances of the disease; and internal remedies will sometimes be necessary, not to correct the acrimony of vitiated fluids, but to depress or raise the general action of the system, and to extinguish the morbid action of the skin itself.

2 In

* De Re Medica.

† Lib. vii. cap. 14. Lib. xix. cap. 29.

‡ A Treatise of Diseases incident to the Skin.

§ "Vulgo retropressus talis herpes, incendio vicinas partes ad ipsum ulceris limbum ferocius adoritur, malumque fit et latius et sævius."—*Lorry.*

In cafes of folitary and circumfcribed eruptions, not attended with much heat and inflammation, aftringent applications are ufeful, and often alone effect a cure, and, on the firft appearance of the papulous areola, fometimes arreft the further progrefs of the difeafe. But when the difeafe is more completely formed, when it is ftill extending, when the heat, tingling, and inflammation, are at their height, fuch applications are to be avoided as ufelefs, and often hurtful. In this ftate, the parts are to be kept cool by the continual application of weak folutions of acetite of lead, and covered in the night-time with the unguentum acetitis plumbi. When the fymptoms have been thus moderated, the more powerful aftringents may be again employed; fuch as, folutions of the fulphate of zinc, the unguentum oxidi zinci, and unguentum gallarum.

When the papulæ are broken, and the inflammation abated, a thin ferous fluid often oozes out from innumerable fmall pores; in this ftage, the beft applications are weak folutions of the muriate of mercury, the unguentum nitratis hydrargyri, and unguentum oxidi hydrargyri cinerei, or one made with lard, and the fubmuriate.

In the active ftate of herpes, a moderate diet, cool regimen, and gentle laxatives, are properly indicated.

Where, however, the difeafe has continued for fome time, and refifted the applications commonly ufed, when the patient is fubject to repeated eruptions, it becomes neceffary to employ other general remedies, which may change the morbid difpofition of the fkin.

A change of diet, regular exercife, and bathing, are often fufficient. The decoctum guaiaci, antimonials, and fmall dofes of the muriates of mercury, are commonly prefcribed, and fometimes are very effectual in obftinate cafes.

The natural fulphureous and chalybeate waters have alfo been much reforted to for the cure of herpes.

K,

PART

PART III.

CRITICAL ANALYSIS.

I.

Ricèrche ſulla Quina. Di GIOVANNI FABBRONI.

THIS eſſay, for a copy of which we are indebted to its celebrated author, ſeems to have been printed in ſome periodical work, as it wants the characteriſtic mark of a ſeparate publication, a title-page. Whether our conjecture be right or not, is of little conſequence; but it was neceſſary to account for the imperfect manner in which it is announced.

Cinchona was in uſe among the Peruvians, when their country was diſcovered by Europeans: that of the fineſt quality grows upon the mountains of Huayaquil and Cajama, in the neighbourhood of Loxa, and on the mountains of Caxanuma, Uritaſinga, and other lofty mountains in the preſidency of Quito, at a barometrical height of 28 inches, and never on the plains. The reputation and conſumption of its bark in Europe became ſo great, that even in 1788, when Condamine was there, there were no old trees in Caxanuma, and even young ones in the neighbourhood of Loxa were ſcarce; ſo that, to ſupply the increaſing demand, various other barks were ſubſtituted for the true cinchona, the variety of whoſe effects tended to bring it into diſcredit. From motives of humanity, and of ſupporting a trade ſo uſeful to their colonies, the Spaniſh Government in 1777 ſent out a committee of learned men to make inquiries concerning it on the ſpot. They diſcovered that there were various ſpecies of the genus cinchona. Ruiza and Pavon deſcribed 15 which they found in Peru, which, added to thoſe of Vahl and Tafalla, make 25. But this valuable genus is not confined to the ſouthern hemiſphere, for ſeven ſpecies, ſome of them officinal, have been found by Mutis in the neighbourhood of Santa Fé, where that celebrated botaniſt has reſided ſince 1783, as director of the exportation of cinchona.

The ſpecies of cinchona deſcribed in the Quinologia of Ruiz, in the order of their virtues, are,

1. C. nitida, *Ruiz;* only a variety of the C. lancifolia, according to *Zea,* fuppofed to be the C. officinalis of Condamine.
2. C. tenuis, *Quinol.* C. hirfuta of the *Flora.*
3. C. glabra. C. lanceolata of the *Flora*
4. C. anguftifolia, *Ruiz;* C. lancifolia, *Mutis.* This furnifhes the yellow bark of the fhops.
5. C. magnifolia, *Ruiz* and *Pavon;* oblongifolia, *Mutis.* This urnifhes the red bark of the fhops.
6. C. glandulifera, *Flor. Peruv.*
7. C. purpurea, *Flor. Peruv.;* C. ovata, *Ruiz;* C. officinalis, *Linnæi.* This furnifhes the palè bark of the fhops.
8. C. lutefcens, *Quinol.;* C. magniflora; C. oblongifolia, *Mutis* and *Ruiz.*
9. C. pallefcens, *Quinol.;* C. ovata, *Flor.*
10. C. fufca, *Quinol.;* C. rofea, *Flor.*
11. C. colorata (Peruviana.)
12. C. califaja, *Flor Peruv.*
13. C. eleifolia.
14. C. micrantha, *Tafalla.*
15. C. dichotoma, *Flor. Per.* Zea excludes this fpecies entirely from the genus cinchona.
16. C. acutifolia, *Flor. Per.*
17. C. lanceolata, *Flor. Per.*
18. C. grandiflora, *Flor. Per.*
19. C. pauciflora, *Tafalla.*
20. C. macrocarpa, *Vahl;* C. ovalifolia, *Mutis.* The white bark of the fhops.

Ruiz admits only two of the feven fpecies defcribed by Vahl, and rejects his floribunda, anguftifolia, longiflora, and fpinofa. He alfo rejects the caribbea of Jacquin and Wright, the corymbifera of Fofter, and the philippica of Cavanilles, but does not agree with Zea in confidering Nos. 2. 7. 9. and 14. as mere varieties of the cordifolia, and Nos. 1. 3. 4. 10. 12. and 17. of the lancifolia. It therefore appears, that although the knowledge of this valuable genus has been much extended by the Spanifh botanifts, much ftill remains to be afcertained; but Tafalla and Manzanilla are now exploring the woods near Loxa, and Mutis ftill refides at Santa Fé.

Although Ruiz will not allow the cinchona of Santa Fé to be equal in value to thofe which grow in the much more elevated regions of Loxa, efpecially the nitida, ovata, and magnifolia, ftill the greater facility of exportation renders the difcovery of valuable cinchona in North America highly important. Of the feven fpecies found in Santa Fê, four only are faid to be officinal, which may be named from the relative colour of their barks,

barks, the red, the orange, or yellow of the ſhops, the pale of the ſhops, and the white.

The orange or yellow of the ſhops was firſt diſcovered. Its effects are truly ſpecific, a doſe of two drachms, given before the fit, cutting ſhort intermittent fever, as if by a charm; but unfortunately it is extremely rare, at leaſt at Santa Fé, not one tree being found for one thouſand of the other ſpecies. It is the bark of the C. lancifolia of Mutis, which is called by the natives quina naranjada, and is probably the ſame tree with the C. anguſtifolia of Ruiz. Zea ſays, that it is the ſame with that called, in commerce, calliſaya, and known in Spain by the name of huanueo. Ruiz aſſerts that it is a diſtinct ſpecies from the nitida, fuſca, and officinalis of Vahl and Condamine. It is thus deſcribed: Surface ſcabrous, with tranſverſe chinks, more or leſs abundant; epidermis tawny, with black, cineritious, or white ſpots; internally more or leſs honey-coloured; from half a line to two lines in thickneſs; moderately heavy; difficult to break, although not ſolid, but ſpongy; fracture exhibits many ſharp, delicate, unequal, longitudinal fibrils; gummy reſinous matter diſcernible, with a lens, although not very abundant; aromatic odour ſenſible, when boiled; taſte bitter, pungent, unpleaſant, ſlightly acid, not aſtringent; ſcarcely tinging the ſaliva, however long chewed.

The pale bark, the quina amarilla of the Spaniards, is next in febrifuge virtues, but partakes ſomewhat of the properties of the red, being alſo purgative. It is the bark of the C. cordifolia of Mutis, of the C. officinalis Lin., and which, probably, is the ſame with the ovata of Ruiz and Pavon. Its external ſurface is ſmooth; its colour, internally, cinnamon; its thickneſs, upwards, of a line; light; fracture, with ſome fibres drawn out; ſmell ſlight, but ſenſible and agreeable during decoction; taſte bitter, ſlightly acid, auſtere, reſembling that of a dried roſe.

The red bark of Santa Fé was at firſt received with enthuſiaſm on account of its ſenſible qualities being ſtronger; but its uſe was followed with diſguſtful nauſea, ſevere vomiting, inſupportable colic, and other effects highly injurious to patients of a ſanguine, bilious temperament, and of a rigid fibre; ſo that it would have been entirely laid aſide, had not Ruſhworth diſcovered its ſpecific virtue againſt gangrene. It is produced by the magnifolia of Ruiz and Pavon, and the oblongifolia of Mutis, the quina roxa of the Spaniards, and is one of the moſt common ſpecies at Santa Fé. The exact deſcription of this ſpecies is accidentally omitted, but the following particulars regarding it are mentioned. Its internal ſurface has a reddiſh cinnamon colour; it contains little gummy reſinous matter; it has the

4 bitter

bitter taste common to all the species, but in a weaker degree, and is austere, causing an evident constriction of the lips, tongue, and fauces.

The white bark of Santa Fè was found by Mutis to be an useful drug, and its efficacy on the glandular system was confirmed by Clarke. It is the bark of the cinchona ovalifolia of Mutis, the macrocarpa of Vahl, and is not found in Peru. It has a whitish cinnamon colour, has little gummy resinous matter, and its taste is rough, with an almost imperceptible acidity. Fabbroni perfectly imitated the colour of the powder of the three first species by the following mixtures, with the view of affording some standard of comparison.

	Red.		*Orange.*		*Pale.*	
Lamp black	0	8	0	6	0	4
Gamboge	29	2	23	1	23	2
Dragon's blood	70	0	46	0	26	7
Licopodium	0	0	30	3	49	8

Our knowledge of the active and soluble principles of cinchona has been summed up by our author in the following abstract.

1. The different species of cinchona require different quantities of water to extract all their soluble principles; 360 parts the red, 240 the orange, and 480 the white.

2. The most powerful febrifuge cinchona is not that which contains either the largest or smallest quantity of principles soluble in cold water.

3. Cinchona infused for some hours in a sufficient quantity of cold water yields to it all its active constituents; 30 pounds of cinchona, exhausted in this manner, scarcely furnished one ounce of insipid earthy extract, by long ebullition in water.

4. Cinchona loses its solubility, and consequently its activity, by long exposure to the air, and by pulverization considerably protracted, with the view of rendering it as fine as possible. From $\frac{11}{100}$ to $\frac{16}{100}$ are obtained from bruised cinchona, which, in fine powder, yields only $\frac{6}{100}$ or $\frac{7}{100}$.

5. The solubility of the extract is diminished during its formation. About one half of dry extract is not soluble again in water.

6. The bitter of cinchona is soluble in warm as well as in cold water.

7. Cinchona boiled successively in seven portions of water gave a bitter taste to an eighth.

8. The infusion, when allowed to stand long, after having been boiled, or even slightly scalded, acquires a deeper colour, and deposits a matter apparently resinous, but only partially soluble in alcohol. The remainder has a very deep colour, and is also soluble in water.

9. The infusion is more aromatic, the decoction bitterer.

10. The infusion on boiling loses its astringent taste with a little volatile oil, but retains its bitter.

11. The sulphate of iron is precipitated of a blackish green by the infusion of cinchona, and still more strongly by the decoction.

12. Lime water produces a more copious precipitate in the recent decoction than in the recent infusion.

13. The alkalies cause a precipitate, which, when added in excess, they redissolve.

14. Cinchona infused in wine prevents it from turning sour, and, in a few days, throws down the colouring matter as charcoal and nutgalls do.

15. Infusions of cinchona ferment spontaneously in summer.

16. Cinchona destroys the emetic property of the supertartrite of antimony, without losing any of its febrifuge virtues.

17. The alcoholic tincture of cinchona is bitter, and precipitates iron from its solutions.

18. Cinchona, after having been subjected to 22 successive infusions in water, yields to alcohol a bitter matter, without astringency.

19. Water extracts more astringent than bitter matter from cinchona previously acted upon by alcohol.

20. Sulphuric acid destroys the bitterness, but not the astringency, of the infusion and decoction of cinchona.

21. Alcohol extracts more from cinchona than water does.

22. By distilling, with a gentle fire, cinchona with water, aroma, with some traces of volatile oil, are obtained.

23. Two drachms of genuine febrifuge cinchona, administered in substance, completely prevent the access of intermittent fever. (Mutis and Zea.)

24. The decoction of two ounces is inadequate to produce that effect.

25. The cold infusion is more powerful than the decoction.

26. The cold infusion and short decoction of good cinchona have the same density, and contain the same quantity of extractive matter.

27. The extract of cinchona is less efficacious than the powder.

28.

28. The residuum of a first infusion of cinchona, although it has lost somewhat of its bitterness, &c. produces the same febrifuge virtues with fresh cinchona, provided it be given in larger doses.

From these facts the following useful conclusions are drawn:

1. That cinchona is partially decomposed even by simple pulverization.

2. That it is decomposed by boiling.

3. That, therefore, a cold infusion is preferable, or rather its administration in substance.

4. That the soluble principles of cinchona being somewhat of a resinous nature, it is advisable to add alcohol to the cold infusion, as some pharmacopœias prescribe, or to infuse it in wine, as was done by the celebrated Pringle, and the empiric Talbot.

5. That cinchona contains the astringent principle, and hence the nutgall was tried as a substitute for it, but without success.

6. That the febrifuge virtue does not belong essentially and individually to the astringent, the bitter, or any other soluble principle, as the quantity of these increase by long boiling, while the virtues of the decoction decrease.

7. Neither does the febrifuge virtue reside in that principle which destroys the emetic property of antimony, or precipitates iron, since the decoction contains more of it than the infusion, while its virtues are evidently less.

8. That cinchona, by boiling, loses its aroma, a small quantity of volatile oil, and a substance which, by new combination, becomes inert; it is therefore probable that it is owing to this separation that the extract is less efficacious than the decoction, and this than the infusion.

We shall pass over our author's account of the analysis of cinchona by Fourcroy and others, and proceed to notice his original experiments. In consequence of a chemical theory of the mode in which cinchona acts on the living system, our author ascertained the relative affinity of different cinchonas, and some other substances to oxygen, by putting in similar vessels a drachm of each in powder, with an ounce of nitric acid, of 35° of Baume, and accurately measuring the greatest degree of heat produced, and the time necessary for its production. The temperature of the air was 18° R, and it rose in each mixture respectively to the annexed degree in the number of minutes prefixed.

3. Genuine pale cin. of Loxa,	34.	10. Licoperdon,	27.
4. Orange cin. last powder,	34.	7. Laucocerasus leaves,	26.
6. White cinchona,	32.	5. Angustura,	25.
4. Orange cinchona,	31.	7. Quassia,	25.
6. Orange cin. first powder,	31.	8. Gall-nuts,	24.
7. Red cinchona,	31.	4. Oak-bark,	23.
12. Spurious cinchona,	29.	1. Colomba,	20.

The

The remainder of this essay has little reference to the practice of medicine, but is almost purely chemical; and although the author modestly apologizes for its imperfections, it contains several curious views and important facts. The constituents hitherto detected in cinchona are, according to Fabbroni,

1*st*, *Mucilage*, probably insipid, soluble in water, decomposible by fermentation.

2*d*, *Ferment*, soluble in alcohol, separable by water, and decomposible by fermentation.

3*d*, *Extractive*, subacid, astringent, soluble in alcohol, and in water.

4*th*, *Resinoid*, strongly attracting oxygen, insoluble in alcohol, and in water, when in a certain degree of oxygenation.

5*th*, *Lime* and *magnesia*, in the states of malate and carbonate.

6*th*, *Vegetable acid*, probably malic.

7*th*, *Volatile oil*, rendered soluble, probably by the extractive.

8*th*, *Fixed oil*, which, united to the picra, resinoid. extractive, and oxygen, is rendered soluble in various menstrua.

9*th*, *Aroma*, of a peculiar nature, very fugitive.

10*th*, *Woody fibre*, finally decomposible into oxallic acid.

11*th*, *Acid not vegetable*, in various states of combination.

We do not know whether Fabbroni has accidentally omitted from this enumeration, or has included under extractive, the bitter principle which he denominates *Picra*, which is characterized by being soluble in water and in alcohol, and tinging animal substances of an indelible yellow colour. The presence of tannin was also indicated by the copious precipitations with solutions of gelatine and muriate of tin; but our author does not seem inclined to admit tannin as a peculiar principle, but rather to consider it as his bitter principle, or picra, united with extractive, ferment, oil, &c.; in proof of which, he adduces Chenevix's experiments on coffee, which, in its raw state, according to our author, yielded picra, but, when roasted, exhibited the properties of tannin, in consequence of the combination of picra with the oil developed by roasting. Our author's experiments on cinchona, subjected to fermentation, and to the action of nitric acid, are new and interesting. He found that, by the latter, the mucilage is converted into oxallic acid, and the ferment, aroma, and volatile oil, destroyed or decomposed, while the picra and supposed tannin remain unaltered. But, notwithstanding the great attention which has been paid to the analysis of this important drug, much still remains to be done. We have repeated the experiments related by Dr Duncan jun. in Nicolson's Journal, vol. vi. p. 225, and are perfectly satisfied of the peculiarity of the principle called by him cinchonin; for gelatin,

gelatin, albumen, and ſtarch, the only other ſubſtances which, ſo far as we know, are precipitated by an infuſion of galls, are inſoluble in alcohol, as well as their precipitates; whereas both cinchonin, and the precipitate it forms with an infuſion of galls, are very ſoluble in alcohol. But we are inclined to conſider theſe precipitates leſs ſimple than they are commonly ſuppoſed to be; for a decoction of cinchona is precipitated both by gelatine and galls, and, when ſaturated by either of theſe reagents, it is ſtill acted upon by the other. Now, if gelatine deprived the infuſion of galls of no other principle than tannin, it would follow, that an infuſion of cinchona contained both tannin and another principle precipitable by tannin, which can ſcarcely be the caſe; and, indeed, we do not at preſent ſee any other way of accounting for the facts, but by ſuppoſing that the infuſion of galls and cinchona contain, each of them, tannin, and another principle of a different nature, in each, not precipitable by tannin, but by each other; and as an infuſion of galls, after being ſaturated with gelatine, does not act on an infuſion of cinchona, it would ſeem that the gelatine throws down from an infuſion of galls not only the tannin, but the other principle precipitable by cinchonin.

II.

Medical Collections on the Effects of Cold, as a Remedy in certain Diſeaſes. With an Appendix, containing an Account of ſome Experiments made with a View to aſcertain the Effects of Cold Water upon the Pulſe. By JOHN EDMONDS STOCK, M. D. &c. 8vo. pp. 200. Longman & Co. 1805.

THE mental habits of man are as incorrigible as his corporeal habits. When the tenor of opinion has been long and uniformly directed in one channel, and the views of a ſubject have been long of a ſimilar complexion, the mind does not readily accede to a different and almoſt oppoſite mode of thinking, whatever the evidence in favour of the latter may be. A collection of facts, numerous and well authenticated, may be ſet before us; by a proceſs of the moſt legitimate induction, a ſeries of incontrovertible inferences may be obtained; additional evidences may be accumulated from the moſt reſpectable authorities; yet we ſhrink from the dereliction of habitual tenets; and it is by gradual ſteps, and not without reluctance, that we ſuffer the derangement of our accuſtomed trains of thought.

Nay,

Nay, after a certain degree of conviction shall have been imposed upon the mind, we have still seen, in the very instance to which we more particularly allude, a considerable hesitation in proceeding to apply it in practice. On the subject of cold, as a remedy in febrile diseases, the habits and prejudices of the public still resist the evidence of experience and philosophy; and while practitioners, under the same influence, recommend its application with an air of diffidence and doubt, as a new remedy,—an experiment, it is not likely that its reception will soon be general. Although Dr Stock, therefore, pretends to no originality of evidence, his work will, we doubt not, be of considerable utility, by repeating the call of attention to the subject; and thus, by contributing to new habits of thought, "it may at once tend to sooth the apprehensions of the patient," and to give confidence to the medical practitioner.

The author commences his work with some observations on the general effects of cold upon the human system, followed by some remarks on the history of its medical application, and its more particular effects, and then proceeds, with Dr Cullen's nosology as a text-book, to point out those diseases in which the expedient is or is not advantageous, according to a well-selected store of evidence from the most respectable sources.

It is chiefly in regard to the first point that we feel any difficulty in assenting to the doctrines maintained by Dr Stock. At the same time, it must be observed, that any trivial difference of opinion upon these speculative topics does not tend, in any degree, to invalidate the particular practical inferences which have been deduced from multiplied observation and experiment.

Some confusion and apparent inconsistency are observable in the opinions of medical writers, in respect to the general effects of cold on the living body. It has been classed among stimulants, and sedatives, and tonics; and it has been recommended by Dr Cullen himself, as the means of moderating the violence of reaction in one class of diseases, and of obviating debility, by supporting and increasing the action of the vascular system, in another. Now, we agree with the author, generally, that both these effects may be explained by the sedative powers of cold; the former being the direct effect of the abstraction of the stimulus of heat, the latter the indirect effect of the same abstraction more transiently operating, according to the general fact stated by Brown and Darwin, of accumulating excitability under such circumstances. The five arguments in favour of this opinion, recounted and illustrated by the author, are sufficiently satisfactory.

"They are derived, 1st, From the paleness and contraction

tion of the skin, which succeed the application of cold; *2dly*, From its diminishing or weakening the action of the heart, and arteries; *3dly*, From the debility and inactivity observable in the inhabitants of cold countries; *4thly*, From the gradual diminution of the vital powers, which commences with its first application, and which, if its operation be long continued, terminates in their entire extinction, either in particular parts, or in the whole body; and, *lastly*, From the accumulated excitability which it induces to the stimulus of heat."—P. 3.

The author thence attempts to controvert a position of the late excellent and lamented Dr Currie, that the principal operation of cold is, in certain instances, stimulant which he affirms that Dr Currie admits, in consequence of being "unconvinced by the ingenious theory of the author of *Zoonomia*." It surely did not require five arguments to prove that the abstracting of a stimulus must be a sedative operation; and Dr Currie allows it to be incontrovertible, that "cold, in extreme degrees, is a powerful and *effectual* sedative."—See his Reports, 2d edit. p. 72. But he justly contends, that the application of cold operates upon two of the sensorial powers, upon *sensation* as well as upon irritation. The application of cold is not a simple abstraction of heat, the stimulus of the irritable fibre; it is also a shock to the sensible fibre; and the powerful *sensation*, which is thus excited, is a stimulus of no inconsiderable influence. It is not easy to conceive that Dr Stock should remain unconvinced by these observations of Dr Currie, and that he should still ask, "Would not the sprinkling of a few drops of tepid water," from its *mechanical* impetus, "rouse a person in syncope, as rapidly as the same quantity drawn from the coldest spring?" We would recommend an experiment to the author, upon the result of which we will rest our ultimate opinion. Let a mug of water be poured into his bed on two successive mornings during his repose, the one tepid, the other ice-cold; and we doubt not that he will be roused from his dreams with a rapidity by no means proportionate to the quantity of the fluid, and inversely proportionate to the quantity of heat which it may contain.

Other *sensations* are resorted to by the practitioner, in the instance of syncope, as inlets to the sensorial power, through the medium of which its activity may be reanimated. A fetid or pungent *odour* applied to the organ of *smelling* produces the same effect on the torpid system, as the sudden impression of cold. The two expedients have nothing in common but the vivid sensation which they excite; to the sensation, therefore, the stimulation must be attributed. This is so perfectly consonant with Dr Darwin's doctrine, that it is difficult to explain why he overlooked

overlooked the operation on the sensation; and considered the application of cold as a simple abstraction of the stimulus of heat. The phenomena of the living body are somewhat more complicated than the chemical mixtures of the laboratory, and the mutual operation of its powers bids defiance to the attempts at simplification which some modern theorists have pursued.

The author considers it as unnecessary to say much with regard to the use of cold in typhus, a subject which has been so fully and philosophically illustrated by Dr Currie. But he gives ample testimony of the efficacy of cold applications in a fever improperly classed by Sauvages and Cullen among the varieties of typhus, namely, the yellow fever. He observes, that however various and contradictory the opinions of the different writers on that subject were, they all agreed in recommending the use of cold water and cool air; and he adduces some observations from Dr Rush, and other physicians, in proof of the salutary effect of the application of cold, even during the exhibition of mercury. He believes, however, that the long-continued application of it is preferable to the simple affusion, especially in those cases in which the heat of the skin is excessive, constituting the true *causus*, and in which the reaction might be so great as to endanger the patient.

Of the utility of cold applications in the various inflammations of the viscera, which are designed by names terminating in *itis*, the author has been able to collect but little testimony. In phrenitis, cold applications to the scalp are probably of some advantage. In one case of enteritis, where the abdomen was exceedingly hot, and exquisitely painful to the touch, Dr Stock ordered it to be bathed with wet napkins wrung out of cool water, with evident advantage and relief to the patient. Hysteritis is the only remaining visceral inflammation in which he has any evidence of the efficacy of cold.

We are satisfied, from our personal observation of the use of cold water in febrile complaints, that the cold affusion or ablution is not attended with any unpleasant consequences, where great determinations to the different viscera occur; and that the fears which exist as to the probable mischiefs which may result from the practice, under those circumstances, are but remains of the old prejudices of our predecessors. The extent of the *advantages* of the practice remains, however, to be proved by future experience. The author has adduced satisfactory testimony, that, even in the different forms of pneumonia and catarrh, it does *no harm*.

In respect to gout, the author is disposed to believe in the safety and efficacy of the local application of cold, as recommended

mended by Dr Kinglake and others; and he has collected some additional facts in favour of it. We are satisfied that, in numerous instances, the practice is efficacious beyond all other expedients; and we have resorted to it frequently, with decided utility, in those local attacks of inflammatory rheumatism which are often denominated rheumatic gout. Nevertheless, we cannot doubt of the occasional *retrocession* of the disease, in consequence of the local suppression; and some satisfactory criterion, which would enable us to anticipate, with considerable certainty, the result of cold applications, is yet a desideratum.

Dr Stock next examines the *exanthemata* and the hæmorrhagies, in all of which the use of cold is shown to be advantageous. In regard to scarlatina, in which the external application of cold water has been proved to be an effectual remedy, in the most decided and unequivocal manner, by Dr Gregory and Dr Currie, Dr Stock suggests, upon principles well understood, that the continued application of the remedy by sponging and washing would be still more efficacious than the affusion, after which the heat of the skin so speedily returns.

In the *comata* the external application of cold is frequently useful. In sanguineous apoplexy, it has been recommended to the head, and, in *apoplexia hydrocephalica*, Dr Rush applied vinegar, in which ice had been dissolved, to the head, with evident advantage. A curious case, illustrative of the efficacy of cold immersion, in removing the apoplexy of drunkenness, is related from Dr Currie, and a long quotation is introduced from a dissertation by Dr Johnson, in proof of its utility in the *apoplexia venenata*, or *asphyxia* produced by the fumes of charcoal.

In respect to the *spasmi*, the efficacy of cold affusion in the cure of *tetanus* has been amply illustrated during the last few years; we have ourselves witnessed its beneficial effects. In *chorea*, epilepsy, and some other spasmodic diseases, it has not been found to possess much power. In colic, *cholera*, and *hysteria*, the author has collected proofs of the utility of cold applied in different modes.

The efficacy of cold, used in various ways to the head or body of maniacs, has been illustrated by many examples, and its employment is recommended, under certain circumstances, by most writers on the subject. Among the *cachexiae*, which are connected in general with a condition of debility and languor, little can be expected from the sedative powers of cold. *Tympanites* is the only disease of this order in which its application can be useful. In *ischuria*, the beneficial effect of cold applied to the lower extremities has been frequently recorded. Dr Stock quotes three pointed cases of suppression of urine, of considerable fiderable duration, in which, after the failure of diuretics, opiates, glyfters, emollients, &c. cold water applied to the legs and abdomen fpeedily removed the difeafe.

On the fubject of burns, the author does not pretend to decide as to the comparative merits of the cold treatment, or of the ufe of turpentine, recommended by Dr Kentifh; but he adduces feveral pointed teftimonies in favour of the former, one of which we fhall tranfcribe.

" Many years ago (the reporter received the facts from the perfons concerned), two brothers, apprentices to a hatter, were employed in taking hats from a boiler, and rinfing them out in a very large tub of cold water. Some difpute arifing, one of them lifted the other in his arms, and feated him directly in the boiler; but being inftantly ftruck with terror at what he had done, without lofing his hold, he again lifted him from the boiler, and feated him in the tub of cold water. The youth, who had been thus hurried through thefe extremes of temperature, had on a pair of wide linen trowfers, and received no other injury than a narrow blifter, which was formed directly under the waift-band, and encircled his body."—P. 167.

The work is terminated with a general fummary of the facts, and an attempt to deduce, from this review, fome general principle, upon which the whole of the operations of cold may be explained. The author is of opinion, that it is, in all inftances, either directly, or through fome fympathetic connexions, a fedative operation, confequent on the abftraction of the ftimulus of heat. In general, no doubt, this is the cafe. But we have already offered fome reafons for concluding, that, through the medium of *fenfation*, its action is fometimes directly ftimulant, (we confine the ufe of thefe much-abufed terms to the *obvious* depreffion or excitement of the living powers;) and we apprehend that, in other inftances, the operation is not purely a fedative abftraction of heat. Cold wafhing will not arreft a typhus in its commencement. This, it appears, can only be effected by the *fhock* of affufion; *i. e.* by a ftrong impreffion on the fenforial powers. Other expedients, which have fcarcely any property in common but that of exciting a vivid impreffion of this fort, accomplifh the fame purpofe. In the inftance of ifchuria, when the fuppreffion arifes merely from over-diftenfion, or a temporary paralyfis of the fibres of the bladder, occafioned by long retention of the urine, we do not fee how a fedative operation of any kind, and more efpecially how the abftraction of the ftimulus of heat from the legs, can roufe the languid actions of the bladder. We cannot help attributing fomething in this cafe to the *ftimulus of fenfation.*

 But,

But, in truth, we deem these speculations of trivial utility. Dr Stock has presented us with a judicious view of numerous and important facts, in which he is fully borne out by the most authentic records of medicine. He has nowhere shown a disposition to overrate, in the slightest degree, the virtues of the remedy whose powers he has undertaken to illustrate; but has evinced equal discrimination and candour in his statements. Many of his facts, however, are confessedly not of modern production, and we almost wish that he had consigned a larger portion of his work to the use of cold in febrile disorders; a subject not only more novel in its nature, but against which a host of prejudices still remains to be conquered.

III.

Cases of Pulmonary Consumption, &c. healed with Uva Ursi; to which are added, some practical Observations. By Robert Bourne, M. D. Aldrichian Professor of the Practice of Physic in the University of Oxford, &c. &c. 8vo. Lond. 1806. pp. 293.

The practical physician will no doubt sit down to the perusal of this, as of every other treatise on pulmonary consumption, without any sanguine hopes of receiving much useful or efficient instruction. A short experience will have been sufficient to convince him of the general inefficacy of medicine in any stage of true phthisis; and an observation of the mass of morbid structure, which presents itself to the eye on the exposure of phthisical lungs by dissection, will have satisfied him of the extraordinary obstacles which, in the latter stages, medicine has to encounter. But we apprehend his hopes will receive an additional depression, if possible, in the present instance, in consideration of the remedy which is recommended on this forlorn occasion. The sensible qualities of *uva ursi* are extremely slight; its medical powers are summed up in a trifling degree of astringency; and, as a remedy in those diseases, in which it has been extolled as efficacious, or indeed in any other, we believe the general opinion deems it almost entirely inert. Great, however, as may be the reasons for viewing a work of this nature with a sceptical eye (and we have not enumerated them all), candour and philosophy suggest a suspension of our judgment until the result of experience be adequately reviewed, and the series of facts be carefully investigated.

Dr Bourne was led to make trial of *uva ursi* in pulmonary consumption, in consequence of the success with which he had exhibited it in a case of apparent ulceration of the bladder, attended with hectic and emaciation. In this instance, the formula employed by Dr Ferriar was followed, viz. about ten grains of *uva ursi*, rather more than that quantity of *bark*, and half a grain of *opium*, three times in the day. Dr B. had previously used the *uva ursi* in two nephritic cases, in the dose of half a drachm, as recommended by De Haen, with the same want of success which physicians in this country have usually acknowledged.

After this preliminary notice, the author proceeds to relate the particulars of sixteen cases of apparent phthisis, fourteen of which occurred in his own practice. In the observations which he afterwards makes on each case, he arranges them under four heads: 1. He considers the first eight as cases of apparently true pulmonary consumption in its first stage, or before purulent expectoration had taken place: 2. The three following as cases of the same in its last stage, being attended with expectoration of *pus*: 3. The 12th and 13th as cases of an affection of the lungs, in which there was purulent expectoration, but which were, nevertheless, not true phthisis: and, 4. Cases of hectic, in which the lungs appeared either not to have been primarily affected, or not at all, including the three last cases. Of these 16 cases, it appears that three died, two while under the remedies, and one in the succeeding winter; nine recovered, and four were apparently relieved. One observation occurred to us with respect to those cases which terminated favourably; they all began to take medicines in the spring and beginning of summer, and were in a state of convalescence before the approach of winter. Now, if there is any one circumstance which appears to possess an influence over the consumptive, it is a warm or mild temperature.

The eight cases of incipient consumption will, we think, be perused with some degree of doubt. The difficulty of ascertaining the presence of phthisis, in its early stage, is universally acknowledged. There is no pathognomonic symptom. In irritable constitutions, we have often seen teazing catarrhal coughs wasting even the strength and flesh of the patient, and accompanied by a marked hectic; yet the ordinary remedies have completely succeeded in removing it, and no future similar attack has occurred. We know, too, that, in female habits especially, a dry cough, with dyspnœa, emaciation, &c. is frequently the concomitant of that languid state of the system which conſtitutes the principal feature of *chloroſis* and *amenorrhœa*, but which occurs alſo independently of theſe ſymptoms. A cough of this ſort is likewiſe an occaſional attendant of ſome forms of *dyſpepſia*, ariſing apparently from irritations in the viſcera adjacent to the lungs or trachea. We do not mention theſe facts as circumſtances of which Dr Bourne requires to be informed. His obſervations evince that, both from perſonal obſervation, and an acquaintance with the records of medicine, he has poſſeſſed himſelf of no inconſiderable ſhare of medical accompliſhments. But we mention them as circumſtances which will influence the opinion of the ordinary reader, but which may be not ſufficiently adverted to by one who is conducting experiments with the hopes of attaining a particular reſult, and whoſe conviction may be modified by his wiſhes. We ſhall quote Caſe III. as an example, chiefly on account of its brevity.

"S. M. who lived in a village near Oxford, an unmarried woman, 28 years of age, rode over to me for advice on May 31, 1803. She had had a cough for ſix months, during the former part of which time it was troubleſome in the day only; latterly it had been ſo both night and day, and had been accompanied with fever. The cough was dry. For the laſt fortnight ſhe had had profuſe morning perſpirations. When ſhe applied to me, ſhe had loſt fleſh conſiderably; her tongue was white; her appetite indifferent; her breath ſhort; her pulſe frequent; and ſhe had ſome pain under the right breaſt. She menſtruated regularly.

I preſcribed ſeven grains of uva urſi, a quarter of a grain of opium, and three grains of liquorice powder, thrice in the day, to be taken in milk

June 21. Cough much better, hardly at all troubleſome in the night. But little fever. Morning perſpirations much abated. No pain under the breaſt. Breath leſs ſhort. Tongue clean; appetite improved. Pulſe leſs frequent. She had taken her medicines very regularly.

She was directed to go on with the powders; but the uva urſi was increaſed to eight grains, the opium to the third of a grain.

July 3. She ſent me a very favourable report. *The uva urſi was now increaſed to nine grains.*

July 30. The cough and all other unfavourable ſymptoms were gone; her looks approached to thoſe of health; ſhe had gained conſiderable ſtrength.

She was adviſed to take one of her powders, night and morning, for ſome time to come."—Page 18.

On March 31, 1804, this patient continued well.

We

We believe that moſt practitioners will be ſatisfied that caſes of this nature not unfrequently occur, and yield to, or at leaſt recover under the uſe of, the ordinary remedies. At the ſame time, it will be admitted, that it is not eaſy to ſhow that ſuch caſes ſhall not terminate in genuine phthiſis. But the circumſtance is ſufficient to excite great diſtruſt of the powers of *uva urſi*.

Of the three caſes which are ranked under the ſecond head, of confirmed phthiſis, with purulent expectoration, two terminated fatally. The third is related in a letter to Dr Bourne from an apothecary at Banbury. A labouring man, aged 51, was attacked with hæmorrhage from the lungs, after conſiderable exertion, and loſt about a pint of blood. An inceſſant cough ſucceeded, with expectoration occaſionally ſtreaked with blood. Two months after the attack (viz. in May 1804), he applied to the reporter of the caſe. "He was much emaciated, his appetite bad, pulſe 120, and his breath ſo extremely ſhort, that it was not without difficulty he could get up ſtairs to bed; his fever uſually came on about ſix or ſeven o'clock in the evening, ſucceeded by profuſe night perſpirations; and the expectoration, which was apparently purulent, amounted generally to a full pint in the courſe of twelve hours. He began taking the *uva urſi* on the 14th May, in doſes of ten grains, twice a-day, combined with a ſmall quantity of *opium*, and he regularly perſevered in it for the ſpace of three weeks, with evident advantage: he now omitted the medicine for a ſhort time; but finding that his cough was worſe, and his complaints on the increaſe, he was glad to have recourſe to it again. He then continued its uſe, with great regularity, till the 6th of July, when I had the pleaſure of ſeeing my patient nearly well; his pulſe was only 86, his appetite remarkably good, and he had in a great degree recovered his fleſh: his breath was ſo good as to allow him to walk up a very ſteep hill; and I can now add (September 4. 1804), he is quite recovered, and enabled to purſue his uſual employment of a common labourer," page 62. Of this caſe Dr Bourne has heard nothing farther. From a ſingle caſe little can be inferred; ſo far as it goes, it appears to mark a connexion between the uſe of the medicine and the alleviation of the ſymptoms. But it may be remarked, that in a man of 51 years of age, who is neither ſaid to have had any conſtitutional tendency to phthiſis, nor to have been ſubject to cough before, the conſequences of a pulmonary hæmorrhage, accidentally produced, are not ſo difficult of alleviation or removal as the ulceration which occurs in phthiſical conſtitutions after the rupture of pulmonary veſſels. Dr Bourne himſelf does not per-

 emptorily

emptorily decide whether it is " rightly arranged" under the ſecond head. Although fully aware of the diſcouraging appearances which generally preſent themſelves in the diſſection of phthiſical patients, he has dwelt at length upon the propriety of not ſuffering all hope to leave us in the more early ſtages of the diſorder. The miſchief, he affirms, is not always ſo extenſive as the quantity of *pus* expectorated would lead us to believe; and the greater part of it frequently takes place only a ſhort time previous to death, during which the progreſs of the diſeaſe is rapidly accelerated.

The 12th and 13th caſes rank under the third head. In commenting on theſe, the author diſtinguiſhes them from thoſe caſes of ulcerated lungs which conſtitute the ordinary form of phthiſis, as well as thoſe which ſucceed to pneumonia. In the two inſtances in queſtion, a large abſceſs had *inſidiouſly* been formed in the lungs, with little previous indiſpoſition, and with no one ſymptom that could indicate the extent of the miſchief which was going on. The author had ſeen three ſimilar caſes previous to his adoption of *uva urſi* as a remedy, all of which terminated in death. He remarks that, in four of the five, the matter diſcharged differed from that diſcharged from abſceſſes formed in ordinary phthiſis, or after pneumonic inflammation, in being extremely fetid; in four, alſo, the complexion was ſallow and duſky, and four were males. They were all above 23, and under 26 years of age.

As the three remaining caſes were confeſſedly not pulmonary conſumption, we ſhall not detain our readers with any account of them. The author is of opinion that, by fair analogy, they afford encouragement for the trial of *uva urſi* in all caſes of incipient or recently formed hectic, whatever be the part of the body wherein the local affection, on which the hectic depends, is ſeated. And he is hence led to ſuggeſt the probability of its remedial powers in ſcrofulous diſeaſes.

We cannot but wiſh that the author had accumulated a more ſatisfactory evidence in favour of theſe hypothetical ſuggeſtions, before he gave them to the world. From the experience of *three* caſes of hectic, connected with ſome irritation in the region of the uterus, of the lungs, or liver, he arrives not only at the ſweeping concluſion that all morbid ſtates of all the viſcera, which are accompanied with hectic fever, are probably curable by the ſame means, but alſo that other great and important organic actions or changes in the glands, or other parts of the body, will probably yield to the ſame drug. This is not the careful and clear mode of induction by which alone ſcience can be advanced with firm and ſteady ſteps, and by which ſome departments of medicine

medicine have of late years received the moſt material and irrefragable illuſtrations. Nor do we conceive it to be the beſt mode of ſatisfying the public of the efficacy of any remedy, nor of laying a claim to the merit of an uſeful diſcovery.

In his laſt chapter, the author proceeds to make ſome "pharmaceutical and practical obſervations" on the medicine in queſtion. He conſiders that the powder of *uva urſi*, which is often, if not commonly, ſold in the ſhops, is ill prepared, and not poſſeſſed of the full medicinal powers of the plant. The *green* leaves alone ſhould be ſelected and picked from the twigs, and dried by a moderate expoſure to heat. "The powder, when properly prepared, is of a light-brown colour, with a ſhade of greeniſh yellow. I have often met with it of a light-brown, without the greeniſh-yellow ſhade; and, when this is the caſe, I ſuſpect either that the leaves from which it was made were not duly ſelected, or that they were expoſed to too great a heat to render them pulverable. The expoſure to too great a heat is certainly the worſe fault; but neither fault is very venial, where health, perhaps life, is concerned. The powder has nearly the ſmell of good graſs-hay, as cut from the rick; to the taſte it is, at firſt, ſmartly aſtringent and bitteriſh; by and by theſe impreſſions on the palate ſoften into a liquorice flavour." We quote this more particularly, becauſe Dr B. affirms, that he "never ſaw a good ſpecimen of the powder which was not prepared in Oxford, or the neighbourhood;" and alſo to caution our readers that they pay particular attention to the medicine which they uſe, in order that their concluſions may be ſatisfactory even to the moſt faſtidious examiner.

We do not acquire much or very accurate information from the author's experiments. The principal concluſion which they afford is, "that water extracts from *uva urſi* nearly all that proof ſpirit is able to extract, and proof ſpirit nearly all that water is able," p. 208. Another is, that it contains the "aſtringent acid;" for a drop of the infuſion or tincture in a ſolution of ſulphate of iron produced a precipitate. Dr Bourne has not attempted to avail himſelf of the accurate means, which chemiſtry would have afforded him, of aſcertaining the quantity of this acid which it contains, nor of tracing the medicinal powers to any particular conſtituent part, the mucilaginous or reſinous for inſtance, of the plant.

With reſpect to the medicinal powers of *uva urſi*, he is of opinion, that even in the ſmaller doſes above ſpecified, it has now and then a very ſenſible effect on the nervous ſyſtem, producing occaſionally lowneſs, headach, or ſlight vertigo; that it has, in one or two inſtances, occaſioned an intermiſſion of the

 pulſe;

pulse; and that occasionally the pulse becomes preternaturally small during the use of it. These effects are by no means stated as being so general as to be very obviously connected with the administration of the medicine; and, what is somewhat extraordinary, they do not seem to be greater, from a dose considerably larger than those which Dr B. was in the habit of using.

On the whole, the sceptical disposition with which we commenced the perusal of this treatise, has not been greatly diminished by a careful and serious execution of our task. In a disease, however, of a tendency so generally fatal as is that of pulmonary consumption, every expedient, which promises even a chance of success, should be examined by the test of cautious experiment, until the full extent of its powers be clearly ascertained; and we trust that no *à priori* opinions will induce a neglect of the suggestions of Dr Bourne.

In an appendix, Dr B. has related six cases more, in which he has had an opportunity of using *uva ursi* in apparently threatening consumption, and which terminated favourably.

IV.

On Epilepsy, and the Use of the Viscus Quercinus, or Misletoe of the Oak, in the Cure of that Disease. By Henry Fraser, M. D. 8vo. pp. 96. London. 1806.

We necessarily open a treatise like the present with some degree of scepticism. The numerous remedies which have been confidently recommended for the cure of epilepsy, but subsequently employed as mere palliatives, or abandoned altogether as inefficient, immediately recur to our recollection. Nor can we forget the frequency of organic causes in producing the disease, or its general obstinacy even under the plans of treatment most generally adopted. We confess, too, that this scepticism is farther excited, in the present instance, by an impression on our minds that the *misletoe* is rather inert as to any medicinal properties; and that its recorded efficacy was rather the result of the superstitious associations belonging to it, than of any innate powers. Dr Fraser recommends it, however, not as a decided remedy, but as one which has been attended with so much success in eleven cases of epilepsy, in which he prescribed it, as to render

render it worthy of a more extensive trial. He has enumerated the names of eighteen authors who have mentioned its efficacy in this disease, from the age of Pliny to the present time; but the majority of them, we fear, will not be deemed more satisfactory authority than the credulous Roman himself. The account of the cases in which Dr Fraser experienced the powers of the viscus is very brief and uncircumstantial, and is preceded by a systematic view of the symptoms, causes, &c. of epilepsy, somewhat after the model of an inaugural dissertation, and abounding with references to authors. To most readers this detail is unnecessary; and it would appear that the object of the author would have been more effectually accomplished by a simple and circumstantial relation of the instances in which the remedy proved serviceable. The following is the sum of his detail:

"The first case, in which I employed the viscus quercinus in the cure of epilepsy, was that of a gentleman in the 23d year of his age, who had been the subject of epilepsy from the third or fourth year of his birth. The case was hereditary, and had gradually increased upon the patient, until it was become so considerable as to threaten his intellectual faculties with destruction. On the 5th March 1802, he began to use the misletoe, by taking two scruples of the powder in a draught of camphorated emulsion twice daily, and the use of this medicine (the dose of the powder being gradually increased to two drachms) was continued without intermission till the 21st of June. The violence and frequency of the paroxysms experienced no visible abatement before the expiration of the first month from the commencement of the use of the misletoe; but, after this period, they became considerably milder, and about the middle of June he bade farewell to his almost constant but disagreeable companion."

Of the 2d and 3d cases we are merely told, that the disease continued for a considerable length of time, and, after valerian had failed, it was cured by the viscus, given twice a-day for three months. The patients were in the prime of life. The 4th was a delicate female, who had been subject to epilepsy five years. The 5th, 6th, and 7th cases occurred in two boys of twelve and fifteen years age, and a girl of nine. "These cases were neither hereditary nor violent, and were speedily cured by the misletoe, after a combination of bark and valerian had proved ineffectual."

"The 8th case was the most violent I ever witnessed. The patient was apparently a robust man of 30 years of age, 22 of which he had been at various times the subject of epilepsy. The paroxysms in this case did not occur very frequently,

quently, nor even ever without giving warning of their approach; but, when occurring, were excessively violent and long continued. The plethoric state of the patient naturally led to the employment of the antiphlogistic plan of treatment, by a rigid perseverance in which, he was twice reduced nearly to the grave, without reaping the least benefit in his complaint. This patient continued the use of the misletoe at stated intervals for nearly six months, and, during this period, he drank, regularly every second or third morning, half a pint of tepid water, in which two to three drachms of sulphate of magnesia had previously been dissolved. By persevering in this plan of treatment for the length of time before-mentioned, and by studiously avoiding irregularities in living, and excessive exercise, he has been fortunate enough to shake off his complaint."

"The 9th case was similar to the 4th."—The 10th proved fatal: it occurred in an elderly lady, and was complicated with a paralysis of the right side.

Though we speak sceptically on the subject, we by no means intend to be guilty of a dereliction of those principles of philosophical inquiry, by which alone medicine, in common with the other sciences, can be successfully cultivated;—the matter cannot be determined but by cautious experiment; and we think with the author, that the success which he has described is sufficient to recommend the further trial of the remedy. The powder of the viscus quercinus, he informs us, may be obtained by applying to Mess. Allen and Wood, *Plough-court, Lombard-street*, or Mess. Jackson, Manley, and Eldridge, *Paternoster-row*.

V.

Darstellung der Gallschen Gehirn-und Schädel-Lehre, von Dr C. H. Bischoff, *ausserordentlichen Professor am Koenigl. Colleg. Medico--chirurgico, und practischem Artzte zu Berlin: nebst Bemerkungen über diese Lehre*, von Dr C. W. Hufeland, *Königl. Preuss. geheimen Rath, wirkl. Leibartzt, Director des Coll. Med. Chirurg. &c.* 8vo. Berlin. 1805.

"*Etwas über Herrn Doctor Gall's Hirnschädel Lehre dem Berliner Publicum mitgetheilt*, von J. G. Walter, *erstem Professor der Anatomie und Königl. geheimen Rath.* 2 *Theile.* Berlin. 1805.

Every body has heard something about the celebrated Dr Gall and his doctrine of cranioscopy; but every body does not know that some curious anatomical discoveries have been made the

the basis of such fanciful conjectures. It will not be risking too much to make such an assertion, since we find in the work before us the indisputable testimony of several learned and respectable men, in favour of the truth of many of Gall's observations. But there have been opponents as well as advocates, (for what subject can be started in Germany without having writers on both sides?) and we have selected the work above mentioned, and the two pamphlets of Professor Walter, in order to lay before our readers a full and fair view of the arguments and reasoning employed by both parties. The two authors, whose names are prefixed to the title-page of the book of which some account is first to be given, are actuated by the laudable ambition of giving a correct notion of the doctrine of cranioscopy, and no one can doubt their qualifications for such a task, inasmuch as *Dr Bischoff* is a professor of anatomy and physiology, and attended Gall's lectures and demonstrations; and *Hufeland*, whose name is well known, became a convert to some parts of the doctrine, after having seen the anatomical illustrations, and heard the author himself expound his system. However, it appears not unworthy of remark, among the swarm of publications upon this subject, of the host of expositions, refutations, criticisms, and explanations, not one is the work of Gall's own hands. This way of making known his theory and discoveries is singular. A doctor of medicine gives public lectures, is praised for having made sublime discoveries, is accused of gross mistakes and falsehoods, is charged with gaining so many disciples by his truths or his blunders, that the safety of church and state is endangered; and yet, when any person writes against him, or any government forbids his lecturing, he chooses to remain silent, and allow others to answer the attacks made upon him. If he were truly desirous of insisting upon the discoveries he has made, if he had confidence in his ability to vindicate his opinions, why not pursue the manly and open course? Why not give a detailed account of his observations, and, instead of the poor excuse of saying his opponents do not understand what he means, why does he not furnish arguments which cannot be misunderstood? Instead of such plain and honourable conduct, Dr Gall is determined to take all advantages of public clamour and partial applause: he screens himself by a stratagem which every man of true science, every lover of truth, would never have recourse to. He probably finds it more profitable and more pleasant to travel about from place to place, and to give lectures, than to write and to print. Restrained by no delicacy, such inexorable abstinence from the press appears extraordinary, and naturally excites some suspicion with respect

to

to the motives. There is some allusion to a great work which the author is said to be preparing for publication, but, till that appears, the public must be content with oral tradition, and with the copies of the lectures printed by his pupils. Many objections started against Dr Gall's theory have been founded on topics not at all essential to the discussion, and much wit and ingenuity have been wasted on questions, not unfit, indeed, to be mixed with the subject, but quite unnecessary for its illustration. The outcry and stale stories against necessity, free-will, and materialism, may be passed over, without troubling our readers either with a repetition of the different arguments, or the refutation.

We shall give first an abstract of the principal contents of Dr Bischoff's book, which may be looked upon as a correct epitome of Gall's lectures; afterwards we shall give the result of Dr Hufeland's critical remarks, and then state some objections to the doctrine itself, partly suggested by Professor Walter's pamphlets, and partly such as have occurred during the perusal of various fugitive pamphlets upon this temporary topic of writing and conversation.

Dr Gall was led to consider the brain as a membrane, and not a pulpy substance, as hitherto supposed, from observing that the intellectual faculties remained unimpaired in cases of hydrocephalus internus, where a quantity of water is collected in the ventricles, and the whole substance of the brain becomes sometimes distended to a membrane scarcely a line in thickness. Other pathological facts, such as the paralysis of the extremities, in consequence of injuries done to the hemispheres of the brain, induced him to remark, that an uninterrupted connexion must exist between these parts and the spinal marrow. With the view of tracing this connexion, and at the same time to demonstrate the membranous structure of the brain, he engaged in a series of anatomical researches for many years, till at last he had the satisfaction of finding his conjectures verified by anatomical discoveries. He attributes his success to his manner of dissecting the brain from the lower parts, beginning with the cerebellum and spinal marrow, and going upwards, instead of following the usual custom of beginning the demonstration at the external superior parts, and slicing downwards; and, instead of a knife, which cuts and destroys the relative situation of the several parts, he employs the handle of a dissecting-knife, or some blunt instrument, and unravels, as it were, the different circumvolutions of which the cerebrum and cerebellum are composed.

The result of his researches is so minutely detailed in the communication with which we have been favoured by Professor Rosenmuller,

Rosenmuller, that, to avoid repetition, we have suppressed our analysis of this part of Dr Bischoff's work, and shall content ourselves with observing that the principal points of the anatomical discoveries seem reducible to the three following assertions :

1st, The origin of the medullary substance of the cerebrum and cerebellum is derived from the spinal marrow.

2nd, The cortical substance is the superficial ganglion of the cerebrum and cerebellum.

3d, All the excurrent nerves terminate in the outer surface of the cortical substance on which the pia mater rests, and all the recurrent nerves take their origin at this place.

Anatomists have usually taught, that the medulla oblongata, the medulla spinalis, and pons Varolii, are formed by elongations of the substance composing the cerebrum and cerebellum. Gall asserts directly the reverse: it is true, he goes the very opposite way to work, to demonstrate this intricate structure; and it is important to prove thus much, because the rest of the physiological reasonings hinge upon these three principal facts. He derives all the chief nerves, too, from the spinal marrow, which is said to consist of bundles of fibres; eleven have been already discovered, and he has traced the corpora pyramidalia through the pons Varolii, crura cerebri, into the substance of the brain. If these circumstances be all true, they are curious, and demand farther examination. Professor Walter declares, there is no truth in what Gall pretends to have found out; the preparations displayed, and the structure talked about, are only the fictions of his fancy, and he protests he saw nothing of what was said to be so clearly proved. Other persons, equally capable of judging, and perhaps more quick-sighted, not only saw what Gall proposed to show, but do justice to the accuracy of his observations, by acknowledging their firm conviction of their truth. In the work before us, we find the names of Loder and Reil, two very eminent men in the university of Halle, brought forward to support the claims of Gall. Loder writes in terms of great praise, and communicates a case, illustrating a part of Gall's new observations, at the same time acknowledging the want of a sufficient number of facts to confirm the theory of the different organs, and declaring himself a champion in the pursuit of truth. This is high authority. Whatever may be the final result of all the noise and rout, some of the principal circumstances are now under trial. The controversy is, in some degree, in the hands of those best qualified to judge its merits ; by the observations of distinguished anatomists, the whole fabric of fame and future utility must stand or fall, and the reputation of Dr Gall

Gall must soon be correctly estimated, in order that the scientific part of the world may put him on the same shelf with Willis, Varolius, and Haller, or class him with another far-famed part of our fraternity, Drs Faustus and Sangrado.

In the second division of his explanatory essay, Dr Bischoff has endeavoured to give a precise definition of what is meant by the doctrine of the skull, and organs of the brain; or what, to use a new term for a new subject, he has denominated *cranioscopy*. It was noticed, in the former part of the exposition, that every one of those nervous streaks, perceived in the great ganglion of the brain, makes a particular circumvolution of the hemispheres, and is to be considered as the organ of a particular function of the mind; *i.e.* each streak may be looked upon as a part on which the mind operates according to a determined degree of force, and its structure is so organized as to receive the impressions communicated to it. A knowledge of these organs, acquired by observing the protuberances and depressions which they make upon the bones of the cranium, consequently a knowledge of the predisposition of the brain for particular actions, constitutes the object of *cranioscopy*. After this definition, however, it is acknowledged, that we cannot perceive the real disposition or already developed faculty of the mind by mere observations made on the skull; the tendency only, or the aptitude, or possibility of any particular intellectual quality in any individual can be discovered; and, besides, all the predispositions cannot be detected by looking at the skull, because many of the supposed organs cannot influence the shape of the bones, in consequence of their remote situation. All the organs, hence all the predispositions, both in men and animals, are said to be innate. The functions of the brain are threefold; 1*st*, Organic life; 2*d*, Sensitive life; 3*dly*, Intellectual life. A particular part of the brain is assigned to each of these functions; it is only in consequence of the size of the hemispheres (the part appropriated for the last of these functions) that man has the largest brain, and not because the size of the human brain is greater in proportion to the rest of the body, as hitherto generally supposed, nor on account of the comparative thickness and strength of the nerves, as *Soemmèring* has remarked. To prove that the organs of thought are placed in the hemispheres of the brain, these parts are said to be larger, and to be more completely developed, in different classes of animals, in proportion to their intellectual faculties; and they are most perfect in man. As each faculty of the mind has its peculiar name, its particular organ, like each of the five senses, so the brain is not to be considered as one whole organ of intellect, common to all the mental operations,

rations, but as a collection or assemblage of organs, a spot in which all the different organs are united together. This hypothesis, of a separate and distinct part of the brain being adapted for each different faculty of the mind, is very old: it is to be found in the writings of Boerhaave, Haller, Van Swieten, Soemmering, Prochaska, &c.; and the Academy of Dijon long ago proposed, as the subject of a prize question, to determine the situation of the different organs. It is necessary, however, first to demonstrate the existence of such a variety of organs; and here we find a series of propositions, which are called certain and convincing proofs. To us, indeed, they appear but very insufficient reasons, being only a mutilated repetition of the common arguments employed on this very difficult question.

Next follows an enumeration of the different organs, to which Dr Gall has the merit of assigning a local habitation and a name. These are classed under three divisions: The *first* includes those organs by whose means man is enabled to act directly upon the objects around him, and are no less than eleven in number.

1. Sexual love.
2. Parental tenderness.
3. Friendship, or faithful attachment.
4. The organ of fighting.
5. The organ of murder.
6. The organ of cunning.
7. The organ of stealing.
8. The organ of goodness or benevolence.
9. The organ of the faculty of imitation.
10. The organ of ambition or vanity.
11. The organ of constancy or firmness.

The *second* order comprehends those organs which place man in closer relation with surrounding objects than he can be by the aid of his external senses, and these amount to eleven more.

1. The organ for acquiring a knowledge of things. 2. Of places. 3. Of persons. 4. Of colours. 5. Of sounds. 6. Of numbers. 7. Of calculations. 8. Of languages. 9. Of arts. 10. The organ of prudence. 11. The organ of high-mindedness and elevated sentiment.

Under the *third* division are placed those organs connected with the highest operations of the human intellect:—1. The organ of the power of comparison. 2. Of metaphysical penetration. 3. Of wit. 4. Of religion.

"The first in this list, the organ of the sexual passion, is seated, we are told, in the cerebellum, and discovers itself upon the cranium, at that part of the occipital bone which is below the linea

linea semicircularis inferior, towards the great occipital foramen. In the living subject, this organ can only be detected by the large size and thickness of the nape of the neck. Its existence in the cerebellum is proved by the following reasons: 1. The cerebellum, and the parts of the skull corresponding to it, develope themselves more and more with age, and with the growth of the passion for the sexes, and not at all in proportion to the other parts of the brain and head. 2. In animals of the most simple organization, in insects, the whole mass of brain only consists of two small nervous knots which constitute the cerebellum. Even these two knots are not found in animals which do not propagate their species by copulation. Bulls and stallions, &c. have the cerebellum more completely developed: hence the back-part of their heads is larger, and their neck thicker. In general, males have the neck thicker than females: the cerebellum in females is smaller, and placed nearer to the occipital hole. Those animals, whose ears stand at a wide distance one from another, are selected for the stud. Mules have their ears close together, and a very small neck, and have no procreative faculty. 3. Castrated animals have a thin neck. The ox, for instance, has the hinder part of his head and neck narrower and smaller than the bull. The horns grow larger in the ox, because the process of ossification increases as the size of the brain diminishes. If the horns of a deer, the formation of which depend likewise on the cerebellum, be cut towards the rutting season, the animal becomes impotent; but becomes fit for procreation the following year, if the horns be left. Gall declares, he found a lady's neck one day very hot, remarkably swelled and painful: the neck was extraordinarily thick in this case; it was a patient affected with *nymphomania*. The weakness of the intellectual faculties, which follows excessive sensual indulgence, the pain, heat, and spasms of the neck, show not only that the brain in general, but the cerebellum in particular, is concerned in the function of generation. Lascivious girls, according to the report of libertines, put their hands to their necks when strongly excited. Injuries done to the nape of the neck are followed by impotence. Another decisive proof of the organ of sensual love being seated in the cerebellum is furnished by a pathological fact observed in hydrocephalus. The faculty of generation is often the only one which remains unaffected, because the cerebellum suffers less than any other part from water collected in the head. This organ of sexual love is double, as the testicles and kidnies, according to the law, that all the organs of animal life are in pairs."—P. 900.

Take another specimen, gentle reader, from another place.

"The organ which is the seat of the disposition for acquiring a knowledge of places (*Organ des Ortsinns*) is situated on the forehead: it is double, and occupies just half the superciliary arch on each side towards the nose. It announces a susceptibility for receiving strong impressions from a survey of particular places, so as to recal them easily to memory, and find them again. This organ is indispensably necessary to many animals, because they inhabit particular places, and often wander to a great distance. By the periodical action of this organ, various birds are instigated to take long flights; the dog is enabled to travel many hundred miles home, and find out his old master; pigeons can serve the purpose of a letter-carrier, and birds which migrate can return to their former habitations. This organ for finding places does not depend on the sense of smelling, because a dog has been known to have crossed the sea, and found his way home, and pigeons return home too from considerable distances, which has never been ascribed to the delicacy of their noses. Persons, who have this organ in a great degree, are fond of travelling, and they know how to find their way any where. General officers, fortunately provided with this organ in perfection, are capable of forming plans and military projects, and can take advantage of positions and local situation. This is particularly exemplified in the case of General Mack, who has this organ strongly marked. Captain Cook also had it in a striking degree." P. 99.

These two extracts are literally translated from the book before us, and therefore may be taken as a fair sample of the substance of the lectures. No doubt, they will be thought particularly profound and instructive. From the latter quotation, we learn several circumstances which, in the phenomena of nature, have hitherto been difficult to explain. The annual migration of birds, we are now informed, is in consequence of the spontaneous and periodical action of a portion of their brain situated over their eyebrows;—the singular instances of sagacity observed in dogs returning to their former masters, especially the fact alluded to (for which Dr Gall's authority is vouched), of a dog going down to the water-side, to Gravesend we will suppose, embarking in a London trader bound to Hamburgh, in order to return to his old master, perhaps at Berlin. Furthermore our countryman, Captain Cook, was led to make his memorable voyages of discovery in consequence of a lump upon his forehead; and the illustrious General Mack, it seems, has the organ of finding places (*hiding-places probably*) in a most astonishing degree. For this last illustration every body must do justice to the critical acumen of the cranioscopist. Some

 doubts

doubts may be fairly entertained as to the rest of his explanations; but it is plain now why Mack took such a position at Ulm, and why he did nothing else but avail himself of this place-taking organ It is to be feared this occupied too large a portion of his brain, to the exclusion of some other equally useful part.

There is a similar commentary upon each of the organs already enumerated; but it would be trespassing too much upon the patience of our readers to enlarge the quotation; and still more would it be an insult to the judgment and good sense of any scientific men in the united kingdoms to think any refutation necessary Dr Gall allows the brain to be the organ of all intellectual operations: This is modest at least, though no very great discovery; for nobody has ever doubted, from the time of Epicurus down to the present day, that men think by means of their heads, as they walk by means of their heels. With regard to the discovery of particular organs existing in particular places, there appears hitherto no foundation for such an hypothesis, in so far as Gall has examined the subject; for he confesses he can assign no particular organ for reason, volition, conscience, or memory. These faculties, he says, are common to all parts of the brain; no residence is assigned for them; yet if there be any chance of discovering the seat of particular faculties, associated with the healthy condition of particular parts, memory would soonest be found out, because the loss of it by paralysis, by injuries done to the head, and the remarkable degree of its existence in some men and certain animals, seem to point out some clue for our inquiries. Supposing it proved that particular portions of the brain are organized for the expression of particular passions and feelings, it is impossible that such a structure should be visible, or could be detected upon the outside of the bones of the skull, bec use the delicate soft texture of the brain itself could only slightly influence some parts of the internal layer of the bone, and that is often not in contact with the outer. One faithful example would be worth fifty fanciful or forged illustrations. Has any person, born deaf and dumb, shown any particular signs on the external form or internal structure of his head? Has any difference been observed even in the organ of hearing in every instance? We doubt the fact. What, then, shall be said to the pretended discovery of the seat of friendship, or of the propensity for theft or murder? Gall acknowledges his ignorance of the precise situation of all the organs; and accordingly we observe a large space of terra incognita still left unexplored upon the charts which he has given of the cranium. It is also allowed that an organ may exist, and not show itself, nor display its energy, notwithstanding it may be strongly marked. Persons have lost by external accidents considerable portions of the brain, of course several organs, according to Gall's doctrine, without suffering any loss or diminution of their intellectual faculties. This single circumstance is enough of itself to invalidate the whole theory.

Professor Walter, in his animadversions upon the doctrine of cranioscopy, is very bitter against the author. The wrath of the venerable anatomist is sometimes quite laughable; he surely might have refuted his antagonist without abusing the object of his lectures, and without referring to the fatal consequences of his opinions, supposing them to be true. Such reasoning avails nothing in physics or in metaphysics. The professor would have done better not to have run so often out of his museum to pick a quarrel with people in the street. The pages of both these pamphlets are filled with dull attempts at wit, partly copied from newspaper scribblers, and partly written for the occasion by Professor Walter himself. He declares that Dr Gall is completely ignorant of anatomy; that much was promised, and very little performed; that he saw no such parts as were pretended to be shown; and was not at all satisfied with the artificial wax-preparations and sarcastic jokes which astonished the gaping multitude, and still less with the answers sent to some queries submitted in the form of a round-robin. For it appears that Gall condescended to enter a little in explanation in a newspaper, in order to appease his opponent, and to satisfy the public. The truth of the matter seems to be this: Gall's lectures tickled the fancy of the people of Berlin; he gave no less than six courses there: they became the universal topic of conversation in every society and in every place, from the palace down to the post-house, and, like other much talked-of things, they became a subject of party-spirit. Professor Walter thought himself called upon to decide for the *Berlin publicum*, as he says in his title-page and preface; and he has signalized himself rather as a vain and vexed controversialist, than as a sound reasoner and formidable adversary.

The '*Remarks*' by Dr Hufeland are very different in their tone and temper from those just alluded to. Although not particularly new or striking, they betray good sense and candid judgment. He says, no one could be more prepossessed against Gall's doctrine than he was himself, before he became acquainted with the author; and only by attending the lectures and demonstrations, by being convinced from what he saw, he has become a partizan. Such a confession is authorized by an appeal to facts, and is published from his desire of expressing

2 the

the truth under any shape. The anatomical is properly separated from the physiological part of the lectures: to the former nothing remains to be added to Dr Bischoff's detail, which is approved both by Hufeland and by Loder. It is only necessary to have eyes, and to open them, to be convinced of what Gall demonstrated concerning the direction of the nerves, the crossing of the corpora pyramidalia, &c. In order to see this structure, the brain must be dissected after Gall's method, beginning at the medulla oblongata, and following the parts from below, upwards, through all their ramifications. With regard to the discovery of their being two distinct sorts of nerves, one going to the circumference of the brain, and the other returning to the centre, and these two sets always being found together, Hufeland expresses his want of faith. He has not distinctly seen these nerves running in opposite directions, and remarks, that no arguments can be drawn from one set being accompanied by arteries, and the other by veins, because, wherever arteries are found, veins are found also. He objects still further to the idea of the different organs being placed upon the external parts of the brain. The two tables of the skull are not parallel in their whole extent, as may be easily found by making a vertical or horizontal section. If it were true that the eminences upon the outside of the bones of the head were produced by the figure of the different parts of the brain, the internal shape of the cranium ought to correspond precisely with the external. A mould of wax or plaster, cast in the inside of the skull, ought to represent the same appearances, only on a smaller scale, as the outside. This experiment has been made several times, and the difference was very obvious and remarkable. Hufeland has met with several persons of his acquaintance, whose imaginary shaped heads do not correspond in the least degree with the real state of their intellectual faculties and disposition.

He concludes the result of his examination in the following words: "I admit the doctrine of Gall, inasmuch as it makes the brain the organ of the intellectual functions, and assigns particular functions to particular and differently organized parts; but I deny that these different organs always show themselves on the surface of the brain by eminences, and still less can I allow the eminences observed to have been formed solely by the action or developement of these organs, so as to lead us to infer the existence of certain intellectual qualities. The doctrine, therefore, seems theoretically true, but by no means demonstrated; or, in other words, *organology is fundamentally true, but organoscopy is doubtful.*" P. 147.

In

In the concluding part of his remarks, Hufeland considers the utility and the application of the doctrine. He discusses its influence upon our speculative opinions, and its practical application to the science of physiognomy, to morals, to jurisprudence, and to medicine. The easiest reply to the question *cui bono* appears to be, that it is an absurdity calculated to do neither good nor harm among people of sound sense and reflection. Many of the observations made by the judicious commentator are only calculated for the place where they were written, and for the people for whom they were intended. At Berlin, Gall himself carried his system too far, for he was induced to pay a visit to the prison and house of correction, and displayed his critical tact upon the skulls of the unfortunate culprits. An account of Gall's visitation is given in a periodical journal called "*der Freymuthige*," said to be written by one of the chief magistrates who accompanied him. The whole history is curious and entertaining, for more reasons than one. Gall was attended by several distinguished magistrates, professors, and literati. About two hundred prisoners were submitted to his touch, and, without knowing any thing previously of their crimes or their character, he discovered their whole history by fumbling their foreheads. He pointed out a great resemblance in the shape of all their heads, especially the young rogues, when put in a row; these were so much alike, that the whole party could almost believe they belonged to one family. The organ of theft was strongly marked in them all, and the protuberances characterizing the great and noble feelings were very deficient. So erudite and refined was the doctor's touch, that, it is asserted, he not only detected the great rogues from the petty rascals, but declared, by feeling their skulls, who were confined for theft, and who were imprisoned for more heinous offences!

High-German doctors are not so much in fashion in this country as formerly; yet such exhibitions as these, and such talking, with the aid of a pea-green coat, a gold-laced hat, and a hand-organ, might do something even at this day, perhaps, in country-towns, and at Bartholomew-fair. In other respects, there is no danger of Gall's theory making much progress in this quarter of the world. It seems probable that he has observed some hitherto unnoticed parts in the brain, and detected some eminences and depressions on the bones of the head among men and animals: he seems to have discovered also some curious instances of structure corresponding with the manners and habits of different animals, and, by the aid of a fertile imagination, he has worked these insulated facts into a sort of system, intended at first merely to amuse a circle of friends, but found at last sufficiently attractive to gain money and fame. "*Mundus vult decipi, decipiatur,*" seems to have been Gall's motto, and with this he has travelled about Germany with great success. If he should stray to Goettingen, we would advise him to look at the collection of skulls of different nations in Blumenbach's museum; he would there find, perhaps, that other causes, besides the supposed organs of the brain, contribute to modify the shape of the bones of the head. The action of the muscles attached to different parts of the cranium, the particular dresses among different tribes and particular employments, have considerable effect in varying the shape of the skull. This circumstance seems to have been overlooked, for there is no allusion to the odd-shaped heads of different races among mankind in the several accounts given of the lectures. Not having had the advantage of hearing the lectures delivered by the author, nor seen his demonstrations and preparations, we must be content with what is published by the best authority; and, from all hitherto published, we must confess our prejudice and creed not at all changed. Considering the doctrine as a good quiz, we readily accede a due portion of praise to the ingenuity of Doctor Gall. As to his observations on the structure of the brain, we must suspend our judgment till further investigations and more impartial inquiries are made; and at present we must look upon the whole matter as one instance, among many, of that absurd love of systematic novelty which is so prevalent in Germany, and carries so many people away from the plain and useful path of observation and experience.

VI.

Observations on Abortion; containing an Account of the Manner in which it takes place, the Causes which produce it, and the Method of preventing or treating it. By JOHN BURNS, Lecturer on Midwifery, and Member of the Faculty of Physicians and Surgeons in Glasgow. London. 1806. 8vo. pp. 139.

THE author of the little volume now before us is already favourably known to the profession by his dissertations on inflammation, and by a small work on the gravid uterus; and, with

with the latter, the ſubject of the preſent treatiſe is in ſome meaſure connected. The ſubject of abortion is one of conſiderable practical importance, and, in many points of view, highly intereſting. There are few ſituations in which the intelligent practitioner can give more uſeful advice than when conſulted in caſes of habitual and of threatened abortion; nor, when we conſider the alarm, and ſometimes danger, which attends the progreſs of actual abortion from ſudden and profuſe floodings, is there any which requires more prompt and active aſſiſtance. Even when this firſt danger is over, when the abortion has been completed, and the hæmorrhage ſuppreſſed, the patient is often left in a ſtate of weakneſs, and ſometimes of diſeaſe, which claims the attendance of the phyſician. But the principles of our conduct in theſe caſes are neceſſarily grounded on a knowledge of the anatomy and of the functions of the ovum and gravid uterus, and of the cauſes of thoſe deranged actions which bring on abortion. Theſe general principles, and the prevention and treatment of abortion, are perſpicuouſly explained by Mr Burns under the following heads: The formation of the ovum. The manner in which abortion takes place; The cauſes giving riſe to abortion; The prognoſis; The prevention and treatment of abortion.

The obſervations of our author on the ſtructure of the ovum, and the view he has taken of the formation of ſome of its parts, are new and intereſting. He deſcribes the decidua as entirely of vaſcular formation, tracing its origin to an elongation of the veſſels of the fundus uteri, or to a new efflorefcence or growth of delicate veſſels ſhooting perpendicularly from the uterine ſurface. From theſe primary veſſels, again, there ſprings, according to Mr Burns, a fine vaſcular tiſſue, in the oppoſite direction, or parallel to the uterus; and this ſecondary production conſtitutes what has been called the decidua reflexa. But as this account of the formation and ſtructure of the ovum has already been laid before our readers in the Fifth Number of our Journal, it becomes unneceſſary to offer any farther remarks on theſe ingenious obſervations of our author in this place.

The manner in which abortion takes place includes the account of its phenomena and ſymptoms. When it happens within three weeks after impregnation, the ſymptoms differ little from thoſe of menorrhagia; there is a copious diſcharge of blood and coagula; but, as the vaſcular ovum has not at this early period deſcended into the uterus, the characteriſtic mark of abortion is wanting; the primary veſſels are ſo ſmall, that they cannot be detected in the diſcharge. But though nothing

thing but coagula can be perceived, the discharge, we are told, generally continues till the small vesicle passes out of the fallopian tube; then it stops, and an oozing of serous fluid finishes the process. Mr Burns does not inform us how this passing of the vesicle out of the fallopian tube has been discovered, or may be known, otherwise than by the cessation of the hæmorrhage. When, indeed, the vesicle has come into the uterus before abortion takes place, it may sometimes be detected in the first discharge of blood, at an early period of gestation. The distinguishing features of abortion in the more advanced period of gestation, between the second and third month, are, uterine pain and contraction, discharge of blood, of the fœtus and secundines.

These symptoms, and the various appearances, are accordingly marked and well distinguished by Mr Burns. But there are also some precursors or signs of the cessation of the action of gestation very material for the practitioner to be acquainted with. On this subject Mr Burns remarks, "There is generally, for a longer or shorter time before the commencement of abortion, a pain and other irregular actions of the neighbouring parts, which give warning of its approach before either discharge or contraction take place, unless it proceeds from violence; in which case the discharge may instantly appear." We wish Mr Burns had been more particular on this subject, for there is danger that these symptoms be confounded with the more chronic ailments that accompany pregnancy. Pain and irregular actions in the neighbouring parts are common at this period in many women, who yet carry well, and go on to their full time. Are there, then, no signs which, together with these, announce that the fœtus is blighted, that the action of gestation has ceased? We know not why Mr Burns has omitted the sudden and premature cessation of the morning sickness, and softness of the mammæ, which, when they do occur with pain and irregular action, are regarded as signs that the action of gestation is over, that the fœtus is blighted, although no more palpable signs of abortion may have appeared. The state of the cervix uteri may afford also useful information.

The causes giving rise to abortion are very fully and ably investigated. Those of accidental abortion are often sufficiently obvious. But the causes of habitual abortion, and of those cases which are not purely accidental, are involved in much greater obscurity. A predisposition to abortion in some individuals must be allowed to exist. This predisposition is referred by our author generally to an imperfect mode of uterine

action,

action, induced by age, former miscarriages, and other causes, as by an immoderate and indiscriminate use of venery. A change of structure also in some part of the uterus may render it unfit to continue the action of gestation, and give rise to premature expulsion. It is easy also to conceive how a general weakness of the system may interfere with the perfect discharge of the uterine functions; or the uterus may be affected by sympathy, with some other organ weakened or deranged, and thus lay the foundation of abortion. Thus, the loss of tone, or diminished action of the stomach, produces amenorrhœa, and it may also induce abortion. Some important facts, connected with these sympathies, are engrafted by Mr Burns on a particular theory which he had formerly endeavoured to establish in his dissertations on inflammation. The leading principle of this theory seems to be, that, when the action of any organ is increased, other parts must be deprived of a portion of their energy; or, to use the author's own words, "We have a certain quantity of action present in the system at large, and properly distributed amongst the different organs, forming an equilibrium of action; and if one organ act in an over degree, another which is connected with it, will have its action lessened, and *vice versa*."

Applying this doctrine (which it is not our business to examine) to the cases of abortion under consideration, Mr Burns observes, "There being increased action of the uterus in gestation, requiring an increased quantity of energy to support it, we find that the system is put, *pro tempore*, into an artificial state, and obliged either to form more energy, which cannot be so easily done, or to spend less in some other part. Thus the function of nutrition, or the action by which organic matter is deposited in room of that which is absorbed, often yields or is lessened, and the person becomes emaciated, or the stomach has its action diminished, or the bowels, producing costiveness and inflation. If no part give way, and no more energy than usual be formed, gestation cannot go on, or goes on imperfectly. Hence some women have abortion, induced, by being too vigorous; that is to say, all the organs persist in keeping up their action in perfection and complete degree." Another source of tendency to abortion is found by our author in the too readily yielding of other organs, allowing the uterus to act too easily. The intestines may yield too easily, and, becoming torpid, induce costiveness; or the muscular system may yield too much, and become enfeebled. Mr Burns considers this doctrine to be of much practical importance in directing the means of correcting habitual abortion. "Much attention should be paid to the

state

ſtate of the principal organs of the body; for, if we confine our attention merely to the uterus, we ſhall often fail, when otherwiſe we might ſucceed; and it will be neceſſary to remember that the chain of ſympathies in geſtation is often extenſive and complicated." The ſtate of the ſtomach, for example, may give riſe to headach, toothach, &c. and often it is dangerous to remove theſe remote effects. It throws too much energy to the uterus and may be productive of abortion, as the pulling of a pained tooth ſometimes reſtores the menſes in caſes of obſtruction.

After having fully examined the prediſpoſing cauſes, or thoſe which lay the foundation of habitual abortion, our author proceeds to ſtate and to explain the operation of the various remote or exciting cauſes of abortion. Theſe are ſuch a degree of violence from falls, blows, violent exerciſe, and the like, as may injure the child, and detach the ovum; the death of the fœtus from diſeaſe peculiar to itſelf, or to its placenta; ſtrong paſſions of the mind; ſtimulating, emmenagogue, and purgative medicines; the acceſſion of morbid action or inflammation in any important organ, exemplified in eruptive diſeaſes; mechanical irritations of the os uteri; tapping the ovum, and eſcape of the waters. But for many ingenious obſervations and uſeful remarks, connected with the examination of theſe cauſes, we muſt refer to the work itſelf.

The medical treatment of abortion embraces the means of prevention when anticipated, the method of checking it when immediately threatened, and the proper method of conducting the woman through it, when it cannot be avoided.

On all theſe ſubjects we can promiſe the ſtudent much information, and the practitioner many uſeful hints, from a peruſal of the work of Mr Burns. We ſhall content ourſelves with noticing one or two examples of what appears to us new in the opinions or practice of our author.

" I have already mentioned that abortion is ſometimes the conſequence of too firm action, the different organs refuſing to yield to the uterus, which is thus prevented from enjoying the due quantity of energy and action. Theſe women have none of the diſeaſes of pregnancy, or they have them in a ſlight degree. They have good health at all times, but they either miſcarry, or have labour in the ſixth, ſeventh, or eighth month, the child being dead; or, if they go to the full time, I have often obſerved the child to be ſickly, and of a conſtitution unfitting it for living. We may ſometimes cure this ſtate by giving half a grain of digitalis, and the eighth part of a grain of the tartris antimonii, every night at bed-time, which diminiſhes the ſtomachic action. Bleeding is alſo uſeful, by making the organs more irritable. Exercife, fo as to prove tonic, is hurtful in this fpecies of abortion; inftead of wifhing to increafe the action of any organ, our object is to diminifh it, and make the different parts more eafily acted on."

The digitalis feems a favourite remedy with Mr Burns, and is recommended by him under every circumftance of abortion and flooding, where it is our indication to diminifh vafcular or organic action. This doctrine, too, and practice of attending to the ftate of the fympathizing organs, and of lowering or raifing their action, is applied in a variety of cafes. We agree with Mr Burns that the hæmorrhage which attends abortion can do no good, and that, in every cafe, it is our bufinefs to moderate and reftrain it. The principal means of effecting this is by the application of cold, by plugging the vagina, and by the ufe of digitalis. But we do not altogether fubfcribe to Mr Burns's profcription of manual affiftance. We are decidedly of opinion that no violence is to be ufed; but we know that the flooding is often protracted by the retention of the whole or part of the ovum or fecundines, which it is fometimes in our power to reach with the finger, and to remove to the great advantage of the patient. We do not recommend any attempt to dilate or force the os uteri in abortions of the earlier months; but, when the flooding is protracted from retention, the practitioner fhould examine, and, if within the reach of his finger, he may attempt, and will fometimes eafily accomplifh, its removal.

While we have much to praife in the plan and execution of this treatife, we regret to obferve the carelefs manner in which it has been printed, a circumftance we muft attribute to the diftance of the author from the prefs. Moft of the typographical errata are noted and corrected; but others have efcaped notice. There is one error in the dofe of digitalis, page 132, to which we efpecially requeft the reader's attention.

The receipt fhould be thus corrected:

℞ Tinct. Digitalis ʒ ifs.—*for* ℥ ifs.
——— Hyofciami ʒ i.—*for* Extract. Hyofciami.
Emulf. Camphorat. ℥ iv. mifce.

VII.

VII.

An Essay on the Effects of Carbonate of Iron upon Cancer, with an Inquiry into the Nature of that Disease. By RICHARD CARMICHAEL, Member of the Royal College of Surgeons in Ireland, and Surgeon of St George's Hospital and Dispensary. Dublin, 1806. 8vo. pp. 116.

A REMEDY which promises the cure or even the alleviation of so formidable and hopeless a disease as cancer, and which is announced under the sanction of a respectable name, cannot fail to interest the public. The experience, however, of others must determine whether or not Mr Carmichael have been mistaken in his observations. We know that some trials, which have been made of the carbonate of iron in his quarter have not been successful, and are disposed to doubt of the nature of those cases which have been cured by Mr Carmichael; indeed, we do not think they have the character of real cancer. Another remark on these cures is calculated to inspire still farther reserve; we mean the very sudden relief, and the rapidity with which these ulcerations healed under the use of the remedy, so unlike what we know of the history and progress of cancer. But, that our readers may judge for themselves, we shall quote one of these cases.

"A very young lady, who, in the year 1799, was attacked by this complaint, afforded an uncommon proof of the efficacy of the carbonate of iron. A small pimple first appeared at the side of the nose, which, by frequent irritations, degenerated into that species of ulcer termed *Noli me tangere*. Many experienced practitioners were consulted, who informed her friends of the inveterate nature of her complaint, and at the same time prescribed cicuta, calomel, arsenical lotions, and the other remedies employed in cancer, but without any beneficial effect.

On the 10th October 1805, in the sixth year of the progress of the disease, carbonate of iron was first applied; at which period the ulcer was irregular, with high-erected edges, and discharged a thin ichor, while redness and induration extended over the greater part of her nose, so that there were serious apprehensions that the cartilage and bones were engaged in the disease. But, on the use of iron, the pain in a few hours ceased, and the application, not having been disturbed for two days, formed a scab, which fell off at the end of that time, leaving

ving the sore evidently amended, and discharging healthy-looking matter. The rust was applied daily till the 16th instant, when a dry crust formed, which dropping off in a few days left the parts completely healed."

Thus this young lady was cured of a disease in six days, which had obstinately withstood, for as many years, the most powerful remedies heretofore employed in this disorder. Now, all the cases related in the text are similar to this. They are all cases of phagedenic ulceration either in the face or legs. In a postscript, indeed, there are some cases more like to cancer, in which the preparations of iron were employed with good effect. A carcinomatous ulcer of the breast was cicatrized, a case of supposed cancer of the womb was relieved, and some other more doubtful cases appear to have received benefit from the remedy.

The connexion between local diseases and the general constitution has not escaped the observation of surgeons. Every day's experience must convince them how unavailing every special application is, unless the general disorder of the system be at the same time corrected. The carbonate of iron, by improving the general health, and invigorating the constitution, may contribute to the cicatrization of phagedenic ulcerations. Its specific powers upon cancer we are disposed to doubt. "Sed adhuc sub judice lis est."

The carbonate of iron is employed by Mr Carmichael both externally and internally. It is applied in fine powder to the sore, sometimes it is made up into an ointment; and he uses also, as a lotion, the solution of the sulphate of iron, while the carbonate is given in large and repeated doses internally.

The discovery of the preparations of iron, as remedies against cancer, was not accidental; and it is curious to observe the analogy, however loose, which will sometimes lead to the employment of something new. Mr Carmichael maintains, with Dr Adams, the doctrine of the independent life of cancer, and, knowing that iron was effectual in destroying intestinal worms, it occurred to him that it might be equally destructive of other parasitical animals, and why not of the carcinomatous? The trial was accordingly made, and his success more than answered his expectations.

Mr Carmichael has bestowed considerable pains on this tract. His observations on cancer may be read with advantage. He has made good use of the labours of former writers, especially of those of Dr Adams and of Mr Abernethy. Introductory to his own illustrations, he engages in a short examination of the opinions of the ancients and moderns concerning

cancer;

cancer: an inquiry is then instituted into the nature of the disease, in which the appearances and structure of cancer are explained according to the latest observations; and this leads to Mr Carmichael's grand object, the evidence of the independent life of cancer.

But although he agrees generally with Dr Adams in attributing to cancer an independent existence, he dissents from him in some particulars. He refuses to the cysts described by Dr Adams, containing a yellow-greenish fat, the power of vitality, and consequently denies the existence of the carcinomatous hydatid. The carcinomatous animal of Mr Carmichael is a kind of zoophite or polypus; for it is to the cartilaginous septa, and processes which radiate in every direction amidst the surrounding cellular substance and glands, that Mr Carmichael attributes an independent vital existence.

"The substance resembling softened cartilage, with its cavities and annexed roots, which I conceive alone to form carcinoma, has no connexion, by communicating vessels, with the parts in which it is imbedded, and strongly resembles the gelatinous texture of the polypus and other zoophites."

This opinion, our author thinks, is strengthened by striking and conclusive arguments, and the above quotation is placed first in the order of arguments, as the most in point; for the others are founded chiefly on the vague supposition, that parts least endowed with life are the most favourable to the lodgment and growth of animalcules, and that such parts are chiefly subject to carcinoma. We are not satisfied that the mammæ, uterus, ovaria, and testicles, are parts naturally endowed with a small portion of life. But the whole argument founded on this consideration is too frivolous to merit farther notice.

"The origin of carcinoma first commencing in a point, the formation of cysts in its texture containing a fluid, those cysts evincing a contractile power, by a forcible expulsion of their contents on being punctured, and the peculiar pain of this disease, are all circumstances which strongly impress the idea that carcinoma is possessed of individual life." It is somewhat singular, and rather unfortunate, that the cysts containing a fluid, and *their contractile power*, should be here brought forward by Mr Carmichael as an argument for the individual life of carcinoma, after having, in another place, destroyed its whole force, by refusing vitality and independent existence to this portion of carcinoma.

"But these appearances seem to be merely the effect of the deranged actions of the animal economy, except the one evincing a contractile power in what he terms capsules, but which, notwithstanding

notwithſtanding repeated inveſtigation, I never could perceive."—P. 42.

But the cyſts of which Mr C. now ſpeaks are probably the larger cavities of the cartilaginous ſubſtance which conſtitutes his carcinomatous zoophyte; and theſe cavities, when opened, ſpurt out their contained fluid with more force, it ſeems to Mr C., than the ſimple elaſticity of the part is capable of effecting. Upon the whole, it appears to us that the proofs of the independent vitality of cancer are woefully deficient. We are at moſt diſpoſed to regard it as an ingenious though fanciful hypotheſis. Yet Mr C. is ſo perſuaded of its truth that, although Mr Nooth might inoculate himſelf with impunity with the matter of cancer, he would not anſwer for the conſequences, had he *engrafted* the ſame limb with a *ſlip* of the cartilaginous ſubſtance of carcinoma.

In ſpeaking of the treatment of cancer, our author takes a view of the principal remedies, palliative as well as efficient, which have been employed; and theſe, he is of opinion, afford a further preſumption of the independent life of cancer. Even the preparations of iron appear to have been employed as efficient remedies in cancer by others. Fabricius recommends a rude form of that medicine, the powder collected from grinding-ſtones upon which iron inſtruments have been ſharpened; Mr Pouteau, a ſolution of the metal in a mineral acid; and Mr Juſtamond, the flores martiales. Iron, then, is concluded to act as poiſon to the carcinomatous zoophite. Mr Carmichael thinks, from ſome coarſe experiments he has made on white-blooded animals, that the carbonate and oxydes of iron are deſtructive to their lives. "It is obſervable that cancers, hydatids, tæniæ, worms, and other extraneous bodies, that are more or leſs endowed with the principle of vitality, and whoſe life is deſtroyed by the preparations of iron, are altogether void of red blood, but that on other animals, whoſe blood is red, it never acts as a poiſon."

PART

PART III.

MEDICAL INTELLIGENCE.

Some Account of the "Medical Topography of Berlin," with a List of Diseases at the Public Hospital in that place.

BERLIN, the capital of Prussia, is situated in a wide sandy plain on the banks of the river *Spree*, 52° 30° north lat. and 31° 10 long.—The surrounding country is quite flat, interrupted by no hills and no woods, except a little rising-ground and a few plantations, chiefly of fir-trees, in the neighbourhood of the town. During the continuance of warm weather, the dust is exceedingly troublesome, in consequence of the soil being so very light and sandy. There are no regularly prevailing winds: the most common are south-west, west, and north-west; east and south-east seldom blow, and only in stationary warm weather. In general, the east wind brings dry weather, and the west wind ushers in wet weather. West winds prevail most, and these are said to purify the atmosphere more than any other gales. The seasons vary in different years, as in other places. In the spring, there is commonly frost, snow, and rain: sometimes, however, clear warm days prevail in the month of March, but these do not continue long without being followed by cold and rain. Not more than from 65 to 70 clear days can be reckoned in the whole year upon an average, and perfectly clear days, when not a cloud can be seen in the sky, are very rare; they do not amount to more than two or three in a year; sometimes a greater number of such days are perceived, from 15 to 18 in particular seasons. Thunder-storms are frequent, but seldom violent. The quantity of rain and vapour that falls in twelve months may be reckoned, on an average, as equal to $19\frac{1}{4}$ inches. In London it amounts to $18\frac{1}{3}$, in Paris 17, in Petersburgh $20\frac{11}{12}$, at Abo $23\frac{1}{4}$.—The average height of the barometer at Berlin is 27 inches; the thermometer usually rises to 92 deg. Fahrenheit in the month of July, and falls to 16 deg. in January. Changes in the weather are very common; indeed, it seldom continues long the same; the vicissitudes are sudden, cold evenings generally succeed to hot days, so that the thermometer rises or falls ten or twelve degrees in the space of a few hours. The air seldom continues dry for any length of time; both in summer and winter it is oftener moist, and, on that account, not remarkable for its salubrity.

The principal hospital for the reception of the sick poor is called "*La Maison de Charité.*" It is a large handsome building, three stories high, containing about twelve hundred beds for three classes of patients, which are separated into three divisions: *1st*, The Medical and

and ſurgical caſes; 2d, The lunatics; 3d, Lying-in women and their children The lunatics have been placed at this hoſpital ſince the houſe, in which they were confined, was deſtroyed by fire in 1798. The funds for the ſupport of this eſtabliſhment are derived partly from ſome lands belonging to the charity, partly from the intereſt of ſome monied capital, and partly from an annual gift preſented by the King. In conſequence of the numerous applications for admiſſion, and the inadequate ſtate of the funds to meet fully the yearly expences, the wards are at this time too much crowded with patients, and there is not ſuch cleanlineſs and internal accommodation as the managers wiſh, and propriety and good order demand. Two ſurgeons reſide in the hoſpital as penſioners; beſides, an army ſurgeon, and nine other ſurgeons, take charge of the patients, under the inſpection of two phyſicians and a ſurgeon-major. The celebrated *Hufeland* is ſuperintendant of the hoſpital and the different departments, and *Dr Fritze* reſides as phyſician in ordinary at the inſtitution. Medicines are furniſhed *gratis* by the apothecary of the court, and all the other charitable inſtitutions are ſupplied in the ſame manner. Pupils in the different branches of the medical art are admitted to attend the patients, and aſſiſt at operations. There is a clinical eſtabliſhment attached to the hoſpital, and every perſon who graduates at any univerſity, and wiſhes to ſettle as phyſician in the Pruſſian dominions, is obliged, by ſome late regulations, to attend the clinical wards at Berlin, and to take two or three patients under his care, and examine and treat them in preſence of the principal phyſician, before he can be admitted to paſs his examination for a licence to practiſe. In addition to the ordinary clinical ſchool, there is a ſchool for ſtudying midwifery, and women are regularly inſtructed in the principles and practice of this art. The variety and the proportion of the moſt prevalent diſorders will beſt be ſeen by a reference to the following liſt, which may be looked upon as a ſummary of the diſeaſes admitted into the hoſpital during a period of four years.

Account of Diſeaſes at "La Charité," *from January* 1801 *to December* 1804.

	NUMBER OF CASES.			
	A. D. 1801.	A. D. 1802.	A. D. 1803.	A. D. 1804.
Inflammatory Fever, -	1	8	5	—
Nervous and malignant Fever,	154	323	364	320
Hectic Fever, - -	61	51	93	45
Catarrhal Fever, -	40	16	22	94
Simple mild Fever, -	60	11	—	3
Intermittent Fever, -	30	39	53	164
Inflammation of the Lungs,	26	10	48	77
Rheumatiſm, -	97	30	24	101
Inflammation of the Kidneys,	1	—	—	—
Small-Pox, -	1	—	1	—
Scarlet Fever,	17	17	35	10

Hyſteria

	NUMBER OF CASES.			
	1801.	1802.	1803.	1804.
Hyſteria and Hypochondriaſis,	17	—	6	14
Mental Derangement,	179	200	238	200
Paralyſis, - -	28	20	10	26
Suffocation,	10	3	6	3
Colic, - - .	6	27	11	4
Poiſon of Lead, -	21	4	7	37
General Debility, -	117	112	91	105
Pain in the Stomach,	9	4	8	17
Epilepſy, . - -	24	30	27	9
Spaſm and Convulſions,	16	23	16	26
Triſmus, - -	2	—	—	3
Apoplexy, -	4	13	16	8
Spitting of Blood, -	8	10	12	15
Hæmorrhoids, -	10	2	1	6
Suppreſſed Menſtruation,	4	—	—	—
Obſtruction in the Inteſtines,	14	4	4	8
Chronic Diarrhœa, -	24	16	30	12
Dyſentery, -	6	—	—	10
Iliac Paſſion,	1	1	2	3
Indigeſtion, - -	3	1	4	5
Chronic Catarrh,	61	29	31	29
Pulmonary Conſumption,	169	173	278	225
Gout, - -	53	86	142	56
Aſthma, -	4	22	13	18
Suppreſſion of Urine,	3	3	11	9
Obſtructions in the Urethra,	4	5	3	3
Itch, - -	806	277	884	831
Lues Venerea, -	687	680	623	626
Dropſy, - -	58	45	43	75
Cachexia, - -	16	13	1	7
Jaundice, - -	7	4	6	6
Tabes, - -	4	12	4	5
Debility from old Age,	61	104	66	76
External Diſeaſes.				
Inflammation, -	44	53	75	—
Tumour, - - -	50	59	70	—
Aneuriſm, - -	1	—	1	—
Hydrocele, - -	7	6	9	—
Cataract, -	5	7	3	—
Specks on the Cornea,	4	6	4	—
Ulcers, - -	297	384	466	—
Fiſtula, - - -	11	4	15	—
Wounds, - -	12	16	30	—
Fractures and Contuſions,	38	50	59	—
Diſlocations, -	11	4	5	—
Rupture, - -	9	17	9	—
Amauroſis,	9	6	7	—
Caries Oſſium, -	25	15	35	—

The tables, from which thefe refults are extracted, give a minute detail of the number of patients admitted each month of the year, with each particular difeafe mentioned in the lift, and fhow how many are cured, how many died, and how many are difmiffed incurable, or fent to other charitable inftitutions. There feems every reafon to believe thefe accounts accurate and authentic, becaufe the lifts are made out every month, and efpecially becaufe moft of the patients are fubmitted to clinical lectures and clinical practice. The number of patients admitted in the year 1801 amounted to 4726. Of thefe 3150 were cured, 472 died, and 294 were difmiffed without being cured, or remitted to other inftitutions. The proportion of deaths in the whole of this number is as 1 to 10, which is by no means confiderable, when it is known that many patients are brought to hofpitals in a dying ftate, and expire a few hours after their admiffion. By comparing the reports of other medical inftitutions, which are well known, the mortality is lefs at Berlin than elfewhere. In the general hofpital at Vienna, the number of deaths, compared with the whole number of patients admitted during the year was as 1 to $9\frac{2}{3}$. In Frederick's Hofpital at Copenhagen, the average proportion of deaths, during five years, was as 1 to 10. What a ftriking difference thefe reports furnifh, when compared with the fame and other fimilar inftitutions in former times! On comparing particular difeafes, the number of deaths is found to be confiderably lefs in fome than in others; as, for inftance, in nervous and malignant fevers, and, on the contrary, in confumption and dropfy. Of 154 cafes of typhus fever, 25 died; and the greateft part of the patients, at leaft one-third of the whole number, are carried off by pulmonary confumption. Malignant and contagious fever is very rare in the hofpital at Berlin. The refident phyfician, Dr Fritze, has only feen a fever of this fort once during the eight years of his being there, and thefe cafes occurred in the wards fet apart for patients with the itch.' The cafes put down under the clafs of fevers are comparatively fmall, when we confider that this hofpital is a general houfe of reception for the paupers among a population of 160,000 perfons; and the nervous fevers are in general lefs violent and lefs dangerous than what are obferved in large towns in this country. Dropfy and dyfpeptic complaints are fmall in number, when compared with the reports of hofpitals and difpenfaries in England, Scotland, and Ireland. This difference points out fome ftriking peculiarity in the phyfical habits of the lower orders of fociety. The general fobriety and abftinence from the abufe of fpirituous liquors may account for this circumftance. Another fingular variety is the fcarcity of difeafes of the kidneys and urinary organs. Gravel and ftone in the bladder occur fo feldom, that no divifion is even allotted to fuch complaints in the long lift of human infirmities. The hiftory of mental diforders affords fome curious refults; under the general title of *Mental Derangement (Gemüthfkranken)* are placed all patients affected with melancholia, mania, and fatuitas, and they form a very numerous clafs. The proportion of men to women is as 104 to 56, nearly double the number of males to that of females; and this excefs

 is

is obſerved to increaſe in the increaſing numbers of this claſs of diſeaſes for ſeveral years paſt. What can be the cauſe of ſuch a difference? Does it depend upon any difference or any change in the moral and phyſical habits of the female ſex? Is it the ſame in other inſtitutions for lunatics? Farther inquiries would throw light on theſe queſtions. Out of 334 caſes of mental derangement 105 were cured, the third part, certainly a great proportion, and more worthy attention, as, it is ſaid, this ſucceſsful treatment was owing to very ſimple means, viz. the external application of cold water. The greateſt number of patients admitted was in the months of January, February, March, and July, and the ſmalleſt number in June. Nervous fevers were more frequent in May, and leſs ſo in October and November. Rheumatiſm moſt common in July, and the greateſt number of mental diſorders appeared in June; at leaſt, ſuch was the ſtate of the admiſſions in 1801. It ſeems probable, *cancer* and *ſchirrus* are claſſed under the heads *tumour* and *ulcers*, becauſe both theſe diſorders are very frequent on the continent, and, of late years, more common than formerly, eſpecially *cancer uteri*. What can be the reaſon for the frequent occurrence of ſuch a formidable malady? Intermittent fevers were unuſually frequent in April, May, and June, in 1804, owing to the cold wet ſpring and ſummer. Many trials were made with gelatin, which cured them, and the reſult of theſe experiments will be given to the public.

On the Treatment of Hooping-Cough.

We are informed that a paper has been preſented to the Medical and Chirurgical Society of London, by Dr Richard Pearson, on the treatment of the hooping-cough. After bearing teſtimony to the advantages to be derived from a reſtricted uſe of emetics, he ſtates that he has failed of ſucceſs when he has attempted to cure this diſorder by vomiting-medicines alone, agreeably to the directions of Dr Fothergill; he has, therefore, had recourſe to other meaſures. After bringing away the phlegm by an antimonial emetic, he preſcribes a medicine compounded of opium, ipecacuanha, and prepared natron, (carbonate of ſoda). To a child a twelvemonth old, he gives one drop of tinct. of opium, five drops of ipecacuanha wine, and two grains of prepared natron, made into a ſmall draught with ſyrup and water, and repeated every fourth hour. This medicine appears to have an antiſpaſmodic and diaphoretic operation. When, by its uſe for ſome days, the hooping-cough paroxyſms are rendered leſs violent and leſs frequent, he directs the ipecacuanha to be omitted, and the gum myrrh, in ſufficient doſes, to be ſubſtituted in its place; the proportions of opiate tincture and alkaline ſalt remaining the ſame. The myrrh is uſed not as an expectorant, but as a tonic; as ſuch, he has found it preferable in this diſorder, eſpecially where the patients are very young, to the Peruvian bark. On what principle the alkaline ſalt acts, he does not pretend to explain; but he aſſerts that the ſame beneficial

neficial effects are not produced by the opium and ipecacuanha, or opium and myrrh, when it is left out. He adds, that costiveness is to be prevented, during the use of these medicines, by proper doses of calomel and rhubarb.

Extracts from Letters from Mr Wilkinson, on the Decomposition of Water by Galvanism.

Since I had the pleasure of seeing you at Edinburgh, the celebrated experiments of Pacchioni have excited our attention, repeated with every possible care as to the water being distilled and freed from every impurity, and after having decomposed as much as to produce me 18 cubic inches of gas; yet I have not discovered the least trace of muriatic acid, nor does the soda, as mentioned by Mr Peele appear, if the decomposition be effected in vessels when no soda enters into their composition.

Dublin, 11*th June,* 1806.

The Experiments of Pacchioni and Mr Peele.

You have requested me to state to you what experiments I have made relative to the experiments of Pacchioni and Mr Peele. From my results, I am persuaded, these gentlemen must have fallen into some error. Mr Peele says, he reduced 16 ounces of water to six ounces, by the decomposing power of Galvanism, and discovered muriatic acid in the residual water. Accustomed as I am to Galvanic experiments on a large scale, yet I cannot comprehend what power must have been employed to have decomposed so much water. I find 600 plates in 30 hours will not decompose more than two drachms. Hence such an apparatus, even acting with considerable force, would require seven weeks to decompose such a quantity. If so long a time was devoted to it, there would be a greater probability of muriatic acid being absorbed by the water from various sources. At Dublin, I procured from Dr Barker, chemical lecturer at the University, some distilled water. Muriate of barytes, and nitrate of silver, had been introduced into separate portions, to prove that no sulphuric acid were present in any form. After decomposing two drachms, a solution of nitrate of silver gave to the residual water a white cloudy appearance, or evinced the appearance of muriatic acid. Since then I repeated the experiment with my apparatus so arranged as to prevent any absorption whatever. With these precautions no discoloration took place. I am persuaded, that, in the first experiment, the error arose from the muriatic acid entering into the composition of the acid employed for Galvanic experiments.

Cork, 28*th March,* 1806.

The MEDICAL COMMITTEE of the SOCIETY for INVESTIGATING the NATURE and CURE of CANCER, consisting of Drs Baillie, Sims, and Willan; Mess. Sharpe, Home, Pearson, and Abernethy, and Dr Denman, Secretary, circulated in 1802 a set of Queries for obtaining information regarding these. Since that time they have been republished, with Observations explanatory of their object. In reprinting a *Brochure* of so much intrinsic value, we hope both to preserve it, and to forward the views of so laudable an Institution.

EVERY person must be sensible of the various difficulties attending the establishment of a new institution, and of the much greater and more numerous difficulties which beset our first steps in the acquisition of knowledge on a subject of which, it may be said, we are even at this time totally ignorant *. But, in order to form a basis of inquiry, in which the nature and cure of cancer, it is presumed, may be pursued with all the advantages of reason and experience, the Medical Committee very early drew out and distributed the following queries, for the consideration not only of the corresponding members, but of all medical men, to whom opportunities of answering them might, by study or by accident, occur. A satisfactory answer to any one of these queries would, in itself, be of great importance, and might probably lead to an explanation of others. It is therefore earnestly requested, if any new observation or discovery respecting cancer should be made, that it may be communicated to the secretary of this institution; and, if any progress in the investigation of the nature and cure of cancer be made by or imparted to them, it will, without delay, be laid before the public by the Medical Committee. It may be necessary to observe that the promoters of this institution have never entertained the idea of creating the jealousy, or of interfering with the interests, of those who are engaged in institutions of a similar kind; their intention being solely that of co-operating in the laudable endeavour to lessen the mass of human misery, by calling for the assistance of others, and by exerting themselves to obtain a remedy for a most painful and dreadful disease, against which all the medicines and methods of treatment hitherto proposed and tried have been unavailing.

The queries above-mentioned are expressed in as plain terms as the nature of the subject would allow; but it has been thought that some benefit would accrue from a short comment or explanation of the aim and purport of each query in the following manner:

QUERY 1st.—*What are the diagnostic signs of cancer?*

It is very much to be wished that we had an exact definition of cancer, those of the nosologists being very imperfect and insufficient. It has accordingly happened that a disease, which has been denominated

* It is scarcely necessary, in this place, to refer the reader to an excellent Treatise on Cancer, by Mr Pearson, surgeon of the Lock Hospital.

nated cancer by one medical man, has not been allowed to be such by another; and painful and hazardous operations have been performed by some, which were not thought necessary, or likely to be successful, by others. Hence an opening has also been made for false pretensions and impositions; and, though no person conversant in practice thinks that a true genuine cancer was ever cured, there is an abundance of cases in which cures of this disease are asserted with the greatest confidence. If a just and exact definition of cancer cannot yet be formed, we must be satisfied with such a description as a correct history of the disease will afford. This, it appears, has never yet been judiciously and accurately done; though it would probably enable us to discriminate the various forms of the disease, and its distinction from other diseases. Till, therefore, a precise definition, or a competent description be formed, it will be incumbent on us to mark all the symptoms peculiar and incident to cancer, and the order in which they arise, together with the varieties of this and similar diseases, and the effects of the medicines which may be tried under all the different circumstances, that we may be able to say something more satisfactory than that it seems to us to be cancer; or that it is cancer, because it is an indurated, painful, and unequally enlarged gland, terminating in ulceration; or that every ulcer, in certain parts, which resists the common modes of treatment, or methods of practice, is to be regarded as cancerous. It is much to be wished that we may no longer be deceived by ambiguous words and phrases, or consider them as conveying to us any essential or practical knowledge.

QUERY 2d.---*Does any alteration in the structure of a part take place, preceding that more obvious change which is called cancer; and if there be an alteration, what is its nature?*

It might first be asked, Does any disposition to cancer in any part take place previously to any physical alteration or change of structure in the part? or are there any symptoms, local or constitutional, which denote that cancer is about to be formed? Then we may consider how the first alteration in the structure of a part disposed to become cancerous is to be distinguished from the structure of a part perfectly sound and healthy, or from the structure of parts disposed to other diseases. To such questions it might be answered, by the aspect; by the touch; by dissection; by corrosion of parts; by maceration; by boiling, or otherwise subjecting them to the operation of fire; by a chemical analysis of the component parts; by putrefaction; and by all the various methods used to detect the structure and other qualities of any part generally, or of its distinct component parts. Nor should this investigation cease with the beginning disease, but it ought to be conducted through the different stages; and this subject is now so open, both with regard to experiment and to the correction of what has been before said and done, that it is scarcely possible

4

possible for any one to employ their thoughts upon it without improvement.

One great consequence of obtaining an answer to this query would be, that though we are unable to cure cancer in an advanced stage, we might extinguish the disposition to it, or suppress it completely in an early stage, whether the disposition or the progress consist in increased or new action of a part, or in a change of structure.

Some pains have been taken to discover, by the properties of the discharge from cancer, the nature of the disease. Through a long series of writers, from the time of Galen, *atrabilis* was considered as the cause of cancer; some thinking that it was of an acid, and others that it was of an alkaline quality; and those of each persuasion have attempted to cure the disease by opposite remedies and applications, with different effects, perhaps, but eventually with the same termination. It is not, however, yet ascertained that the discharge from cancer is different from similar discharges, whether serous, sanious, or purulent, made from parts affected with totally different diseases.

QUERY 3d.—*Is cancer always an original and primary disease; or may other diseases degenerate into cancer?*

This is a question which has been very much disputed; at least there have been many different opinions concerning it. It does not imply that all the changes which take place from the commencement of the same disease, through its progress to the time when it is acknowledged to be indubitably a disease of a certain kind, should bear an exact or close resemblance: but it relates to the absolute change in the essence of one disease to that of another, with which it had originally no resemblance or affinity. We must, therefore, leave this query to be determined by future experience and observation; and if the latter clause of it should unexpectedly be decided in the affirmative, we must then inquire what kind of disease, and under what circumstances of the part, or of the constitution, there exists such aptitude to degenerate into cancer.

QUERY 4th.—*Are there any proofs of cancer being an hereditary disease?*

Whether cancer or any other disease be, strictly speaking, hereditary, has, like many other opinions, been positively asserted, and as positively denied. Whether children born of cancerous parents be more liable to cancer than others, from any structure or organization of the body, or any rooted principle of the constitution, may, by attentive observation, be discovered; and, if it should be so proved, we might be led to the prevention of cancer by medicine, by well-regulated diet, or a circumspect manner of education, and of living. If it be proved, on the contrary, that cancer is not hereditary, the minds of many would be relieved from the distress of perpetual apprehension.

QUERY 5th.—*Are there any proofs of cancer being a contagious disease?*

This query certainly requires some explanation. Does it imply a possibility of cance being conveyed from one person to another by the breath, as in the hooping-cough, and, as some have suspected, in consumption? or by effluvia exhaled from a body afflicted with this disease, as in infectious fevers? or, by the breath passing over an ulcerated surface, as in cancer of the mouth or lip? The opinion of cancer being contagious having been advanced, it is become necessary to discuss it, as far as we can, by observation, by experiments, and by casual occurrences. Now we are endeavouring to collect all the *incidentia cancro*, the most apparently trifling fact, if duly authenticated, should not be suffered to pass without notice, as it may direct us to the knowledge of things of great importance.

QUERY 6th.—*Is there any well-marked relation between cancer and other diseases? If there be, what are those diseases to which it bears the nearest resemblance in its origin, progress, and termination?*

Whether there be any relation or affinity between cancer and other diseases acknowledged not to be cancerous, as is the case with all unproved assertions, has been by some affirmed, and by others denied. The second part of this query is equally unsupported and maintained. Some have been assured of the affinity between cancer and scrophula, and others of that between cancer and syphylis: but neither of these opinions have been proved or well supported by a just statement of facts, by regular induction, nor by any collateral circumstance accompanying methods of cure, or the use of any particular medicine. Many of the terms given to disease by the ancients seem not to have been precisely used; yet they made some distinctions of similar diseases, with which few people at the present time seem to be exactly acquainted. For instance, by Cancer, or Carcinoma, they meant a spreading ulceration of a schirrous tumour; by the term Lupus, an inveterate and corroding ulcer; and, by *Noli me tangere*, probably they meant to denote in general what the words imply; tumours, which, while they remained easy and at rest, should not be disturbed. They gave also names according to the part affected, but without any difference in the nature of the disease. But more particular inquiry should be made on this part of our subject; for Mr Home has given a very interesting account of his having removed large portions of the tongue, in diseases of that part, which were allowed to be cancerous. Is it proved that cancer of the breast is exactly the same disease as cancer of the tongue, or that of the uterus? or that, in every case of cancer, in any part, the same method of treatment will be proper? The distinction of similar diseases is very necessary, because medicines, which may be of service in one of these, may be injurious in another. Let us hope that, when precise distinctions are made between cancer and resembling diseases, and between the various kinds of cancer, appropriate and efficacious methods of treatment

ment of each disease will follow, to the great benefit and relief of the afflicted, and to the credit of the profession.

Mr Hey of Leeds, in a late publication, has given an account of a new or hitherto imperfectly described disease, which he calls *Fungus Hæmatodes*, which, as it is incurable, we have no better way of classing than as a species of cancer.

Now we are speaking of the terms used by the ancients, it will not be amiss to observe that, from the time of Galen to the present, there seems to have been little or no difference between the medicines given, and the applications used, for the cure or relief of cancer.

Query 7th.—*May cancer be regarded at any period, or under any circumstances, merely as a local disease? Or does the existence of cancer in one part afford a presumption that there is a tendency to a similar morbid alteration in other parts of the animal system?*

An answer to this query would be highly important, as it is the *experimentum crucis* of many operations which have been performed for the extirpation of cancerous parts. In cancer of one part, perhaps, all similar and sympathizing parts may be affected; perhaps the whole constitution. A surgeon, who is said to have great skill and success in removing cancerous breasts, has said, that in many truly cancerous affections of that part, he had found, on examination, that the uterus exhibited marks of the same disease, and that the state of the uterus was his guide in determining him to extirpate or to avoid operating upon diseased breasts. If the uterus was discovered to be affected, he refused to perform the operation, having constantly found it unsuccessful under such circumstances; yet it does not follow that all extirpations of the breast will be successful, if the *uterus* be free from disease. When operations fail to remove the whole disease, which is in some cases impracticable, the sufferings of the patients are aggravated, and their lives shortened, by operations; of course they ought not then to be performed. Tumours in the breast, of a considerable size, will often remain in a quiescent state for many years, even to the close of life, if not disturbed by injudicious treatment or extraneous injuries, of which the ancients were well aware. It therefore appears as improper to extirpate these as it does to suffer them to remain, when they begin to be disturbed, and can be wholly removed. It appears that more caution than has been usually exercised seems necessary in these operations. It is also requisite to decide, by repeated trials, whether the extirpation of cancerous breasts by the knife or caustic be preferable, as far as relates to the operation, or a prospect of a return of the disease. In practice, we must distinguish between the extirpation of a diseased part and the cure of the disease; the latter of which is the object of these queries, as many parts which do not admit of extirpation are liable to cancer. Certainly many breasts, which were not cancerous, have been extirpated by a painful operation, often through the want of some criterion of cancer, and sometimes, it is feared, from motives of self-interest, or a cupidity to acquire undeserved reputation. It is worthy of observation *to determine* whether any cancerous sore in the breast, or any other part, had ever more than one opening, and whether external injuries ever give rise to cancer, or merely aggravate and put in action a disease which before existed. In the *Lock Hospital*, there is at this time a case of cancer of the *penis*, apparently occasioned by external injury alone. The same fact has been often asserted in cancer of the breast.

QUERY 8th.—*Has climate or local situation any influence in rendering the human constitution more or less liable to cancer, under any form, or in any part?*

There is a considerable variety in the diseases to which human beings are liable in hot and cold climates, and in damp or dry situations, or in those which are low or exposed. The *Goitre* has not been found, or very rarely, in warm and flat countries, nor the *Yaws* in cold ones. The *Lepra*, of every kind, is infinitely more frequent in some countries than in others, and more virulent. With regard to cancer, it is not only necessary to observe the effects of climate and local situation, but to extend our views to different employments, as those in various metals and manufactures; in mines and collieries; in the army and navy; in those who lead sedentary or active lives; in the married or single; in the different sexes, and many other circumstances. Should it be proved that women are more subject to cancer than men, we may then inquire whether married women are more liable to have the *uterus* or breasts affected; those who have had children or not; those who have suckled, or those who did not; and the same observations may be made of the single. The cancer to which chimney-sweepers are subject is known, but not accurately understood; and none but fruitless observations have yet been made upon it, except such as relate to operations.

QUERY 9th.---*Is there any particular temperament of body more liable to be affected with cancer than others? If there be, what is the nature of that temperament?*

The word *temperament* has been often used by medical writers without any precise meaning. It is here meant to signify any native or acquired habit of body, which may dispose to or resist the influence of cancer. Should this query be answered in the affirmative, having discovered the temperament most liable to cancer, we might be led to the prevention of this disease, as was before observed under query the 4th.

QUERY 10th.---*Are brute creatures subject to any disease resembling cancer in the human body?*

It is not at present known whether brute creatures are subject to cancer, though some of their diseases have a very suspicious appearance. When this question is decided, we may inquire what class of animals is chiefly subject to cancer; the wild or the domesticated; the carnivorous or the graminivorous; those which do, or those which do not chew the cud. This investigation may lead to much philosophical amusement and useful information; particularly it may teach us how far the prevalence or frequency of cancer may depend upon the manners and habits of life. As establishments are now formed

for

for the reception of ſeveral kinds of animals, and as the treatment of their diſeaſes has at length fallen under the care of ſcientific men, it is hoped that the information here required may be readily obtained. If animals which live only on herbs, and never drink any other liquid than water, prove to be the leaſt or not at all ſubject to cancer, ſuch proof may, in many caſes, become a guide in practice.

Trees and other vegetables are ſubject to diſeaſes which in time deſtroy them, if not remedied by art. They are alſo ſubject to injuries from external cauſes. In both theſe caſes, the conſtitutional powers of the plant are exerted as evidently for its preſervation, and for repairing its injuries, as in animal bodies, and in a manner not unlike what has been obſerved in animals, under the ſame circumſtances.

QUERY 11th.—*Is there any period of life abſolutely exempt from the attack of this diſeaſe?*

With regard to the periods of life when human beings are moſt or at all liable to cancer, it ſeems to be generally admitted to be moſt frequent in old or advanced in age; but this is not ſatisfactorily proved. Nor is it certainly known what is the earlieſt period of life at which cancer has been obſerved to take place; though no caſe of that diſeaſe has yet been noticed before twenty years of age; at leaſt not before the time of puberty, when the parts, moſt frequently affected with cancer, undergo a great and conſpicuous change; ſo that ſome connexion may poſſibly be obſerved between puberty and this diſeaſe. The ſame may alſo perhaps be obſerved at the time of the final ceſſation of the menſes. Among large bodies of children collected together in charity and other ſchools, or of adults in hoſpitals, in convents, and in monaſteries, opportunities of anſwering this query muſt certainly occur. There is, however, at this time, a young woman in the inſtitution with cancer of the tongue. She is in the eighteenth year of her age, full grown, but has never menſtruated. She never had any glandular or ſcrophulous complaint, but was a very healthy girl, till about ten months ago, when a ſlight ulceration appeared on the left ſide and near the middle of her tongue, which is in great part, at this time, deſtroyed. Her teeth are of a jet black colour. Though ſhe muſt of neceſſity ſwallow conſiderable quantities of purulent matter from the ulcerated cancer, her health is, in all other reſpects, perfectly good.

QUERY 12th.—*Are the lymphatic glands ever affected primarily in this diſeaſe?*

This query goes to the very root of inquiry with reſpect to cancer, which has been hitherto ſaid always to originate in the glandular ſyſtem, without diſtinguiſhing, however, the particular ſet of glands. In cancerous affections of the eye, it is believed that the ball of the eye is not primarily affected, but the lachrymal gland. In cancers of the breaſt, the lymphatic glands appear to be affected only in a ſecondary way, when the diſeaſe is making progreſs. It is probable that careful attention to the objects of this query would lead to many new obſervations reſpecting the firſt ſeat, cauſe, and effect of cancer.

QUERY

QUERY 13th.—*Is Cancer, under any circumstances, susceptible of a natural cure?*

Many diseases and accidents, to which the human body is liable, are cured or repaired by some process of the constitution peculiarly and admirably adapted to the kind of disease or accident. The principle of this process, or the process itself, has usually been expressed by the term Nature, and, in medical language, more frequently *Vis Medicatrix*. But no instance has ever occurred, or been recorded, of cancer being cured by any natural process of the constitution. It is not, however, unlikely that the enlargement of a part containing the *corculum*, or first principle of cancer, may be in consequence of a process set up by the constitution for confining the effects of the disease to the part where it originally existed: thus preventing its ravages or influence upon the constitution. When, therefore, an indurated and enlarged part of a truly cancerous disposition begins to inflame and to be disturbed, the morbid principle may be considered as having overpowered the shield or barrier formed around it for the defence of the constitution. On this principle, trees, when injured by external or other causes, seem to exude and form an external or adventitious support to supply the deficiency of the part weakened or destroyed. But this is a speculation with which we are not concerned, and by which we are in no degree whatever to be guided in the present inquiry. Facts alone, and those indubitably proved, are in this place to be admitted, till such a number shall be collected as will enable us to establish, by fair induction, a sound practice, no longer the creature of presumption or vain opinions.

In the few instances of cancerous parts becoming gangrened, in the breast for example, though the whole *mamma*, or a great part of it, has sloughed away, the ulcer has remained cancerous, and none of the patients have been saved. It is a curious fact, and worthy of particular notice, that no person with an old ulcer in the leg has ever been known to have cancer, though the ulcer was not suspected to be cancerous. From this observation it is probable that issues have been so often directed, with the view of preventing or retarding the progress of cancer.

On the 24th of June, the SENATUS ACADEMICUS of the University of Edinburgh conferred the degree of Doctor in Medicine on the following Gentlemen, after having gone through the appointed examinations, and publicly defended their respective Inaugural Dissertations.

FROM AMERICA,

John Wragg,	*De Nutrimento Fœtus.*
John Taylor,	*De Hominum Varietatibus.*

FROM ENGLAND.

John Thatcher,	*De Febre Puerperarum.*
Henry Herbert Southey,	*De Origine Syphilidis.*
John Booth Freer,	*De Impuberum Morbis.*
William Winstanley,	*De Hysteria.*

FROM

FROM IRELAND.

Mathew Quinlan,	*De Calculis Urinariis.*
Thomas Hancock,	*De Morbis Epidemicis.*
John Morrifon,	*De Menfibus.*
George Clarke, A. B.	*De Vermibus Inteftinorum.*
Samuel Fergufon,	*De Syphilide.*
James Browne,	*De Febre Puerperarum.*
Richard Hanly,	*De Noftalgia.*
Luke Burne,	*De Anafarca.*

FROM SCOTLAND.

Andrew Halliday,	*De Emphyfemate.*
Alexander M'Donald,	*De Veneno Serpentum.*
David Martin,	*De Typho.*
William Thomfon,	*De Generatione.*
John Haftie,	*De Hæmaturia.*

An Account of the Difeafes treated at the Public Difpenfary, Carey-Street, from 28th February to 31ft May, 1806.

ACUTE DISEASES.

	No. of Cafes.
Synochus	4
Ophthalmia	3
Epiftaxis	2
Apoplexia	1
Pneumonia	1
Peripneumonia Notha	5
Catarrhus	91
Cynanche tonfillaris	5
——— parotidæa	1
Pertuffis	2
Rubeola	5
Scarlatina	1
Eryfipelas	1
Herpes Zofter (fhingles)	2
Peritonitis Puerperarum	1
Rheumatifmus acutus	12
Arthritis rheumatica	3
Gonorrhœa	3
Ifchuria	1
Cyftitis traumatica	1
Dyfenteria	7
Convulfio	2
Dentitio	2

CHRONIC DISEASES.

	No. of Cafes.
Cephalæa	17
Hemicrania	2
Catarrhus chronicus	9
Pleurodyne	34
Afthma and Dyfpnœa	8
Hæmoptyfis	10
Phthifis	10
Dyfpepfia	15
Gaftrodynia	25
Dolores hepatici	4
Icterus	3
Conftipatio	2
Enterodynia	9
Colica Spafmodica	1
——— Pictonum	1
Diarrhœa	14
Afcarides	7
Lumbricus	1
Tænia	2
Marafmus	9
Hæmorrhois	4
Nephralgia	6
Dyfuria	5
Eneurefis	1
Exulceratio Pudendi	2
Hydrops	5
Tympanites	2
Leucorrhœa	10

CHRONIC

CHRONIC DISEASES.	No. of Cases.	CHRONIC DISEASES.	No. of Cases.
Memorrhagia, — —	10	Lumbago — —	3
Amenorrhœa and Chlorosis,	9	Sciatica — —	2
Hysteria, — —	9	Aneurisma Aortæ —	1
Chorea. — —	1	Dysphagia — —	1
Epilepsia, — —	2	Rachitis — —	2
Hemiplegia, — —	3	Scrofula — —	3
Amaurosis, — —	1	Syphilis — —	4
Asthenia, — —	29	Impetigo — —	4
Melancholia, — — —	2	Prurigo — —	1
Dysecœa, — —	1	Aphthæ — —	2
Cancer Uteri, — —	1	Echthyma — —	3
Abscessus Abdom. post Partum,	1	Scabies — —	4
Dolores post partum, —	2	Psoriasis (of washerwomen)	1
Rheumatismus chronicus, —	35	Lichen — —	2

The month of March was ushered in by cool, moist, and variable weather; from the 9th to the 13th it was exceedingly cold and sleety, and there were two heavy falls of snow; the 14th, 16th, 17th, and 18th were rainy days; and the remainder of the month, with the exception of three or four days, was damp and cold. With two similar exceptions, the month of April was cold and damp, with a general prevalence of east and north-east winds, as in March, and on the 12th and 13th much snow fell. May commenced with two days of extremely mild and clear weather, with a south-west wind, succeeded by two of cold and wet, with a return of the N. E.; which has continued to blow through the month, except from the 6th to the 9th, when the heat was considerable, with a westerly breeze, and on the 14th, when a heavy rain fell, with the wind S.W. During the whole month, there have been frequent alternations of warm and cool days, and the mornings and evenings have been frequently cold.

The number of catarrhal complaints has been considerably greater than during any three months since these reports were commenced. They were not only very prevalent in the severe month of March, but continue to prevail at present; without exhibiting those symptoms of debility, however, which were their frequent concomitants in the early part of the winter. The different forms of catarrh constitute about 150 of the 500 cases comprehended in the preceding catalogue.

Two of the cases of acute rheumatism terminated fatally at an early period; the one on the 6th day from the attack, the other a few days later. These are the only instances of the fatality of this disease that have ever fallen under my observation; and I should have considered them rather as anomalies, had not several similar cases been lately recorded by Dr Haygarth. Dr H. justly remarks, that the common observation of physicians, that the acute rheumatism is seldom or never a fatal disease, is true, while it remains in its proper seat, the muscles and joints, and when it is not combined with other

other mortal maladies. "But," he adds, "out of 170 cases, I have found 12 which had a fatal termination, either by a translation of the inflammation to the brain, lungs, kidneys, stomach, or some other vital part, or as being found in combination with other diseases." Seven of the 12 were combined with *phrenitis*; and in one, where the pain and swelling receded from the joints, the patient was attacked with shortness of breath, cough, and spitting of blood, which soon terminated fatally. The two cases above mentioned occurred in strong muscular men, of about 40 years of age. In the one, the pain and swelling of the knees and ancles, after having continued a few days, with little benefit from sudorifics and laxatives, became less troublesome, but did not altogether cease, and the patient complained of a severe pain, returning at short intervals, at the pit of the stomach, and greatly impeding his breathing. He had no cough. The pulse was frequent, but extremely soft and compressible; and there was a considerable tremor of the hands. Opium, with other stimulants, produced a temporary relief; a blister was also applied, but ineffectually; and, the pain and difficulty of breathing rapidly increasing, the patient died. The second, a remarkably stout and heretofore healthy man, was exposed to the rain of the 2d of May, and was seized the same evening with shivering and great pains in all his joints. On the 4th I saw him. He complained severely of the pains in all the large joints; the knees and ancles were slightly swelled. He had also a slight dry cough, and some pain in the chest. The pulse was frequent, full, and strong. Although experience seems to have decided against the propriety of bloodletting, at least in London, in rheumatic fever, yet the congeries of symptoms in this instance and especially the combination of the slight pulmonic affection, led me to order about 12 ounces of blood to be taken away; a sudorific was given at bed-time, and ordered to be repeated in the morning. But he felt himself restless and uncomfortable, and I found him out of bed, with the symptoms apparently more favourable. The next day (6th May), the difficulty of breathing was considerably increased, and he complained little of pain in any part. The pulse was more frequent, but less full and strong. A large blister was applied, but removed in the night, and not replaced till morning. The difficulty of breathing and cough had rapidly increased; there was obviously already a great effusion in the lungs, and he was unable to lie in the horizontal posture. At my next visit, (May 8th), he was dead. It is probable that a more liberal use of the lancet might have been beneficial in this instance; in the former it may be doubted whether it was admissible. These cases tend to confirm the remark of Dr Haygarth, and the still more pointed observation of Professor Callisen: "Rheumatismus externas partes occupans, fixus, periculo carere solet; vagus, internas nobiliores partes petens, *maximas sanitati ac vitæ insidias struit* †.

T. B.

* See a Clinical History of Diseases, part I. p. 61.

† Systema Chirurg. Hodiern, tom. I. p. 228.

TO CORRESPONDENTS.

The Communications of *Senex* and Mr *Coates* arrived too late for this Number.

No. VIII. *will be Published on Wednesday, October* 1. 1806.

EDINBURGH
MEDICAL & SURGICAL JOURNAL.

OCT. 1. 1806.

PART I.
ORIGINAL COMMUNICATIONS.

I.

"*An Account of the Illness and Death of* H. B. DE SAUSSURE, *late Professor of Philosophy, at Geneva.*" Communicated by LOUIS ODIER, M. D. and Professor of Medicine.

MR DE SAUSSURE was accustomed, from his infancy, to mountainous excursions, which had inured him to the influence of the greatest possible range of atmospherical temperature, as well as to bodily fatigue. Nevertheless, he enjoyed a good state of health, until after a journey, made about three years ago, to the Boromean Isles, during which, he ate a large quantity of acid fruits: he was attacked with a long and serious complaint, which seemed to have its seat in the stomach, or pancreas; for a long time he was unable to bear any sort of food, all remedies proving ineffectual, with the exception of Starkey's Soap, from which he received considerable benefit. He henceforth constantly laboured under symptoms of difficult digestion, being frequently troubled with flatulence, and his stomach was so apt to generate acidity, that although, for a number of years, he lived almost entirely upon animal food, carefully avoiding the use of fruits, greens, and acid drinks, he experienced every day, some hours after dinner, a sort of Pyrosis, which obliged him to have recourse to chalk and other absorbents in large quantities, and even to reject a part of the contents of his stomach. Fortunately he had acquired the faculty of voluntary vomiting, which he effected without any effort. When he resisted that urgent propensity to vomit, he felt a great load on his stomach, accompanied with so much anxiety and acidity, that nothing could remove these symptoms except vo-

 miting

miting, to which he was at last obliged to resort. Commonly however, he did not wait till that affection had gone so far, but he selected his opportunity so well, that most of his friends and relations remained ignorant of his infirmity. For the last 15 years he had been subject to frequent attacks of the piles, which sometimes gave a pretty copious discharge of blood. His skin was rough and uneven from an herpetic disposition, common to several individuals of his family. Lastly, he had, some years before his death, a pimple on his nose, which continued many months, and passed into a bad sort of ulcer, with hard and callous edges: of so alarming a nature, that the use of the actual cautery became necessary, which operation he bore with great courage, and it was attended with complete success. An issue was then made on his arm, and kept open ever since.

At the end of the year 1798, after long and laborious efforts to stem or to direct the torrent of our political revolutions, joined to the painful idea of the downfall of his former opulence, which nobody had more right to deplore than he, who had always employed his pecuniary means for the noblest purposes, he was suddenly seized with vertigo, which was followed by a distinct sense of numbness in the left arm and cheek. The vertigo did not last long; but nothing could remove that feeling of numbness or torpor. I resorted to blisters, purgatives, frictions with mustard and with flannel, in vain; and successively, to a number of tonic and antispasmodic remedies. That affection of the arm seemed to be seated rather in the sentient extremities than in the moving fibres, for the patient retained his strength; his arm, could perform all kinds of movements, but he could not distinguish easily what he was touching. It seemed to him as if sand was interposed between his fingers and the bodies. That sensation was even painful to a certain degree, and the excess of sensibility made him fearful of using his hands without gloves. He experienced a similar sensation in the cheek and mouth of the same side, which, on passing his hand over his face, formed, in a most unpleasant manner, a well marked line of demarcation between the right and left side. In other respects, he was well, his general health was not impaired, nor did there exist symptoms either of plethora or of weakness. He retained likewise, for a long time, his presence of mind, and his intellectual faculties, entire. Many months were passed in this state, in the course of which, a great variety of remedies were tried, as cold and warm bathing, elecricity, arnica, valerian, blisters, embrocations, artificial and natural thermal waters, change of regimen, travelling, &c. but all in vain. The complaint became worse and worse, always however by starts; the attacks being more or less

less violent and complete. One of the most violent was occasioned suddenly at Bourbon by a shower-bath employed too warm. The attack produced by it was so complete, that the whole of the left side, from the leg to the tongue, were affected. His pronounciation became by degrees indistinct and unintelligible; his legs, especially the left, became heavy, and lost their flexibility and strength. He observed this, particularly when he tried to walk in a straight line in his room, along the narrow dark coloured boards which crossed the floor of his apartments. Exercise of this sort had been very familiar to him, and by this he had acquired greater facility in climbing mountains along narrow paths on the borders of precipices. But his disorder had rendered it more and more difficult for him. He could not long preserve his equilibrium, nor direct his steps as he wanted. What is singular, after the complaint had deprived him of the power of walking without support, it was in passing through doors, that the motion became particularly painful and difficult. He crossed his room, for instance, with a tolerable steady step; but when he reached the door, although it was wide open, much wider than his body, and quite on a level with the next parlour, it required great exertion for him to get through it. He balanced and quickened his motion as if he had to make a dangerous leap, or a bad step to get over; when it was done, he recovered his equilibrium and usual firmness, crossed the room, but had the very same difficulty to surmount, in order to get into another apartment.

On his return from Plombières, he had a copious herpetic eruption over the eyes and forehead. Hopes were entertained of some possible diversion of his disorder upon this and other occasions. However, the disease went on encreasing; the only remedy that seemed always to have some temporary efficacy in alleviating the symptoms was a blister, and he had recourse to these whenever he experienced any return of headach, vertigo, or flashes of light before the eyes, (*éblouissemens*) to which he became often subject. About 15 months ago, I was led by the reports of Dr Beddoes on the use of factitious airs, to have Mr de Saussure respire a superoxygenated air. Before a convenient apparatus could be procured, he tried water impregnated with a small quantity of oxygenous gas, made under his inspection by his son; but I advised him afterwards to give it up, because it seemed to encrease considerably the quantity of urine, (this excretion amounting to more than his drink) and to aggravate his weakness. The rough feeling of his skin, the œdema of his legs, the acidity to which he had long been subject, his immoderate appetite, and lastly, the thirst, which he experienced

2 also

also at this period, made me suspect the existence of some diabetic affection. To this disorder, he seemed to me particularly predisposed, and this was not to be lost sight of, as he entirely changed his diet for some months past, by the advice of Dr Tissot. Since the paralytic state had been quite established, the vomiting had also entirely ceased, and his food consisted principally of vegetable acid fruits, from the use of which, he did not perceive any inconvenience to arise while the herpetic eruption had been much mended. At any rate, those fears about diabetes were soon dismissed. I had his urine evaporated; it gave but little extractive matter, but a large proportion of saline residue, resembling what is found in hysterical urine; by merely relinquishing the use of fruits and oxygenated water, the diabetic symptoms above described soon disappeared. Some time after, we got the proper apparatus for inspiring superoxygenated air. He tried it, but could never inspire it without efforts which fatigued him; and the continuance of the practice was the more objectionable, as he received no benefit from it. The complaint advanced rapidly by insensible degrees, the intellectual faculties became every day weaker, a troublesome incontinence of urine, a spasmodic contraction of the three last fingers of the left hand, and a gangrenous ulcer on the prepuce came on in succession, till at last death supervened, almost suddenly, to free him from so many infirmities. The evening before his death he seemed to enjoy his supper, but was restless during the night, towards morning his head leaned to one side, he breathed with more difficulty than usual, and expired without agony.

On opening the body, 32 hours after death, the dura mater was found adhering firmly to the cranium, particularly along the longitudinal sinus; but that deviation from the natural structure is often met with, and is of no importance. Between the pia mater and arachnoid coat we found a considerable effusion of a substance, resembling at first sight that gelatinous matter found frequently in the brain of persons who have died of some comatose affection. It had the bluish colour peculiar to that matter. In various places there appeared circular spots of a grey yellowish colour, about two or three lines in diameter: these seemed as if they penetrated into the membranes, though susceptible of being detached from them, like small separate spheres, surrounded by a little circular margin of a dark red. At first view, we took those spots for real hydatids; but, on attempting to separate them from the membranes, we found that red margin was a blood vessel connected with other vessels of the head, and convoluted in the form of circles. There were no separate pouches or solution of continuity in the membranes, only

-ly they were more transparent in those places than in others. The serosity underneath communicated freely with that which was diffused over all the surface of the brain, both having the same colour and qualities. On opening the membranes, the serous effusion ran off like water; we collected two or three spoonfulls of it, and exposed it to the flame of a candle. No coagulation took place; a strong ebullition was continued until the whole of the fluid was evaporated, without leaving any perceptible residue. The effusion existed not only upon the whole surface of the brain, but likewise on that of the cerebellum. In this part, the effusion appeared much more considerable on the right than on the left side. We obsesved, in some blood vessels, bubbles of air mixed with the blood, as is sometimes the case between the globules of mercury in Barometers, into which any atmospherical air has been forced by a shake. The ventricles too were full of the same serosity, their capacity was enlarged considerably by the contained fluid. We estimated the whole quantity at about five ounces. The choroid plexus seemed as if almost entirely made up of hydatids in the form of beads; but that appearance is not uncommon. It is owing to the dilatation of the delicate vessels which compose that plexus, and not to separate hydatids. The examination of the head presented nothing more of importance, except that the brain was flattened at the temples, and deeply furrowed by arteries.

The abdomen presented a very extraordinary appearance. When the integuments and peritonæum were laid open, we could perceive neither the stomach, nor liver, nor colon. The small intestines and the cæcum only could be seen. The latter was of a monstrous size, its circumference measured 14 inches. That of the ileum, on its entrance into the cæcum, was four or five inches. The appendix vermiformis was four or five inches long, adhering, by its extremity, to the posterior surface of the cæcum. The colon, entirely hid by the small intestines, was likewise much dilated, and after ascending on the right side above the liver, to the diaphragm, under the 6th and 7th rib, passed then to the left side, where it ascended again so far as to the 5th rib, exactly under the breast, so as to be contiguous in that place to the apex of the heart, from which it was separated only by the diaphragm, which was pressed upwards by that adaptation of parts. Instead of passing under the liver and the stomach, the colon passed above those viscera. It embraced the stomach at its superior orifice, and compressed it so much the more; because, instead of descending, as in the natural state, on the left side, it turned back obliquely towards the right, so that its sigmoid flexure was next the cæcum. It terminated at length in the rectum, which was itself dilated up the common size of the colon. All the other abdominal viscera were in a sound state: there was no vestige of obstruction, or hardness, or any other mark of disease in the pancreas.

In the cavity of the chest the lungs were found small, but perfectly healthy, so were the heart and large vessels; the diaphragm, however, being pressed upwards. Had the cavity of the thorax been confined to its usual limits, there would not have been room enough for the organs of respiration to play. The lungs had consequently got under the clavicles, rising pretty high on each side of the neck. Time did not allow us to examine minutely the attachments of the pleura and mediastinum, under those peculiar circumstances of internal structure.

From the above dissection, the following consequences may be deduced:

1°. The proximate cause of this complaint, and of Mr de Saussure's death, was the effusion of a large quantity of serum into the ventricles, and between the membranes of the brain, which, by compressing that organ, must necessarily have impaired the energy of all the faculties depending on its action. It is possible the effusion began between the membranes of the cerebellum, since it was there only that we were able to find any difference between the right and left side. The complaint, though general towards the conclusion, was long confined to the left side, which would lead us to conclude, as is commonly supposed, that the right side of the brain was most affected. An effusion similar to the one just described, is a pretty frequent cause of apoplexy; but it usually takes place suddenly, and the duration of the complaint is only for a few days. I have lately seen a man, 60 years of age, attacked with a fit of apoplexy, which terminated fatally after 60 hours; and the same appearances presented, on opening the head, as in the case of Professor de Saussure, whose disease lasted five years. It is singular such an alteration in the natural organization of the brain should have produced so little change in the intellectual faculties. Another thing worthy of attention is, that with the exception of some occasional flashes of light, the eyes were never affected, and the pupil always contracted readily. Its dilatation, we know, is the usual consequence of an effusion into the ventricles, which occurs in the hydrocephalus internus of infants. We may conjecture that the complaint of Professor de Saussure having advanced by slow degrees, the optic nerves were able to habituate themselves to a compression which would have affected them, if the effusion had taken place suddenly. But in the person I mentioned, whose illness did not continue three days, we were equally unable to observe any dilatation of the

pupil

pupil. What may be the cause of such differences? That is at present, and will probably long continue, unknown to us. Disorders of the brain, to all appearance, exactly analogous, often produce very different effects; and effects precisely similar, are frequently owing to very different disorders. In most cases, the cause of the effusion is equally obscure. Here it may be ascribed with sufficient probability to grief, anxiety, and over-exertion of mind, excited in Mr de Saussure, by our revolutionary events. On the other hand, I have heard since his death, that he had a violent fall on a stone stair-case, at the beginning of the year 1793; and we know hydrocephalus is frequently the consequence of a fall, or a violent blow upon the head. Next I have been assured by his son, that his father frequently mistook one word for another long before his death, and was so unconscious of his mistake, as to get angry when not understood. This would seem to indicate a commencement of the disease, prior to the first attack in 1793. Lastly, it might be supposed, that the displacement of the intestines might, to a certain degree, press upon the large vessels, and thus impede the circulation in the head. At any rate, may I be indulged with a conjecture,—in certain cases, the disengagement of some elastic gases in the vessels of the brain may impair the functions of that organ? The well-marked appearance of air-bubbles which we observed in some of those vessels, and the same appearance has frequently struck me in other dissections, has given rise to this idea, the truth of which I leave to further enquiries to ascertain or to disprove.

2°. Passing to the state of the abdomen, we may remark, that the change of situation of the colon and its pressure on the superior orifice of the stomach, easily explain the habitual vomiting of the patient some hours after eating. The extreme dilatation of the large intestines may have been the effect of the keen appetite which the mountainous excursions of Professor De Saussure must have induced, and which he usually satisfied with a coarse kind of food, apt to generate large quantities of fæcal matter, accumulated and hardened by exercise in the whole course of the great intestines. I had long foreseen the dilatation of the rectum, because it produced symptoms of compression upon the vesiculæ seminales, which the patient had often mentioned to me, and I could only account for under a supposition of that sort. Perhaps it was one of the causes of the incontinence of urine, which troubled him during the last six months of his life. Nothing, however, could have enabled me to guess the extraordinary change in the situation of the colon—Was it in consequence of peculiar conformation, or of gradual dilatation? I am rather inclined to the latter opinion. The perfect healthy

4 state

state of the pancreas leads me to think that organ had never been affected (as some eminent practitioners had said), and the symptoms suspected to be seated in that part, were most likely owing to the unnatural situation of the colon, which I conclude to have been displaced at that time. For those symptoms had continued ever since, though attended with less irritation in consequence of habit: while on the other hand, it is difficult to believe, that an affection of the pancreas, so great as was then supposed, should have left no traces of its existence. I must confess, however, an accidental displacement of the colon, and in that direction too, is a phenomenon which I never saw before; it is quite unheard of in the annals of medicine, and apparently contrary to the first principles of physics. These would naturally make us believe, that the weight of matters contained in that intestine, should have depressed its curvature, and brought it nearer to the ossa pubis, instead of removing it farther off under the diaphragm. But we must consider the great muscular strength of Mr De Saussure, and the continual exercise to which he was accustomed, especially ascending mountains, a motion very familiar to him, which, by causing the abdominal muscles to contract frequently, must encrease considerably their tension; these circumstances may have, to a certain degree, counterbalanced the effect of gravity, and forced the intestine to extend, in the upper part of the abdomen, away from the obstacles opposed for its depression.

3°. Lastly. The small capacity of the chest, cannot serve to explain, why the breathing of Mr De Saussure was affected on the top of high mountains. Other naturalists, with a very large chest, supported the rarefaction of the air, with more difficulty than he did, and even at a less height. The symptoms he experienced in those elevated regions are much the same, as those described by the Academicians who ascended the Cordillieres: and it is not likely any of them had the same formed chest as Mr De Saussure. I never saw it but in his case. It is singular, it produced no effect in his usual state; and still more, that the coarse matters which had to pass along the colon so near to the heart, never occasioned the slightest alteration in its movements. I have lately seen a woman betwen 60 and 65 years of age, who has been long subject to violent fits of spasms, the cause of which had never been ascertained. I was called to see her in one of these paroxysms.—I found her stretched on her bed, unable to move, complaining of a sense of pressure at the region of the stomach that rendered her breathing difficult, with constant palpitation of the heart, the pulse beating 180 in a minute, and very irregularly. It was rather a tremor than successive contraction. This state was preceded

ceded for some days by constipation of the bowels, which began suddenly, and lasted 30 hours, when she had a copious evacuation. Immediately after, she became pale, and fainted away; and, on recovering from this syncope, which did not last long, she felt perfectly well. I saw her at that moment, her pulse was then regular, beating 72 strokes in a minute. A few minutes before, I found it just as frequent and irregular, as at the beginning of the paroxysm. That circumstance led me to presume, the cause of the disorder was the sudden accumulation of fæces in some pouches of the colon, which compress the aorta or vena cava at a small distance from the heart, and thus obstruct the whole circulation, until the pouch was emptied, and the compression ceasing, the blood could resume its free course. The sudden occurrence of such a circumstance, might occasion, for a few moments, a disturbance of the equilibrium, which produced fainting. I directed my plan of treatment under that supposition. I advised 1°. To keep the bowels open by remedies capable at the same time of strengthening the intestines. 2°. To give, at the commencement of the paroxysm, some spoonfulls of castor oil Although this method has not completely checked their return, it has succeeded so far as to diminish considerably their intensity, and the length of their duration.

Geneva, Dec. 1805.

II.

Remarks on the White Induration of Organs. By G. L. Bayle, M.D. Assistant Anatomist to the School of Medicine at Paris *

THE white indurations of organs are easily recognized at first sight by a remarkable change in the colour, and consistence of the altered part. But these indurations, which at first sight may seem identical, are in fact very various, and the constant diversity of their progress leads to terminations so disimilar, that it is of the highest importance to mark well the distinguishing characters of each.

These indurations are fibrous, tuberculous, or cancerous. The fibrous are not of themselves dangerous, they pass to the fibro-cartilaginous, or osseous state; but the carcinomatous, or tuberculous terminate in the destruction of the affected part.

As

(* See Journal de Medecine, Vol. 9. An. xiii. page 285.)

As these different lesions are not easily distinguishable at first sight, and have been commonly confounded under the name of scirrhus, we have endeavoured to find, in their structure and progress, the means of distinguishing them from each other. I am now accordingly to describe the common characters, and particular differences, of the tuberculous and carcinomatous indurations.

These two modes of lesion may be included under the name of *chronic albuminous degeneration of organs*. Their common character is a particular alteration in the texture, distinguished by a white or grey colour, and by the property of hardening by the action of fire, by boiling in water, and by immersion in acids.—The most remarkable difference in their progress consists in this, that the tuberculous terminates in a white suppuration, more or less grumous, and not corrosive; while the carcinomatous terminates in an ichorous and sanious suppuration, which excoriates the neighbouring skin.

There are other modes of albuminous degeneration not yet described, which might hereafter form new genera of the order of lesions here spoken of. These will be noticed in a separate memoir. I shall here confine myself to a description of the general characters of tuberculous and carcinomatous degenerations. These diseases which are extremely common, I have had many occasions of observing and comparing with each other, in all their stages.—I have thus been enabled to mark well their particular progress, the characters which distinguish them from other modes of alteration, and those, by which the tuberculous may be distinguished from the carcinomatous degeneration. These characters will be readily understood, by a short description of these two modes of alteration, and by a relation of the progress of each.

Distinguishing Characters of the Tuberculous Degeneration.

In the tuberculous degeneration, the altered part is opaque, and commonly of a dull white, slightly citrine, and uniform. The colour indeed may vary from a dull white to brown; but the opacity is always perfect, and the intimate structure homogeneous.

There are three degrees of this change. In the first, the affected portion seems to differ only from the natural state, by a slight white, or grey colour, which however may be distinguished even in those organs, which are naturally white, because the parts affected with this change of structure, are of a more dead white, and more opaque than the rest of the organ In the second stage, the altered portion becomes still more opaque, it acquires a greater density than the rest of the organ, and becomes at the same time, more firm, and more elastic. It is still, however, manifestly organized granized, and when strongly compressed, it separates into very irregular little masses, between which may be perceived cellular substance, varying in quantity, and closeness of texture, and sometimes also small, but very distinct vessels. To this succeeds the third stage, characterized by the want of every organic appearance, and by the dissolution which proceeds from the interior to the exterior, transforming the altered organic portion into pus, thicker or thinner, in which are commonly found purulent lumps, or solid, softish, irregular, greyish or whitish, and caseous little masses. The surrounding parts frequently become hard, and at length even ulcerate; but they never become tuberculated in consequence of this induration.

Distinguishing Characters of the Carcinomatous Degeneration.

In the carcinomatous degeneration, the altered organ appears at first sight of an uniform dead white colour, but when viewed more minutely even with the naked eye, and still better if assisted by the lens, the degenerated part is discovered to have a texture composed of two substances; the one fibrous and opaque, and the other, which hardly seems organic, is commonly transparent. The fibrous substance consists of laminæ, which are irregular, unequal, of different size and thickness, and disposed in different directions. These laminæ form a great number of different irregular cells, containing the inorganic substance, of a bluish colour, a sky blue, and sometimes sea green, seldom white or red, almost always shining, transparent and crystalline, and at least as firm as the fibres which form the opaque substance.

The carcinomatous like the tuberculous disease has three stages; the first is that which we have just described; the second is characterised by the softening of the transparent matter, or by ulceration proceeding inwards from without, and sometimes from within outwards. The third stage is easily known by a fungous ulceration with unequal and often elevated edges, the surface being more or less deeply furrowed, covering a very firm tumour, which insensibly passes from the second to the third stage, while the neighbouring parts indurate, change their nature, and become scirrhous, then cancerous, and shortly after, dreadful carcinomatous ulcers, which, when they cannot be removed by art, are always mortal.

The first stage of the carcinomatous disease, is the only organic alteration to which the name of scirrhus should be given, it is the only one which becomes cancer, while tubercles, and the tuberculous degeneration not contained in a cyst, and commonly called scirrhus, never become carcinomatous; neither do the fibrous bodies

bodies of the womb, and different other alterations of structure, which have been termed scirrhus, even terminate in real cancer.

Varieties of Tuberculous Affections and of Carcinomatous Affections.

After having described the tuberculous and carcinomatous structures, it is proper to mark the varieties of these genera.

Considering them with a view to pathological anatomy only, several lesions may be arranged under these two modes of organic change.

Amongst the tuberculous affections may be placed:—

1. Tubercles which form in different organs.
2. Tuberculous degenerations not encysted.
3. Accumulated tuberculous matter.

Tubercles are formed by a white or grey matter, but always more or less yellow and compact, contained in cysts generally membranous, and always adhering to the tissue of the organ in which they are placed.

Tuberculous degenerations not encysted have the same appearance as the internal matter of tubercles; they form in the immediate substance of organs, and the diseased texture is not separated from the sound by any intermediate substance or cyst.

Accumulated tuberculous matter is a solid body not organized, formed of a white or grey albuminous substance, which separates the texture of the organ in which it is inclosed, and finishes by softening from the centre towards the circumference, becoming changed into a grumous pus.

Amongst the carcinomatous affections may be placed:—

1. Cancers of glandular organs.
2. Cutaneous cancers.
3. Cancers of mucous membranes
4. Cancers of the muscular coats of hollow viscera.
5. Cancers of parenchymatous organs.
6. Carcinomatous alteration of different organs secondarily affected in consequence of the propagation of the cancers already enumerated.

On former occasions, we have delivered our observations on scirrhus of the stomach (1.); and ulcerations of the womb (2.); we have marked the characters by which fibrous bodies differ from scirrhus (3.); and we have spoken fully of tubercles. (4.)—In our next communications, we shall examine very fully the tuberculous degenerations *not* encysted.

(1.) Journal de Medecine Tom. v. page 72.
(2.) Journal de Medecine Tom. v. page 238.
(3.) Journal de Medecine Tom. v. page 62.
(4.) Journal de Medecine Tom. vi. page 3.

III.

Observations on Tubercles found in the Brain of two Scrofulous Subjects, By F. V. MERAT, M. D. Clinical Assistant at the School of Medicine of Paris.*

I HAVE thought it might be useful to present to the profession examples of a variety of lesion which appears to me not to have been observed, or at least not described, amongst scrofulous affections, and which, in this view, will perhaps appear interesting.

CASE 1.

L. H. æt. 14, had always the appearance of delicate health, without, however having ever been affected with any serious disease. His skin was fair, he spoke slowly, and showed more maturity of understanding than is common at his age; he preferred study to the usual amusements of children. The general character of his constitution was scrofulous, although no symptoms had appeared before the 13th year. At this period, he complained of pain of his left knee, which soon became enlarged, but without change of the colour of the skin—about six weeks before this, he had had an intermittent fever, which was properly treated; and when convalescent he went to the country. The swelling of the knee being deemed scrofulous, was treated accordingly. A celebrated surgeon who was consulted, advised bitters, an animal diet, emollient applications, and afterwards the tepid affusion to the knee. During this treatment, the child could scarcely make any use of his limb; the joint was a little bent, so that he halted. However, after six months, the knee sensibly diminished, especially after having used the pump bath of sulfureous water.

For two months he had complained of severe pains of the head, for which a gentle treatment had been employed without relief, when, on the 5th Prairial last, he was suddenly, and without any obvious cause, attacked with convulsions, which in two days terminated in a comatose state. Leeches were applied to the neck, blisters to the back and legs, and stimulant drinks were given, but ineffectually, and the patient died in an apoplectic state on the 8th day of this attack.

Dissection.—On opening the body, we found the brain large, having the circumvolutions flattened, the vessels turged, and swimming

(* See Journal de Medecine, Vol. x. Vendemiaire, An. xiv. page 3.)

ing as it were in a bed of gelatinous serosity. There were tw or three ounces of water effused in the lateral ventricles; som also was found at the base of the skull, and in the canal of spinal marrow.

Behind the superior part of the medulla oblongata, there wa discovered a fatty body of the size of a wallnut, of a reddish o rather rose colour, appearing interiorly a homogeneous substanc penetrated by little red lines, which were probably small vessel. It was contained in a very fine thin covering, little adherent t the neighbouring parts; in a word, it was a true tubercle. On other tubercle, only not quite so large, was found in the mid of the left lobe of the cerebellum.

In the abdomen, the mesenteric glands were enlarged, and s veral becoming obstructed. In the cavity of the small intestin were found, here and there, ulcerated spots.

Remarks.—This patient died suddenly of a disease, which to have been independant of the scrofulous affection. tumors, however, might perhaps, by compressing the origin of nerves, have been the cause of the convulsions, and of the which succeeded. It is evident, that the severe headachs of wh he complained are to be attributed to the tubercles of the b which compressed the surrounding parts. And the reason is clear why they could not be relieved by any mode of treatment.

Case 9.

A. S. C. æt. 35, of an infirm constitution, and irascible temper, had been subject, during the greater part of his life, to a succession of severe diseases, which hardly left him one moment of tolerable health.

In his infancy he had a malignant small pox, followed by obstinate ophthalmia, and an epistaxis which returned almost every spring. At the age of 13, he had an ague of nine months duration, but cured at length by cinchona and bitters; when 14 years, he suffered from a gleet which continued two years, and yielded at last to saturnine injections; he had at the age of 18 a gastric fever, which lasted six weeks, and enjoyed for some years rather better health; when 24, he was attacked with hæmoptysis, which continued six days, and was succeeded by a cough of six months; at 25, he contracted a fresh gleet, with chancres and buboes, which persisted under different forms for four years and a half, at which time, after an incomplete course, the symptoms were relieved without being radically cured. A.S.C. had now attained his 30th year, and was still affected with scrofulous symptoms. And now having engaged in the military service, he he was employed in a cold country covered with snow, (*le pays de grisons*); after remaining there a month, new chancres appeared on the glans, and several glands of the neck became enlarged. To these symptoms were joined severe pains of the joints, loss of appetite, and prostration of strength. And after some time, he was discharged on account of the shattered state of his constitution. With difficulty he walked to Paris. During his journey, which lasted two months and a half, the cough and oppression of which he had complained, became worse. He was feverish; the glands of the neck which had been obstructed were now ulcerated; the chancres of the glans were extended, the feet swelled, and, to use his own expression, *he slavered blood.* He was received into the Lock Hospital, where he underwent a mercurial course of four months, suspended however, from time to time, on account of the hæmoptysis. The venereal symptoms were cured; but the scrofulous disease continued unchanged.

About a twelvemonth thereafter, new scrofulous symptoms appeared, such as obstructions and glandular swellings, which suppurated; the hectic fever returned. He was received into the Hospital of St Louis. The only relief obtained after remaining there two years, was the healing up of several ulcers; but when dismissed he had still a cough, and a fistulous sore, connected with caries of the second metatarsal bone of the right foot. He remained six months at home tolerably easy; but he was seized last autumn with a catarrhal complaint, for which, on the 18th Brumaire, An. 13, he became a patient at the Clinical Hospital of the School of Medicine. Besides the catarrhal symptoms, he had evident marks of scrofula, of lues, and even of scurvy. But chiefly remarkable was the violent pain of the head, of which for some days he had complained, and which continued unabated till death, notwithstanding every remedy employed. Towards the conclusion of his life, it became so intolerable, that he was obliged to remain motionless in bed, the slightest movement aggravating it to perfect torture.

The catarrhal affection abated; the scrofulous disease persisted; the phthisis ran its course; and, in spite of all the resources of art, A. S. C. gave up the ghost on the 10th Messidor, An. 13. seven months after his admission. The marasmus was complete, and, for a month previous to his death, the odour from the suppuration of the scrofulous sores was detestable.

Dissection.—The whole body was greatly emaciated, and covered with the cicatrices of scrofulous ulcers, and open sores of the same kind. The brain was soft. The lateral ventricles contained about three ounces of colourless serum; there was none at the base of the cranium. At the superior and middle part of the

the right hemisphere of the brain, there was a pretty firm tumour of the size of a pigeons egg. It had a fine reddish coat.—The inside of the tumour was a yellowish substance somewhat of the cerebral colour, but having a very distinct organization. In the anterior part of the left lobe of the cerebellum there was a similar tumour, but twice as large, and more rounded in its outline.

The disorganisations of the throracic and abdominal viscera were such as belong to the highest degrees of phthisis and scrofula.

Remarks.—Again, we must observe to what a troublesome series of diseases this patient was subjected, and how wretched his existence. An observation which ought not to be overlooked, is the age at which the scrofulous affections began to appear in this individual. He had no sign of this disease before the age of 30. Now, although scrofula may appear at any age, it most commonly declares itself in infancy; and even where it remains concealed till more advanced years, there are almost always some appearances to be observed in youth, which anounce the future disease.

Shall we say, that this disease was induced by the venereal virus? This metamorphosis has been admitted by some authors, and the present case, it must be confessed, is favourable to the opinion; for the scrofula did not declare itself till after the patient had been four years and a half afflicted with venereal disease, badly treated, and not cured. In this, as in the former case, the cause of the cephalalgia is evident; but it was much more considerable. It is true, that the tubercles were larger; and also, that they had existed much longer, if we refer their origin to the beginning of the disease, which had continued more than seven months. No remedy, it is evident, could affect these tubercles.

Reflections on these Cases.

Tubercles of the brain appear to me to be of very rare occurrence. I do not recollect to have read of any example of this aflection, even in the latest authors. M. Bayle, who has written a Memorial on Tubercles, makes no mention of them. These cases may, therefore, serve as a supplement to his Memoir.

Some objections may perhaps be made to the name of tubercles conferred on the cerebral tumours which I have described. The little adherence which they have to the organ in which they are found, and their existence, even without the organ, may

may give rise to doubt. It is difficult, however, to assign them any other name.

The small quantity of cellular substance with which the brain is provided, is probably the cause of their slight adherence. I can aver, that placing certain tubercles of the mesentery beside those of the brain, it was almost impossible to perceive any difference. Nor is it so wonderful, that tubercles should be formed in the brain. Scrofula produces them in all the other organs; and probably, it is only because circumstances are there less favourable to their formation, that they are more rarely found in the brain.

These observations lead us to believe, that when very obstinate pains of the head occur in scrofulous subjects, the presence of tubercles may be suspected in the brain. And they demonstrate the insufficiency of art in such circumstances. But relative to the history of scrofula, these cases are not altogether without interest, and are therefore offered to the public.*

IV.

The History of a Case of Diseased Spleen, with the Appearances on Dissection. By NATHAN DRAKE, M. D. Hadleigh, Suffolk.

GENTLEMEN,

I TRANSMIT to you the detail of a series of singular symptoms, and which appear to have arisen from as singular a cause. I consider the case, indeed, as unparallelled in the History of the Morbid Anatomy of the Spleen; at least, after much research, I have not been able to discover, in those authors who have collected the phœnomena of Morbid Anatomy, any instance of similar derangement.

 Mrs

---

* The appearances on dissection in these cases are unusual, but not unexampled. To us, they appear chiefly interesting, as marking a connection between scrofula, and hydrocephalus internus, already observed by others. For we cannot doubt that these patients died of water in the head. The first case is a well marked example of acute hydrocephalus; the tubercles, in all probability, had existed long before the attack of this fatal disorder, and were remotely connected with it.—EDITORS.

Mrs. Newman, aged 49, a widow lady of a corpulent habit, and who had been subject, for many years, to dyspeptic complaints, was, in the afternoon of the 29th of October 1805, shortly after dining heartily on roasted pig, seized with violent sickness, vomiting, and pain, in the region of the stomach, which symptoms, though somewhat mitigated by the evacuation of the contents of the stomach, returned in a few hours with augmented force, accompanied with extreme lancinating pain under the left spurious costæ.

As these distressing complaints continued with few intervals during the night, my attendance was requested on the following day. I found her labouring under frequent returns of sickness, and bringing up, with strong convulsive efforts, a great quantity of thin porraceous bile of an extremely acid odour, and agonized with so much pain in the left hypochondriac region, and more immediately under the spurious costæ, as frequently to occasion her to shriek aloud. Her pulse was 130, neither full nor hard; the tongue white, but not dry; the skin hot and harsh to the touch, and the thirst considerable. Her bowels had been rather in a constipated state for some days previous to the attack; and she had had no motion since the commencement of her present symptoms, although powerful medicines had been given, and other means resorted to for that purpose, by my friend, Mr Bunn, her family surgeon. No hardness was discoverable in the abdomen or hypochondria; the body, however, appeared rather distended and full; and the urine was high coloured, and deposited a copious lateritious sediment. No rigor or shivering had been experienced preceding, during, or since the first attack, and there was no pain or difficulty in breathing.

The irritability of the stomach being so great as to occasion the almost immediate rejection of every thing she took, whether food or medicine, an opiate plaster was applied to the pit of the stomach, effervescing draughts, with a slight opiate, were ordered every two hours, with small doses of calomel in pills, and an opening glyster was injected in the evening. A considerable portion of the draughts and pills was retained; but as no motion had taken place on the 31st, though the tendency to vomiting had abated, pills, with calomel and extractum colocynthidæ compositum, were given every two hours, the abdomen was assiduously fomented, and the enema was repeated. No evacuation having taken place in the evening, and the pain continuing violent, two table spoonfulls of a strong solution of magnesia vitriolata were ordered every hour; she went also into the warm bath, which she bore very well for 15 minutes, and had another enema injected shortly after her return to bed. As no effect, however

ever, was yet produced, and the danger was encreasing every moment, I proposed a consultation, and Dr Clubbe of Ipswich met me early on the succeeding morning. The medicines had, with few exceptions, staid upon the stomach for a considerable time after they had been taken; but the vomiting was, at intervals, excessively violent, and the peristaltic motion of the stomach and intestines appeared to be completely inverted. The pain of the left side was excruciating, and the pulse was more than 130, and feeble. Upon Dr Clubbe's arrival, we agreed to continue the magnesia vitriolata, combined with manna and calcined magnesia, and, with a view to ascertain the state of the circulating fluids, to take four or six ounces of blood from the arm; this, on standing a due time, exhibited a thin, concave, buffy surface; but as the crassamentum was dark, and remarkably loose and broken, and the pulse very weak, we thought it dangerous to push this evacuation any further. The enemata were repeated, the fomentations continued for some hours, and afterwards a blister applied to the whole abdomen. At length, on the evening of the 1st November, after a very large quantity of purgative medicines had been given, a small motion took place, which, in the course of the next 24 hours, was succeeded by 15 more, and a prodigious quantity of black, knotty, and hardened fæces, but with little fœtor, was evacuated. The relief obtained was great; the pain was removed; the irritation of the stomach subsided; and the pulse sank to 80.

We had now great reason to hope, that the seemingly apparent cause being removed, our patient would do well; but in this respect we were unhappily disappointed; the pulse, on the following day, again rose to 100, and though the vomiting at present but rarely returned, an unconquerable degree of acidity existed in the stomach. The pain of the left side was now little felt, whilst the patient was laid upon her back; but there was an inability of lying upon that side, even for five minutes, without an insupportable sensation of weight and dragging. Tonics, bitters, and antacids, both in diet and medicine, were prescribed, and the bowels were kept in a laxative state by calomel and a solution of magnesia vitriolata.

On November the 10th, Dr Clubbe again met me; the vomiting and pain had returned violently, and the pulse was 110; another opiate plaster was applied to the pit of the stomach and a draught, with five grains of ammonia, and three drops of tinctura opii, was taken every four hours; no benefit, however, being derived from this plan, brisk purgatives were ordered the following day, and as soon as the bowels were completely evacuated the symptoms subsided.

It is worthy of remark, that during the whole course of this disease, which was of six months duration, nothing afforded so much relief as purgatives. I was under the necessity of exhibiting them every third or fourth day, for, when longer delayed, distention, flatulence, sickness, vomiting, and extreme pain invariably recurred, and were as certainly removed for a time by their use. The fæces were, in general, natural in their colour, and had always their due portion of bile; they were neither fetid nor acrimonious, and the urine was, during the greater part of the disorder, nearly of an healthy appearance. A torpor of the intestinal canal, however seemed to exist, and no advantage was derived from the constant use of *laxatives*, the intervention of brisk purgatives being essential to relief.

From the 10th of November to the 23d, the symptoms were nearly stationary; the pulse was about 96 in the morning, and 108 in the evening; but no rigor or chill, or regular paroxysm had been experienced: the tongue was foul, the breath fetid, and extremely sour; little pain was felt, except when lying on the left side; she slept tolerably well, but the appetite was greatly impaired, and emaciation proceeded rapidly. Every possible means of removing irritation, and correcting acidity were employed; lime water, the alkaline mephitic water, and the decoctum cornu cervi were alternately used for common drink, and the testacea, alkalies, &c. &c. combined with various bitters, and tonics, vegetable and mineral, were tried in vain; purgatives were the only things that afforded any assistance.

Another consultation was requested on the 23d, and we agreed to try the effect of a diet of asses milk. On again examining the abdomen, though the patient was greatly reduced in bulk, no tension, tumour, or schirrosity of any viscus could be discovered, no symptom of any absorption of bile had occurred; there was no discolouration of the skin, no uneasiness on the right side, nor was the liver felt below the margin of the thorax, neither had there been the smallest indication of suppuration or hectic fever.

Better than a pint of asses milk was taken daily for four days, which, at first, sat well upon the stomach; the pulse dropped to 88, and the strength seemed to encrease; but, at the conclusion of the above period, it turned completely acid shortly after being drank, and it was therefore relinquished for a small quantity of solid animal food for dinner, and a strong decoction of sarsaparilla, with lime water, was ordered every four hours.

This slight appearance of amendment was speedily followed by an increase of the pulse, which rose to 120; and, on December the 6th, the vomiting returned almost incessantly, with great pain at the scorbiculus cordis, and in the left side. The effervescing

vescing draughts were repeated, and blisters were applied to the region of the stomach, and to the side, and the bowels were opened by magnesia vitriolata. The symptoms were, as usual, mitigated by this plan, and the vitriolic acid, and afterwards the nitric was liberally ordered, with a view, from their tonic action, of promoting digestion, and therefore of palliating acidity, but without effect.

The pulse continued to fluctuate between 96 and 120, until December the 16th, when a return of excruciating pain, under the left spurious costæ, occasioned the pulse to mount to 136. The pain extended to the scorbiculus cordis and umbilical region, and gave rise to a spasmodic affection of the diaphragm. Doses of magnesia vitriolata were given every three hours, and a strong volatile opiate liniment was rubbed into the side. The pain was relieved in about an hour, and the symptoms subsided within their usual range soon after motions had been obtained.

As nothing, however, which had hitherto been given, had produced any permanent good effect, I proposed to Dr Clubbe, on December 21st, the introduction of mercury into the system by friction; to this he readily assented, but as the family expressed a wish for further advice, and Dr Maclean of Sudbury, was mentioned, we postponed the trial until Dr Maclean's arrival, which was fixed for the 23d.

After a retrospection of the series of symptoms, and of the medicines and means which had been employed, Dr Maclean united with us in thinking, that, with the exception of mercurial friction, every thing had been done, which was likely to afford relief; he therefore urged the immediate adoption of the mercurial plan, and half a drachm of the strong ointment was ordered to be rubbed into the interior part of the leg and thigh, night and morning; pills composed of aloes, myrrh, vitriolated kali, and calomel, were directed to be taken occasionally, and a volatile opiate liniment to be applied to the left side, which was still painful, and accompanied with a sense of soreness under the spurious costæ, when pressed with the hand.

With regard to the seat of the disease, we differed considerably, whether the orginal cause of derangement had occurred in the stomach, colon, liver, omentum, or spleen, was canvassed at great length; Dr Maclean was inclined to consider it as a liver case, and that the left lobe was the seat of the disease; in this supposition, however, we entirely differed from him; but such had been the peculiarity and intricacy of the symptoms, that an absolute decision was not not only difficult but presumptuous. As we perfectly agreed, however, in the means to be adopted, the pathology was rendered of little consequence, and I shall therefore proceed

ceed to enumerate what was the precise state of our patient's symptoms at this period of her complaint.

The emaciation had gone on rapidly, and Mrs Newman, who, as remarked before, had originally been very corpulent, was now extremely thin and reduced; she was confined to her bed, and only able to sit up in it for a few minutes to take nourishment, which, in very small quantities, she kept down without much uneasiness. The pulse was about 100 in the morning, and 110 in the evening, weak, and its frequency apparently the consequence of mere irritation; for no rigor, chill, colliquative perspiration or diarrhoea, no one symptom, indeed, of hectic fever or suppuration, had supervened. A vomiting of porraceous bile recurred every second or third day; the stools, when procured by purgatives, for without assistance no evacution ever took place, were of a dark appearance; the urine was somewhat high coloured; the skin, as had been the case throughout the whole disease, was dry and harsh; the tongue foul, the breath fetid, much flatulence, and the acidity in the primæviæ great. Upon strict examination no tumour was discoverable in the abdomen, though Dr Maclean thought a little hardness was perceptible to the finger on the left side. The pain of that side frequently extended to the epigastric and umbilical regions; a total inability still existed of lying on it, and sleep was broken and disturbed, but except when the pain was excruciating, the breathing was calm and easy.

In about twelve days a very gentle ptyalism was produced, which continued for a week, and than gradually subsided. The pulse during the action of the mercury was accelerated, but no other effect was induced; the pain, and the necessity for purgatives every second or third day, continuing as usual, and on the total cessation of the mercurial agency, the symptoms were, with the exception of increased debility, exactly what they had been previous to the application of the ointment.

On January 10th 1806, I proposed to Dr Clubbe a trial of the cicuta, which, in the form of a saturated tincture, was taken, for some time, in a strong decoction of bark and sarsaparillá, but without any good effect.

On the 13th of this month a violent pain seized the left ancle, which was shortly transferred to the left knee, and in a few hours the leg and thigh of that side began to swell, and, in 24 hours, were more than double the size of the other limb; the pain, and the frequency of the pulse, which had risen to 140, somewhat abated on the increase of the swelling, which appeared to be the consequence of lymphatic effusion. There was no inflammation on the surface, but the lymphatics on the interior of the thigh were hard and enlarged. I immediately opened the bowels by an active

purgative,

purgative, after which an opiate was given; stimulating fomentations were assiduously applied to the swelled parts, and, on their removal, a volatile opiate liniment was used.

During the violence of this attack, little or no pain was felt in the side or stomach, but on the 16th, the sickness vomiting, and pain under the spurious costæ returned in an aggravated form, these were mitigated by a blister, and the effervescing draughts; and the lymphatic swelling, by the daily use of the fomentations and volatile liniment, began gradually to diminish. Bitters, and tonics, and steel, combined with the effervescing materials, were taken frequently.

On the 28th of January, the pain, which had for some days been greatly mitigated in the side, was felt acutely between the cartilago ensiformis and umbilicus; a blister was immediately applied to the part, and an opiate given in her usual tonic draught. In the morning of the 29th she was perfectly easy, and Dr Clubbe meeting me that day, we advised an issue to be opened on the inside of the left knee, with a view to accelerate the diminution of the effused fluid.

In the month of February, the symptoms preserved nearly their usual routine; the pain of the side occasionally, but not permanently, severe; the sickness, distension and vomiting certainly returning with violence, if the purgative was deferred beyond the third day; emaciation and debility encreasing, yet no tumour or hardness discernible in the abdomen; stools and urine of their natural colour; no hectic symptoms, tongue cleaner, acidity in the stomach great, but the breath not so fetid; has lived for a considerable length of time on beef-tea, gruel, jellies &c. taken frequently in very small quantities; sleeps at night for some hours, but the total inability of lying on the left side continues; the swelling of the left limb has nearly subsided, though it had at one time, however, extended over the left hypochondriac region, and was removed by fomentations and volatile liniment; the skin clear and free from any morbid tint; and has taken, during this month, various preparations of bark, bitters and antacids.

About the middle of March, in consequence of taking a very strong decoction of cinchona and quassia with vitriolic acid, the appetite and strength seemed to increase, and the pain of the side had not been felt for several days. She was able to lie upon her couch for eight hours, and at length, after a week's apparent amendment, to sit an hour in the erect posture, with a pulse reduced to 90.—These flattering symptoms, however, soon vanished; the sickness, vomiting and pain returned with as much violence as ever, and the pulse rose to 130; a purgative, as heretofore, mitigated the symptoms, but, from this period, no hope, even of temporary a-

mendment

mendment could be expected. With a view, however, of ascertaining what effect a purulent discharge from the left side might produce, a seton was introduced immediately under the spurious costæ; it produced, however, excessive irritation, and though endured with great patience, until some evacuation had been effected, no relief was obtained, and it was therefore withdrawn.

The debility, languor, and emaciation, were, at the commencement of April, very great, and cordials, both in diet and medicine, were frequently necessary. The pulse was about 116 in the morning, at night 120 or 125, and sometimes 130, and very feeble.

About the 7th or 8th of this month, Mrs Newman suddenly complained of a swelling at her stomach, accompanied with a sense of great fulness and distension, and, on examination a day or two after, I found a considerable tumour, reaching from the cartilago ensiformis to the umbilicus; it was perfectly circular, prominent, and well defined, and there was a distinct fluctuation. I ordered poultices to be applied every two hours to the part, and requested a consultation, as I deemed an operation essentially necessary as soon as it could be performed with safety. Dr Clubbe met me on the following day, but the tumour had then subsided to half its former bulk, and though a fluctuation was still very evident, we thought it proper to postpone the introduction of the trocar until the swelling should again acquire its former bulk,— The poultices were continued, and on the 17th, when we met again, the tumour had risen even beyond its former dimensions, and the fluctuation was perfectly evident. Its bulk and pressure so affected the stomach, that not a tea-spoonful of any thing could now be retained, even for a minute, and as the anxiety and oppression were rapidly proceeding, the evacuation of the contained fluid was the only means in our power of diminishing suffering, and protracting life. Having obtained, therefore, the consent of the patient, who had resolution adequate to the endurance of any thing which might be deemed necessary for her relief, Mr Bunn, her surgeon, introduced a trocar into the most depending part of the tumour, and drew off two pints of a fluid, resembling in colour thin diluted coffee; it was perfectly free from fœtor, and slightly saline to the palate; when diluted with water it had the appearance of pale Lisbon wine; and when boiled, exhibited a portion of coagulable lymph; it seemed indeed, in every respect, to be merely the serum of the blood, which, by long separation from the fibrine, had acquired its present appearance.

Mrs Newman bore the operation extremely well; and, without any increase of faintness or languor, she was able, almost immediately after the fluid had been withdrawn, to retain the usual quantity

quantity of food upon her stomach, and she passed the evening nearly free from pain, and had some sleep. On the morning of the succeeding day, however, there were present symptoms of much exhaustion; the pulse was very feeble and quick, and the countenance assumed a cadaverous aspect; the breathing also was very short, and sometimes laborious, yet she felt no pain, though it became very evident, that death was approaching with rapid strides. This event, indeed, took place early on the morning of the 19th, without the smallest struggle or appearance of pain.

As soon as I was informed of Mrs Newman's decease, which was about nine o'clock in the morning of the 19th, I thought it necessary, for the satisfaction of all parties, to lose no time in obtaining the consent of the family, that the body might be opened; the request was immediately granted, and Mr Bunn and myself, together with Mr Mudd, an intelligent medical gentleman of this place, began the dissection at twelve, and after minutely examining the different viscera, for nearly four hours, I drew up, on the spot, the following statement of the morbid phænomena.

Appearances on Dissection.

1. The coats of the stomach were nearly three times thicker than usual; its cavity reduced to about one third of the customary size, the rugæ very distinct; the cardia and pylorus in a sound state; but a little above the sphincter pylori there was a quantity, nearly an ounce, of cheese-like matter in a granulated form, adhering to the external coat of the stomach, but not constricting the passage into the duodenum; there were no traces of inflammation either on the inner or outer coat of the stomach.

2. The omentum was greatly enlarged, and entirely covered with cheese-like matter in a granulated state; considerable portions of its substance were thickened to a full inch in depth, and were altogether formed of the same caseous material, which might be rubbed between the fingers into a paste, but somewhat gritty to the touch. The omentum was depressed far below its usual situation, and strongly and extensively adhered to the peritonæum and intestines.

3. The spleen was one mass of disease; half of its proper bulk appeared to be absorbed or wasted, and the organization of the remaining part completely obliterated, and in a state approaching toward solution; the peritonæal coat of its internal concave surface, was dilated into a very large cyst, with blood vessels of an enormous size, ramifying on its inferior part, or fundus. The upper

upper part of the cyst strongly adhered to the whole under surface of the stomach, and the lower part to the upper edge of the great arch of the colon. The diameter of the cyst was full six inches, and it contained more than a pound and a half of dark, dense, coagulated blood, several portions of which, nearly as large as a man's fist, floated in a brown coloured serum, of which there was better than a pint. We have already related that two pints of a similar fluid had been drawn off, previous to death, and the capacity of the cyst, was such as to admit of considerably more than four pints. The bottom and sides of this bag were covered about an inch deep, with a black tenacious matter of the consistence of congealed honey, and when examined with the fingers, was found interspersed with masses of the same caseous substance, which covered the omentum. The great size of the cyst pressed the stomach high up, and close to the diaphragm, and the arch of the colon was, from the same cause, thrust down many inches below its natural situation, and was contracted in that part of its course to the size of a small intestine. There was no communication from this cyst with the liver, stomach, or intestines, and there was no fœtor, and no pus in any of the diseased viscera.

4. The liver was pressed high up by the bulk of the cyst, its lower edge being considerably within the margin of the thorax. It was perfectly sound and healthy in all its lobes, not a mark of disease appearing, either externally or internally. It was rather smaller than usual in size, and the left lobe could not be said to pass into any part of the left hypochondriac region, owing probably to the magnitude of the cyst. The lobulus spigelii was also in the most perfect state, and the gall bladder was distended with bile, and of its proper colour.

5. The intestines, with the exception of the arch of the colon, were nearly free from disease, but compressed into a very small compass, and adhering to the omentum. The blood vessels upon the arch of the colon were turgid, and part of the mesocolon was as much diseased as the omentum, being thickly interspersed with cheese-like matter in a granulated form. The arch of the colon was so reduced in bulk, and compressed, that when the body was opened, it projected like a chain of very small bladders.

6. The kidneys, uterus, and bladder, were in a sound state.

7. The thoracic viscera were also perfectly sound.

Case

V.

Case of successful Amputation of the Uterus. By Joseph Clarke, M. D.—Dublin.

In the month of June, 1803, I was consulted by a very young lady, who had been about eleven months delivered of her first child, and whose health had since been in a most precarious state.

The history that she gave me, was, that she had been attended in her lying-in by a midwife, who boasted of having received her instruction in the Lying-in Hospital. Soon after delivery, she was affected with severe pains, and excessive floodding. While she was fainting, and supposed to be in great danger, her obliging attendant ran to the house of a neighbouring physician, who prescribed something which afforded temporary relief. By wearing bandages to support what was supposed to be a falling down of the womb, and by taking strengthening medicines, this lady became tolerably well, insomuch, that she was once able to walk to a neighbouring market to buy dinner for her family; and, on reflection, she thinks this the only occasion, during eleven months subsequent to her delivery, on which she could say she was well.

Soon after this event, she went from Dublin to a distant part of the country, and became subject to very profuse uterine hemorrhage, for which she took the opinions of many medical men, and swallowed drugs in large quantities, with very little effect. Some of her medical attendants in the country told her the womb was inverted, but made no examination to ascertain the fact.

Under these circumstances, I did not hesitate to propose an examination by the touch, to which, in her reduced and bloodless state, she made not the slightest opposition. I found a round fleshy tumour, hanging low in her vagina, about an inch and half, or two inches from the os externum. On the anterior part of this tumour, I thought I could perceive the os tincæ in a dilated state; but on the posterior part nothing like it could be distinguished.

Not doubting that this tumour was the cause of her distress, I desired to have a consultation with a surgeon of eminence next day, adding, that I rather suspected the tumour to be of the polypous kind. Having stated the circumstances as they occured and appeared to me, the surgeon, after examination, thought my conjecture about the nature of the disease most probable. Some decisive effort was necessary to rescue the patient from impending destruction. We agreed to pass a ligature on the tumour, in the usual manner, as in cases of polypus. During

ing the first, and indeed many succeeding nights and days, it gave great pain, occasioned severe vomitings, and much watchfulness. We gave opium freely, and kept the bowels open with glysters. The patient was very heroic, and determined, if possible, to get rid of what had so often reduced her existence to the lowest ebb. After tightening the ligature frequently, as far as we judged prudent, at the end of a fortnight we took it off, in despair of success by this mode of proceeding; still, however, giving her reason to hope, that after so much pressure, it might fall by an effort of nature.

When released from pain and sleepless nights, her health mended rapidly; the extensive uterine hœmorrhages ceased; she bathed in the open sea, and considered herself getting quite well, when, in consequence of some extraordinary effort, a tumour shot suddenly out at the os externum, of considerable size. She returned to town, and it was now manifest the tumour we had inclosed in ligature was the uterus, then partially, and now completely, inverted. On a further consideration of all the circumstance, and encouraged by the event of a case recorded in the Edinburgh Medical Annals for the year 1799, by Mr Hunter of Dumbarton, we agreed on the propriety of amputating the prolapsed tumour.

Before proceeding to a step so unusual, we deemed it prudent to submit our opinion to the consideration of two of our professional brethren. Their opinion coincided with ours; and, on the 18th day of November, a ligature of small tape was tied tightly, almost an inch above where our former ligature had made its indentation, and, with a scalpel, the tumour was removed before the patient had an idea that the operation was begun. Her recovery was rapid and complete. In six weeks she was able to walk nearly as well as ever; these were her own words. Her husband died soon after her recovery, so that I have had no means of ascertaining any circumstances relative to their subsequent cohabitation. After three years absence from town, she called on me in the end of March of this year, is grown fat, and altered so much in her appearance, that at first I did not recognize her. She complained only of bad appetite, and that she had never *changed since*, which I assured her, was no uncommon occurrence after such operations, and I begged of her not to be anxious on that score, so long as her health was reasonably good.

This case seems to me, to justify several important conclusions.

It proves, that the partially inverted uterus will sometimes bear considerable pressure from ligature, without producing fatal effects.

It

It affords strong probable evidence, that such pressure is capable of restraining those violent and wasting discharges of blood which have hitherto, in general, proved, sooner or later, fatal in inversions of the womb.

It tends to confirm the propriety of Mr Hunter's bold practice, who, unaided by consultation, and without encouragement from modern authors, ventured successfully to deprive the female constitution of one of its most important organs.

And, lastly, It suggests, *most forcibly*, the necessity of examining accurately the state of the os tincæ, whenever excessive hemorrhage and pain supervene speedily to the expulsion of the secundines.

Inversions of the uterus, and especially if partial, when speedily discovered, are generally reducible. I have myself seen, in consultation, one case of this kind; and practical writers contain many such. Keeping this melancholy example steadily in view, may all practitioners, in future, make enquiry precede prescription.

I offer neither excuse nor apology for my erroneous first judgment in this case. On the contrary, I trust it will increase my claim to the gratitude of the liberal reader. The patient would probably not have submitted with so much fortitude, nor should we perhaps have applied so much pressure, had we been certain of the nature of the tumour. The surgeon who regulated the ligature, is, in my opinion, entitled to much credit, for having proportioned so well his efforts to the patient's strength. To this hour, I believe, our patient thinks she was only deprived of a polypus, and it would be an act of very wanton cruelty to undeceive her.

Conceiving the circumstances of this case to be important and instructive, I thought it a duty to endeavour to prevent them being lost to the medical world.

Rutland Square,
DUBLIN, 27th June, 1806. }

To Dr Clarke's case, the following extract from Voigtel's instructive Manual of Pathological Anatomy, forms an important addition.

" Examples of the extirpation of the uterus, either from ignorance or as a surgical remedy are not rare. Many of these terminated unfortunately (*a*), but many succeeded. Thus Wolf (*b*) amputated

(*a*.) *Peyer*, Misc. Nat. Cur. Dec. ii. An. i. Obs. lxxxiv. p. 198. *Bartholini*, Hist. anat. rar. Cent. ii. Obs. xci. Tom i. p. 334. Journal für Geburtshelfer, 1787. St. I.

amputated a prolapsed uterus with the happiest consequences. Volkamer (*c*) relates a similar example. Figuet (*d*) tells of an ignorant accoucheur, who mistook an inverted uterus for the child's head, and tore it quite away with the crotchet. Faivre (*e*) put a ligature around a prolapsed and inflamed uterus, which could not be reduced, and was almost gangrenous; on the 27th day it separated, and the woman recovered speedily. Wrisberg (*f*) relates an example, in which, an ignorant midwife, after a natural birth, cut away the uterus, which she had drawn out, yet the woman survived. Laumonier (*g*) describes the successful amputation of an inverted uterus, which was mistaken for a polypus. Hunter (*h*) cut entirely away an inverted uterus, and the patient was cured in a month, without any bad symptom. Several other examples of excision of the uterus, without proving fatal, may be read in Schenkius (*i*), Rousset (*k*), Moinichen (*l*), Slevogt (*m*), Dietrich (*n*), Zwinger (*o*), and Cavallini (*p*).

VI.

Case of Chorea St Viti cured by Purgatives. Communicated by GEORGE KELLIE, M. D.

THE account given of this curious disease by Dr Hamilton, has exposed its pathology in a new point of view, and laid the foundation

---

(*b*.) Miscell. Nat. Cur. Dec. ii. An. ix. Obs. xciv. p. 161.
(*c*.) Ibid. Dec. i. An. vi. Obs. lxxiii.
(*d*.) Journal de Medecine, Tom. xli. Janvr, p. 40.
(*e*.) Ibid. Tom lxviii. August. p. 195.
(*f*.) Commentatio de uteri mox post partum naturalem resectione non lethali. Gott. 1787.
(*g*.) In Fourcroy Medec. eclairée. Paris, 1792. Tom iv.
(*h*.) Duncan's Annals of Medicine for 1799.
(*i*.) Lib. iv. Obs. ccciii. sq. p. 711.
(*k*.) Hysterotomotocia Basil, 1688, p. 100.
(*l*.) Obs. Med. Chirur. cum Annot. Lanzoni Dresd, 1691. Obs. iv. p. 17.
(*m*.) Diss. de utero per sarcoma ex corpore extracto, postmodum resectò. Jenae, 1700.
(*n*.) Rede von einem wahren Vorfalle und glücklicher Absetzung der Gebährmutter. Regensb. 1745.
(*o*.) Neue Sammlung für Wundärzte, St. iii. p. 218.
(*p*.) De felici in quibusdam animantibus uteri extractione, Flor. 1768.

foundation of a more rational and more successful practice, than that generally pursued by physicians. The evidence brought forward by Dr Hamilton, in support of the utility of purgative medicines in chorea, is so complete and satisfactory, that I should have deemed it quite unnecessary to record any observation of my own, or case in favour of the practice, which might have occurred since the publication of his valuable book. A higher authority, however, and stronger testimony, because much less suspicious, in favour of any new method of treating a disease, is that which may sometimes be deduced from the history of cases related by preceding writers, who, unbiassed by any relative view, have deviated as it were accidently from the usual routine, and stumbled on that method, which experience afterwards establishes as a rule of practice. This is a kind of evidence, which Dr Hamilton has not rejected, which he has very properly produced when it could be found; and in this disease, he has even endeavoured to extort it from the practice of Sydenham. I cannot therefore refrain from offering to the Edinburgh Medical and Surgical Journal, the following very interesting illustration, which I have met with in a clinical work not much known in this country, the Ratio Medendi of Maximillian Stoll, the successor, I believe, of the better known De Haen.

" A young man of 16, was on the 23d May 1779, affected with sickness and giddiness of the head; being in other respects well enough. On the following days, the head was still more affected, and he complained besides of heat, and a sense of opression about the præcordia, distention of the hypochondria, subacid eructations, nausea, retching, feverishness, a kind of rheumatic pain, with a sense of prickling of the left arm, immediately followed by startings and momentary convulsions of that extremity. His nights were disturbed.

26th May. The gesticulations and motions of the left arm more and more irregular, and less obedient to the will. The other symptoms as before.

27th — Became irrascible. The left leg also affected, and its motions irregular. The other symptoms worse.

28th — The tongue covered with small pustules. The mouth drawn somewhat to the left side.

30th — A few pustules have also appeared on the face: All the former symptoms aggravated. He was blooded both on this and the following days, without experiencing any relief. Nights very restless.

" With these symptoms, he was received into the hospital on the 1st June.—The tongue was white; and the belly was, as it had been all along, very costive. Some opening saline medicines being premised, he had an emetic—what he vomited was bitter. The fever and uneasiness of the præcordia disappeared, and the limbs became steadier. Purgative medicines were afterwards given; and thus by the 7th of June, he was so far cured, that he complained of nothing but the rheumatic pain of the left shoulder and arm. A blister was applied between the shoulders, and a diaphoratic draught was administered. But on the following day, without any obvious cause, he began to weep, and talk very foolishly, and every limb, the trunk of the body, the head even, and the muscles of the face, were affected with inordinate gesticulations. The disease advanced under

under the use of the fetid gums, and became still worse after the administration of camphor. Now the mouth was clammy and foul, and the teeth covered with sordes.

"At length the symptoms were relieved by saline laxatives, but the disease was not cured.

"The extract of belladona was tried, but occasioning vertigo, headach, and delirium, it was omitted, and then it was thought best to purge the bowels with rhubarb, neutral salts, and the oxymel of squills. He passed slime, and one lumbricus, and he said that he had formerly discharged others. The belly was moderately but daily purged; and thus his tongue became clean, his limbs strong, and the other symptoms disappeared, so that by the end of the month, he returned home cured."

"Another case of Chorea S. Viti I have treated in the same way. The patient was a girl subject to rheumatism, which being neglected, terminated spontaneously in chorea; she was cured by solvents, eccoprotics, rhubarb, arcanum duplicatum, (sulphate of potass) and oxymel scillicum—Stimulants, belladona, the flowers of zinc, and electricity, have appeared hurtful in that species of chorea, which arises from pituita, and worms of the intestinal canal."

M. Stoll—Ration. Medendi, pars 3tia. page 219.
Observat. vii. *and* viii.—*Edit. Paris* 1787.

No examples can be more decisive than these cases, and none surely could more happily illustrate the pathology and treatment of chorea recommended by Dr Hamilton. For first, we remark, as precursors of the disease, symptoms of disordered and loaded bowels, heat or oppression of the præcordia, acid eructations, nausea and vomiting, and costiveness; next, the inefficacy of antispasmodic and stimulant remedies; then relief from laxatives, and disorder from narcotics; and lastly, the speedy completion of the cure, on the administration of medicines evacuating the bowels moderately, but daily.

Leith, 10th July 1806.

VI.

Letter on the Application of Galvanism, in the Cure of Congenital Deafness. By ALEXANDER VOLTA, Professor of Natural Philosophy in the University of Pavia.*

I FORMERLY wrote to you, that the many cases related of deaf and dumb persons, who have received their hearing, by means of

---

* See Annali di Chimica e Storia Naturale, di L. Brugnatelli. Tom xxi, p. 200, 8vo. Pavia, 1802.

of the Galvanic pile, especially at Tevers, in Westphalia, with the ingenious apparatus, contrived and employed by Mr Sprenger, were more than sufficient to convince the most incredulous, that its use is by no means to be neglected, but merits, at least, to be tried by others.

This I myself accordingly resolved to do, although my doubts exceeded my hopes, and, for the last 15 days, I have been employing Sprenger's method, in our Orphan Hospital, with a girl of 15 years of age, who was born deaf. I cannot say that hitherto I have been very successful; but it is not to be denied, that she has so far acquired the sense of hearing, as to perceive various sounds, even though not very loud, and at the distance of some feet. It was observable, that she began to hear on the commencement of the third day, that is, after it had been applied eight or nine times to each ear, for ten minutes at a time, in shocks repeated every second. On the succeeding days, some slight progress has been observed. It is curious, that obtuse and hollow sounds, such as beating on an empty wooden box, or clapping the hands, were those she first perceived; a fact also noticed in the experiments made at Tevers; but for some days past, she also hears other sounds, such as various instruments of music, the ringing of a bell, the human voice, but apparently very obscurely, confounding often one sound with another. I shall continue for 15 days more to galvanize each ear at least four times a day, in the same manner; that is, by applying a small button at the end of a metallic wire, connected with the positive extremity of the apparatus, alternately for a minute, to the tragus, for two, to the meatus externus, and for another minute behind the internal ear to the mastoid process, and giving frequent shocks, by touching every second the negative extremity with a metallic rod, held in the moistened left hand, when the right ear is galvanized, and vice versa. The experiment will thus last a month, the longest time employed by Sprenger in the worst cases of deafness; but I have great doubts of succeeding as well, for it has been repeatedly published, that more than 40 cases have been cured by him, besides various other cases by other practitioners. I am doubtful that my patient will be enabled to discriminate articulate sounds. She has certainly gained something, as she did not perceive the strongest sounds with either ear, and she now hears moderate sounds, particularly with the right; but she is still far from that delicacy of hearing, which is necessary for hearing the human voice little raised, and to distinguish the articulation of words sufficiently for learning the art of speech. But even if it were possible to attain that fineness and perfection of hearing, we know

not

not how long it would last, since we are told in the history of the prodigious cures performed in Germany, that several of them, though not all, have, after a time, relapsed into their original deafness; and of the others, we know not if many, or few or any of them, have learned to speak, since we have had no account of them posterior to the month of June, when a sufficient time had not elapsed after their cure. I am told, that for some time past, they have been making experiments at the deaf and dumb institution at Paris, but I know not in what manner, or with what success. In Germany, where the experiments have been made in so many places, and by so many individuals, and where there have been published so many cases, and so many valuable works, on the application of Galvanism, they boast of many other cures of weakness of sight, even of amaurosis, of paralyzed limbs, &c. and it is curious, that some have acquired the sense of smelling, which they previously wanted entirely, by merely galvanizing the ears in the manner described. But this is not wonderful, since almost all the internal parts of the head feel these shocks, and are penetrated by the galvanic current, and even many of the external parts, as is evident from the contractions of the temporal and zygomatic muscles on each shock.

VII.

Explanation of a supposed Case of Small Pox, after Vaccination. By HENRY JOHNSTON, Fellow of the Royal College of Surgeons, Edinburgh.

AT a time when the progress of vaccine inoculation is threatened with some interruption and disrepute, particularly about the Metropolis, the following statement may perhaps not be unacceptable. It appears to me useful in this respect, that it points out the great propriety of medical men using every endeavour in tracing the history of those cases where it is alledged that vaccination has not proved a preventive of small pox.

Some time ago I inoculated the child of a gentleman in this city, with vaccine matter. The infection took place, and went through the usual course. From the pustule I inoculated the infant of the hired nurse who suckled the child. This also succeeded

ceeded, but as it lived at two or three miles distance from Edinburgh, I had not an opportunity of seeing it through the whole progress of the affection; however, I was so satisfied with the appearance about the 8th day, that I desired the child might not be brought back again, as it was very inconvenient the doing so. Some months after, I was sent for by the gentleman whose child had been first inoculated, and found the family in a state of great anxiety, in consequence of having learnt, that the nurse's child had been seized with small pox, as well as three other children in the same house, all of whom were said to have had the cow pox. I was requested by the gentleman to visit them, which I readily did, not doubting to find an instance of chicken pox; I found, however, all the children severely suffering under the real small pox, in different stages of this loathsome disease, except the infant which I had vaccinated, which had very few pustules, *and had not been perceptibly sick.* The mother of the other children stated positively, that they all had had the cow pox. As I was about leaving the house, a good deal perplexed and mortified, I accidently inquired who had inoculated the children. This led to a most satisfactory explanation; they never had been inoculated, but according to the mother, had all taken the infection from wearing some article of apparel, belonging to another child under vaccine inoculation. This you know is considered as hardly possible. I now examined more particularly the child whom I had inoculated, and found, that the few pustules upon it were confined chiefly to one side of its face, neck, and one arm, and appeared to me to be quite analogous to the local pustules which take place on the breasts and arms of nurses, when suckling children in small pox; the child having slept constantly in the same bed, and, I dare say, in contact with one of the others. I am persuaded, that if every case of alleged failure of cow pox, as a safeguard against small pox, were traced with care, similar errors to the above would be detected. I assure you the above instance made a considerable noise and clamour in the place where it happened, and I am not sure, that my endeavours to represent the matter in its proper light, and to shew, that the whole circumstances were in favour of vaccination, were successful.

Before concluding, I would leg leave to observe, that the practice of vaccine inoculation, is beginning to be held by far too light; any body is supposed capable of performing an operation so trifling. Every surgeon knows how frequently he produces an inflammation of several days standing with a pustular appearance, without supposing he gives constitutional infection, and security against small pox. I fear such a simple affection of the arm, is too often considered as the real and necessary infection.

I am led to make this observation, from finding my own apprentices, when of very short standing indeed, frequently trying their skill in this way.

PRINCE'S STREET,
24th July, 1806.

VIII.

Case of Epilepsy cured by Trepanning. By HENRY COATES, of the Royal College of Surgeons in London, and Surgeon to the Salisbury Infirmary.

JAMES GODDARD, ætat. 33. a gentleman's coachman, was admitted a patient into the Salisbury Infirmary, July 28th 1804. He stated, that about four years before, as he was driving his master's carriage under a gateway, (not stooping sufficiently), the crown of his head struck against a beam; this at the time was not followed by any other symptoms, than a slight headach for a few days, and an inconsiderable swelling of the part, which soon subsided. Nothing occured to remind him of the accident, till, about a year afterwards, when a small tumour appeared on the part on which he received the bruise, which (to use his own language), continued to swell without much pain, and at last burst. The wound was afterwards dilated by a surgeon, and healed with difficulty in about six months, and he says, that he continued perfectly well for about six months afterwards, when he was attacked with an epileptic fit while on the coach box; and has since had repeated attacks of them at intervals of from a week to a month. He now complains of extreme pain in his head, loss of vision of his left eye, numbness and coldness of the left side, particularly of the foot; his general health and appetite are otherwise tolerably good. On examining the scalp, I perceived several small puffy ulcerations about the centre of the coronal suture, which, on pressure, give him pain. He was directed to take some opening medicine.

July 29th, The appearance of the scalp indicating some further disease, I determined to ascertain the state of the bone, for which purpose I made an incision of about 3 inches in length in an oblique direction, beginning an inch in front of the sagittal suture and running backwards. The bone at the anterior part of the incision was found roughened, and a portion of it about the size

size of a shilling, porous, with a sinus in the centre, which readily admitted a probe being passed to the dura mater.

My friend Dr Fowler being desirous of seeing the state of the case, and not being able to attend at this time, I deferred attempting any thing further for the present, and the wound was slightly dressed. I saw the patient again in the evening, when he informed me he thought he felt rather less pain in his head, which I attributed to the loss of blood in the operation.

July 30th.—The wound looked very well, and was dressed as before.

July 31st, The wound appeared perfectly healthy, he was free from pain or fever, but said he felt as if he should have a fit before the end of the day. I now determined to remove the diseased portion of the bone, and applied a trephine, the crown of which was sufficiently large to include the whole of it. The operation was tedious from the extreme delicacy of the part, and care required in the use of the instrument. It was, however, completed without accident, and on extracting the bone, its internal surface had an honeycomb appearance. The dura mater was detached, but perfectly healthy. The skin was brought into contact in the manner recommended by Mr Minors, and retained by adhesive plaster, with light superficial dressings. He was put to bed, and an opiate draught was ordered.

I saw him again in the evening, and found him remarkably well, he thought he could see better with his left eye, had scarcely any head-ach, his pulse but little quickened, and his foot much warmer, with more sense of feeling in it.

August 1st. He had passed a very good night, felt quite comfortable and free from pain. I ordered some opening medicines, and to be kept on low diet.

August 2d—Examined the wound, found it very healthy, union by the first intention had in part taken place, and there was but little discharge. It was dressed as before. Nothing occurred worth notice the remaining part of the time he was in the house, and he was discharged the 1st of September, cured.

It is now 18 months since the operation was performed, and I have seen him several times lately; he continues well, and follows his usual occupation; he has had no return whatever of the fits. The numbness and coldness of his left side is quite removed. The vision of his left eye is better, though not quite recovered.

IX.

Cases of Idiopathic Tetanus, with Observations. By C. L. Mursinna, Chief Surgeon to the Charité of Berlin.*

A Soldier of the regiment of Mollendorff, aged 26, of a stout habit of body, the day before his return to the regiment, from a furlough, overheated himself very much while exposed to the burning rays of the sun, by violent exertion at rough field work; in the evening, when dropping with sweat, he exposed himself to a current of cold air, in order to refresh himself, and drunk cold beer to allay his great thirst. After he had spent an hour in this way, he suddenly felt great bodily weakness, and an inability to open his mouth.

He was put into a warm bed, and took some warm beer with ginger. After passing the night sleeping and sweating alternately, he found himself in the morning somewhat easier, but still unable to walk or move his limbs voluntarily. He was, therefore, laid upon a cart, and brought to the garrison at Berlin, the 16th October 1802. I saw him the following morning, in the Lazaretto. The battalion surgeon, Mr Fisher, ordered him elder tea, with spirit of Mindererus every hour, from which he sweated much during the night. In the morning, however, I found the under jaw so strongly drawn up towards the upper, that I could only with difficulty get in one finger between the teeth. At the same time, he complained of difficulty in swallowing, and stiffness in all his limbs. I found all the fleshy parts around the neck, hard and preternaturally tense, so that the patient was quite unable to move his head. The pulse was soft, small, and slow, giving only 65 beats in a minute.

From all these symptoms, it was sufficiently clear, that the disease consisted in a violent asthenia, and that the vital power (or according to the new language, the excitability,) was weakened, or rather, to speak more plainly, the nervous energy was oppressed. Hence arose the great bodily weakness, conjoined with a considerable degree of insensibility of all the fleshy parts; from the same cause arose also the preternatural contraction of the muscles of the jaw, and neck, and of most of the fleshy parts of the body. All these, clearly indicated a deficiency, and partly a total annihilation of the nervous influence on the muscles and vessels, and consequently a paralysis of them. The most urgent indication, therefore, was to excite their action, to remove the paralysis, and

* See Neues Journal, für die Chirurgie, Arzneikunde und Geburtshülfe, von C. L. Mursinna. Erstes Stück, 8vo. Berlin, 1803, page 92.

and lastly, to restore the natural state. The remedies for fulfiling this, must be strong and penetrating, and consequently of a stimulating nature. The more volatile they are, the more easily they penetrate, and the quicker is their effect. According to the best and most accurate experience, all this is accomplished by the internal use of opium, and most effectually, when combined with spirituous remedies.

For these reasons, I ordered the patient to take tinctura opii crocata, and spiritus sulphurico-æthereus, mixed in equal parts, every two hours, ten drops for a dose, in water, and at the same time, daily to be put into a warm soap bath for a quarter or half an hour. Externally, I caused all the hard and preternaturally tense parts, about the jaw, neck, and spine, to be frequently and smartly rubbed with a liniment of camphor oil, tinctura opii crocata, and the liquor ammoniæ causticæ.

The 17th, in the morning, the patient was much worse. He had not only not slept any, but passed a very restless night. He complained of an indescribable anxiety which impeded his breathing, and rendered his sufferings unbearable. I found him quite stiff, and all the muscles of his body, more especially those of the neck and spine, drawn together and hard, so that he had not the motion of a single muscle in his power. The head likewise was rigid and drawn somewhat backwards, and the mouth so much contracted, that the teeth touched each other. In a word, the patient was affected by the greatest degree of trismus and tetanus. His face was also red and much distorted, like that of a strangled person.

I ordered 20 drops of the above medicine to be given every hour, and an ounce of the kali causticum to be added to the soap-bath.

All this was given, indeed with difficulty, but faithfully, and in the intervals, as often as possible, water, soup, and wine, were exhibited. The 18th, in the morning, there was no change, which I conceived to be a favourable symptom. For, if this disease does not hourly increase, there is great hope of recovery.

I now prescribed 20 drops of the tinctura opii crocata alone, to be taken every hour in water. Externally I ordered equal parts of camphorated spirits and laudanum to be rubbed into the tense muscles round the neck, jaw, and spine, as often as the patient could bear it; and twice a day, I had him put into the soap-bath with kali causticum.

In the evening, the patient was much relieved. The sweat flowed without interruption from the surface of his whole body; the breathing was free, the anxiety much diminished, and he was able to move his head a little.

Next morning all the symptoms were in their old course, and the patient extremely low and dejected. This was a very natural consequence of an interruption of the medicine. I learned, that no medicine had been given him during the night. I therefore appointed a surgeon to watch during the night, with instructions to give him the medicine every hour, whatever might occur.

In consequence of this, on the 20th, the disease was much alleviated. The sweat flowed very freely, the mouth was so far opened, that a finger could again be easily introduced, of course, the deglutition was also easier, and the head again more moveable. As, for these four days, he had had no evacuation of his bowels, an emollient glyster was given, which produced a motion. After the bath, the patient complained of greater anxiety, and was evidently stiffer and more dejected. The kali causticum was therefore in future omitted, and the soap-bath alone employed. As this relieved all these symptoms, it was employed twice every day as long as it was agreeable to him, which was for the most part about half an hour.

The 22d, he was completely convalescent. He had slept now and then, for the first time, during the night, and had likewise sweated very freely, and with great relief, which he still continued to do. The pulse beat 75 in a minute, soft and full. The hardness of the muscles had remarkably diminished, so that the head could not only be moved freely, but the patient was able to raise himself up without assistance for the first time. The mouth was opened more than an inch, and the deglutition and breathing almost quite natural. He also expressed a desire for food, and he was allowed a good nourishing diet, and wine to be given at intervals, in small quantities. On account of the costiveness, an emollient glyster was again exhibited, which produced a full evacuation.

With regard to the treatment, I did not yet venture to make any change, but ordered him to take every hour 20 drops of laudanum, both day and night; the fleshy parts, especially around the neck and on the spine, were still rubbed frequently with camphorated spirit and laudanum, and two warm soap-baths were employed daily.

From this date, the improvement was daily greater, so that on the 26th, he was able to walk about the ward, and open his mouth almost completely.

I now reduced the laudanum to ten drops, and ordered only one warm bath daily.

On the 28th, the patient was again rather worse, the jaws less capable of being opened, and the deglutition, as well as the appetite,

appetite, diminished. I prescribed 15 drops of laudanum every hour, with instant relief, and at last perfect recovery. From the 1st November, I diminished the dose of laudanum again to ten, and on the 3d, to five drops.

On the 6th, I omitted the laudanum and baths entirely, and ordered him a decoction of one ounce of bark, and four drams of valerian, with vitriolic æther. After he had used this for some days, he was dismissed the 10th, completely cured. He is at present perfectly well, and does his duty as usual.

A Girl, 26 years of age, of a good habit of body, who had been hitherto healthy, stout, and of a chearful disposition, was taken suddenly ill on the 10th April 1803, and at once, so severely, that she could not remain out of bed. The scarlet fever having been very prevalent here during the winter, and the girl complaining especially of her throat, caused the family in whose service she was, to apprehend this dreadful disease, and they therefore sent for me immediately. I instantly perceived, that the girl was affected with trismus and tetanus. The mouth was drawn so close, and at the same time so painful, that a spoon could only with difficulty be brought in between the teeth. The muscles of the neck, also of the breast and spine, were stiff, and strongly contracted, of course, the head and the whole upper part of the body were perfectly immoveable. The pulse, in this case, was feverish, which in these diseases, at least in the beginning, has seldom been observed.

In order to discover the cause, I inquired into the mode of life, and particularly, into what she had been doing the preceding days. And I then learned, that the day before, she had scoured the rooms of the house, with open windows and doors, and had perspired very much. To avoid this, and at the same time to rest herself, she had laid herself several times over the window, though only for a quarter of an hour at a time, and again resumed her work with greater vigour.

It was sufficiently clear, from this account, that she had been very much heated after severe bodily exertion, and as she had exposed herself during the breaking out of the sweat to a cold stream of air, that she had caught a severe cold. In the course of the same evening, she felt herself weakly and sick, and had therefore gone earlier to bed than usual, without any supper. From her great weariness, she had indeed got a little broken sleep, but became still worse, and awakened in this wretched state.

As

As I distinctly recognised this disease, and was acquainted with its proximate cause, I concluded, both from its origin, and all appearances, that it had a very great resemblance to the case just described; therefore, that it belonged to the same genus, and of consequence, that it could be cured by the same means. I therefore prescribed four ounces of cinnamon water, a dram of Sydenham's laudanum, and one ounce of syrup of white poppies, of which she was to take a table spoonful every hour, and likewise ordered water and white French wine for common drink.

In twelve hours, after this mixture had been all used, the patient felt herself so far easier, that she could move the head a little, and could open her mouth some lines wider. The sweat flowed in great quantity from the whole surface of the body. The more this annoyed the patient, the greater hope I thence conceived of her recovery, as in this disease I had always found so violent a sweat alleviating and salutary. I therefore exhorted her to patience, and to a light but equable covering, and positively forbid the changing of the linen of the bed.

I continued the same medicine day and night, and gave her as much strong soup with wine and water, as could be got down.

The 3d day, I found her in every respect worse. The head was more immoveable, the deglutition more difficult, and the anxiety insupportable, although the sweat flowed as before, and an exposure to cold could not well be suspected. However willing I might have been to employ the warm bath, yet it was impossible in this situation. The appetite was quite gone, so that nothing but fluids could be given, and that with difficulty, and partly by force, as the patient began to despair, and would take nothing more. The pulse was soft and quick, and between 90 and 100. The belly was, as usual, costive, and the urine flowed sparingly, and with great pain. These are the effects of the opium, which under these circumstances, at least at first, always follow, and need not alarm the physician. In order to promote the flow of urine, a decoction of chamomile flowers was applied very warm over the pubes, and the whole abdomen frequently rubbed with oil, camphor, and laudanum. This had the effect, as in similar cases, to make the urine pass easily, and without pain.

The relapse proceeded merely from the medicine having been omitted during the night. In the morning, also, she could only be induced to take it, from the fear of being sent to the hospital. Being now unable to swallow without great difficulty, and having a great aversion to every thing sweet, I made her take every hour, five drops of laudanum in white wine. This was given her day and night, by a careful nurse, and in the intervals, as often as possible, alternately, strong soups, wine, and also beer.

Externally,

Externally, the camphorated spirits with laudanum were rubbed into the muscles of the neck and spine.

Next morning, the pains were more bearable, and all the symptoms easier, but the aversion to all medicine, and even to wine, was extremely great. We could only induce her to take the medicine every two hours. The consequence was very striking and convincing. Such violent anxiety followed during the night, that her end was expected every moment, therefore all medicine was left off, and only a little water with difficulty poured down. In the morning, I not only found her quite stiff, and every limb immoveable, but the mouth also firmly drawn together, every muscle of the face distressed, and the anxiety insufferable.

As she had had no evacuation during this disease, I now ordered her a glyster of decoction of chamomile with honey, which procured a copious stool, with evident relief. Immediately after it, I ordered her to take every hour, ten drops of laudanum in a little Madeira, and a tea spoonful of the latter to be poured in in the intervals. This was done most accurately, though it could, with difficulty, be introduced, and with still greater difficulty swallowed. Towards evening there was an evident change. The anxiety was much diminished, as also the stiffness of the whole body, and the mouth could again be opened an inch. The sweat flowed from the whole surface of the body. As the deglutition was also much easier, the medicine and the wine were continued during the night, without interruption. Although the patient had slept none during the night, yet I found her so changed in the morning, that I declared her convalescent. She was sitting in bed, all the limbs were moveable, the mouth fully open, and the pulse natural. From this moment, she had a return of appetite, and a great desire to leave her bed. The first I allowed her to gratify sufficiently, but the latter I opposed, because she still sweated extraordinarily, I dreaded her catching cold, and accordingly kept her still in bed, although less covered. The last medicine was now given every two hours.

This night, for the first time during the whole disease, she enjoyed a refreshing sleep for six hours, and, in the morning, she was quite well. I then ordered a decoction of bark, and a good nourishing diet. In a few days she was quite restored to her natural state, and she still enjoys steady good health.

About the same time, I was called to a man, who was attacked by similar symptoms. He was 40 years old, and had hitherto, for the most part, led a healthy life. He now complained very much of a difficulty in swallowing, and an inability to open his mouth. Except those, he had the full use of all his limbs, a

natural

natural pulse and appetite: he only felt himself very weak, and in very bad humour, and the surface of his whole body was cold.

After the most accurate enquiry, I could not discover any other cause of his disease, than exposure to cold. On account of his poverty, he had been working very hard for some weeks, and the day before he was attacked, had caught a severe cold. Immediately thereafter, he had felt himself unusually weak, and observed a difficulty in swallowing, and the drawing together of his mouth. Being in want of every thing, he had only sipped a little warm beer, and kept his bed.

I ordered him every hour five drops of laudanum, in a table spoonful of white French wine, and also to drink it mixed with water, and to take as much white bread as he could eat. All this the man followed most punctually.

In the morning, I saw, with pleasure, that the deglutition was relieved, his mouth more opened, and the skin warmer and moist, particularly over the breast. No change was made, except, that at the same time, his landlord gave him some strong soup. As he was accustomed to the use of brandy, and had a great desire for it, I allowed him also a little.

On the third day, a copious sweat broke out, and completely removed all his sufferings.

I made him take the laudanum for two days more, though not so frequently, and, in general, continued the practice already described. In eight days he was not only quite well, but much stronger than ever.

From these cases, it is sufficiently evident, that opium alone is capable of removing the whole of the morbid state; but that it must be given often, and without interruption, and that particular attention must be paid to increase the dose gradually, which can only be regulated by its effects. A small quantity of opium may cure a slight degree of this disease, as is proved by the third case. But if the disease is more severe, a greater quantity of opium is required, and especially the frequent and unremitted exhibition of it, as appears particularly from the first case. As soon as its use was omitted, during the night, all the symptoms returned with greater violence. And this also happened, if the opium was given in too small doses, or too long continued at the same quantity. As it cannot be fixed, to a certainty, how much opium is necessary for overcoming this disease, it is therefore right, in every individual case, to give it in a small quantity; for example, five drops of laudanum every hour in any convenient fluid. If, in three hours, no evident amendment follows, this dose may be doubled, and so on, every three hours, until some salutary effect is perceived. When the disease is very violent,

lent, a greater quantity must be given from the first, even ten or twenty drops, and gradually increased. If this is neglected, or if, from the very first, in a *very* high degree of this disease, we do not immediately proceed to such a dose of opium as is requisite to diminish this spasm, all is lost, and the patient is found dead next morning, or in so dangerous a state, as seldom to allow any chance of recovery, as I have had the misfortune to see in some cases, in which I was too timid in the use of the opium.

Sometimes it is necessary to go so far with the use of the opium, that 50, or even a 100 drops of laudanum, may, and must be given, every hour, in order to subdue this dreadful spasmodic affection, and to save the life of the patient.

X.

On the Plan for Medical Reform.

IN the 'Medical Intelligence' of your sixth number, it appears that an association for a medical reform has been established under the most respectable auspices, so far as patronage goes. I wish with all my heart, success to the reformers, and to the object of their reformation; but I have lived long enough to know, that nothing short of a miracle, or even a succession of miracles, will accomplish any sudden change in the manners, propensities, and prejudices of the people. Wherever quacks and pretenders are preferred to well informed and regularly educated men, it is because the former do, or what amounts nearly to the same thing, are supposed to do, as much and perhaps even more good, than the latter. It is not with medical men, as with that exorbitant tribe of paupers and beggars, who are legally supplied with the necessaries of life, squeezed from the more industrious and useful classes of the community. No parliamentary interference has yet been deemed necessary to support the learned or unlearned fraternities; no parish assessments are likely to render medical men independent of their own industry, of the good will and confidence of their neighbours. Should that time ever come, when such coercive measures must be resorted to, there might then be grounds for mending the rules concerning the qualifications requisite to constitute a doctor, a surgeon, or an apothecary. But till such a period arrives, I must enter my protest against any reform, tending to make the rate of expences the pro-

per

per criterion of fitness for medical practice. A set of men would thus be forced upon the public, whose merits stand sometimes in the inverse ratio of their pecuniary means; it is to make them believe, that attending two or three years at an University, that is to say, eating, drinking, and talking with men of the same age and pursuits as their own, or having their names inscribed on the college books, for even a longer period, is quite sufficient to constitute a regular education. Lest I should be thought a prejudiced London-bred man, one of those sprigs of insignificance and temerity, who would sell their penultimate shirt, in order to walk a full three months pupil at an hospital, with the expectation of rising one day from the camp or the cockpit, to the bright station of an eminent practitioner in the metropolis, I beg it to be understood, that I have run my medical career in the old regular way, beginning with studying three years at Edinburgh, and afterwards frequenting a London hospital, to see whether I could recognise, in the one place, any of my nosological friends, with whom I was so proud to become acquainted with at the other. I observed then more accurately, because I had comparative experience to direct me, that men do not differ so much on the two sides of the Tweed, as not to substitute and confound, in many cases, forms for realities. Attendance for three months in a large hospital, under good teachers, will generally prepare young men for the army and navy with a proper stock of firm feelings, so as not to faint at the sight of blood, nor shrink from doing their duty. With regard to the useful part of their services, their superiors by the aid of their experience will ward off some mischief, while nature and chance will do the rest. University men spread themselves through the kingdom, where they enjoy credit and consideration proportionate to their gentlemanly appearance, the charms of their conversation, and behaviour. As to the strict performance of their duties as physicians, success, and success alone, will establish their fame in that respect. Now I ask, what can possbly establish the reputation of low-bred uneducated men? Is it not, that the common people are unable to pay the higher classes of the profession, stand in awe of them, on account of the great difference of their manners, and so far as their contracted experience goes, the high minded men are not more successful in their practice than the others. Cases are quoted of the unskilful, almost brutal conduct, of those town and country quacks in the different branches of medical art; but is it very certain, that no such cases could be recorded from the secret annals of regular practitioners? We are shocked by the plain ignorance, as well as by the plain and open vices of the lower classes of the community, but an easy apology is found for the genteel blunders,

the

the delicate immorality of the rich, and powerful. I distrust that tendency to condemn, or at least to endeavour to stifle, by force, a class of men, who are openly supported by a great number of their fellow creatures, for whom personal sensations must be equally good guides, and personal experience an adequate rule of conduct in all that relates to their own preservation and bodily welfare. Let well educated men receive with gratitude the humble offerings of the poor, let them behave towards their inferiors, with that gentleness, and that spirit of active benevolence, which commands affection and respect, instead of fear and painful humility, then the tide of public opinion will be turned, even under the supposition, which I trust is nothing more than a bare assumption, that their professional success is not greater than that of their self taught competitors. Instead of obliging young men to go to London, or to an University, to be taught at a vast expence, why should not medical seminaries be appointed in different parts of the country, where good hospitals are already established?—Their number would excite emulation among country professors, which could not fail to benefit them, as well as the charitable institutions entrusted to their care. Young men, destined for the army and navy, would acquire at less expence, a much more complete education and better morals, than they can possibly boast of, under the present circumstances of our medical schools. London and regular Universities would enjoy the same prerogatives, so far as public opinion goes, which they do now; but every district in the country having its centre of an inferior though regular education for medical practice, would have its own local attachments for the pupils taught there, whose merits would be better appreciated, and the public at large would be less subjected to the influence of men, of whom the best that can be said in many instances is, that nobody knows, and therefore nobody can say, any thing about them.

From the foregoing remarks, it may have already been guessed, that I am no advocate for any interference of the Legislature with our private concerns. Such an interference seems to be in the first place, ridiculous, amounting to nothing less than an attempt to make fine well bred gentlemen of us all, which naturally leads to the second part of the argument, respecting the impossibility of accomplishing a reform of that kind. For if the premium bestowed freely by society on learning and manners be not sufficient to raise their professors out of the crowd, I am really afraid, Parliament will lose its time in discussing a plan for enlarging the understandings of the medical and unmedical part of the nation; and the Right Hon. Chancellor of the Exchequer will do better (if my information be correct), to postpone raising the sum

of

of nearly half a million on medical practitioners to be drawn indirectly from the public, until every other taxable object be exhausted for raising the annual supply. Monopolies of all sorts, intellectual as well as commercial, are bad, and will always be the last resource of an enlightened government, and I sincerely hope will never be resorted to by our Imperial Parliament.

SENEX.

THE INQUIRER. No VII.

On the Study of Mental Pathology.

WHEN we consider the many opportunities which the physician enjoys for acquiring an accurate knowledge of the human constitution, we cannot avoid being surprised, that so little advancement has been made in the theory of those diseases, which ar generally referred to the mind. This, in some measure, must have arisen from the intricacy and obscurity of the subject. But it is not less true, that our progress in this branch of knowledge, has been very much obstructed by many circumstances which, ere this time, might certainly have been removed.

In their inquiries into this subject, medical men seem to have been too much attached to that system, which imagines philosophy to consist in a knowledge of causes. Hence have arisen their unprofitable and obscure discussions concerning the qualities and existence of mind. Hence also, their vain attempts to explain the nature of sensation, whether by the intervention of animal spirits, the vibrations of nervous fibres, or by any other means, In a medical point of view, it is of no importance, whether the phænomena of mind be accounted for by the agency of an independent immaterial substance, or on the principles of organization. All that is necessary is to record those facts which daily present themselves to our observation, and to endeavour to refer them to their general laws. But hypotheses like those already hinted at, without in the least degree promoting our knowledge of mental pathology, have been productive of many bad consequences, by introducing into medical language a degree of vagueness and ambiguity, which has much embarrassed and impeded the progress of the science.

In

In the present imperfect state of medicine, it would be unreasonable to expect that its language should always be precise and well defined. Innumerable expressions however, which have obviously sprung from the distempered imagination of some enthusiastic theorist, are still retained in use, though the theory itself has long since sunk into oblivion. Were such expressions invariably restricted to one particular sense; were they considered merely as terms of art, employed to mark the unknown causes of known effects, no good argument could be urged against their use. Instead, however, of this being the case, every individual who employs them, thinks himself at liberty to give them an interpretation suitable to his own views. But the evil does not stop here; by many, these empty and unmeaning phrases are believed to afford an explanation of some obscure and otherwise unintelligible phænomenon; and thus, by imposing upon the understanding, they retard the cause of truth, and under the appearance of instruction, serve only to plunge us deeper into error and ignorance.

Besides these prejudices, medical men have been too much accustomed to associate the term disease, with some palpable change in the state of the body. Many of them apply their remedies with as great indifference, and speculate concerning their operation with as little discrimination, as if the animal machine were subject to no other laws, than those which regulate the attractions of a chemical mixture, or the motions of an hydraulic apparatus. But the opinions and reasonings of such men can have no influence with the physician, who has just views of the object of his profession; and who is aware, that the healing art cannot be successfully practised, without an accurate knowledge both of our moral and physical constitution. Important as this fact undoubtedly is, it has been long and shamefully neglected. I know there are many, who laugh at the idea of a disease of the mind, and, who think it absurd to conceive, that an immaterial and incorruptible substance should be affected by the gross and subordinate changes of matter. Such unphilosophical jargon, which even at this day is still too prevalent, has evidently arisen from mistaken notions of the proper objects of our inquiries. Of the nature either of matter or spirit we know nothing, and we are equally ignorant of all those changes, which take place in the brain and nerves during the time of sensation, or which appear to be subservient to the developement of all the varied phænomena of intellect. Enough, however, is it for us to know the results of these changes, to investigate their laws, and to discover, how far it is in the power of man to increase his comfort and happiness, by seeking for those objects, which give rise to agreeable sensations, or by avoiding those which produce a contrary effect.

No one can doubt, that the principles of metaphysics, and of moral philosophy have been much advanced in modern times.— But that branch of the subject, which respects mental pathology, chiefly from the causes already mentioned, has not made a similar progress. It nevertheless comprehends many interesting and important inquiries, which seem calculated, if properly conducted, materially to improve the happiness of man. These inquiries may justly be considered, as falling particularly within the province of the medical philosopher. It is his business, not only to examine the pains which arise from the disordered states of our moral and intelectual faculties, and the influence which these exert on the physical constitution; but likewise to investigate the various modifications and combinations of these faculties, which result either from a peculiar conformation of the body, or from the diseased states of its functions.

To obtain satisfactory information on these subjects, we must, to a luminous theory of the human mind, add all that accurate and extensive knowledge, which is to be derived from an attentive observation of man, in the greatest possible diversity of circumstances. We must trace him from the lowest stage of barbarism, to the highest pitch of cultivation and refinement, and endeavour to ascertain the principles of his character, and the changes which it undergoes, whether from habit, education, or any other cause. By thus presenting a connected view of our moral and physical constitution, and of their reciprocal influence on each other, we shall be able to investigate all the sympathies of our nature, to discover the origin and effects of the passions, and to illustrate and decypher the ever varying motives of human action. But the chief advantage which would result from these inquiries to the physician, would be to enable him to classify and arrange the different branches of mental disorders, by discovering the causes from whence they originate, and the nature of the constitution of those individuals in which they are most liable to take place.

The importance and necessity of such a mode of proceeding, must at once appear, when we consider the great degree of disorder and confusion which attend all our discussions on these subjects. To a set of symptoms, collected from individuals of the most oposite characters jumbled together without order or discrimination, we find the terms mania, melancholia or hypochondriasis promiscuously applied. While in the histories of these affections, we discover none of those accurate investigations into the previous state of the patient's associations, which not only modify all the impressions which he receives, but likewise determine the effects which result from them. To another class

of

of diseases, which have a most material influence on the happiness and comfort of a certain description of men, little or no attention has been paid. Sometimes indeed, they are most *significantly and pertinently* characterised by the names, "low spirits, vapours," &c. The poor patient is held out to public view as an object of ridicule and contempt, and is considered as unworthy of all sympathy and regard. The causes and effects of his disease are confounded together, and all are ascribed to the creative powers of a diseased fancy.

Nothing can be more repugnant to every principle of sound reasoning, than this popular but unmeaning declamation, which may easily be traced to faulty and imperfect views of the nature of the imagination. It is the province of this power, to form new combinations among the objects which are presented to its observation.—The facility with which these combinations are made, and the pleasure or pain with which they are attended, depends principally on the cultivation which this faculty has received, and the associations which we are led to form in early life. By these associations, we are directed in the estimations which we form of the value of surrounding objects. To them also are to be refered, most of those errors and prejudices which so often embitter this life, and give rise to a great proportion of mental disorders. It should always be remembered, however, that the most extravagant flights, and most monstrous combinations of this faculty, are determined by the previous state of the mind or body; as every succeeding thought, is the result either of some new impression, or of an association with the preceding. In all these cases, therefore, where a diseased state of the imagination exists, we must endeavour to trace the links in the chain of events, from which it has arisen. If it depends on the disagreeable impressions which a bodily disease engenders, it must first be removed. On the contrary, should the mind become affected, "without the body's fault," we must endeavour to introduce new associations, either by a change of studies and occupations, or by "diversions, hurry, and a restless life."

In many cases it is extremely difficult to ascertain, whether the primary affection originates from the body or the mind.—Many individuals are affected with different varieties of mental disorders, without the bodily functions undergoing any material change. In cases of this kind, it will generally be found, that the patient is endowed with a sound and vigorous physical constitution, which in some measure resists the effects of the mental disease. In other cases, when the bodily organization is of a more delicate texture, the slightest mental irritation produces different consequences. The organs of digestion are almost instantaneously affected, and the patient is tormented with all the miseries of dyspepsia. Again the effects which result from diseases of the body, are modified by the previous state of the mind. Many diseases of the former, produce little effect on the minds of those men, who are engaged in some active employment, and whose character has not been softened by domestic sympathies, or polished by a refined education. Thus we perceive, that the organization of the body has considerable influence in moderating the effects which are apt to arise from affections of the mind. While the previous state of the mind (from whatever cause originating), in a great measure determines the consequences which are to result from diseases of the body.

Were these speculations pursued to their utmost possible extent; were the laws which regulate the connection between mind and body traced with sufficient care and accuracy, we should be able to foretell with almost unerring precision, the effects which would necessarily take place from diseases of either. As pertaining to the same subject, it would be necessary to investigate the changes in our moral affections, which take place during the time of certain varieties of maniacal attacks. From what has been said, it is evident these changes must vary in every individual in proportion to the nature of the cultivation which his faculties have received, and the causes from which his disease has originated. Facts are probably wanting to enable us to form a correct theory on this subject. Were it, however, investigated with that attention, which it well merits, we should not only be able to reconcile many of those events which appear at present so anomalous and discordant, but also to shew, that they are the necessary consequences of the circumstances in which the patient was placed. It would be vain to attempt to illustrate this subject at present. As connected, however, with the foregoing remarks, it may be worth while to make a few observations on the mode of reasoning, which is generally adopted, when talking of some of the causes of mental disorders.

These have been divided with sufficient propriety into moral and physical. Among the former are ranked the passions, and all those other calamities, which tend to disturb the harmony of our constitutions; that love, hatred, revenge, fear, grief, &c. have given rise to different mental disorders, no one can doubt. But it may be observed, that from such mutilated and imperfect information, very little addition is made to our stock of knowledge. An object which will excite fear, or love, or hatred, in one person, will produce no such effects on another. Whence does this arise? Whence does it happen, that *the same event* which will strike terror and dismay into one man, will only stimulate

mulate another to more arduous exertions? Whence does it happen, that an event which will overwhelm one man with grief will have no such influence on a person of a different character!— These, and many other questions of a similar nature, which naturally present themselves, on considering this subject, have been totally overlooked by medical writers. They seem altogether to have forgotten, that the effects of the passions, in individuals of different moral constitutions, must vary according to the different circumstances of the combination. Thus the effects of anger will be different, when combined with cowardice or bravery, envy or hatred, and in short, with any other, either of our benevolent, or malevolent affections. The same remark holds equally true, when applied to our physical constitution. Fear in some cases, it is said, occasions paleness, diarrhœa, syncope, &c. A greater degree of fear, instead of giving rise to such consequences, sometimes produces events of a perfectly opposite nature.— Speech has been restored to the dumb, and strength to the paralytic! It is needless to multiply instances, in order to evince the confusion which has arisen from want of attention to these facts; and the hints which have been thrown out, may perhaps be sufficient to suggest a more scientific arrangement of the passions, than that which is commonly adopted.

After these cursory remarks, it might have been proper, shortly to state the advantages, which are likely to accrue from examining the brain, and other organs, of those persons, who have been affected with mental disorders. But this field comprises so many important topics of discussion, that little benefit could be derived from any thing, which could be advanced here. Some of the principles, however, which should guide our researches into this subject, may probably be inferred from several of the preceding speculations.

I have thus attempted to give a rough outline of a great and important subject; a subject, which not only involves consequences peculiarly interesting to the practical physician, but to every man who is anxious to acquire a scientific knowledge of human nature.

3 J. B.

PART III.

CRITICAL ANALYSIS.

I.

" *Manuel de Médecine pratique, ou Sommaire d'un cours gratuit donné l'an vii. et l'an viii. de la Republique Française aux officiers de Santé du Département du Léman.* Par LOUIS ODIER, Docteur et Professeur en Médecine, á Geneve; de l'Imprimerié de la Bibliothique Britannique, et se trouve chez J. J. Paschaud Libraire. An. xi.

DR ODIER was a pupil of Dr Cullen, and retains his nosological arrangement. It is a remarkable fact, that Geneva is almost the only spot on the continent, where the sound principles of British medical education, and of regular practice, have become popular, under the patronage of those Genevese physicians, who have been able to estimate the comparative value of the different methods adopted here and abroad. The various improvements which are introduced, from time to time, into our practice, to be confined to the libraries of Germany, or overlooked by the supine indolence of the French, seem to be duly appreciated by the Genevese college. The city of Geneva, and the surrounding country, are highly indebted to Dr Odier, for his gratuitous endeavours to disseminate the results of his experience among a set of men, whose practice has been hitherto unguided by rules, and unassisted by any acquaintance with the progress of their art. Young men likewise, who intend to lay some foundation for subsequent methodical studies, will derive from one or two preliminary courses of this sort, a great advantage over those who fall plump upon University benches, where they lose a year at least in the act of reconnoitering the place. The purpose of this publication is expressed by the author himself, in the following words;

" After 30 years spent in the observation and treatment of a vast number of " diseases, I have thought, that if by consulting only my own experience, con" fining myself to the diseases which are most common in the department where " I live, describing them such as I have seen them, and laying down the basis " of the treatment which I have found most successful, I might be of some " service

"service to those among my professional brethren, who are in need of assistance, " or rather possess zeal and knowledge enough to become desirous of new in- " formation in the exercise of their art."

The work is a sort of syllabus to a very limited course, consisting of 24 lectures only. It will be sufficient to make a few observations on such of its contents as are most deserving of attention.

The author makes, and perhaps with great propriety, only one species of the numberless varieties of continued fevers, viewing those varieties, as founded on a difference of symptoms, which originate entirely in accidental causes. Our typhus gravior, the ship, or jail fever, had remained almost completely unknown to the practitioners of Geneva, until very lately, when it made its appearance in the public jail, imported there, it is presumed, by the military passing through the town. The endemical fever of Geneva, is vulgarly known there, under the name of bilious fever; it is frequently epidemical, especially in the country, but very rarely contagious, and the symptoms of malignity, when they do occur, come on usually, during the progress of the complaint. Those fevers begin commonly towards the end of January, or the beginning of February, with some symptoms of catarrh, anorexia, nausea, and vomiting, sometimes accompanied with gripes and diarrhoea. The catarrhal symptoms cease usually after a few days; but the others go on throughout the duration of the complaint, which is very uncertain. The treatment consists in evacuating first by a gentle emetic the contents of the stomach, afterwards keeping the bowels open, and ending the cure with some tonic. It appears to be nothing else but the common synochus of this country, modified by the season of the year, in which it usually prevails.

Accidental symptoms are treated by particular means; those of malignity, besides the internal remedies generally known, are successfully attacked by cold washing, repeated several times in the day. "I do not know, says Dr Odier, any thing, whose effects are more rapid in abating the feverish heat, arresting delirium, and inducing a gentle natural sleep."

Nephritis, in Geneva, is often the consequence of a gouty or rheumatic affection, but never, as is the case elsewhere, of a stone, or the gravel, which are complaints almost unknown in that country. This observation is worthy of attention, when it is considered, that Geneva lies in the centre of vineyards, where sourish wine grows plentifully, for common use; and we are informed, that the same remark applies to the whole range of the banks of the Rhine, whence the acid Rhenish wine is brought over to this country.

Rheumatic affections are extremely common throughout that part of Switzerland, lying confined between the chains of high mountains, which cause sudden and considerable changes in the temperature, the common exciting cause of those painful disorders. Dr Odier distinguishes three species of rheumatism. The first species affects the muscles, rather than the ligaments and tendons. The pain resembles that produced by fatigue, luxations, or contusions, is very fugitive, goes off immediately by rest, and frequently disappears, entirely of itself, after a few days. There is commonly no fever present, although sometimes it comes on with great violence; but the patient remains very liable to be affected by the least change of temperature, and thereby apt to relapse. Warm or stimulating applications are usually sufficient. The best prophylactics are flannel shirts, and the cold bath. Under the head of this species of rheumatism, the author treats of the toothach, and mentions a remedy, which he has often employed with advantage in his own case. He swallows slowly mouthfuls of cold water, which he allows to grow warm in his mouth, before passing down; after he has drank in that way three or four pints, he has some slight febrile sensations, which carry off the pain.

In the second species, generally known under the name of acute rheumatism, the joints are red, painful, and swelled; the pain and swelling fly from one joint to the other; the pulse is quick and strong, the periods of the relapses are much more distant than in the preceeding species, and in the intervals, the patient is not more liable than any body else, to suffer from exposure to cold and moisture. The treatment consists in promoting the different secretions, and quieting the irritation of the vascular and nervous systems, by drinking copiously sour milk, or sugar of milk, by the use of tartarised antimony, of nitre and magnesia, by anodynes made slightly diaphoretic, and by sedative, or stimulating frictions. If the patient be robust and plethoric, one or two venesections may be used at the commencement of the attack. Among the various symptoms which are apt to supervene on acute rheumatism, and to degenerate afterwards into a chronic complaint, Dr Odier mentions an affection of the heart, the prominent features of which is a species of hectic fever, originating in a slow inflammation of that viscus, commonly of the rheumatic kind. Its characteristical symptoms are frequency and irregularity of the pulse, oppression, and cough. It is frequently accompanied with anasarcous swellings, and ends either with sudden death, or with the usual colliquative symptoms

toms. The chief remedies are rest, a proper regimen, and cooling medicines, such as nitre and acids, and diuretics against the dropsical swellings. When head-ach and delirium accompany the rheumatic fever, leeches to the temples; a large blister to the nape of the neck; a bladder filled with ice, and applied over the head are recommended; a practice equally successful in maniacal phrenzy, but surely not to be advised in that violent inflammatory affection, commonly called *phrenitis*. We hint at this ground of distinction, because it is our decided opinion, that acute rheumatism cannot be considered as a genuine inflammatory disease.* In chronic rheumatism, which constitutes the third and last species, the pains are fixed, and permanent, accompanied with a sense of coldness; they continue for weeks, months, and years, without any fever, and terminate often by anchylosis, contractions of the limbs, and sometimes by palsy. The general indication is to stimulate the small vessels of the whole system, and especially those of the parts affected. The plan of strong sweating has succeeded with Dr Odier in cases of chronic rheumatism, which had resisted a number of other remedies. It usually excites a strong fever, and sometimes a general miliary eruption, similar to that produced by some thermal waters used for the same purpose.

Under the head of eruptive fevers, we see, with pleasure, that the vaccine inoculation is gaining ground very generally in that part of the Continent, where our author resides; and we have heard from another quarter, the difficulty of procuring small-pox matter there, amounts, at present, nearly to absolute impossibility. The desquamation in scarlatina, lasts, says Dr Odier, five or six weeks; if during that time, the patient exposes himself to cold, moisture, or merely to the open air, he is in danger of becoming anasarcous, or even of being suddenly carried off by a rapid effusion into the cavities of the brain, or of the chest. That, however, never happens, when the patient secludes himself from the access of air for forty days, or till the desquamation is completed. It has been sometimes observed, the author adds, during epidemics of scarlatina, that persons, without any appearance of fever, of redness, or desquamation, were suddenly seized with symptoms of anasarca or oppression, as if they had had the scarlet fever, and had imprudently exposed themselves to the open air. The treatment is very simple; the antiphlogistic regimen, with a steady temperature, is sufficient. If the angina presents, either from

* See Edin. Medic. and Surg. Journ. No. 8, p. 157, &c.

from the beginning, or during the course of the complaint, symptoms of malignity, antisceptics, and especially cold air, with fumigations of nitric acid, directed on the ulcers of the throat, have been found to answer well. This last method, Dr Odier observes, has had the most complete success, during a late epidemic in and about Geneva. The use of cold washing and affussion in the common scarlet fever of this country, has been found not only harmless, but one of the best remedies to lessen the violence of the symptoms, to crush it even at its commencement, and to diminish the danger of its contagious influence. We do not wish to invalidate any conclusion deduced from actual experience; and what is good practice here, may turn out to be bad elsewhere; but Dr Odier will allow, perhaps, the practice which he supports, to be indentically the same with that of Sydenham, grounded itself upon a piece of theory. "Cum hic "morbus nihil aliud mihi videatur quam mediocris sanguinis "effervescentia à prægressæ æstatis calore, aut alio aliquo modo "excitata, nihil quicquam molior, quo minus sanguis sibi despumando vacet, et materiæ peccanti, quæ satis promptê abjungitur, "per cutis poros ablegandæ. Quamobrem satis habeo ut æger à "carnibus in solidum abstineat, et a liquoribus spirituosis qui-"buscumque, tum ut neque usquam foràs prodeat neque se per-"petim lecto affigat."—Observat. Medic. circâ morb. acut. Sect. vi. cap. 11.

To Sydenham, however, we remain indebted for this incipient amelioration, in the treatment of our eruptive disorders, had he generalised his ideas on small-pox, by extending his mode of practice to other constitutional affections of the skin, he might have been accused of being nothing else than a presumptuous theorist, and have deprived himself of the pleasing reflection, that he had done much in preventing the fatal effects of one of the most dreadful contagions, which has ever assailed the human race. It was reserved to the late Dr Currie to complete, in a better age, assisted by a vigorous genius, and supported by his enlightened zeal for the good of his fellow creatures, the task of his illustrious predecessor. Prejudice may oppose, reason may struggle, but the broad basis is laid, on which a simple, but majestic edifice will gradually rise, to teach us, that good sense in the art of the physician, as in that of the moralist, goes hand and hand with sound philosophy, and can never be separated from it. But to return to Dr Odier, even if we admit the propriety of his practice, when the complaint is once established, and the natural functions of the skin considerably impaired, still the use of the cold affusion, to destroy at once the feverish symptoms, and thus to prevent the consolidation of the disease, might be recommended in those cases, where confinement is likely to prove inconvenient to the patient.

The author distinguishes two species of dyspepsia, one proceeding from atony, the other from irritability. This latter kind is very common in Geneva, and Dr Odier thinks he has observed, that the motion of the arms disposes particularly to it; perhaps it is more probably the consequence of the sedentary life led by that class of people, females especially, who work with the hands alone. It differs from the dyspepsia atonica, by the absence of loathing for food, and a sense of pain supervening two or three hours after a meal, accompanied with cramps, which terminate usually by nausea and vomiting After having tried, with little success, various tonic and antispasmodic medicines, the author discovered in 1786, a new remedy, which, in cases not otherwise complicated, succeeds much better than any other, and is never attended with any inconvenience, viz. the *white oxide of bismuth*, in a dose of from six to twelve grains four times a-day.

In the 16th lecture, Dr Odier treats of mental disorders, and reckons *incubus* in the number; he mentions the case of a gentleman between 25 and 30 years of age, who could not go to sleep in his post-chaise, when in motion, without beeing soon awakened suddenly, by a most painful sensation, as if an enormous weight had fallen on his brain. His head bent forwards under that imaginary weight, he was unable to speak, and his whole body was seized with a convulsive tremor, which lasted some time. He did not experience these sensations, either when sleeping at rest, or when he could resist sleep in his chaise. As his business obliged him to travel frequently by night, he wished much to get the better of this disorder. Several antispasmodic medicines were tried in vain; it was, however, entirely removed by the petals of the *cardamine pratensis*, recommended by Sir George Baker in nervous asthma, in the dose of two or three drachms every day.

Under the head of slow fevers, and of atrophy, the ingenious author points out a cause of the *marasmus infantilis*, well deserving our attention. "Infants at the breast, says he, are "sometimes seen to decline without any apparent reason; "their countenance becomes pale and wrinkled; giving them "the appearance of diminutive old people. Infants suckled by "mothers, endowed with great sensibility, are, as far as my personal observation goes, more subject to that sort of decline "than others. It is probably owing to some change in the quality of the milk, occassionally produced by a maternal attachmant too exalted or ill directed." For it is usually sufficient to deliver the child to a nurse of calmer affections, or to wean it altogether,

altogether, in order to restore it in a few days to its natural plumpness and vigour. And what is more, the same milk that disordered one child, will agree perfectly well with another, for whom the nurse does not feel the same degree of anxiety; she may even return after a few days to her own infant, when her mind is become more composed; so that a temporary exchange of nurses, and of nurslings, will frequently stop the progress, and remove permanently the causes of the disorder in question. The author has evidently omitted a species of atrophy *(atrophiâ lactantium)*, which, in Great Britain, at least, is a growing evil, especially among the lower classes. The frequency of nervous disorders in his own place of residence, which he himself confesses to be rapidly increasing; the tendency to premature decay, which is commonly observed in females of mountainous countries, and the habit of suckling their own children, surely very common in a city, inseparably associated with the lessons and the name of the author of Emile, must render this complaint still more common in that part of Switzerland, the diseases of which, Dr Odier now professes to review. The proper mode of treating it would have been highly acceptable to that class of medical practitioners, for whom these lectures are avowedly intended.

A case is related of Tympanites, produced by an accumulation of feces in the intestines, in which the operation of entereotomy was successfully performed. A patient aged 70, after a diarrhœa which had lasted four months, became constipated to a great degree, the strongest purgatives were exhibited without effect, the belly swelled, and became painful. Evident symptoms of gangrene soon supervened, and death seemed unavoidable. Under those circumstances, it was determined, that the operation should be tried. Mr Fine (an eminent surgeon in Geneva), cut into the most prominent part of the swelled abdomen, and retaining the intestine on the surface of the wound, by means of a thread, which was passed through the mesentery, and fixed on the sides of the belly with sticking plaster, he opened the intestine, by means of an incision, long enough to give passage to the feces, which issued from it in great abundance.

The tympanitic swelling, and symptoms of gangrene, became less, and soon after disappeared completely. The intestine adhered to the sides of the wound, so as to render the thread useless: an artificial anus was the consequence, and the feces issued from it, not continually as expected, but once or twice a-day only, with a sense of previous warning, which enabled the patient to prepare the proper apparatus for cleanliness. With the exception of that inconvenience, the person was well enough for a whole year to walk about, and to attend to all her usual business.

She

She then became dropsical and died; on opening the body, a hard tumour was found, compressing the intestinum rectum at its origin, so as to obliterate it completely.

Bronchocele is considered as an obstruction and swelling of the thyroid gland, which frequently increases so much, as to render respiration difficult; on dissection, it offers the same appearance as that of the breast. It sometimes passes into a state of ulceration, which, however, is never phagedenic nor painful. The causes of this disease called *goître*, are very obscure: It is endemical in some countries, especially in *Valais*. Some persons think, that it is owing to the difficult circulation of air in valleys; others ascribe it to the quality of the waters. Dr Odier inclines to the latter opinion, because it has appeared to him, that distilled water prevented the increase of the tumour, and even tended to lessen its bulk. Women are more subject to it than men; and it is more particularly during their lyings-in, that it makes a rapid progress. It is cured in Geneva by burnt spunge, exhibited in powder, or infused in wine, and combined with purgatives, to prevent the cramps of the stomach, which sometimes accompany the disappearance of the swelling. Muriate of barytes has likewise been recommended.

We have thus picked up at random, some specimens of Dr Odier's practical notions: In perusing this book, we have felt more at home than is usually the case, when examining such of the continental productions as relate to the practice of medicine. Our author's general mode of treatment, is neither systematically passive, nor rashly active; he knows well, that patients do not call physicians to their bed-side to be looked at and rest satisfied with draughts of patient expectation; if it were for no other purpose, than to raise the spirits and confidence of the sick, the physician must take upon himself the direction of nature, and lead her as well as he can, to a favourable issue. For such is the weakness of human nature, such is the tendency of the generality of men to a species of superstition, that they must have medical priests and ceremonies to attend them through life, and to help them to die.

II.

Observations on the Utility and Administration of Purgative Medicines in several Diseases. By JAMES HAMILTON, M. D. Fellow of the Royal College of Physicians, and of the Royal Society of Edinburgh; and Senior Physician to the Royal Infirmary of that city. *Second Edition, corrected and enlarged,* 8vo. *p.* 349. *Edinburgh,* 1806.

THE principal additions which have, in this new edition, been made to the former observations of the author, are a chapter on hysteria, and another on tetanus. And these, for the convenience of the purchasers of the first edition, have, with their corresponding appendixes, been published also in a separate form. The whole work, however, has been revised, and some less important additions made to the general text. It is unnecessary to recall the attention of our readers to the subjects we have already so fully examined, when reviewing the first edition of this useful work, in our fifth number. It will be sufficient here, very shortly, to notice the additional chapters on hysteria and tetanus.

Chap. 7.—*Observations on the Utility and Administration of Purgative Medicines in Hysteria.*

After premising a short history of the disease, in which the symptoms are narrated in the order of their occurence, Dr H. remarks, that the most constant and invariable of these, are pains of the abdomen, flatulence, constipation, the hysteric globe, acid and fetid eructations, vomiting and sometimes purging, all indicative of considerable derangement of the stomach, and alimentary canal. This affection of the stomach and bowels, he considers as primary, and the other multifarious symptoms of hysteria, as depending upon it. According to this view, he employs purgatives in hysteria, with the same limitations as in chorea, and other diseases already treated of.

" I have not been disappointed in my expectations in thus treating hysteria, my success has been equal to my wishes, and the source of much satisfaction to me. Yet my experience is not so complete as to enable me to say to what extent purgatives may be employed in hysteria, exclusively of other medicines. Within certain limits, I accordingly call in the aid of fetid and tonic medicines; but, in my estimation, they are merely subsidiary, and, on some occasions, might be altogether overlooked, as they were in the treatment of Sarah M'Millan and Isabel Black, whose cases are inserted in the Appendix, No VIII. In particu-

lar

lar cases, where great anxiety prevails, recourse may be had to wine in moderate quantity, till such time as relief is obtained by purgatives.

"I may add, by way of caution, that in hysteria as well as in chorea, chlorosis, and hæmatemesis, the full exhibition of active purgatives is necessary to procure even moderate evacuations from the bowels; and that this exhibition must be continued from day to day, till such time as the feces are natural, and till the disease ceases.

"The first purgative that we use, may seem, on some occasions, to aggravate the symptoms, but the practice must not be deserted on that account. The additional irritation, which purgatives may give in the first instance, soon passes away, and the perseverance in the use of them, removes that irritation which gives rise to the disease, which of course, disappears in proportion as the bowels are relieved of the oppressive mass of accumulated feces."

We believe there is much truth in the doctrine, and much good in the practice of Dr Hamilton. But, we cannot help thinking, that he all along keeps one indication too much in view, that his practice is too exclusively purgative in some cases. We must recollect, how successfully we have seen chlorosis treated by the preparations of iron, and how often we have combated hysteria by tonics, and antispasmodics, and recollecting this, we cannot, all at once, part with them in the treatment of these diseases. But the lesson given us by Dr H. to unload the bowels, is not the less important. And the utility of purgatives in hysteria, might, if necessary, be largely confirmed by other documents.

Chap. 8.—*On the Utlity of Purgative Medicines in Tetanus.*

Hitherto Dr Hamilton has had experience for his guide; his opinions have been founded on observation, and his practice has been confirmed by extensive experience. His observations on the utility of purgatives in tetanus, are more hypothetical and analogical. But the result of the investigation certainly encourages the fair trial of these medicines in a disease, the treatment of which has been hitherto so hopeless. In tetanus, the bowels are obstinately constipated, there is uneasy sensation and tenseness of the præcordia; it occurs in those climates and seasons in which derangement of the hepatic system, and of the alimentary canal prevail; chorea and hysteria are spasmodic diseases, accompanied with disorders of the bowels, and with costiveness, and are relieved or cured by purgatives; the tetanus of children, or trismus nascentium, is cured by free purging; lastly, besides there presumptive circumstances, Dr H. has endeavoured to support his opinion by shewing, that where purgative medicines have been given in tetanus, whether by design or not, they have proved eminently useful, and that some examples of cures may fairly be attributed to the purgative operation of some of the remedies employed, an opinion which is corroborated by Mursinna's cases, inserted in this number of our Journal, p. 435. Cases from his own practice are also adduced of tetanic affections cured by purgatives.

III.

Practical Observations concerning Sea Bathing. To which is added, Remarks on the use of the Warm Bath. By A. P. BUCHAN, M. D. of the Royal College of Physicians, London. P. 207. 8vo. London, 1804.

THE enlightened practitioner, whose information has kept pace with the progress of science, will not perhaps find any thing very new in this little volume. But, an attempt to embody, and render more accessible, the knowledge which has gradually sprung up, is at all times acceptable; and a treatise on a subject so popular as the present, cannot fail to be useful. While persons of every temperament and predisposition, and invalids of every description, are annually flocking to the sea coast, in search of pleasure and of health; there must be reason to apprehend, that a remedy so powerful, and so useful in some diseases, cannot be of universal application, and must be hazardous and pernicious in others. And in truth, we know but too well, that sea bathing is much abused in this, fully as much as the warm bath is abused in other countries. Misled by the popular theory of the general tonic, and invigorating powers of the cold bath, our countrymen are inclined to regard it as an universal remedy adapted to every case of debility and disease. A similar prejudice has condemned the warm bath as relaxing and debilitating. But, even when sea bathing does suit the disorder, when it has been advised by an experienced physician, the patient is very generally sent to the sea coast, ignorant and uninstructed. He is to bathe indeed, but he has no just notion of the remedy, he has no rules for his direction, he knows not how, in his particular case, he may bathe with safety and advantage. It is certain, however, that the effects of the cold bath not only vary in different constitutions, and in different states of disorder, but that they vary also in the same individuals, and in the same case, with the manner and circumstances of using it. It produces, even in a healthy individual, very different effects, when taken before or after meals, before or after exercise, when the body is cool, temperate, or heated. These varieties of effect are still more remarkable in a debilitated or or diseased system; and should therefore be fully understood, and duly appreciated, in each individual case. For just notions of these, we are especially indebted to the much lamented Dr Currie, whose valuable work has destroyed a host of prejudices entertained on the subject of cold bathing. In general, the effects of temperature on the animal body, and the operation of the various modes of bathing, are better understood than formerly. We have general principles and experience to direct our future observations; and the way is cleared of those prejudices which obstructed the progress of improvement. Dr Buchan aims not at novelty, he professes only to be useful, by diffusing those philosophical opinions, respecting the important objects of health and life, among persons who might be deterred from the perusal of a work professedly medical. But, though the design of his undertaking be popular, even the medical student may peruse it with advantage. The general principles are laid down in a clear and scientific manner, and many of Dr Buchan's practical observations and illustrations are deserving of notice. It is, upon the whole, a good compendium of the most material facts and doctrines relating to the subject of sea bathing.

Dr Buchan has divided his work into eight chapters. In the first, entitled General Observations on Cold Bathing, he gives an account of the immediate effects of plunging into cold water, explaining the phænomena as he goes along, the shock, the convulsive respiration, the action of the heart and arteries, the rigors, and the glow which takes place on resuming the usual clothes, the presence of which glow, is the best criterion of the eventual utility of bathing.

"If immersion in the bath, be not succeeded by this glow on the surface of the skin, bathing should by no means be persisted in. The absence of it is a proof, either that the water has been too cold, or immersion in it too long continued, relatively to the vigour of the constitution; and that the powers propelling the blood have not sufficient energy to overcome the temporary torpor of the superficial vessels. Head-ach, indigestion, cold, and appearance of deadness of the extremities, will be the certain consequences of persisting in the use of the bath, by individuals, in whom this salutary symptom does not occur; their systems being too feeble, either naturally, or from the effects of disease, to derive benefit from this remedy. From these observations may be deduced the reason why bathing in the sea is salutary to many persons who are injured by the lower temperature of a bath supplied by a cold spring; and also, why the thermal baths at Buxton, in Derbyshire, are beneficial to many delicate or debilitated invalids, who are unable to bear the greater cold of the open sea."

The remote effects of sea bathing, are to invigorate the constitution, and render it less susceptible of disease. In a more particular manner, Dr Buchan is anxious to prove, that the practice of of cold bathing prevents catarrhal affections, or what is usually termed, catching cold. These complaints are the effects of atmospherical variations of temperature, and are most prevalent during autumn and spring. The more tenderly any individual is brought up, the more susceptible he becomes of disease from those variations. Those who accustom themselves to heated rooms, and warm cloathing, are the most subject to colds; while those, on the contrary, who have been used to go thinly clothed, can bear the vicissitudes of the weather, with much less risk of disease. The powers of the living body are much under the influence of custom; and much may be done, by accustoming ourselves to the vicissitudes of temperature. A habit, in this respect, will render us much less susceptible of cold, and the occasional use of the cold bath, by inuring the body to a wider range of temperature, tends to diminish the danger of those sudden transitions from heat to cold, and the contrary.

" After having bathed in the sea, during a few weeks in autumn, I have observed," says Dr B. " with respect to myself, as well as in many other instances, that persons prone to catarrhal affections, are much less susceptible of them, during the ensuing winter. By the occasional use of the cold bath, the perspiring vessels of the skin are also invigorated, and accustomed to perform their functions in lower temperatures, their susceptibility of slighter alterations is diminished, and perspiration becomes firm and regular, while the danger of disease, from suppression of this function, is diminished. As a proof, that the organs of perspiration are rendered more vigorous, by occasional exposure to cold, I have known many examples of people who never failed to catch cold, as it is called, on having their feet in the slightest degree wet; who, in consequence of adopting the habit of washing their feet regularly every morning with a cloth dipped in cold water, or what is preferable, in a solution of common salt in water, have entirely overcome this delicacy of constitution."

The lower the temperature at which the organ of perspiration is accustomed to perform its functions, the less it is maintained, will be the risk of its due action being interrupted by the inconstancy of our climate, and this view leads our author into a considerable digression on the abuse of cloathing.

" The habitual use of flannel garments, by accustoming the exhaling vessels to perform their functions in a certain high temperature, in like manner diminishes their natural energy, and renders them liable to become torpid, by the slightest abstraction of their usual warmth; and thus gives rise to colds, rheumatism, and other complaints, arising from checked perspiration, which much clothing, is commonly, but erroneously, supposed to prevent."

We have no doubt, that the flannel shirt, like every other good, may be abused. The general experience of its good effects, however, has recommended, and supports its use. A person who wears a flannel shirt, will not, in this country, be overheated by it, it, but the transition from a warmer to a colder air, will be less sensibly felt. And spite of the dogmatism of Dr Trotter, our sailors and soldiers are as sensible of the benefit of a flannel shirt, as the most luxurious and self-indulgent of our countrymen.

A saline incrustation is formed on the bodies of those who bathe in the sea, and Dr Buchan is inclined to think, that part of the good effects resulting from bathing in salt water, may depend on its saline impregnation exciting, in some measure, the action of the cutaneous vessels. Certain it is, that sailors and fishermen are convinced, that they are less liable to be injured by being wet with salt water, than with rain; an observation, which may be partly explained by the slower evaporation of water impregnated with salt, and partly by the excitation of the skin, by the saline particles.

Chap. 2. *On the Time of Bathing.*—Chap. 3. *On the Manner of Bathing.*

There are many popular prejudices of a dangerous tendency entertained on these subjects. It is believed, that it is impossible to bathe too early in the morning; that it is best and safest to bathe with an empty stomach; that the body should be perfectly cool, and the circulation calm, not hurried by heat, exercise, or other adventitious stimulus.

It is undoubtedly not safe to bathe with a full and loaded stomach, immediately after meals; digestion is disturbed by plunging into the cold bath. And this observation, or perhaps motives of convenience, have suggested the morning, as the fittest time for bathing. It may suit, well enough, the healthy and vigorous, but it is, upon the whole, the most improper time of the day, for the debilitated invalid.

"I have frequently been shocked, at seeing delicate invalids of both sexes, apparently just risen, and before the vital functions had resumed their proper energy, standing pale, and shivering on the bleak beach, or waiting in a bathing room, chilled by streams of cold air rushing through opposite doors and windows, and expecting, apparently with a degree of horror, their turn to go into the water."

This is but too true a picture; from bathing in this state, no possible advantage can be derived. Such invalids should have the energies of their systems roused by a slight breakfast, and such a degree of exercise, as may produce a general sensation of warmth over the whole body, before plunging into the cold bath.

Noon, or a little after it, is therefore, by far the best time for general sea bathing; the sea is also warmer at this time, than it is in the morning. Our author has found the temperature of the sea, when high water occurs about two or three o'clock in the afternoon, to be from 10 to 12 degrees above what it was at low water, at eight o'clock in the morning.

Before bathing, the body should be perfectly cool: The very reverse of this, which is commonly inculcated and acted upon, by bathers, would be a safer general rule. Infirm persons should use such exercise before immersion, as may excite some increased action of the heart and arteries, with some increase of heat, and no one should plunge into the sea, with feelings of languor, lassitude, and chilliness. It should be generally understood, that it is safer to plunge into the cold bath, like Falstaff, hissing hot, than when the body is chilly and cold. Generally, let the system be sufficiently warm and vigorous, to be able to resist the shock of the cold bath, and to secure that salutary reaction, which is distinguished by the succeeding glow.

Many important lessons are comprehended under this rule. For the general doctrine connected with it, we refer our readers to the writings of Dr Currie. But we quote the following very pertinent remarks from Dr Buchan:

" Many of the circumstances, which perhaps, unavoidably precede the present mode of bathing, seem calculated to induce a state of the system, the very reverse of what has just been insisted on as the most proper, with which it is eligible to enter the water. The machines, as they are called, which are provided for conveying bathers into the sea, are frequently composed of canvass; at least, the extensive awning with which they are in some places furnished, and which, as subservient to the purposes of shelter and decency, they certainly ought never to be without, is always constructed of this material. Being necessarily exposed to all kinds of weather, they are occasionally so completely pervaded by rain, that several days of sunshine are required to render them perfectly dry. They will, moreover, be found, in general replete with moist exhalations, arising from wet clothes and damp boards, the perpetual evaporation of which, is so productive of cold, that I have frequently observed the thermometer indicate their temperature, as being from three to five degrees under that of the open air.

" Of these vehicles, such as they are, a sufficient number is never to be found in readiness to accommodate the bathers in uninterrupted succession. As persons are only entitled to a machine, in the order in which their names are set down, numbers must necessarily be always waiting in expection of their turn. This interval is generally passed in loitering in an apartment rendered cold by the exclusion of the rays of the sun, the exhalation of moisture from various sources, and a perpetual thorough draught of air. The apprehension, which many timid people have of going into the sea, is further increased by the abatement of spirits, consequent to that kind of slight disappointment, which arises from not having an opportunity of bathing at the moment when the mind was made up to it. All these circumstances tend to impair the energies of life, and consequently, to diminish the advantages to be expected from the cold immersion. Such inconveniences do not perhaps admit of being completely corrected; it is, however, proper to point them out, in order to put the more delicate, and especially invalids, on their guard; to prevent them from imputing evils to sea bathing, which in fact, originate from their own improper conduct; and at the same time,

time, to enable them to use such precautions as are within their power, in order to obviate those evils.

"By continuing a due degree of exercise, the heat of the body should be kept up to its highest point, till the moment of entering the bathing machine. If the clothes be taken off too soon, an interval elapses between the time of undressing, and of immersion in the water, during which, the body is liable to be chilled by exposure to the air. But the preferable plan is, after undressing as quickly as possible, immediately to wrap the body in a large dry flannel gown, which should not be laid aside, till the very moment previous to plunging into the water. By this means, the shock of immersion will be diminished, and the occurrence of the salutary glow, which ought always to succeed bathing, may in general be insured."

Bathers are guilty of other dangerous imprudencies, which are well exposed by our author. But, for many other just observations, and useful cautions, we must refer our readers to the work itself.

We pass over the 4th Chapter, on the complaints in which sea bathing is beneficial, as containing nothing of sufficient novelty or importance, to detain the medical reader. We wish, for the benefit of those to whom this volume seems more immediately addressed, that Dr Buchan had extended his observations "on some of the bad effects of sea bathing," the subject of his 5th Chapter. We agree with Dr Buchan, that sea bathing is a remedy not very useful, and sometimes prejudicial, in diseases of the skin We believe, that much more benefit is to be derived from the warm, than from the cold bath, in cutaneous disorders. But we cannot agree with him, when he asserts, that ulcerations of the legs are, without exception, injured by the contact of sea water. These are often connected with general disorder of the health, and we have frequently known such ulcers heal very rapidly, under a course of sea bathing.

Many delicate people, who in other respects agree with the cold bath, are observed to have their ancles swelled, and œdematous. These slight œdematous appearances, are speedily removed by the warm bath.

Sea water is not used as a bath only, it is taken also internally, as a medicine, by those who frequent the coast for the recovery of their health; and some farther benefit may perhaps be derived from change of air by those invalids who come to the sea, from interior and elevated situations.

Two more chapters are, accordingly, added by Dr Buchan, the one on the internal use of sea water, the other on sea breezes.

Sea water is used as a purgative and alterative, and thus may prove beneficial in some chronic disorders, in scrofula and in glandular obstructions. Our knowledge of the medicinal effects of sea water is, however, not very precise. Our author assures us, that it answers particularly well as a purgative, when the bowels are loaded with viscid phlegm, and that the use of it frequently restores health and appetite. "But in irritable, hectic, and what are termed bilious habits, it heats the body, and occasions considerable, and sometimes permanent, disorders of the digestive organs."

It is sometimes useful in worm cases, and in the beginning of mesenteric obstruction, or the early stage of the atrophy of children, and in cutaneous complaints.

In popular language, we hear much of the purity and salubrity of sea breeze, and our philosophy, some time ago, supported the opinion. The air was washed and purified by the water of the ocean; the fixed air, the product of animal respiration, and of combustion, and other noxious effluvia, were absorbed by the sea, and the atmosphere purified. Dr Buchan seems firmly persuaded of all this, and has amused himself with experimenting, fruitlessly enough, on the absorbing power of sea water. He quotes, too, the eudiometrical experiments of Ingenhouz; but these have not been confirmed; and the most correct observations, with improved eudiometrical instruments, lead us rather to believe, that the constitution of the atmosphere is almost every where the same, at least, that the proportion of good respirable air is not greater on the sea coast, at sea even, than elsewhere. Whatever benefit, therefore, may be derived from sea breezes, this is not to be attributed to the greater purity of the air.

The density and pressure of the atmosphere is greater, indeed, on the coast, than in more elevated situations in the interior; the sea breeze is cooler than the air of large and populous towns; it is frequently loaded with vapour, and even with saline particles. And these are the only sensible qualities to which we are, at present, able to refer any peculiarity of effect it may have on emigrants. The subject of change of air is an obscure, but curious one. The effect of changing the air, as it is called, is in some complaints too striking to be denied. But the inhabitant of the sea coast will experience the same benefit from emigrating to the interior, which the invalid, from the country, reaps from a journey to the sea coast, and that, too, under the same condition of health.

Our author having now discussed every thing relating to the subject of sea bathing, closes his volume with a few remarks on the use of the warm bath. He briefly exposes those prejudices which are entertained, with regard to the effects of warm bathing, and to the time and manner of using it; and lays down those juster opinions, which science and observation have developed. Properly used, the warm bath is not relaxing and debilitating, but

invigorating

invigorating and refreshing to the invalid, and to those exhausted by previous fatigue. Nor is there that danger of catching cold after immersion, that is commonly apprehended. The fittest time, therefore, for warm bathing, is not in the evening, before going to bed, but an hour or two before dinner. A very few practical observations are added, on those disorders in which the warm bath has been found peculiarly beneficial.

IV.

Surgical Observations.—Part the Second; containing an account of the disorders of the health in general, and of the digestive organs in particular, which accompany local diseases, and obstruct their cure:—Observations on diseases of the Urethra, particularly of that part which is surrounded by the prostate gland:—And observations relative to the treatment of one species of the Nævi Materni. By John Abernethy, F. R. S. &c. *London*, 1806.—8vo. Pages 245.

If Surgeons of the present age, were indeed as ignorant of medecine, as Mr Abernethy would have us believe, or if entirely occupied hitherto with their knives and saws, ointments and plasters, they had paid little or no attention to the general health of the system, had overlooked the influence of internal disorders on local diseases, and the reciprocal action of external diseases on the vital and natural functions; or if having remarked what indeed was too obvious to escape observation, they still were unable to prescribe a dose of physic in a surgical case, without the advice and authority of the physician, we might with Mr Abernethy regret this evil consequence of the artificial division of the healing art into the medical and surgical departments. We think much more favourably, however, of the attainments of our surgeons, and on this side the Tweed at least, we cannot complain of their attention being so exclusively directed to their own art, as to have rendered them either unwilling, or unable, to undertake the medical treatment of their own patients. But Mr Abernethy would insinuate, that from this artificial division of the healing art, the effects of local disorders upon the constitution have been too little attended to; "and indeed" he adds, "I know of no book, to "which I can refer a surgical student for a satisfactory account "of those febrile and nervous affections, which local disease pro-"duces, except that of Mr Hunter."—Yet the doctrine and treat-

 ment

ment of symptomatic fever are laid down in almost every surgical work, that is not a mere book of bloody operations; and no well educated surgeon can be ignorant of those various febrile affections of the system, of their influence on local diseases, or of the indications arising from a knowledge of the reciprocal action of constitutional and local disorders. Who, in truth, is ignorant of the use of those general remedies, of venesection, and the antiphlogistic regimen; of clysters, cooling laxatives, and occasional purging; of wine, opium, bark, and mercury; of good air, appropriate diet, and exercise, in the treatment of local diseases? Or what surgeons need be told, that blows on the head, and injuries of the brain, bring on sickness and vomiting; or that wounds of the omentum are attended with hiccup, retchings, and other symptoms of disorder of the primæ viæ; that the irritation of a sordid ulcer will affect the general health; or that a white and furred tongue with inappetency and other dyspeptic symptoms, indicate derangement of the digestive organs, and that these and costiveness are relieved by purgatives, and bitters; or that these symptoms often accompany local disorders, and react upon them?

We do not mean by this exordium, to bring discredit on Mr Abernethy's book, or to insinuate, that he has written an useless, or unnecessary one; but we think, he has depreciated the previous state of our knowledge of this subject, with the view of enhancing the value of his own observations, and attributed, unjustly, the imagined ignorance of surgeons of the mutual influence of constitutional and local diseases, to the too exclusive practice of their own art. We allow to Mr Abernethy, the merit of having taken a more comprehensive view of the subject, of having traced pathologically the steps of connexion between local and general disease, and of having laid open to the profession, a field of new and interesting observation and inquiry. He has embodied our looser knowledge into a more compact system, and enriched the whole by his own observations. Mr Abernethy's general theory seems to be, that the irritation arising from local disease, through the medium of the sensorium and nervous system, produces often great disorder of the digestive organs, which reacts on, aggravates, and keeps up the local disease, whence this general derangement originally proceeds.

The symptoms characterising this disorder of the chylopoietic organs are those which belong to dyspepsia; diminution of appetite and digestion, flatulence, unnatural colour, and fetor of the excretions, costiveness; a dry, foul, and furred tongue; pain of the epigastrium on pressure; and turbid urine. On each of these symptoms, Mr Abernethy comments at considerable length; and he he particularly calls the attention of his reader to the state of the tongue, and the colour, and other sensible appearances of the alvine discharge. The inspection of these last will furnish, to the practitioner, indications of the state of the biliary system so often interested in this disorder, and of the degree of the failure of the digestive and assimilative processes. "The colour of the alvine ex-"cretions in these disordered states of the viscera is various.—"Sometimes they appear to consist of the residue of the food, "untinged, in the least degree, with bile. Sometimes they are of "a light yellow colour, which denotes a very deficient quantity "of healthy biliary secretion; they may also be of a deep olive, "of a clay brown, and of a blackish brown; all which shew a vi-"tiated state of the biliary secretion."

These disordered states of the chylopoietic viscera, to which our author invokes the attention of the surgeon, as accompanying local diseases, and obstructing their cure, may subsist without any organic change taking place. Mr A. has examined the bodies of a considerable number of those who have died of local diseases complicated with this disorder of the primæ viæ, in which the secretion of the bile had been altogether suppressed, or faulty in quality, without discovering any alteration of structure. In other cases, however, where the disordered state of the bowels had been of longer duration, he has found the villous coat of the intestines swoln, pulpy, turgid with blood, apparently inflamed, and sometimes ulcerated. The liver has also been found diseased and tuberculated.

The general inferences are thus summed up:—

1. "Sudden and violent local irritation will produce an equally sudden and vehement affection of the digestive organs.

2. "A slighter degree of continued local irritation, will produce a less violent affection.

3. "This affection is a disorder in the actions, and not a disease in the structure of the affected organs; although it may, when long continued, induce evident diseased appearances, both which circumstances are proved by dissections.

4. "A similar disorder of the digestive organs occurs without local irritation, and exists as an idiopathic disease, in which case, it is characterized by the same symptoms.

5. "There are some varieties in the symptoms of this disorder, both when it is sympathetic and idiopathic.

6. "The disorder probably consists in an affection of all the digestive organs in general, though in particular cases, it may be more manifest in some of those organs, than in others.

7. "That disorder of the digestive organs frequently affects the nervous system, producing irritability, and various consequent affections. This is proved by the effects of blows on the belly in persons previously healthy; and the same consequences are often observed, from whatever cause the disorder originates.—

At

At the same time, weakness must be produced from imperfect digestion; and from the combination of these causes, viz. weakness and irritation, I deduce the origin of many local diseases, and the aggravation of all."

Such disorder of the chylopoietic viscera, whether idiopathic or induced by the irritation of local diseases, is productive of a great variety of morbid symptoms, abolition of the functions of the brain, delirium, muscular weakness, irritation, and pain, tremors, and palsies, and aggravation of existing local diseases; and in particular, from continuity of surface of the stomach, local diseases of the throat, mouth, lips, nose, ears, and skin, may be orginally caused, or aggravated by this complaint.

In the treatment of these disorders of the digestive organs, which are connected with surgical diseases, Mr Abernethy, considering the disordered parts to be in a state of irritability and weakness, directs his measures to diminish the former, and allay the latter. A simple regimen, and that diet which best agrees with each patient, moderate exercise, and a due regard to former habits, are recommended. Regularity of the alvine discharge is included—And nature, when necessary, must be assisted by laxative medicines. The object is to excite the peristaltic motion of the bowels without purging. In giving purgative medicines, he endeavours to combine them, so as to excite, and strengthen at the same time. Thus, rhubarb, colombo, and kali vitriol. are given together, or an infusion of gentian with senna, or tincture of rhubarb, or the following draught twice or thrice a day.

Rec. Infus. Gentian. comp.—Unc. unam.
Infus. Sennæ.—Drachm. duas.
Tinct. Cardamom. comp.—Drachm. unam.

When the biliary secretion is defective or faulty, it is to be corrected by such small doses of mercury as do not irritate the bowels, and are not likely to affect the constitution, even though persevered in for a considerable time.

In short, the general remedies employed in dyspeptic complaints are useful in this; tonics, the bark and chalybeates, are of the number—and with regard to the vegetable diet-drinks often used in local diseases, Mr A. observes, that it is by amending the disorders of the stomach and bowels, that they are efficacious.—"When diet-drinks fail to correct the disorders of the digestive organs, they also fail to produce any amendment on local diseases."

In illustration of the general doctrine, Mr Abernethy next relates a variety of cases. These are classed in different sections:

1st, Cases of paralytic and other affections of the nervous system, connected with disorder of the digestive organs, and relieved or cured by the restoration of these functions.

A young lady whose stomach and bowels were disordered, complained of pain in the loins, and weakness of the lower extremities, and perceived no relief from blisters applied to the spine; the bone however was not diseased, and she recovered by general treatment.

A young man, whose limbs were palsied, had been previously subject to severe disorder of the bowels, after which had supervened headach, imperfect vision, paralysis of the lower extremities, and of the bladder, impaired speech, and weakness also of the arms. When admitted into the hospital, there was complete paralysis of the lower extremities, and great debility of the upper; the bowels were also much disordered. Two grains of calomel, with eight of rhubarb, were taken twice a week; and infusion of gentian with senna occasionally. At the end of three weeks, the bowels became regular, the biliary secretion healthy, and his appetite good; the eye sight was much improved; the hands and arms became nearly as strong as ever; the functions of the bladder were restored; the speech became articulate; there was no amendment however in the state of the lower extremities.

The next case was also one of palsy of the lower extremities, supposed to originate from disease of the spine; she was subject also to attacks resembling epileptic paroxysms; the bowels were greatly disordered—She was attacked in the hospital with fever, and died.

There was no diseased appearance detected in the brain, and no disease of the vertebræ. The intestines were inflamed and ulcerated, and the bile was of light green colour, and very fluid.—Such cases Mr A. is led to believe, from his own observations, are very frequent. In such, there is no organic disease of the brain, and the nervous affections seem rather to depend on the disorder of the digestive organs. Cases also of wasting and imbecillity of the limbs, of muscular affections, and nervous pains of the nature of the tic douloureux, Mr A. has known cured, by correcting the unhealthy state of the digestive organs. He suggests too the propriety of attending to the state of the bowels in tetanus

2d, Cases in which Local Disorders of the Head, produced by blows are kept up, and aggravated, by affections of the digestive organs

The sympathy existing between the head and the stomach, has been long observed. Vomiting, and other symptoms of disorder of of the last, are the immediate consequences of injury done to the first. And the cases produced in this section are intended to show that this disturbance of the stomach, even when moderate in degree, will often re-act upon the head, so as to occasion an irritable state of the injured parts, and impede their recovery.—The secondary symptoms, which are recorded in these cases as seperverning to blows on the head, sometimes after the first accident had been forgotten, and conected with symptoms of disorder of the stomach and bowels, are nearly the same which accompany the slow inflammation of the brain, and membranes, or contused and necrosed bone, consequent to such accidents. But here the symptoms seem to depend rather upon irritation, communicated by the disordered state of the digestive organs, than on local disease of the head: This Mr Abernethy at least thinks may be fairly inferred from their ceasing so immediately when the disorder of the digestive organs is corrected. Such symptoms then may be the effect of local inflammation, and disease, or of sympathetic irritation only. But we see no grounds for discriminating the cases, except what are derived from the result of the treatment.

The last case was a recent accident, and appears to us an example of pure concussion; the man was very freely and repeatedly bled, and then purged with calomel and rhubarb. He passed much highly offensive feculent matter, of a light greenish yellow colour. By persevering in the use of purgatives, till the discharges became healthy, the man got well. Purgatives we believe are very commonly given in such cases. We have often employed them with the best effects.

3d. Already Mr Abernethy has called the attention of practitioners, to certain diseases of an equivocal nature, in appearance venereal, yet, in the apprehension of some celebrated practitioners, not syphilitic. Already we have stated our opinion on this subject. And we have not yet been able to learn from Mr Abernethy, what are the circumstances that determine him to consider this a syphilitic, and that a pseudo-syphilitic case, unless it be the declaration of the patient himself, and the event of the disease, ceasing without the assistance of medicine. In the 3d section of the book now before us, he states, that a disorder of the digestive organs constantly exists in those pseudo-syphilitic diseases of the throat, skin, and bones, and produces, or at least aggravates, and protracts, a state of weakness and irritability of constitution; to which the origin of the disease must undoubtedly be referred.—Of the cases which are now brought forward, we remark, that in some, mercury had been employed with good effect, particularly in the first; and that in others, the recovery cannot fairly be attributed

buted to the treatment directed merely to the bowels, as the disease is by petition one which exhausts itself, or which ceases spontaneously. And it is still a question how far the venereal disease itself may be modified in particular constitutions, so as to get well without mercury.

4th, The next class of cases is that of unhealthy indurations, abscesses and sores, local diseases which often break out in succession, in different parts of the body; and this, it is remarked, is a circumstance strongly presumptive of their being connected with some error of the health in general. Accordingly, Mr A. states, that he has observed that they are seldom unattended with disorder of the digestive organs. "I can confidently affirm" he adds, "that those diseases in general become tractable, in proportion as "the disorder of the viscera is corrected; and that frequently no "new local symptoms occur, after some attention has been paid "to the state of the digestive organs."—Several cases are related in illustration of this remark:—Cases of spreading ulcerations, cutaneous affections, ulcerated tubercles, carbuncles; scrofulous affections, sequelæ of small pox, painful indurations of the breast, and other diseases of a like kind, which had resisted the usual local treatment, but appearing complicated with disorder of the viscera and biliary secretion, were relieved or cured by general treatment, by small doses of mercury, occasional laxatives, and infusion of gentian.

5th, *Disorders of parts which have a continuity of surface with the Alimentary Canal.*

The cases and observations given under this head, are spasmodic strictures of the œsophagus, of which an interesting example is communicated; diseases of the mouth and throat, carbuncles, ulcerations, and herpetic eruptions of the nose, ozæna, ophthalmia, herpetic, and other diseases of the skin: Such cases often appear connected with the disorder of the general health, and more especially with that derangement of the digestive organs, the influence of which, on local diseases, it has been the object of our author to investigate.

6th, *On the causation of other diseases, by those of the digestive organs.*

Apoplexy, palsy, and epilepsy, are commonly direct diseases of the brain, from morbid alteration of its stricture. Yet these diseases do sometimes take place, without any visible change in the structure of that organ being detected on dissection. The experience

rience of Mr Abernethy has amply confirmed the observation; and he concludes, therefore, "That disorder, and abolition of the nervous functions, may take place, without any organic affection of the brain." The connection between the brain, and the stomach, and the mutual influence, and reciprocal action of disorders of the brain, and chylopoietic viscera, have been long observed, and acknowledged. And we are thoroughly convinced, that physicians would do well to keep this constantly in memory. We believe, that much light may thus be thrown on the pathology of some obscure diseases; and that important practical applications may be deduced from a careful observation of the connexion, between primary disorder of the chylopoietic viscera, and cerebral diseases.

The interesting observations on the marasmus of childhood, and youth, delivered by Dr Hamilton, in his book, on the administration and utility of purgative medicines, must be fresh in the memory of most of our readers. He has there advanced, that this which is originally a disorder of the digestive organs, is not only often attended with symptoms resembling those of hydrocephalus internus, but may, on some occasions, actually give rise to that disease, by impairing the vigour of the constitution, and by favouring the effusion of water, into the ventricles of the brain. In our review of that publication, we have stated our opinion, that derangement of the biliary organs is particularly interested in the causation of this disease. Knowing therefore, the full importance of the subject, we have been much gratified with Mr Abernethy's general observations, and shall quote, without farther comment, that passage which more particularly relates to the doctrine in question.

"I have examined the bodies of six patients, in whom disease most certainly began in the abdominal viscera, and was continued in them, to the conclusion of their lives. Nevertheless, the patients seemed to die rather of nervous disorder, than of disease of the parts first affected. One of the patients died, affected with apoplectic symptoms, and five with hemiplegia."

"In all these cases the liver was greately diseased, and the bowels also exhibited a diseased appearance. In three of the cases, there was considerable inflammation of the membranes of the brain; and a good deal of water in the ventricles. In two of them, no morbid appearance of the brain was discovered. I have also examined a child, who was supposed to have died of the hydrocephalus, accompanied by great disorder of the stomach, and bowels. In this case, the bowels were inflamed, the liver sound, and the brain perfectly healthy in appearance; yet there had been so great a diminution of sensation and motion, as to leave no doubt of the existence of hydrocephalus."

These observations on the influence of disorders of the digestive organs, are brought to a conclusion, by a few remarks on their relation to pulmonary complaints, and diseases of the heart and arteries. The connection between pulmonary affections, and disorder of the liver, was first suggested to Mr A. by Mr Boodle of Ongar, in Essex. The observations, and dissections, made by Mr Abernethy, have also tended to prove, that the chylopoietic viscera were the seat of the greatest and most established disease, and that the pulmonary affection was a secondary disorder. The liver was greatly diseased, and the lungs were also beset with tubercles, yet a considerable portion of those organs was sound.

We learn also from Mr A. that Dr Curry, of Guy's Hospital, has prosecuted the same tract of investigation, and we are happy to understand, that he is now preparing to lay before the public, his "Observations on the Influence of the Hepatic Functions, on various forms of Disease."

On Diseases of the Urethra, particularly of that part which is surrounded by the prostate gland.

THE disease described under this title, is characterised by dysuria, and the common signs of irritable bladder; there is often a sense of torpor and pain of the perinæum; the bougie is arrested at the neck of the bladder, occasions great pain, and when withdrawn, its point is covered with blood and mucus. In these cases, there is stricture and irritability of that part of the urethra, which is surrounded by the prostate.

Sometimes the prostate is, at the same time, diseased, and enlarged. It may be complicated also with strictures in other parts of the urethra, or with disease of the bladder itself; but more frequently it exists as an original and independent disease. The stricture is removed, and the irritable state of the parts subdued by the introduction of the bougie; but sometimes the symptoms are rather aggravated by it, and at others, it fails to produce the expected relief—warm bathing of the perinæum is also recomended.

The species of Nævi Materni, described by Mr Abernethy, is that congenital deformity which consists in a cluster of enlarged vessels, filled, and occasionally distended, by the influx of blood, from numerous surrounding arteries. Two cases are related. The one a monstrous enlargement of the vessels, distributed every where beneath the fore arm, from the wrist to the elbow, so that the diseased arm was twice the size of the other. The vessels were large, and, contorted, and according to the expression of the child's mother,

mother, they resembled the entrails of a pig. The skin was of a dusky hue: pressure forced the blood out of the vessels, and temporarily diminished the bulk of the limb.

Continued pressure by the adhesive bandage, and cooling applications to the limb, were attended with complete success. The arm was reduced to its natural size, and the contorted vessels felt like solid chords interposed between the skin and fascia of the fore arm. In the other case, this unnatural state of the vessels was in the orbit of the eye. The clustered vessels projected out of the orbit, forming a tumour, as large as a walnut. The disease was upon the increase when Mr A. was consulted. Pressure could not be used in this case; but he recommended that folded linen, wetted with rose water saturated with alum, should be bound on the projecting part, and kept constantly damp. Under this treatment, the tumour gradually shrunk, and eventually disappeared. In some instances, however, such marks disappear spontaneously, and without the assistance of art.

V.

Pepinieren zum Unterricht ärztlicher Routiniers, als Bedürfnisse des Staates, nach seiner Lage wie sie ist. *Vom* Professor Reil, 8vo. *Halle*, 1804, p. 140.

At a time when the propriety and practicability of a medical reform are agitated so generally, and so keenly, the pamphlet now before us has peculiar claims to attention. It is written by one of the most enlightened medical philosophers in Germany, and its object is to prove, that in Prussia at least, seminaries, or institutions, for the education of what he calls *Medical Routiniers*, are requisite in the present state of society. It is addressed in a pointed dedication to the celebrated Hufeland, as the chief of the Medico-Chirurgical College of Berlin, and calls upon him to exert the influence connected with his situation, so that medical instruction be freed from whatever is obsolete, and be carried to the same degree of perfection, as other branches of scientific education.

In society, there are rich and poor citizens; individuals who practice medicine as a science, and others, who exercise it as a trade; universities, and less dignified seminaries. The wealthy citizen, and scientific practitioner, suit each other exactly. The one commands the best assistance, and the other receives an adequate

quate reward for his knowledge. But how small is the number of the opulent compared with the poor? The multitude pay their medical attendants ill, or not at all, and cannot do otherwise. But who would advise a young man possessed of talents, and capable of turning them to good account, to devote himself to an art, the study of which is expensive, and the exercise fatiguing, to spend his labour unrequited on the poor, to suffer both in body and mind, to lose both capital and interest. As a citizen, the medical practitioner contributes his proportion towards the legal support of the poor. If, from humanity, or any other motive, he also attends them *gratis*, he does more than the state can require of him. But the natural desire of self-preservation makes the poor, when sick, as well as the rich, seek for medical advice, for which they are, therefore, forced to have recourse to a variety of unqualified persons. The state is thus obliged, on the one hand, to connive at these irregularities and abuses, and on the other, feels its want of power to apply a radical remedy to the evil. What is to be done in these circumstances? It has been proposed to defray the expence of medicines for the poor, and to provide district physicians to attend them. But can this be required of the state, any more than the unconditional support of the poor in general? Could the state even do it, if it were willing? Allowing but one physician to a thousand people, how much would Prussia have to pay for medicines and medical attendance, for nine millions of people? Since, therefore, the poor cannot pay a scientific practitioner, and since there is none else to pay for them, are we to rest satisfied with what has already been done for them? Certainly not. The state has considered it as its duty to institute universities for the education of scientific physicians for the rich. And, it is surely not unreasonable to demand, that seminaries should also be instituted, in which *routiniers* should be educated for the service of the multitude.

Instruction in any art can be communicated in two ways only, either both the theory and practice are taught entire and undivided, or only the mechanical part of the art, without the principles, is imparted to the pupil, with the same limitations as the sphere in which he is in future to act. All other distinctions, as into military or civil, medical and surgical schools, are either false or injudicious. All attempts at uniting universities and seminaries are abortive, and perish from the incongruities of their constitutions. The same instructions are not united to the scientific and mechanical pupil. They must either be unintelligible to the one, or uninteresting to the other. What, it may be objected, is it seriously proposed to erect seminaries for the education of empiricks, who, from want of science, may commit murder? Is it in-

 tended

tended to sanction such institutions by public authority? Even By this arrangement, individuals may perish, whom more skillf physicians might have saved. But even now they perish, and tho sands besides. Let the many be saved in the first place, and th the few. While we look with indifference on the present state of poor, routine practitioners are not to be despised. Instructed *routi niers* are surely preferable to the numbers who now practice wi instruction, more especially, when we consider, that althoug there are many learned physicians, there are none truly scien fic, whose theory and practice are one and indivisable. What that power in nature which imparts life to animals, and motio to the universe? What the process which each moment wastes the individual, and, by the same act, recruits him; which excites and removes diseases, and by which external nature, and of course remedies, operate on organization? Till these questions be answered in a satisfactory manner, with regard to the individual to be treated, all pretensions to perfect rationality in practice must be renounced. This deficiency is the reason why experienced empiricks so often practise better than superficial theorists. The medical science of both is on a level; but the latter do not act so well as the former, because they mistake the glare of hypothesis for the light of truth. But in recommending the formation of *routiniers*, it is by no means conceived, that they alone are sufficient for the necessities of the state. If left entirely to themselves, they would become careless and indifferent, and each succeeding generation, by copying the bad, as well as the good, would be worse than that which preceded it. Men of learning and science are absolutely necessary, both for the formation of *routiniers*, and as active powers in the machinery for improving the art, possessing, in themselves, the means of their own improvement, and capable of approximating the mass to their own standard.

The learned physician, in contradistinction to the *routinier*, is said to be the scientific physician. Scientific, however, he is not, but must have a tendency to become so, and must endeavour, by uninterrupted approximation, to produce in himself his ideal prototype. Let the object of the scientific pupil's exertions be the science itself, with which no reference to its application must interfere. Let him endeavour to develope it in himself, to identify it with his mind, which he is to constitute its living organ inseparable from it. Hence, let the teacher be not merely the instrument of instruction, but rather serve as an example how the whole mind must be devoted to science. Only in this way can he become, what he ought to be, actual proprietor, and not merely tenant of what has been communicated to him; creator

in

in himself of a portrait of nature which shall resemble its original. Let him enter his proper school after he has become possessed of all the literary aids, whose acquisition excites the genius, and renders easy the access to the sources of science, which should be opened to him by philosophy. Let the knowledge of those truths, with which the ancients were acquainted, serve him as means to obtain his ends; and let the history of the errors of the human mind caution him against the numerous paths by which he would in vain attempt to attain his object. But in this, let him guard against excess. For this colossus encreases with the revolutions of time, and absorbs every power which would have had a nobler purpose in the appropriation of real knowledge. So long as science is not developed in its whole extent, only the method to be employed in seeking it can be laid down, but by no means the method of communicating it.

The philosophical physician must combine cautious speculation with pure empiricism. The latter will take up the facts at the limits beyond which speculation cannot penetrate, while the former will guide him from generals to particulars, from principles to phœnomena. Operating thus in harmony with each other, empiricism will compare the laws developed by ratiocination with experience, while each fact promulgated by experience will find a philosophical sanction in speculation. The philosophical physician is himself the prototype of the school in which alone he can be educated. Its organization must be on a level with the state of the science itself, and keep equal pace with it in its progress towards perfection. To science and art it must unite learning. This triad is exclusively the right and the duty of Universities, in regard to the education of scientific physicians.

The medical *routinier* is characterized partly by his practice being mechanical, partly by being confined within the sphere in which he is employed as an instrument. Like the scientific physician, he must possess sufficient natural endowments. He must represent to himself an object and the means of obtaining it; but only as a psychological automaton, who, like the land-surveyor and arithmetician, knows the rules according to which he acts, but is ignorant of the principles from which these rules are derived. He must be able to distinguish the varieties of disease by the symptoms, although he does not comprehend their causes, and know the effects of remedies against them, although he is ignorant of their mode of action. He is occupied with art, not with erudition; with what is, not what should be; with the fact, not the cause; with the existence, not the possibility; with the individual, not the genus; with what is real, not what is ideal.

ideal. The *routinier* is merely a means employed in the service of others, and his education must therefore be limited to its object. By carrying it farther, he may indeed become more useful in himself; but in reality, less useful for the purpose to which he is destined. *Routiniers* must therefore be classed according to the degree of their perfection, and be appointed to corresponding situations. An arrangement must be made of the applications of medicine, the most indispensible being placed in the centre, the least necessary and general in the circumference, so that the studies of the *routinier* may be confined within a narrower circle or extended, according to circumstances. But this arrangement must not have any reference to the division of medicine into several branches, but merely to the degree of dexterity. For the *routinier* must be a healing artist in the most extensive sense of the term, and in possession of all the means of curing. He must be physician, surgeon, accoucheur; for the poor, for whose service he is destined, cannot afford to pay different individuals for different species of assistance. Lastly, in his appearance, manners, language, and mode of thinking, in short, in his manner of communication, he must exactly resemble the common people, that he may not be offended by their coarseness, and may react upon them with greater energy. Thus will he gain their confidence, and contribute, more than the learned physician, to crush quackery.

According to this plan, since the practice of the *routinier* is confined within a certain sphere, he will in a short time acquire an uncommon degree of dexterity, and become eminently useful, if, in his formation, natural abilities, and adequate instruction be united; and from this sketch of him must the organization of his school be deduced. For the good of the state, academies for *routiniers* are more necessary than universities for learned physicians. The latter may be educated abroad, the former must be instructed at home. These academies must not be situated in the same place with a university, lest the routinier be excited to envy, and to depart out of his sphere. The teacher in these academies requires more power and self command, than in universities. He must be a philosopher, and a scientific physician: He must possess a microscopical accuracy in elucidating particulars, as well as a mind capable of comprehending the whole. His mode of delivery must be positive, not argumentative; dogmatical, not critical; popular, not learned. He must be acquainted with the sphere of his action, and allow nothing to draw him out of it. He must possess peculiar talents, and must have been instructed how to apply them. The state must reward him according to his deserts; but he must devote himself to instruction, and be interdicted from writing for his bread, or practis-

ing

ing, except in the hospital, or engaging in any other occupation whatever.

The education of the routinier must be limited to what is practically useful. He has nothing to do with the history or literature of medicine, with medical police or jurisprudence, comparative anatomy, the veterinary art, and many other subjects of the like nature. The course of instruction must therefore be fixed according to the future destination of the *routinier*. After an adequate preliminary education, he must be taught the natural philosophy of man in its healthy state, comprehending anatomy and physiology; the same in its morbid state, in conjunction with therapeutics, and the means of cure. These may be divided into mechanical, physico-chemical, and mental. Of the latter, he must learn only what is most indispensable. He must be made acquainted with the indigenous and officinal plants, and learn something of poisons and their cure. He must collect the officinal plants for the hospital, and prepare them for use, that he may be accustomed to cheap remedies, such as the poor can afford. With materia medica, chemistry pharmacy the art of writing receipts and dispensing medicines are connected. He should prepare the chemical medicines for the hospital. With the rare and difficult operations he has nothing to do; but he must be well instructed in the treatment of wounds, ulcers, dislocations and fractures, in the art of applying bandages, and in the taxis of hernia. He must be versed in the diagnosis and treatment of easy and quick labours, but must call in assistance in the difficult. His dietetical information must be directed to the field in which he is to act. It would be preposterous to caution the postillion against the danger of getting wet, or the poor against indulgence in eating; but let him exterminate their prejudices, and instruct them in the attentions due to the sick.

There is an absolute want of books proper for the use of the *routinier*. They ought to be published under authority, and written according to a positive plan, by the professor of the institute, in the pure spirit of empiricism, and with a reference solely to the mechanism of practice. They will serve to direct the professor in his instructions, and as manuals to the pupils, who must not be permitted to take notes in the lecture room: There must be an hospital connected with the institution for practical instruction, where the pupil may be exercised in bathing, rubbing with the flesh brush, and other parts of the mechanical treatment of the sick. The course of instruction may last from three to five years, and may require four professors.

The institution must be placed under the superintendance of the state, which must support it. But the hospital will serve as a poors hospital, and the pupil, or his parish, should pay so much of his necessary expences, as may excite his industry, but not be disproportionate to his future income. Universities must be prohibited from receiving pupils from the institution, lest it should encourage desertion, and excite *doctromania*. But occasionally the most distinguished may be sent to them, not arbitrarily, but according to fixed regulations.

There must be daily examinations and exercises; and, at the termination of each division of the course, a more formal examination, of which the result must be recorded. At the completion of the whole, is the final examination, when the pupils are to be divided according to their merits into classes, to which there are corresponding posts. He who deserves most should earn most; and the parish which can afford most, has a right to demand most. This is but reasonable for both parties. On his leaving the institution, he must get a suitable collection of instruments, and of practical books, written in the style already observed, for which an adequate price must be paid.

The state must be divided into districts, such as a *routinier* is capable of attending; but he must neither be tied down to his district, nor his district to him, despotism in matters of health is worse than any other despotism. Monopolies extinguish, competition awakens genius. If the treatment of the parish poor forms part of his duty, he must be paid for it by the parish.

"Where *routiniers* and scientific physicians practise in the "same place, the public may chuse which of them it will, as "now it chooses between the physician and corporation surgeon. "Can we, without being guilty of an absurdity, grant or refuse "leave to practise to the same individual, because it happens to "be in the country or in the town? Must not, in both places, the "rules of practise be the same? Must not rational beings, of "equal rank, be every where treated in the same manner? Phy- "sicians who must be protected by external aid, are not worth "protection. Let them maintain their own superiority. This "mutual relation will awaken an emulation advantageous to the "art, and to the public. Over the shallow pupil of the barber's "shop, the physician easily triumphs, but he will be afraid of the "able *routinier*, lest he get the better of him, if he be indolent or "incapable. In like manner such institutions will excite the uni- "versities to greater exertion, that they may preserve their superi- "ority, and rise above the sphere of empiricism."

We have thus endeavoured to give an abstract of Dr Reil's opinions; but of our success, we are extremely doubtful. The eloquence, the enthusiasm of his style, cannot be transfused into a tame analysis, as ours necessarily has been, while his faults, the

occasional

occasional insufficiency of his arguments, and the want of arrangement, are not concealed. We have purposely avoided giving any opinion on the merits of the plan. Its boldness and originality cannot be denied; its practability, and even its utility, may be doubted. Medical reform is so vast, so intricate a subject, involving so directly, not only the undoubted privileges of so many corporate bodies, but the interests of the whole profession, indeed of the whole community, that we must candidly confess our opinions regarding it, are as yet unsettled and unsatisfactory, even to ourselves. Since, however, the question has been agitated, it should not be relinquished, until it has undergone a thorough and deliberate investigation, both as a subject of abstract speculation, and as having a direct reference to the rights and privileges, the prejudices and opinions, which already exist. To this investigation we shall impartially afford every facility in our power, convinced as we are, that the advocates for, and opposers of, medical reform, have the same objects in view, the good of the community, and the advancement of the profession.

VI.

Versuche und Beobachtungen über die Würksamkeit der thierischen Gelatina zur Heilung intermittirenden Fieber. Vom Dr Giuseppe Gautieri delegato Medico des Departements von Ancona. Uebersetzt und mit Anmerkungen begleitet vom Dr Bischoff Arzt zu Berlin.*

It would be unjust, as well as illiberal, not to acknowledge with gratitude, the many improvements in science, for which we are indebted to our rival neighbours the French, but we must also be upon our guard, not to be misled by the exaggerated praises they bestow on every discovery, however trifling, which they ascribe to any of their countrymen, and by the zeal with which they propagate these as widely as their language is understood. Indeed, to this spirit of nationality are the French sçavans, as much indebted for their celebrity, as their generals for their victories. Of the truth of this remark, the essay before us is a striking example. Seguin anounces the discovery of a fact, and draws from it

* See Journal der practischen Heilkunde herausgegeben, von C. W. Hufeland, 18ter Band, 3tes Stück, 8vo., Berlin, 1804.

it a conclusion, which leads him to adopt a particular remedy in intermittent fever, and his praises are echoed from Ancona to Berlin. Let us examine how far they are merited. The fact is simply this, an infusion of genuine cinchona bark is precipitated by an infusion of gall-nuts, but to the merit of discovery, in this instance, Seguin's pretensions must be set aside. It was previously published by our countryman Dr Maton*. Seguin, however, was certainly the first to conclude from this re-action, that cinchona contained gelatine, and that to this gelatine its febrifuge powers were owing. Now, as it has been proved, that cinchona contains no gelatine, the whole merit of Seguin's reasoning founded on that false conclusion, falls to the ground. But he was led by it to propose the use of gelatine as a substitute for cinchona, in the cure of intermittents; and as truth sometimes springs out of error, he may have thus accidentally contributed to the advancement of the healing art. Even here, however, we are not disposed to allow him credit for originality, or the skillful application of an accidental discovery. For surely no one will pretend, that Seguin was the first to prescribe light animal food in agues; and most certainly it is no improvement in its exhibition, to substitute for beef-tea, gravy soup, portable soup, and calf-feet gelly, or even for the more homely, but not less wholesome dishes, cow-heel, and ox-cheek, a nauseous and disgusting solution of carpenters glue. Instead, therefore, of agreeing in opinion with Dr Gautieri, who thinks, if gelatine and glue shall be proved capable of curing even slight intermittent fevers, Seguin's name worthy of immortality, and who classes him as an inductive philosopher with Bacon; we can only allow Seguin the praise of having extended, by a series of blunders, the opportunities for observing the effects of animal jelly in intermittent fevers.

In this point of view, the essay before us is not without interest, although many circumstances conspire to prevent us from relying implicitly on our authors accuracy. It were needless to enumerate the Italian villages in which, or the Italian doctors by whom, this remedy was found to be successful, in all the varities of Febris Tertiana, Quartana, Quotidiana, Subcontinua, and Continua; it is sufficient to quote our authors conclusions from them. "Such a variety of facts, and the unanimous testimony of so many impartial physicians, irrefragibly controvert all the arguments of those who are disposed to deny the great efficacy of glue. Who would have believed, that in the space of four months, and in this department alone, above 250 intermittents should have been

* Medical and Physical Journal, Vol. V. p. 35.

been cured by means of glue; in many cases, concentrated glue not only equals, but surpasses cinchona in point of efficacy."

As might have naturally been supposed, other animal jellies were found to be as efficacious as the fetid and nauseous carpenters glue, but we must confess, that we should not have been led by analogy to trust the cure of a double tertian to gum-arabick, which, however, we are here told was effected by Calatroni, with only two doses of half an ounce each. We could have wished, that the immediate effects of these substances on the animal economy, in its sound and morbid state, had been detailed with greater perspicuity, and in a more judicious arrangement, but the wildest hypotheses are so intermixed with facts, and the grossest ignorance so combined with observation, that it is not easy to separate the one from the other.

Sthenic intermittent fevers, he informs us, when treated with glue, assume a continued type, as do also asthenic intermittents when they are nearly cured. But this continuity lasts only one or two days, and generally ceases towards mid-day, when it seems to take on the character of synocha, which disappears without further aid. But only those sthenic intermittents treated with glue became continued, which had been previously treated with cinchona. The disease then not only assumes a more dangerous type, but is much more obstinate, and continues for several days or weeks.

"In these cases, the effects of cinchona and glue are almost identical. Both suspend the cold fit, interrupt and destroy the regularity of the paroxysms, and at last put a stop to them, as the patient approaches to a state of convalescence. I consider it is a certain indication of the action of the glue, when the cold fit is suspended, and as a harbinger of reconvalescence, when the fever becomes obviously continued, which also not unfrequently takes place, under the use of cinchona. This fever is often so inconsiderable, that the physician only, and not the patient, is aware of it. It is, however, observed that the patient is disposed to sleep, is unwilling to be disturbed, and when awaked, yawns and stretches himself, the pupils are unusually dilated, and the eyes sensible to light, sweat appears on the forehead, and moisture over the whole body, the hair shines from sweat, the countenance is unusually pale, the tongue whitish and furred at the sides, the patient complains of uneasiness, drowsiness, and want of appetite, and the pulse is small and soft, but frequent. It very seldom happens that the fever entirely abates, and suddenly disappears."

Instead of being satisfied with the fact, that glue, like cinchona, suspends the regularly of intermittent paroxysms, Dr Gautieri loses himself in a long digression, in which he attempts to explain how an animal substance should have the same action with a vegetable, and at last solves this important problem by discovering, *risum teneatis amici*, that both cinchona and glue contain a large proportion of tannin!

Glue

Glue and cinchona, we are told, both act powerfully on the stomach. As soon as glue is swallowed, an agreeable sensation of warmth diffuses itself over the stomach, and from that, not unfrequently, over the whole surface of the body. Both injure the appetite; both suppress the febrile rigors, and promote the perspiration; both operate a certain depression, and procure quiet sleep; both taken during the hot fit, rather increase it, and cause unpleasant symptoms, which are avoided when they are taken, however shortly, before the cold fit; both cause a lasting antipathy to acids, especially vegitable acids, so that those who use them during their convalescence are apt to relapse. Fevers cured by both are apt to terminate in a critical eruption about the lips, or in some other cutaneous affection; and lastly, both require the co-operation of the physician, patient, and reconvalescent, to support the powers of the stomach, and the cutaneous transpiration in their natural state.

We have also a long digression to prove, that intermittent fevers are occasioned by an *anomalous* state of the stomach and skin, and to suggest, that the superoxygenation of the gastric juice, is the cause of the periodical type of fevers; that cinchona and glue cure them by absorbing this excess of oxygen; and that the hot fit is caused by caloric being rendered free during the combination of oxygen with the constituents of the body, especially the animal gluten, and absorbed fat. "From what has been said, it appears that we are warranted in concluding, that an increased flow of oxygen to the stomach is the cause of the return of the febrile paroxysms, and therefore, in employing remedies not only to expel or absorb it, but also to neutralize it by substances containing much carbone, or azote, and lastly, to prevent the secretion of it altogether, and restore the equilibrium with the skin."

Glue is more active in proportion as it contains less water, and therefore, the patient must not be allowed to drink for some time after taking it. Seguin orders one ounce and three drachms of glue to be dissolved in two ounces of water, and this solution to be divided into three portions; the first of which is to be taken half an hour before the paroxysm, but the second 10, and the third 20 minutes after it. This is, in general, sufficient to prevent the recurrence of the paroxysm.

"Calatroni and Borsalini are perfectly satisfied, that they can prevent a second fit as certainly with glue, as with cinchona; and lastly, the observations of Raggi, Calatroni, Borsalini, Cappa, Cantone, Sant Agostino, and others, as well as my own, have sufficiently proved, that glue has cured intermittent fevers in fewer days and hours, than could have been done with cinchona, or any other known remedy."

We

We shall pass over the remainder of this prolix essay, shewing the advantages to be derived to the state by the substitution of glue for cinchona, and refuting the objections which our author thinks may be brought against it, and conclude by translating, as less exceptionable authority in its favour, an appendix written by the German translator, Dr Bischoff.

"It must be interesting to our readers to learn, that a considerable number of experiments, made by Dr Fritze, in our large hospital the Charité, on intermittents of various kinds, which have happened to be very frequent during the last few weeks, partly with gelatine prepared from fresh bones, partly with common carpenters glue, have hitherto been perfectly successful, and have completely confirmed the substance of the preceding essay. This most important subject has already attracted the notice and benevolent activity of the enlightened head of our College, and a committee of able practitioners has been appointed to investigate it thoroughly, and to publish the result of their investigation, which will soon appear in this Journal. As this remedy, which was found so active in Italy, and during the summer months, does not fail with us, and in the opposite season of the year, it is not to be doubted that it will every where effect what is expected of it, and what we have already witnessed. We therefore solicit also the physicians of other countries actively to unite with us in investigating thoroughly this important subject."

VII.

Alexandri di Humboldt et Amati Bonpland, Plantæ æquinoctiales, per regnum Mexici, in provinciis Caracarum et novæ Andalusiæ, in Peruvianorum, Quitensium, Novæ Granatæ Andibus, ad Oronoci, fluvii Nigri fluminis Amazonum ripas nascentes. In ordinem digessit Amatus Bonpland, Vol. I. Fasc. 1. & 2. Fol. imp. Lutetiæ Parisiorum, 1805.

WE fully participate in the general interest excited by the travels of Humbold and Bonpland into the interior of America. Few countries were more worthy of being explored by men of science, few travellers have united to a spirit of observation and variety of talents, so much zeal and courage, and seldom has an undertaking of so much difficulty been so completely successful. Their exertions, however, have not been suspended on their return to Europe, but they are equally indefatigable in communicating to others their observations and discoveries. The manner in which they have chosen to do this also appears judicious; for, instead of combining into one enormous work a vast mass of heterogeneous materials, and interrupting the general narrative to describe

describe a plant or an animal, they have resolved to devote to each department of their subject a separate work, so that, without increasing the expence of the whole, the discoveries in each science may be had separately. Their travels, properly so called, which will include every thing relating to the general physics of the country, the origin of its inhabitants, their manners, intellectual culture, condition, its antiquities, commerce and political economy, are delayed to the last. In the mean time, to satisfy public curiosity, they proceed with the following works.

1. An abridged account of travels into the interior of America during the years 1799, 1800, 1, 2, and 3.
2. A collection of astronomical observations and measurements.
3. An essay on the geography of vegetables.
4. Equinoctial plants.
5. Observations in zoology and comparative anatomy.

The first fasciculi of the two latter publications have reached us, and we hasten to communicate to our readers the most interesting part of their contents. In a preface to the equinoctial botany, written by Humboldt, we are informed that it is chiefly the work of his able coadjutor, who, in the midst of all their fatigues, and often at the expence of his night's rest, prepared and dried sixty thousand specimens of plants, many of which Humboldt found time, notwithstanding his other occupations, to delineate on the spot. The number of new species and genera they have discovered will not appear surprising, when we consider, that they traversed the interior of America, from the Caracas to the frontiers of Brazil, through a great extent of territory which had never before been visited by any botanist. In transporting such extensive collections many thousand miles by land, the difficulties appear almost insurmountable, and yet they only met with one loss of consequence, in a vessel which was shipwrecked on the coast of Africa. In these splendid fasciculi, they do not follow any arrangement, but give in succession delineations and descriptions of such plants as they have sufficiently compared with those of the same family already known. Each fasciculus, except the first, will contain ten plants, and ten fasciculi will form a volume. When this work, in which the detail is very minute, shall be sufficiently advanced, they propose to publish, in Latin, in 8vo, and without plates, an abridged description of all the plants they have brought with them, in the manner of Smith's Flora Britannica.

In the first fasciculus only one plant is described, constituting a new genus of the family of Palms, to which they have given the name *Ceroxylon*, from its singular property of affording wax. It is only found on the mountains of Quindiu, consisting of granite and micaceous schistus, in 4° 35′ north latitude. Its habitation

tion is a singular phenomenon in the geography of vegetables. Tropical palms, in general, do not grow at a greater height than 500 toises above the sea, but the wax palm is not found below 900 toises, and grows abundantly at 1450, where the mean temperature is from 66° Fahr. to 68; or 1000 toises higher, and at a temperature 30 degrees lower than the rest of the same family. It is also, perhaps, the tallest tree in the world, rising even to 180 feet, and having leaves 20 feet long. But the most remarkable circumstance about this elegant palm is, the secreted substance with which its trunk is covered, to the thickness of about two inches. According to Vauquelin's analysis, it consists of two-thirds of resin and one of wax. It is extremely inflammable, and is used by the natives, melted with one-third of tallow, for the manufacture of candles.

The second fasciculus contains the Matisia cordata, Jussiæa sedioides, and natans, Myrtus microphylla, Freziera reticulata, canescens, sericea, and nervosa, and the Cinchona condaminea. The last of these is so interesting an article of the Materia Medica, and even yet so much involved in ambiguity, that we transcribe its description.

"Cinchona Condaminea. Pentandria Monogynia *Linn.*
"Ordo Naturalis, Rubiaceæ, *Juss.*
"Character Genericus. *Juss.* p. 201; *Schreb.* Gen. Plant. 301;
"*Gaert.* De fruct. et sem. p. 167, t. 33, f. 4; Flora Peruv. et Chil. t. 2, p. 50.
"Synonymia. Quinaquina, *Condam.* Act. Paris. 1738; Cinchona officinalis *Linn.* Spec. edit. 2, p. 244; Syst. veget. edit. 10, p. 929; *Lam.*, Encycl. pl. 164, f. I.; *Lambert*, A description of the genus Cinchona, fig. I.; *Wild*, Spec. plant. p. 957.
"Foliis ovali-lanceolatis, nitidis, infra ad axillas nervorum scrobiculatis; corolla limbo lanato; staminibus inclusis; capsulis ovatis.

"Arbor procera, elegans, foliis semper ornata, sectione ex undique succum luteum, adstringentem, exhibens. Truncus erectus, bi-aut tri-orygalis et ultra, quindecim unciali diametro, cortice rimoso, cinereo. Rami teretes, decussatim oppositi, erecti, brachiati; junioribus ad nodos obsolete quadrangularibus. Folia nitida, ovali-lanceolata, tripollicaria, petiolata, in axillas nervorum inferne scrobiculata. Petiolus folio sexies brevior, superne planus, inferne convexus. Scrobiculus liquore aqueo adstringente scatet, orificio pilis subclauso. Stipulæ duæ, acutæ, sericeæ, adpressæ, caducæ. Panicula terminalis, brachiata, foliosa, trichotoma. Pedunculi et pedicelli pulverulento-sericei, teretes. Flores albo-rosei, bracteolati. Calix campanulato-globosus, quinque-dentatus, pulverulento-sericeus; pariter ac pedunculi, dentibus acutis, brevissimis, adpressis. Corolla subhypocrateriformis, calice sexies longior; tubo obsolete pentagono, sericeo, sæpius roseo; limbo rotato; laciniis ovalibus, tubo multo brevioribus, supra lanatis, niveis. Ovarium globosum, disco epigyno, quinque tuberculato, coronatum; stylus vix exsertus; stigma bifidum. Capsula ovata, lignosa, longitudinaliter lineata, dentibus calicinis coronata, bilocularis, polisperma, opposite bisulcata, a basi ad apicem, bivalvis. Semina plurima marginata, sursum inbricata. Receptaculum subcarnosum, elongatum, compresso-tetragonum, marginibus valvularum intro flexis longitudinaliter affixum.

"Habitat in Peruviæ Andibus, prope Loxam et Ayavacam."

The

The plant, so accurately described, was ascertained to be the very Cinchona delineated by Condamine, and is characterized by the pits or holes at the roots of the large nerves of the leaves. The genus was established by Linnæus in 1742, in the second edition of his genera. This was the only species then known, and he gave it the trivial name of *officinalis*. But since 1767, when he published the 12th edition of his Systema, no less than four different species have been confounded under the same name; the *C. officinalis*, Linn. (1.); the *C. Macrocarpa*, Vahl. (2.); the *C. pubescens*, Vahl. (3.); and lastly, the *C. nitida* of Ruiz and Pavon (4.). This ambiguity was originally occasioned by Linnæus himself supposing that a specimen of *C. pubescens*, sent to him in 1762, belonged to the species described by Condamine; and although the latter is that which furnishes the bark most esteemed in commerce, and known by the natives under the name of *Cascarilla fina*, yet, as several other species are also officinal, we think that our authors have done right in rejecting altogether the ambiguous epithet of *officinalis*, and designating this species by the name of its discoverer.

We are almost sorry that our authors have delayed the curious particulars which they have collected respecting so inseresting an object of the Materia Medica, until they have completed the collection of materials which they are making for a monography of the genus, which we sincerely hope no accident will prevent the publication of. We are here, however, told, that there is annually exported from America 12,000 or 14,000 quintals of Cinchona bark. Of these, the kingdom of Santa Fé furnishes 2000, which are sent from Carthagena. Previous to 1779, Loxa furnished 4000, but at present only 110 are cut, which are sent to Spain for the use of the king. The provinces of Huamanga, Cuença and Jaen de Bracamorros, and the thick forests of Guacabamba and Ayavaca, furnish the rest, which is sent from Lima, Guayaquil, Payta, and other ports on the south sea. The *Cinchona Condaminea* always grows on micaceous schistus, and is found at as great a height as 1282 toises, and as low as 975 toises above the level of the sea, so that it occupies a zone of 307 toises.

(1.) Mat. Med. p. 66. Syst. nat. edit. 10, p. 929. Spec. edit. 2. p. 244.

(2.) Act. Soc. hist. nat. Hafn. 1. p. 20. t. 3, exclusis synonymiis; *Lambert*, p. 22. t. 3; *Wild*, Spec. plant. p. 598. exc. Syn.

(3.) Act. Soc. hist. nat. Hafn. 1. p. 19. t. 2; Symb. bot. pars 2. p. 37. *Lamb.* p. 21. t. 2. *Wild*, Sp. pl. p. 958; Cinchona officinalis, *Linn.* Syst. nat. edit. 12. p. 164; Syst. veget. edit. 13. p. 178; Supplem. p. 144; *Gaertner*, de fruct. et sem. t. 1. p. 169. t. 33. f. 4.

(4.) Flor. Peruv. et Chil. t. 2. p. 50. t. 191. Cinchona officinalis *Ruiz*. Quinol. art. 2. p. 56.

PART III.

MEDICAL INTELLIGENCE.

Medical Reform.

THE following Advertisement has repeatedly appeared in the London Newspapers, and both on account of the high authority from which it comes, and of its immediately affecting the interests of the whole Medical Profession, it merits a conspicuous situation in this department of our Journal.

THE ROYAL COLLEGE OF PHYSICIANS in London, having received accounts from various parts of England, complaining of the number of irregular Practitioners, calling themselves Physicians, who exercise the Profession of Physic without authority, and in many instances without due Qualifications, feel it their Duty to apprize the Public of the legal Provisions to obviate this evil, and to refer them to the List annually printed by the College, (which in future they will take care to have properly circulated), in order that the Names of all those may be known, who, having been examined by the College according to Law, have been deemed competent to practise as Physicians.

Extract from the Acts of Parliament 14th and 15th of Hen. VIII.

" That it may be Enacted in this present Parliament, that no Person " from henceforth be suffered to exercise or Practise in Physic through " England, until such time that he be examined at London, by the said " President and Three of the said Elects, and have from the said President and Elects Letters testimonial of their approving and examination: except he be a Graduate of Oxford or Cambridge, which hath " accomplished all things for his form without any Grace."

By Order of the College,

JAMES HERVEY, M. D. Register.

June 25. 1805.

Highly as we esteem the talents of the Fellows of London College, and their characters as individuals, we must candidly confess, that to us the object and tendency of this act of their corporation, are not very apparent. Complaints have been made of the number of irregular practitioners in medicine throughout England, and the Royal College feel it their duty to apprize the public that *all* practitioners, who have not been licensed by them, except the graduates of Oxford and Cambridge, are irregular, and

and exercise their profession in defiance of the laws of the land, and that they will circulate a list of those whom they have deemed competent to practise as physicians. Do they conceive that they have fulfilled their duty, in merely apprizing the public of the alleged legal provisions to obviate the evil; or do they mean to enforce them? Do they hope to be supported in this attempt at monopoly by the public; or do they expect, that physicians, whose talents the public has been accustomed to revere, will now petition for leave to exercise them? Of their intention to give greater publicity to the names of their fellows and licentiates, no one can disapprove; but we have very great doubts, indeed, whether, in law, they are legally intitled to designate all other physicians as irregular practitioners.

Their powers in regulating the practice of medicine within a circle of seven miles round London, are much more unlimited than over the rest of England. Although, by partial favour, they never refuse admission into their corporation, to graduates of the English universities, they still have the right of refusing it, and of prohibiting them from practising in the vicinity of London. Beyond that circle, however, their charter, 10th Henry VIII., gave them no powers, and when, by the subsequent statutes of the 14th and 15th, Henry VIII, they acquired the superintendence over all England; it is most expressly stated, that they shall have no controul over the graduates of Oxford and Cambridge, which exemption, we conceive, according to the articles of Union between England and Scotland, must be extended to every graduate of any of the universities in the united kingdom, which hath accomplished all things for his form, *without any grace.*

Art. 4th, "That all the subjects of the United Kingdom of Great Britain, shall, from and after the Union, have full freedom and intercourse of trade and navigation, to and from any port or place within the United Kingdom, and the dominions and plantations thereunto belonging; *and that there be communication of all other rights, privileges, and advantages, which do or may belong to the subjects of either Kingdom,* except where it is otherwise expressly agreed in these articles."

25th, "That all laws and statutes in either kingdom, so far as they are contrary to, or inconsistent with, the terms of these articles, or any of them, shall, from and after the Union, cease and become void, and shall be declared to be so by the respective Parliaments of the said Kingdom."

Of the question at issue, these extracts are decisive, the right of practising medicine acquired in an university in either Kingdom is extended to the other, and in this liberal manner, has the treaty of Union always been understood by the Royal College of Physicians of Edinburgh, who expressly concede to the Graduates of the English Universities, the rights conferred in their charter exclusively on those of Scotland

Association

Soho Square, August 9, 1806.

At a numerous meeting of the Faculty, held this evening at the house of the Right Honourable Sir Joseph Banks, Bart. K. B., President of the Royal Society, Dr Harrison laid upon the table the answers he had received to the different circular letters transmitted to the Public Bodies, &c. and Individual Practitioners of the United Kingdom, in pursuance of a former resolution. He then presented the following Plan for better regulating the Practice of Physic in its different branches; which being read and considered, the subsequent resolutions were entered into:

PLAN.

"1st, That no person shall practise as Physician unless he be a graduate of some university in the United Kingdom, and has attained the age of twenty-four years; that he shall have studied the different branches of physic in an university, or other respectable school or schools of physic, during the space of five years at least, two of which shall have been passed in the university where he takes his degree.

"2dly, That no person shall practise as Surgeon under three-and-twenty years of age, nor until he has obtained a diploma or licence from some one of the royal colleges of surgeons or other chirurgical corporations of the United Kingdom; that he shall have served an apprenticeship of five years to a practitioner in surgery, and afterwards have spent at least two years in the study of anatomy and surgery in a reputable school or schools of physic.

"3dly, That no person shall practise as an Apothecary until he shall have served an apprenticeship of five years to some regular apothecary, or surgeon practising as an apothecary; that he shall have studied the different branches of physic in some reputable school or schools during the space of at least one year, and shall have attained the age of twenty-one years.

"4thly, That no man shall practise Midwifery, unless he has attended anatomical lectures twelve months, and received instructions for the same term from some experienced accoucheur, and shall have assisted at real labours.—And that no female shall practise midwifery without a certificate of fitness and qualification from some regular practitioner or practitioners in that branch.

"5thly, That no person shall follow the business of a retail Chemist or Druggist, unless he shall have served an apprenticeship of five years to that art.

"6thly, That none of these restrictions be construed to affect persons at present regularly practising in the different branches of medicine.

"7thly, Whether Physicians shall be entitled to recover their fees by the usual legal means?

"8thly, That a register shall be kept of all medical practitioners in the United Kingdom, and every person in future entering upon the practice of any branch of the profession, shall pay a fine on admission, the amount and disposition of which to be settled and specified hereafter."

Resolved,—1st, That it appears from the returns to the circular letters, that the abuses complained of do exist to a great degree in every part of the United Kingdom; and that the necessity for adopting regulations for their correction is universally admitted.

2dly, That it seems to be expedient that the plan proposed by Dr Harrison be adopted as the basis of regulation; subject, however, to such alterations as may hereafter appear to be necessary.

3dly, That Sir Joseph Banks and Dr Harrison be requested to wait again upon the Right Honourable Lord Henry Petty, to state to him the progress of the undertaking, and to consult him upon further measures.

4thly, That the following gentlemen be appointed a committee to confer and correspond with the different public bodies of the United Kingdom, upon the subject of the proposed regulations; that they be requested to report their proceedings from time to time, and to take such other steps as they may judge necessary.—Sir John M. Hayes, Bart.; Sir Walter Farquhar, Bart.; Doctors Blackburn, Harrison, Garthshore, G. Pearson, Stanger, Willan, and Clutterbuck *(Sec.)*.

5thly, That a voluntary subscription of one guinea each be received from the town and country practitioners by any member of the committee, to enable them to prosecute the important objects in which they are engaged. (The names of subscribers to be published hereafter.)

6thly, That Dr Harrison be requested to circulate the above Plan and Resolutions of this evening among the Faculty of the United Kingdom, in the manner of the former circular letter.

7thly, That since persons of every rank and occupation in life are deeply interested in the proposed regulations, the Faculty are particularly requested to submit them to the principal inhabitants of their respective districts, by convening meetings, or in any other mode which they may think proper.

8thly, That the thanks of this meeting be given to the Right Honourable Sir Joseph Banks, for his continued attentions to the Association, and the important objects of their pursuit.

August 25, 1806.

At a meeting of the Committee held this evening, at the house of Dr Garthshore, the following letter addressed to the Royal College of Physicians, and, *mutatis mutandis*, to the different Universities and Incorporated Medical Bodies of the United Kingdom, was read and approved; and Dr Harrison was requested to transmit the same, with the Plan and Resolutions as above stated.

"*To Sir Lucas Pepys, Bart., M.D., F.R.S., President, and to the Fellows of the Royal College of Physicians, London*

"Gentlemen,

"I am requested by the Committee nominated at a late numerous meeting of the Faculty at the house of the Right Honourable Sir Joseph Banks, to transmit for your consideration a copy of the proceedings and resolutions then agreed to, on the subject of a proposed medical reform.

"The Committee are decidedly of opinion, that the object in contemplation can by no means be so effectually accomplished, as by their acting in conjunction with the Royal College of Physicians of London, and

and the other incorporated medical bodies in the United Kingdom, the rights and privileges of which it is, they think, highly desirable to maintain, and perhaps to extend by legislative provisions, as far as may be necessary to attain the desired purposes. I am, therefore, also requested by the Committee respectfully to desire, that the College will depute two or more of their body to confer with an equal number of the said Committee; at such time and place as may be convenient, in order to consider of a plan of procedure, which, while it preserves inviolate the rights and privileges of the different corporate bodies, shall afford protection to the regular Faculty throughout the United Kingdom, against the ignorant and unskillful; and insure, in future, to the community practitioners qualified, both by education and knowledge, for the respective important stations they shall assume.

"I have the honour to be, Gentlemen, your most obedient humble servant, E. HARRISON."

"*Some Account of the* General Hospital *and* Medical School *at Vienna.*"

VIENNA is indebted to the active benevolence of the Emperor Joseph II., for the establishment of this large and useful institution. Formerly a poor-house, or charitable institution for invalids and orphans, founded by Leopold I., and enriched by successive endowments, stood in the situation where the General Hospital is now placed. These were removed into two separate houses, in the year 1780, when the Emperor Joseph carried into execution his plan for building a very large hospital, capable of receiving all the sick, under one general establishment. The scale on which this is founded, is extensive, and it is considered one of the first institutions of its kind in Europe. To one unaccustomed to see such splendid establishments for the sick and infirm poor as are to be met with in every part of the British dominions, the hospital at Vienna must indeed be very striking. But there is something so irreconciliable with our ideas of a perfectly neat and well regulated hospital, in the attachment to dirt, and the neglect of propriety and cleanliness, so universally prevalent among the lower orders of people on the Continent, that an Englishman must be allowed to retain his national prejudice, and to speak warmly in praise of any charitable institutions of Germany, only by comparing them with one another, or with those of any other country but his own. Cleanliness seems to be habitual to the lower class of society only in England and Holland; hence it becomes extremely difficult to procure and to preserve that constant attention to neatness, so necessary to the healthy, and seemly internal economy of a public hospital. What strikes a stranger as most objectionable, in the generality of hospitals on the Continent, is the bad ventilation of the rooms, in which a number of patients are crowded together. There are seldom any fire-places in the wards; but these are heated by means of stoves, or ovens, and animal effluvia seem not only to accumulate more in such rooms, warmed by stoves, but to ferment more easily and more quickly, than when open fires and chimnies are employed, which burn them very soon, or allow them to escape. The General Hospital at Vienna is upon a very good footing, and the domestic arrangement is well conducted. The benefits of it are not merely confined to the sick poor; persons of the middle class of society, in easy circumstances, who wish to be away from their own houses in case of illness, may be admitted into the hospital, and for this purpose, the patients are divided into four classes. The first class consists of those who have a room and a nursery entirely to themselves, they are taken care of, boarded, lodged, and attended for one florin (about 2sh. English money) per day. Patients of the second class are put several together into one room, they enjoy all the other privileges of the first class, and pay only half a florin a-day. The third class includes all the sick people, who belong to public charities or foundations, and the hospital claims the ordinary allowance which the patient used to receive, from the time of his or her admission. The fourth class is that of the poor of both sexes, who come provided with a certificate of their indigence from the minister of their parish. Servants from private families are admitted, and attended in the hospital for 10 kreutzers, (4d. English) a-day. Every patient has a separate bed, without curtains, at the head of which a wooden tablet is hung, marking the number of the bed and ward, the name of the disease, the remedies prescribed, the hours for administering them, the diet ordered, and the daily report of the symptoms. The building is two stories high, situated in an airy part of the suburbs, on a wide space of ground, including seven courts, or squares, planted with trees. There are 111 rooms, 26 feet long, 17 feet wide, and high in proportion: 61 of these wards are for men, and 40 for women, the rest are applied for other purposes, as warm and cold baths; an apothecary's shop, a chapel, and every thing useful for an establishment of such magnitude. The number of patients in this general hospital, on the last day of December, 1804, amounted to 417 men, 473 women. In the course of the year 1805, were admitted - - - - -

- - - -	men	7331	women	6847
Discharged -	——	6176	——	5748
Died - -	——	1050	——	1048
Remained on the books	——	522	——	524

An

An asylum for lunatics is attached to the general hospital, and the building is placed adjoining to it. The shape of this place of confinement is somewhat remarkable; it is a perfectly round tower, the elevation was probably more to gratify the emperor's whim, than for any particular advantages belonging to such a structure. It is three stories high, and each story is divided into 28 rooms, of different degrees of comfort and accommodation, appropriated to each patient, according to the class in which he is placed, and the price that he pays. Four distinctions of ranks are made, the same as in the hospital. At the end of the year 1804, were 170 men, and 144 women in the lunatic asylum, in the course of 1805, were admitted - - -

- - - -	men 117	women	94
Discharged -	—— 104	———	70
Died - -	—— 42	———	32
Remained -	—— 141	———	136

The proportion of males to females is as considerable, even from this report, as was observed in the history of the number of cases of mental derangement at Berlin; and the difference would here be greater, if a certain class of patients, which in most places is very numerous, were not excluded. Ecclesiastics are not admitted, because another similar institution for patients of this holy order is under the superintendence of the charitable brothers, who have another large hospital in another quarter of the town.

The 'General Hospital' is under the direction of one principal physician, and one principal surgeon, besides a number of assistant physicians, surgeons, apothecaries, and pupils, who have each a separate department allotted to them. Free admission is allowed to patients of every description, at every hour. Great regularity is observed in the management of the various concerns of so great an establishment, and the relative duties of the medical attendants, and the nurses are upon the whole scrupulously, and faithfully fulfilled. The clinical department is admirable, and merits all the commendation bestowed upon it. To the munificence of the Emperor Joseph it owes its origin, and to the judicious exertions of *Professor Frank*, must be ascribed all its usefulness, its merit, and its fame. In the middle of the great court-yard belonging to the hospital, is a handsome building, appropriated as a dwelling-house for the Clinical Professor, and the requisite accommodations for clinical lectures, and clinical practice. Two large and lofty rooms are allotted to patients, selected from the whole number of those who present themselves for admission; each chamber contains 20 beds, placed at a considerable

able distance from one another; the bed-steads are made of wood, no curtains are allowed, and for an upper covering, sheets and counterpanes are used instead of a feather-bed, which is usually employed in Germany. By the side of every bed, a board is hung with the name and age of the patient, the day of admission, the character of the disease, and the remedies administered written down upon it. The history of the disease, and all the circumstances of the case, are accurately taken down in Latin, on the patient's admission, by one of the candidate's for a doctor's degree, and this is read aloud at the bed-side, in presence of the Professor and the pupils, when the young man undertakes the treatment of the case, under the superintendence of the Clinical Professor, and undergoes a public examination, every day, in answering questions relative to the diagnosis, prognosis, and cure of the patient before him. The hour of visiting the patients is from eight o'clock to nine in the morning, and after every visit, the Professor delivers a short lecture in a room appointed for that purpose, stating the reports of the different cases under his care, and illustrating the practical injunctions by general remarks, deduced from his own experience, or by a reference to the best authors. Adjoining to the lecture-room is a museum, principally consisting of morbid preparations, which was bought by the Emperor Joseph, from the celebrated *Soemmering*. It contains many useful pathological histories, and its value increases every year, by the additions it receives from the occurrences in hospital practice. A collection of morbid anatomy ought to be made in every large hospital, and not merely the finely injected vascular preparations preserved, but an accurate detail of all the peculiar circumstances of the case. The Clinical Professor is appointed by the Emperor, and has a house, firing, &c. granted to him, with an allowance of 200l. sterling per annum. His assistants reside at the hospital as well as himself, and they, and the other medical attendants, receive a salary from the government. Besides the clinical establishment for the practice of medicine, there are two others attached to the hospital, one called the medico-chirurgical clinic, and the other, the chirurgical clinic. Six wards are appropriated for this more general clinical practice. In the regular establishment already described, the pupils who attend, are preparing to graduate, and the examinations and lectures are in the Latin language; in these others, the examinations and reports are delivered in the German language, and they are attended by those who practise as surgeons and apothecaries. The manner of proceeding in the Surgical Clinical ward is much the same, for those students who are to take a surgeon's diploma; but the lower class of students only frequent the wards where

medical

medical and surgical cases are mingled together, where they can have an opportunity for acquiring some knowledge of the other infirmities of the human body, besides that of having a beard, which it is their daily occupation to remove. The inferior class of surgeons at Vienna still shave, and draw teeth, and bleed; but there are some men of eminence who are attached to the hospital, and have very good private practice in the town, both as regular physicians and surgeons. *John Peter Frank* was invited from Pavia, to take the charge of the Clinical School, and he exerted himself very successfully in making an useful arrangement, and attracting a vast concourse of students from different parts of the Austrian empire. He was considered as the father and the founder of that systematic mode of teaching the elements of practical medicine, and was very highly esteemed by all his pupils, and much admired by the wisest and best of his contemporaries; but by the chicanery, and low tricks, and intrigues, of courtiers and court-physicians, he found himself placed in a situation too despicable for an independent and high-minded man to endure, with any sort of patience. His plans were thwarted, and his requests rejected by his own sovereign, when the present Emperor of Russia made him very advantageous offers, and flattering proposals, to go and settle at Petersburgh. Thus *Frank* resigned the Clinical Professor's chair; he left his country and his friends to seek that fame and fortune, which, in an happier age, he might have found in the favourite spot of his reputation, in the school of Vienna. After his departure, Dr *Joseph Frank*, his son, became his successor at the hospital; but he soon followed his father, and is now at the University of Wilna. Several intelligent men, who had long been the favourite assistants and pupils of *Frank*, quitted their situation at the hospital with disgust at the banishment of their master; and the celebrity of the Clinical wards is now talked of, as one of those things which *has been*. The name of the present Professor is *Bridel*, he has a friend at court, to whom he is indebted for the appointment; and it is said, he is, in every other respect, directly the reverse of his distinguished predecessor. *Professor Harn* conducts the surgical clinical department, and *Professor Rheinlein* the medico-surgical, both these men are highly spoken of, and they are followed by many pupils.

Before leaving the description of the General Hospital, it would be wrong to pass over without notice, the Lying-in, and the Foundling Hospital, which make a part of the establishment. Any female may gain admission to the lying-in wards at any time, and remain unknown, and after her delivery she can leave her child to the care of the hospital for foundlings, or take it

4 away

away with her. Although any woman may be admitted under an assumed name, she must deliver her real name in a sealed packet, which is returned to her unopened, on her leaving the hospital, but is opened in case of death. Accommodations are provided for three classes of patients, who pay a small sum of money in proportion to their means, or they are received *gratis*; and if the child be left behind, the parent must pay 24 florins, (about 28 shillings) in order to get it put into the Foundling-Hospital. Pupils of both sexes attending the hospital are allowed to frequent some of the lying-in wards, but others are kept quite secret. On the last day of December, 1804, according to the report published last year, there were 107 women, and 21 children in the Lying-in Hospital; in the course of the year 1805, the number of women admitted, amounted to 2112; discharged, 2084; died, 9; remained, 126 women, and 26 children. This statement only refers to the wards for the delivery of pregnant women, an annual report of the Foundling Hospital is not published. If accurate details were yearly published of every Foundling Hospital in Europe, it is likely, a very melancholy picture of mortality would be unfolded. The policy and expediency of such places is very questionable. Experience has shewn, that the number of objects multiply, in proportion to the provision made for them, and such receiving-houses as this at Vienna, without the risk of any discovery, must operate as a sort of bounty on vice and seduction, and the exposure of infants. Take away all sense of shame, remove the fears of any deviation from the paths of virtue and chastity, being detected, and you take away the grand barrier, that serves to counterpoise the suggestions of sensual passion, and thus encourage, instead of alleviating, the evils incident to the female sex, in a crowded, and consequently corrupt metropolis.

Account of the Diseases treated at the PUBLIC DISPENSARY, *Bishop's Court, near Carey-street, from May 31st to August 31st,* 1806.

Acute Diseases.

	No. of Cases.		No. of Cases.
Hydrocephalus acutus	2	Febris infantum	4
Phrenitis	1	Ophthalmia	3
Typhus	1	Cynanche tonsillaris	5
Synochus	13	——— parotidæa	1
Quartana	1	Pneumonia	4

Acute

ACUTE DISEASES, *continued.*

	No. of Cases.		No. of Cases.
Peripneumonia notha	7	Dysenteria	12
Hæmoptysis	8	Enteritis	1
Catarrhus	57	Nephritis	1
Tussis post rubeolam	2	Hysteritis	1
Erysipelas	5	Ischuria renalis	1
Variola	2	Pertussis	3
Rubeola	3	Dentitio	4
Scarlatina	7	Apoplexia	1
Urticaria	2	Rheumatismus acutus	13
Hespes zoster	1	Arthritis rheumatica	6
Cholera	4	Hectica adolescentium	2

CHRONIC DISEASES.

Cephalæa	14	Chlorosis et amenorrhœa	13
Tussis chronicus	17	Dysmenorrhœa	2
Gastrodynia	14	Menorrhagia	17
Dyspepsia	13	Leucorrhœa	8
Hepatitis chron.	2	Prolapsus uteri	1
Enterodynia	10	Cancer uteri	3
Diarrhœa	13	Aphthæ	2
Constipatio	1	Ascites	3
Verminatio	2	Anasarca	2
Tænia	1	Hydrothorax	2
Tabes mesenterica et marasmus	7	Scrofula	4
Tympanites	2	Paralysis	3
Hæmorrhois	1	——— saturnina	1
Nephralgia	12	Asthenia	45
Hæmaturia	2	Aneurysma aortæ	1
Catarrhus vesicœ	1	Varicæ cruris	1
Dysuria	3	Plethora	2
Phthisis	13	Lichen	1
Asthma	4	Prurigo	5
Pleurodyne	3	Psoriasis	4
Rheumatismus chronicus	34	Pityriasis	1
Lumbago et sciatica	7	Impetigo	13
Epilepsia	5	Porrigo	3
Hysteria	2	Scabies	8
Chorea	1	Ecthyma	2

The temperature of the air has been moderate during the last six or eight weeks; there have been several heavy rains, and three or four unusually severe thunder storms. Hence, probably, we may account for the small number of disorders of the biliary system and alimentary canal, and for the multitude of catarrhal

tarrhal and rheumatic affections. The month of June was almost uniformly warm and dry; on the 10th and 14th the thermometer in the shade arose to 82½°.

The Synochus, or summer fever, seems to be on the increase in this district: it occurs in a mild form, is accompanied with more or less abdominal pain and tension, and is relieved considerably by purgatives. The single case of Typhus succeeded to, and appeared to be, the effect of an over-dose of a hot terebinthinate medicine, which is sold under the name of "Dutch drops." The man had swallowed fifteen times the quantity prescribed, and was seized soon after with head-ach, delirium, and fever, which assumed the form, and went through the common course, of pure typhus.

For the Gastrodynia, which is extremely prevalent among the poor at all seasons, the oxide of bismuth, which was recommended by Dr Odier of Geneva, has been employed both by my colleague, Dr Laird, and myself, with considerable success. It has, in some cases, produced a permanent relief, after the usual tonics and stimulants had been taken with a trifling, and but temporary, advantage. In a dose of about ten grains it sits easy on the stomach, and seems to be generally efficacious. For a minute account of the medicine, and the proper mode of preparing it, the reader may refer to an excellent paper on the subject, in the 6th Vol. of the Memoirs of the Medical Society of London, by Dr Marcet.

Two of the cases of jaundice, in the report of last quarter, were those of middle-aged women, who have before applied to the Dispensary, for the cure of the same complaint. The disease appeared to arise, in both, from the presence of gall-stones, or inspissated bile, in the biliary ducts, as it was accompanied with frequent attacks of acute pain in that region. It was relieved, for a time, by opium, and calomel as a purgative; but in both, the most marked and essential benefit was derived from the use of the nitric acid. In one of the instances, the jaundice was speedily removed three or four successive times by this medicine, having returned when it was omitted for a short time: and, in the other, not only the jaundice, but slight and frequent pains in the region of the liver, were invariably removed by recurring to its use. I have employed this remedy in a few other cases with similar advantage, as well as in some instances of chronic pains referred to the region of the liver; in some of which, perhaps, it may have acted merely as a tonic to the stomach. The hypothesis of oxygenation, with which the practice was coupled, when it was transmitted from the East Indies, has probably contributed to throw discredit on a medicine, which, in some modifications

fications of disease in the biliary organs, possesses, beyond a doubt, considerable remedial powers.

J. Bateman.

London, Aug. 31st, 1806.

Extract of a Letter from Dr Joseph Frank, *Professor of Pathology in the University of Wilna, dated* 19*th May,* 1805.

YOUR letter was sent after me from Vienna, which city we left last September in consequence of an invitation from the court of St Petersburgh. Both my father and myself are appointed to this university, my father as Clinical Professor, myself as Professor of Pathology. Our incomes are considerable; so we have not suffered by the change; and have, besides, the pleasure of contributing to the diffusion of science under the enlightened government of the Emperor Alexander. Wilna lies in that part of Polish Lithuania which, at the last partition of that country, was allotted to Russia. The university has an yearly income of L.20,000 sterling, and the Emperor is about to increase it. I am already appointed my father's successor; in the mean time, I teach pathology not merely theoretically, but I demonstrate the diseases at the bed-side of the sick. For this purpose I make use of one of our hospitals, which I am now endeavouring to put upon the footing of the English hospitals, for I have also got the superintendence of all the hospitals in this place. Among my colleagues I have an old schoolfellow whom you perhaps know. He graduated in Pavia, and was some time in Edinburgh. His name is Sniadecki. At present he teaches chemistry and pharmacy.

Although we are entirely separated from Germany, we still know what is going on there with regard to medicine. The Brunonian System is daily more and more modified, so that it is scarcely to be recognised. You will be astonished to hear that I have deserted it. "What system," you will ask, "have you "then adopted?" None. I consult my own experience, and benefit by all correct observers, whether they belong to the new or to the old school. It is only since I have adopted this method, that I feel as if I were a physician. Perhaps I should have been longer of arriving at this point if I had not travelled through Britain; at least I can say, that it was from reflecting upon what I saw there, that this new light burst upon me. My present mode of thinking is much censured by the young physicians, who

find

find a system so convenient, but is approved of by all real practitioners, and it is only the approbation of the latter that can and ought to weigh with me. In justice to myself, I must, however, remark, that I never was a blind follower of Brown; and that, after more mature consideration and greater experience, I am convinced his principles cannot be adopted as the foundation of the science of medicine.—My father will soon publish the sixth volume of his *Epitome de curandis hominum morbis*. It treats of hemorrhagies.

Extract of a Letter from a Gentleman connected with the University of Wilna, dated Hamburgh, 4th August, 1805.

I BEG your pardon for not having sent you an answer to your letter from London, I was so much occupied there with my departure. During my stay in Hamburgh, I received some communications from our University, which enables me to do it with still more information than I could have done in London; I am therefore very glad that I can fulfill at least part of my promises.

You will find here inclosed two papers, the one is the *Act of Confirmation of the University of Wilna*, the other is an *Extract of some Articles from the Statutes of the University*, relating to the method of election, for vacant places in the University, both translated into French, in order to be communicated to foreign countries.

These papers might have been known in your country 18 months ago, if the gentlemen in England, to whom they were sent by the University, had taken the trouble to insert them in any public Journal, which would have prevented a misunderstanding between some of your learned countrymen and the University, which was intimated to me several times during my stay in Edinburgh.

By the letters which I received from the University, I am enabled to give an explanation of this misunderstanding, partly by sending you the printed papers here inclosed, partly by communicating to you what has been noticed to me by the University: and you will find, that if the method of competition and election to vacant places in the University, prescribed by the laws and statutes, had been known to those gentlemen who had been proposed to the University, there could have been no mistake made. Amongst all these learned gentlemen, only one has sent a paper in the English language, on the subject which he professed; and this paper is now under consideration. One paper more has been

been received from another gentleman, which contains nothing but heads of lectures; and this you will easily perceive, by the § 22 of the "*Extrait du Chapitre,*" does not answer the conditions prescribed by the Statutes of the University. There were a good many more of your learned countrymen proposed, whom the University would have been very happy to have employed; but except these two papers which I mentioned, the University has not received one single line from any British gentleman, as I am authentically informed, up to the 10th May, 1805; therefore, there could be neither consideration nor election.

There are still six places vacant in the University, viz. Natural History, Rural Economy, Moral Philosophy, Political Economy, Universal History, and L'art Veterinaire. These places the University has pointed out to me as vacant, in a letter of the 10th May 1805: sending me at the same time, the two papers here inclosed, in order to be communicated in your country. I know I can send these communications to no better hands than yours, and I am persuaded you will be so kind as to give them a publicity, which will repair the misunderstanding, and keep up the honour of our University, so that I hope we still may have some of your learned countrymen amongst us, which I most heartily wish.

By the unlucky fire at the Central House of the Royal Jennerian Institution in London, the most important of the inclosures mentioned in the preceding letter was destroyed. The letter however, fortunately, renders the loss less important, and at least is sufficient to prevent a repetition of the disagreeable and awkward occurrences which took place here, and perhaps in some other parts of Britain, a year or two ago. Some gentleman misunderstanding the nature of the communications made to them, on the part of the univerfity of Wilna, conceived themselves empowered to dispose of certain professorships then vacant, instead of merely making known the vacancies and the conditions which candidates were required to fulfil. In consequence of their representations, several young gentlemen of promising talents were induced to accept of their offers, and, after putting themselves to very great and serious inconvenience, and being kept in the most awkward suspense until their patience was worn out, found, that their appointments were perfectly unauthorized. The following extracts from the *Act of Confirmation of the Imperial University of Wilna* will give some idea of the encouragement held out to strangers, and of the mode of supplying vacancies:

§ 5.

§ 5. The election of all places and functions in the university, even to the Theological Chairs, shall be vested in the plurality of votes, collected in a general meeting of the university, and presented by its Curator, for the confirmation of the Minister.

§ 15. Foreigners appointed to the university, may quit the country without paying any tax on the exportation of their effects. On their first arrival in Russia, they may bring for their own use, effects to the value of 3000 rubles, without paying duty.

§ 22. The annual appointments of each Professor shall consist in 1000 rubles in silver, for a principal course, and in 500 rubles for a supplementary course.

There are also pensions allotted to the widows and orphants of the professors, and to such professors as from ill health, are rendered unable to fulfil the duties of their chair; besides, after 25 years service, the professors may retire on full pay.

Extract of a Letter from Mr Elder, *Missionary: dated Otaheite, July 24th,* 1805.

We have of late seen two instances of locked jaw, and one of apoplexy; and there is reason to think that these diseases are frequent on the island. We use the cold bath, and large doses of opium for the locked jaw, as directed in Cullen's first lines, and bleeding, &c. in the apoplexy. The natives have got amongst them a dangerous swelling which rises to a great size, but neither comes to any head, nor contains any matter; it is found in the arms, legs, and thighs. They have got an out-striking, which breaks out on the side, and often spreads round the whole body; it has got a white crust, is loathsome to look at, and does not discharge any matter. It is sometimes fatal, and appears to be infectious. I do not think any of these two diseases are described in medical books. I sometimes give those labouring under them cooling things internally, but do not know what external application to make. The venereal is common among them, but whatever is the cause, it appears on this island to be a mild disease. *The first three years I was here, I never saw a chancre or bubo, nor gave to any native mercury, and yet they all got better.* Within these last four months, I have seen three men who had both bubo and chancre, all of them got mercury, one has been cured, and the others are not cured.

Besides the swelling which I have mentioned, they have got another swelling, which attacks their legs and arms, sometimes one

one leg and not the other, and sometimes one arm and not the other; it rises to a great size, seems to contain water, is not attended with pain, never proves fatal, and is much laughed at by the natives. I observed this kind of swelling at Rio Janeiro. There are a great many diseases on this island, but the most common and most fatal is what is called by the natives Hotete. It attacks all ages (perhaps), but particularly the young. It begins like an intermitting fever, the cold fits are not regular, sometimes returning on the third, and sometimes on the tenth day; after two or three months it changes its type, and is more like a continued fever, or perhaps like a hectic. It is very difficult to learn from the natives how it attacks them, and I cannot say positively what are its symptoms. In the beginning I have given some of them emetics, and I think with some success. I have given to some the bark, (some have taken it in very large doses), but I do not know that it ever was attended with any good effects, owing, most likely, to the method of giving it, or to inattention to regimen, &c. in those who did get it. Dr Bass, who was here, (commanding the brig Venus), and who is a very eminent physician, told me, that those dying of the Hotete, are dying of consumption, or, in other words, of scrophula; and I think, with him, (so far as I can judge), that scrophula is the cause of the Hotete. It is certain, that after a person has laboured for several months under the Hotete, it is not uncommon for the back to break, and when the back breaks, they generally get better, although not always

---

Extract of a Letter from a Surgeon on the Madrass Establishment, dated 22d October 1805.

My last letter from —— gave me sad accounts of his health. He is suffering much from excessive use of mercury; and has had, he says, spasms of the diaphragm, and excruciating pains in his skin, bones, and head. It may be news to you, that mercury, in this country, when given in too large quantity, causes sufferings more dreadful than the disease for which it is the specific, and experienced surgeons are cautious never to exceed in its employment. You ask me if the erythema mercuriale is frequent with us? Very lately a brother surgeon here had a case of it in his hospital which terminated fatally; and with the natives, who never can be made to clothe themselves sufficiently, or almost at all, when under the use and influence of mercury, this disease occurs frequently, and often proves destructive.

In

In reply to your query, if any cases of small-pox have occurred here after vaccination, I am sorry to say that some have, in the hands of Europeans, and very many in those of natives, as might be expected from the manner adopted to propagate the cow pock. The latter, at least, became so loose in their practice, that very many of them did not look near their subject from the day of using the lancet, so that it would be more proper to say, Small Pox occurred after *Inoculation*, than after *Vaccination*. The allowance of L.4 per 100 patients tempted them to great impositions; and there was no adequate check on them, either as to practice or discovering falsity in their accounts, so that when you see the accounts of hundreds of thousands vaccinated, you must not give credit to more than a half.

New regulations have been introduced lately to improve and reform the conduct of cow-pock inoculators, not much, however, to the benefit of the practitioners in it.

Original Vaccine Pock Institution. Broad Street, Golden Square, *Weekly Board*, 15th *July* 1806.

The following Propositions were read, and unanimously agreeed to be published:—

I. That it does appear, on adequate evidence, that persons who have gone through the Cow Pock, in the manner commonly believed to give security, have, in the proportion of one in a thousand, subsequently taken the Small Pox, according to the experience of this Institution, up to the present time.

II. That disorders which can be at all reasonably imputed to inoculation, have been observed less frequently after the vaccine than after the variolous inoculation.

III. That considering the slightness of the Cow Pock, and that no fatal case has occurred in the practice of this Institution, vaccination is greatly preferable to variolation; and especially on account of its not being propagated in any way but by inoculation, it is infinitely more valuable to the public.

IV. That it be recommended to every one who has been, or shall be vaccinated, to be re-inoculated with variolous, or vaccine matter.

V. That according to the experience of this Institution, the test of the insertion of vaccine matter (which is perfectly harmless) is to be relied upon equally with that of the variolous.

VI. That there are good reasons for imputing the late mortality by the Small Pox to its having been highly epidemical last year, as well as to the influence by which some writers, opposers of the Cow Pock, were enabled to prevail upon a great number of persons to be inoculated for the Small Pox; thus multiplying the sources of variolous infection.

Note

Note.—It has been urged, that vaccination may only destroy the susceptibility of the Small Pox for a *limited* time; and hence that the second inoculation only affords a proof of the time for which that unsusceptibility subsists. This may be justly redargued.

1st, The failures afford only equivocal evidence of the alleged temporary unsusceptibility.

2d, Such a temporary state is against analogy.

3d, There is no inconsiderable positive evidence of permanent unsusceptibility.

On the 12th of September, the SENATUS ACADEMICUS of the University of Edinburgh, conferred the degree of Doctor in Medicine, on the following Gentlemen, after having gone through the appointed examinations, and publicly defended their respective inaugural dissertations.

FROM ENGLAND.

William Bealey,	*De Epilepsia.*
Richard Byam Dennison	*De Morbis e Graviditate pendentibus.*
John Eyre	*De Vaccina.*
Jonathan Rogers Stokes	*De Erysipelate.*

FROM GENEVA.

Peter Marignac,	*De Urethra constricta.*

FROM IRELAND.

Jeremiah Curtayne,	*De Noxiis alcoholis effectibus.*
Thomas Doxey,	*De Phthisi pulmonali.*
Henry Edgeworth,	*De Exercitatione.*
Patrick Fleming,	*De Apoplexia.*
Timothy Kerin,	*De Peritonitide Puerperarum;*
Samuel L'Estrange, A.B. T.C.D.	*De Epilepsia.*
James Ogilby,	*De Nutrimento Plantarum.*

FROM SCOTLAND.

Robert Briggs, A.M.	*De Antimonio.*
Archibald Campbell,	*De Cerebri compressione.*
Alexander Gardner,	*De Scarlatina Cynanchica.*
Robert Maclean,	*De Cynanche maligna.*

FROM VIRGINIA.

John Wharton	*De Mania.*

FROM WALES.

William Mason,	*De Typho.*

University of Edinburgh.

The classes for the different branches of Medicine will be opened for the ensuing session as follows:

CLASSES.	DAY AND HOURS.		PROFESSORS.
Anatomy and Surgery,	Wednesday, *Oct.* 29th.	1	Drs Monro
Chemistry and Chemical Pharmacy,		10	Dr Hope
Dietetics, Materia Medica, and Pharmacy,		8	Dr Jas Home
Theory of Physic,		11	Dr Duncan
Practice of Physic		9	Dr Gregory
Theory and Practice of Midwifery,		3	Dr Jas Hamilton
Natural History,	- - -	-	Mr Jamieson

Two courses of Practical Anatomy will be given, under the superintendance of Dr Monro, jun. and Mr Fyfe; the one to begin on the 1st November, and the other on the 1st February.

Clinical Lectures on the cases of patients in the Royal Infirmary, by Dr Duncan and Dr Rutherford, upon Tuesday and Friday,—the first lecture by Dr Duncan on Tuesday, Nov. 4. at 5 p. m.

Clinical Surgery by Mr Russell, the first lecture on Monday, Nov. 3. at 5 p. m.

Dr Rutherford will begin a course of Botany in May 1807.

University of Glasgow.

The Medical Lectures in the University of Glasgow will begin on Tuesday the 4th November, at the following hours:

Dietetics, Materia Medica, and Pharmacy, by Dr Millar, at 10 o'clock forenoon;
Midwifery, by Mr Towers, at 11;
Theory and Practice of Physic, by Dr Freer, at 12;
Anatomy and Surgery, by Dr Jeffray, at two o'clock afternoon;
Chemistry and Chemical Pharmacy, by Dr Cleghorn, at seven;
Clinical Lectures on the cases of patients in the Royal Infirmary, by Dr Cleghorn and Dr Freer. The first lecture by Dr Cleghorn, on Tuesday evening the 11th November, at six o'clock
Dr Brown will begin his Lectures on Botany, about the beginning of May next.

Medical

London

The autumnal course of Lectures at St Thomas's and Guy's Hospitals, will commence in the following order:—

St Thomas's Hospital.—Anatomy, and operations of surgery, by Mr Cline and Mr Cooper, Wednesday, October 1, at half past one.—Principles and practice of surgery, by Mr Cooper, on Monday October 6, at eight in the evening.

Guy's Hospital.—Practice of medicine, by Dr Babington and Dr Curry, on Wednesday October 1, at ten in the morning.—Principles and Practice of Chemistry, by Dr Babington and Mr Allen, on Thursday, October 2, at ten in the morning.—Theory of Medicine, comprehending Pathology, Therapeutics, and *Meteria Medica*, by Dr Curry, on Friday October 3, at eight in the evening.—Physiology, or Laws of the Animal Economy, by Dr Haighton, on Monday October 6, at a quarter before seven in the evening.—Midwifery, and Diseases of Women and Children, by Dr Haighton, on Monday October 6, at eight in the morning.—Clinical Lectures on Select Medical Cases, by Dr Babington, Dr Curry, and Dr Marcet, from November till May.—Besides these, during the winter a course of Lectures on the Structure and Diseases of the Teeth, will be given by Mr Fox, Surgeon-Dentist; and one on Veterinary Medicine, by Mr Coleman, Professor at the Veterinary College. These several lectures are so arranged, that none of them interfere with the others in the hours of attendance; and the whole is calculated to form a complete course of medical and chirurgical instruction. Terms and other particulars to be learnt from Mr Stocker, apothecary to Guy's Hospital, who is also empowered to enter gentlemen to such of the Lectures as are given at Guy's.

Medical Theatre, St Bartholomew's Hospital.—The following Courses of Lectures will be delivered at this Theatre during the ensuing winter.—On the Theory and Practice of Medicine, by Dr Roberts and Dr Powell.—On Anatomy and Physiology, by Mr Abernethy.—On the Theory and Practice of Surgery, by Mr Abernethy.—On Comparative Anatomy, and the Laws of Organic Existence, by Mr Macartney.—On Chemistry, by Dr Edwards.—On Midwifery and the Diseases of Women and Children, by Dr Thynne.—The Anatomical Lectures will begin on Wednesday, October 1, at two o'clock, and the other Lectures in the course of the same week.—Further particulars may be known by applying to Mr Nicholson, at the Apothecary's shop, St Bartholomew's Hospital.

London Hospital.—The autumnal courses of Lectures delivered at this Hospital will commence on the 1st of October.—Theory and Practice of Physic, by Dr Cooke.—Chemistry by Dr Hamilton, and Dr Yelloly.—*Materia Medica*, by Dr Frampton.—Theory and Practice of Midwifery, by Dr Dennison.—Clinical Observations on Surgical Cases, by Sir William Blizard, and Mr Thomas Blizard.—Anatomy, Physiology, and the Operations of Surgery, by Mr Headington and Mr Frampton.—Anatomical Demonstrations and Dissection, by Mr Armiger.—Principles of Surgery, by Mr Headington.—Further particulars

lars may be known by applying to Mr Price, apothecary, at the Hospital.

St George's Hospital, *and Great George Street, Hanover Square.* —In the first week of October will commence a course of Lectures on the Practice of Physic, Therapeutics, and Chemistry, in the Lecture Room, No 9, Great George-street, Hanover-square (removed from Leicester-square), at the usual morning hours, viz. the medical lectures at eight, and the chemical at a quarter after nine o'clock; by George Pearson, M.D. F.R.S. senior physician of St George's Hospital, of the College of Physicians, &c. A register is kept of Dr Pearson's Cases in St George's Hospital, and an account is given of them every Saturday morning, at a Clinical Lecture, at nine o'clock.

Mr Home's Lectures on the principal Operations in Surgery, given gratuitously to the pupils of St George's Hospital, will commence in October next, as usual.

Mr Gunning will likewise give Lectures on the Lues Venerea, &c.

Mr Gunning, Surgeon Extraordinary to his Royal Highness the Duke of Sussex, and Surgeon to St George's Hospital, will commence his Course of Lectures on the Principles and Operations of Surgery at his house, 43, Conduit-street, on Monday, October 13, at seven o'clock in the evening.—Further particulars may be known by applying to Mr Gunning, at his house, 43, Conduit-street, Hanover Square.

Theatre of Anatomy, Great Windmill Street.—Mr Wilson will begin the Winter Course of his Lectures on Anatomy, Physiology, Pathology, and Surgery, on Wednesday, October 1, at two o'clock as usual. A room will likewise be opened for Dissections, from nine o'clock in the morning, until two in the afternoon, where regular and full Demonstrations of the parts dissected will be given, where the different Cases in Surgery will be explained, the Methods of Operating shewn on the Dead Body, and where also the various Arts of Injecting and Making Preparations will be taught.—The plan and terms of the Course may be had in Great Windmill-street.

Dr Clarke and Mr Clarke will begin their winter course of Lectures on Midwifery, and the diseases of Women and Children, on Monday the 6th of October. The lectures are read every day (Sundays excepted), at the Lecture-room, No 10, Upper John street, Golden-square, from a quarter past 10 o'clock in the morning, till a quarter past eleven, for the convenience of students attending the hospitals. For farther particulars apply to Dr Clarke, New Burlington-street, or Mr Clarke, Upper John-street, Golden-square.

Mr Carpue will commence his Anatomical Lectures, on Wednesday, October 1, 1806.—The structure of the human body will be explained, as also its physiology. The operations of surgery will be shewn on the dead body.—The Dissection-room will be open from seven o'clock in the morning, till five in the evening. The pupils are here taught the method of operating, as also the art of injecting and making preparations.

Mr Brookes will commence his Autumnal Course of Lectures on Anatomy, Physiology, and Surgery, on Wednesday the 1st of October, at two o'clock, at his Theatre, Blenheim Street, Great Marlborough Street.

Street. The Dissecting Rooms will be open from eight o'clock in the morning till two, where Mr Brookes attends.

Dr Bradley will commence his Autumnal Course of Lectures on the Theory and Practice of Medicine, on Monday the 13th of October next, at Whitehall.

Mr A. Carlisle, F.R.S. F.L.S. and Surgeon to the Westminster Hospital, intends to deliver a Course of Lectures on the Art and Practice of Surgery, in all its branches, during the present season, at his house in Soho-square.

Dr Reid's Winter Course of Lectures on the Theory and Practice of Medicine, will commence on the 20th of October next, at his house, No. 6. Grenville Street, Brunswick Square, where particulars may be had.

Mr Thomas's Autumnal Course of Lectures, on the Theory and Principles of Surgery, will commence, as usual, early in October. Particulars may be known at his house, Leicester Place, or at the Anatomical Theatre, Windmill-street.

Mr Moor, Surgeon Dentist to her Royal Highness the Duchess of York, will commence a Course of Lectures on the Structure and Diseases of the Teeth, some time in November, in which will be explained the complete practice of the Dentist.

Dr Badham's Lectures on Medicine and Chemistry will be commenced on Friday, October 10, at eight o'clock.—15, *Clifford Street, Burlington Gardens.*

Extract of a Letter from Paris.

M. Faujas has just returned from a journey in the Venetian States. He has brought a great collection of Fossil Shells and Bones. He saw the entire skeletons of a rhinoceros and elephant, found on the banks of the Po.

PART IV.

LIST OF NEW BOOKS.

PHILOSOPHICAL Transactions of the Royal Society of London, for 1806. Part I. 4to.

Transactions of the Royal Society of Edinburgh. Vol. VI. Part I. 4to. 9s.

The Transactions of the Royal Irish Academy. Vol. X. 4to. 1l.

Memoirs of the Literary and Philosophical Society of Manchester. Vol. I. of the 2d Series. 8vo. 7s.

Memoirs of the Medical Society of London. Vol. VI. 8vo. 12s. boards.

The New London Medical Dictionary. Part I. 4to. 1l. 4s.

An Address to the Proprietors and Managers of Coal Mines, particularly of those in the neighbourhood of Newcastle upon Tyne, respecting the means of destroying the Fire Damp; in reply to a Proposal, lately circulated by Dr Trotter. 8vo. 2s.

Manual of Health, or the Invalid safely conducted through the Seasons; to be continued occasionally. 12mo. 5s.

The Domestic Guide in cases of Insanity. 12mo. 2s.

A Letter to Mr Birch, in Answer to his late Pamphlet against Vaccination. By a Member of the Royal College of Surgeons. 8vo. 2s. 6d.

The Medical Observer; containing an impartial account of Advertised Nostrums, &c. 2s. 6d.

Surgical Observations on Health. By Mr Abernethy. Part II. 6s. 8vo. boards.

Letters to D. Rowley on his late Pamphlet, entitled, "Cow Pox Inoculation, no security against Small Pox Infection." By Aculeus.

A Recapitulation of several circumstances and arguments contained in the Author's "Outlines," and "Medical Researches," relating to the impropriety of considering Fever as arising from contagion. By Thomas Alder. Part I. 4to. 5s.

A Concise Statement of the most important of the difficulties and imperfections in Medicine; of the causes of them, and of the remedies for them. By T. Alder. 4to. 2s. 6d.

Essays on the Anatomy of Expression in Painting. By Charles Bell, 4to. 2l. 2s.

The Principles of Surgery. Vol. II. in two parts. By John Bell. 4to. 5l. 5s.

A Meteorological Journal of 1805. By. W. Bent. 8vo. 1s. 6d.

Letters on Natural History. By John Bigland. 12mo. 9s. boards.

The

The Vaccine Contest. By William Blair, 2s 6d.

A Compendium of the Anatomy, Physiology, and Pathology of the Horse. By B. W. Burke. 12s. 6d. boards.

Observations on Abortion; containing an Account of the manner in which it is accomplished, the causes which produce it, and the method of preventing or treating it. By John Burns, 4s. 6d. 8vo. boards.

An Essay on the Effect of Carbonate of Iron upon Cancer. By Richard Carmichael. 8vo. 4s. boards.

Practical Essays on the Management of Pregnancy and Labours, and on the Inflammatory and Febrile Diseases of Lying-in women. By John Clarke, M. D. 2 Edit. 8vo. 4s. 6d.

The Modern Practice of Physic. By Edward Goodman Clarke, M.D. 8vo. 9s. boards.

Critical Reflections on several important Practical Points relative to the Cataract; comprehending an Account of a New and Successful Method of Couching a particular species of that Disease. By Samuel Cooper. 8vo. 4s.

A Synoptical Table of Diseases. By Alexander Crichton, M. D. Large sheet, 2s. 6d.

A Letter to Thomas Trotter, M. D. occasioned by his proposal for destroying the Fire and Choak Damps of Coal Mines; containing Chemical and General Strictures on that Work. By Henry Dewar, M.D. 8vo. 1s. 6d.

The Edinburgh New Dispensary, 3d edition. By A. Duncan, jun. M. D. 8vo. 10s. 6d.

A Dissertation on Ischias, or the disease of the Hip-joint, commonly called a Hip case; and on the use of the Bath Waters, as a remedy in this complaint. By William Falconer, M. D. F. R. S. 2s. 6d.

A Sketch of the professional Life and Character of John Clark, M. D. By J. R. Fenwick M. D. 8vo. 2s.

The History and Treatment of the Diseases of the Teeth, the Gums, and Alveolar Processes, with the Operations which they respectively require. To which are added, Observations on other Diseases of the mouth, and on the mode of fixing Artificial Teeth; illustrated with copper plates. By Joseph Fox. 4to. 1l. 1s.

A Treatise on Epilepsy, and the use of the Viscus Quercinus, or Misletoe of the Oak, in the cure of that disease. By H. Frazer, M. D. &c. 2s. 6d. 8vo. sewed.

Observations on Vaccine Inoculation, tending to confute the opinion of Dr Rowley and others. By Henry Frazer, M. D. 2s.

Observations and Experiments on the Humulus Lupulus *Linn.*, with an Account of its use in Gout and other Disseaes, with Cases. By A. Freake. 8vo, 2s.

A System of the Anatomy of the Human Body; illustrated by upwards of 200 tables, containing near 1000 figures, copied from the most celebrated Authors, and from nature. By Andrew Fyfe. 3 vols. 4to. 7l. 7s. half bound.

The Efficacy of Inoculated Small Pox, in promoting the Population of Great Britain. By R. Gillum, M. D. 6d.

Arguments relative to Cow Pock, inscribed to Lord Hawkesbury, and laid before the Board of Health. By R. Gillum, M. D. 6d.

The Metaphysic of Man; on the Pure Part of the Physiology of Man. Translated from the German of T. C. Goldbeck. By S. F. Waddington, M. D. 8vo. 5s.

Remarks on the Ineffective State of the Practice of Physic in Great Britain. By Edward Harrison, M. D. F. R. A. S. S. 1s. 6d.

Observations on the Utility and Administration of Purgative Medicines. By James Hamilton, M. D. 2d edition. 8vo. 7s. 6d.

An Epitome of Infantile Diseases, with their Causes, Symptoms, and Method of Cure. Published in Latin, by William Heberden, M. D Translated into English, by J. Smith, M D. 3s.

Epitome of Chemistry. By W. Henry. New edition, 8vo. 12s.

Cow Pock Inoculation, vindicated and recommended from matters of fact. By Rowland Hill, A. M. 12mo. 1s.

Practical Observations on the Natural History and Cure of the Venereal Disease. By J. Howard. 2 vols. 18s.

Essays, chiefly on Chemical Subjects. By the late William Irvine, M. D. F. R. S. and his son William Irvine, M. D. 8vo. 9s.

A Treatise on the External Characters of Minerals. By Robert Jameson, F. R. S. Edin. 8vo. 4s.

A System of Arrangement and Discipline for the Medical Departments of Armies. By Robert Jackson, M. D. 8vo. boards.

Observations on the Epidemick Disease, which lately prevailed at Gibraltar; intended to illustrate the nature of contagious fevers in general. By Henry Seguin Jackson, M. D. 8vo. 4s.

Cases of the Excision of Carious Joints. By H. Park, and P. F. Moreau, M. D. With Observations by James Jeffray, M. D. with engravings. 8vo. Glasgow 4s. 6d.

The Report, and the Evidence, at large, as laid before the Committee of the House of Commons, respecting Dr Jenner's discovery of the Vaccine Inoculation. By the Rev G. C. Jenner. 8vo. 6s. boards.

A Reply to Dr J. Carmichael Smith, containing Remarks on his Letter to Mr Wilberforce: And a further account of the discovery of the power of Mineral Acids, in a state of Gas, to destroy Contagion. By John Johnstone, M. D. 8vo. 5s.

Vaccination vindicated against Misrepresentation and Calumny, in a Letter to his patients. By E. Jones. 8vo. 1s

A New System of Family Medicine. By W. Keighly, M. D. 8vo. 6s.

An Address to the Medical Practitioners of Ireland, on the subject of Cow Pock. By Samuel Labatt, M. D. 8vo. 3s. 6d. sewed.

Inoculation for the Small Pox Vindicated, and its superior Efficacy and Safety to the practice of Vaccination clearly proved. By George Lipscomb, Surgeon. 2s.

A Manual of Inoculation for the Use of the Faculty and Private Families. By George Lipscomb, Surgeon. 8vo. 2s.

A Dissertation on the Failures and Mischiefs of the Disease called the Cow Pox. By George Lipscomb. 8vo. 3s.

A Treatise on Hernia Humoralis, or Swelled Testicle. To which are added, Remarks on the Opacity of the Cornea. By Thomas Luxmoore. 12mo. 2s.

A Manual of Anatomy and Physiology, reduced as much as possible to a tabular form, for the purpose of facilitating to Students the acquisition of those Sciences. By T. Luxmoore. 8vo. 8s. 6d. boards.

Outlines of the Origin and Progress of Galvanism; with its Application to Medicine. By W. Meade, M. D. 8vo. Dublin. 3s.

A Reply to the Anti-Vaccinists. By James Moore. 2s.

Remarks on Mr Birch's "Serious Reasons for uniformly Objecting to the Practice of Vaccination." By James Moore. 8vo. 1s.

An Examination into the Principles of what is called the Brunonian System. By Thomas Morrison. 4s.

Commentaries on the Lues Bovilla, or Cow Pox. By B. Mosely, M.D. 8vo.

Chirurgical Institutes. By H. St John Neale. 8vo. 6s.

The Cure of the Gout proposed on Rational Principles. By James Parkinson. 5s. 6d.

Admonitory Hints on the Use of Sea Bathing. By J. Peake. 1s. 6d.

A Practical Treatise on various Diseases of the Abdominal Viscera. By C. R. Pemberton, M.D. 8vo. 7s.

Notes on the West Indies. By G. Pinckard, M.D. 3 vols. 1l. 10s.

A Treatise on the Origin, Progress, and Treatment of Consumption. By John Reid, M.D. 7s. in boards.

An Answer to Dr Mosely, containing a Defence of Vaccination. By John Ring, Surgeon. 8vo. 6s. boards.

Cow Pox Inoculation no Security against Small Pox Infection. By William Rowley, M.D. 2s. 6d.

An Illustration of the Anatomy of the Human Ear, accompanied by Views of that Organ, accurately Drawn, of the Natural Size, from a Series of Dissections; to which is added, a Treatise on its Diseases, the Causes of Deafness, and the proper Treatment. By J. C. Saunders. Folio. 1l. 5s.

Observations and Experiments on the Digestive Powers of the Bile in Animals. By Eaglesfield Smith. 8vo. 3s.

Remarks on the Report of M. Chaptal to the Consuls of the former Government of France; with an Examination of the claim of M. Guyton de Morveau to the Discovery of the Power of the Mineral Acid Gas on Contagion. By J. Carmichael Smyth, M.D. 8vo. 1s. 6d.

An Introduction to Botany. By James Lee. A New Edition, corrected and revised by Charles Stewart. 8vo. Edinburgh, 1806.

A Practical Treatise on the Diseases of the Stomach, and of Digestion. By Arthur Daniel Stone, M.D. 8vo. 6s. boards.

A Practical Account of a Remittent Fever frequently occurring among the Troops in this Climate. By Thomas Sutton, M.D. 8vo. 2s.

Commentaries on the Treatment of Scirrhi and Cancer, from the earliest period to the present time; for the purpose of pointing out and establishing a Specific for those Diseases on Rational Scientific Principles. By William Thomas. 8vo. 3s.

Vacciræ Vindicia; a Vindication of the Cow Pock. By Robert John Thornton, M.D. 1s. 6d.

The Naval Surgeon. By W. Turnbull, A.M. 8vo. 9s. 6d.

An Analysis of the Malvern Waters. By A. Philips Wilson, M.D. F.R.S. Edin. 8vo. 2s. 6d. boards.

Observations on the Use and Abuse of Mercury. By ditto. 8vo. 1s.

An Encyclopædia of Surgery, &c. By J. J. Watts. 8vo. 8s.

INDEX.

Page

Abdominal muscles, fatal abscess of 129
Abernethy's, Mr, surgical observations - - - - - 463
Abortion, observations on - 366
Absorption, cutaneous, experiments on - - - - - - - 10
Abscess of the abdominal muscles, fatal - - - - - 129
Acid, sulphuric, good effects of, in lichens - - - - - 59
Air-bubbles found in the vessels of the brain - - - - 399
——, change of, effects of - 462
Albumen in animal fluids, how estimated - - - - - 37
Alkali, fixed, useful in prurigo 61
—————— psoriasis 66
Allen's, Mr, theory of inflammation 78
Alvine discharge, indications from 465
——— evacuation, use of, in idiopathic tetanus - - - 435
Amaurosis cured by Galvanism 426
Amputation successful in tetanus of the extremities - - 204
————— of the uterus, successful - - - - - - 419
Anderson's, Mr, case of teeth and hairs found in the ovarium - 180
Animal fluids, analysis of - 37
Appetite, inordinate, cured by violent exercise - - - - 5
Arthritis rheumatica, observations on - - - - - - - 260
Arteries, natural cessation of hemorrhage from - - - - 224
———, on the best mode of securing - - - - - - 176
Ascites, with hydatids, case of 170
Assafœtida, effects of, in Guinea worm - - - - - - 304
Atkinson's, Mr, case of tumour of the tongue - - - - 318
Atrophia lactantium, observations on 452
Bateman's, Dr, Carey-street dispensary reports, 122, 258, 390, 498
Bathing, practical observations on 456
Bayle, Dr, on the white induration of organs - - - - 401
Berlin, medical topography of - 376
Biliary organs, affected in hydrocephalus internus - - 470

Page

Biography of Dr J. Currie - 46
Biot's experiments on the decomposition of water by Galvanism 118
Bischoff's, Prof. account of Dr Gall's cranioscopy - - 354
—————, on the medical use of gelatine - - 483
Bismuth, white oxide of, useful in dyspepsia - - 451, 498
Board of health, second report of 111
Bonpland's equinoctial botany 485
Books for routiniers, deficiency of 476
Bostock's Dr, analysis of a stearoid tumour - - - - - 14
—————, on the analysis of animal fluids - - - - 37
Bourne, Dr, on uva ursi in pulmonary consumption - - 346
Brain, examination of, in hydrocephalus - - - - - 396
——, scrofulous tumours in 405
——, Dr Gall's discoveries in 390
Bronchocele, observations on - 453
Bruce's, Mr, account of the Guinea worm - - - - 145
Brunonian theory, modification of, by Dr Wilson - - - 76
——————, observations on 499
Buchan, Dr, on sea bathing - 456
Burns, Mr A., on the anatomy of crural hernia - - - 265
Burns, Mr J. on the human ovum 1
—————, observations on abortion - - - - - 366
Cabanis, M. on the revolutions in medicine - - - - 206
Cæcum, enormous size of - 397
Caldwell's, Dr, case of ossified fœtus and uterus - - - - 22
Calomel successfully used in tumour of the tongue - - 318
Cancer, queries concerning its nature and cure - - - - 382
———, effects of carbonate of iron in - - - - - - - 372
Cantharides, tincture of, successfully used in gleet - - 134
Carbonate of iron, effects of, in cancer - - - - - - 372
———— of soda, use of, in hooping cough - - - - 380

Carcinomatoc.

INDEX

Page

Carcinomatous degeneration, character of - - - - 403
Cardamine pratensis, effects of in incubus - - - - - 451
Carey-street-report, 122, 258, 390, 498
Carmichael, Mr, on carbonate of iron in cancer - - - - 372
Catarrhal affections prevented by cold bathing - - - - 458
Catheter male, mode of introducing - - - - - 240
Ceroxylon, account of - 485
Chaptal on unwholesome manufactories - - - - - 290
Chorea Sancti Viti, utility of purgatives in - - - - 106, 422
Chlorosis, utility of purgatives in 108
Chylopoietic organs affected by local diseases - - - - 464
Cicatrization of punctured arteries explained - - - - 229
Cinchona, essay on - - 333
——— does not contain gelatine 480
——— condaminea, description of - - - - - - - 485
Clarke's, Dr, case of amputation of the uterus - - - 419
Clark's, Dr, E. G. practice of physic - - - - - - 81
Clinical institution at Vienna, account of - - - - - 493
Coates's, Mr, cure of epilepsy by trepanning - - - - 428
Cold, a cause of idiopathic tetanus 430
——, body defended against, by the external use of oil - - 199
——, medical effects of - 340
—— affusion, use of, in arthritis rheumatica - - - - 260
——, mode of application in hernia - - - - - - 246
—— washing or bathing useful in preventing catarrhal affections 458
——— useful in endemical fever of Geneva - - 447
—— water swallowed with good effects in tooth-ach - - 448
College of physicians in London, powers of - - - - 487
Colon, uncommon course of - 397
Concussion cured by purgatives 468
Congenital hernia, treatise on - 250
Constitutional diseases affected by local - - - - - 464
Contagion counteracted by oily frictions - - - - - 200

Page

Cooper, Mr A. on hernia - 241
Cow pock, *see* Vaccine.
Cranioscopy, Dr Gall's - 354
Crowther's, Dr, case of abscess in the abdominal muscles - 129
——— syphilitic ulcertion of the skin - 133
Crural hernia, anatomy of - 265
Currie, Dr J., biography of - 46
Curry's, Dr, proposed work on the hepatic functions - - 471
Cutaneous absorption, experiments on - - - - - - - 10
——— diseases, Dr Willan on 56
Cynanche maligna, utility of purgatives in - - - - 104
Degrees, medical, in the university of Edinburgh - - 389, 505
Deafness, use of galvanism in 434
De Carro, Dr, on the state of vaccination on the Continent - 126
Depopulation of Otaheite, causes of - - - - - 284
Diabetes mellitus, case of - 16
———, prize questions concerning - - - - 118
Diet-drinks, mode of action - 466
Digestion disturbed by cold bathing - - - - - - 459
Digestive organs affected by local diseases - - - - - 465
Dracunculus; *see* Guinea-worm.
Drake's, Dr, case of diseased spleen 409
Dropsy, oily friction in - 201
Dubois's M., observations on Guinea worm - - - - 300
Dysentery frequent at Otaheite 286
Dyspepsia, degree of exercise in 5
———, varieties of - - 451
Education, medical, on the improvement of - - - - 472
Egypt, surgical diseases in - 218
Egyptian opthalmia, M. Larrey on 214
Elder, Mr, on the diseases prevalent at Otaheite - - - 502
Elephantiasis common in Egypt 219
Empiricism, judicious, preferable to hypothetical knowledge - 474
Entereotomy, successfully performed - - - - - - 452
Epilepsy cured by trepanning - 428
———, use of viscus quercinus in - - - - - - 352
———, frequent at Otaheite - 287
Epiphora, observations on - 239
Equinoctial botany - - 483

Erysipelas,

INDEX.

Page

Erysipelas, diagnosis between, and erythema mercuriale - 31
———, Chinese, account of 29
Erythema mercuriale, frequent in India - - - - - 503
———, essay on 25
Exercise, degree of in dyspepsia - 5
Extraction of the Guinea worm, how performed - - 148
Fabbroni's, G., researches on Cinchona - - - - - 333
Faulkner, Dr, on violent exercise in dyspepsia - - - - 5
Febrile diseases, treatise on - 72
Fevers, endemical, of Geneva 447
———, frequent at Otaheite - 285
——— at Leghorn, account of 83
Fistula lachrymalis, observations on 240
Flannel shirt, effects of - 458
Fluids, animal, analysis of - 37
Fœtus found in the abdomen of a woman aged 83 - - 19
——— ossified with the uterus 22
Forbes, Mr W. on sulphurated hydrogen in dyspepsia - - 9
Foundling hospital, bad effects of 496
Fourcroy, M. on phosphate of magnesia in bones - - - 262
Frank, John Peter, merits of 495
Frank, Dr Joseph, letter from 499
Fraser's, Dr, case of diabetes mellitus - - - - - 16
———, on viscus quercinus in epilepsy - - - 352
Fritze, Dr, on the medical use of gelatine - - - - 483
Fumigations recommended by the board of health - - 114
Gall's, Dr, anatomical discoveries in the brain - - - - 320
——— cranioscopy, account of 354
Galvanism, use of, in congenital deafness - - - - 424
Gamboge not the produce of the koutam-poulli - - 172
Gautieri, Dr, on the medical use of gelatine - - - 479
Gastrodynia, observations on 259
———, good effects of oxide of bismuth in - - 498
Galatine, in animal fluids, how estimated - - - - 40
———, medical use of - 479
Geneva, state of medicine in - 446
Gillum, Dr, on some good effects of inoculated small pox - 182

Page

Gleet cured by tincture of cantharides - - - - - 134
Glow after bathing, criterion of its utility - - - - 457
Glue, medical use of - - 479
Gonorrhœa, slight at Otaheite 274
Gravel not common in some wine countries - - - - 447
Gregory's, Dr, observations on erythema mercuriale - - 29
Grivel's, M. case of abdominal fœtus - - - - - 19
Guinea worm, account of, by Mr Bruce - - - - - 145
———, by Mr Dubois - - - - - 300
———, cases of, by Mr Paton - - - - - 151
Gum Arabic, successful in the cure of intermittents - - 481
Gun-shot wounds, effects of, in Egypt - - - - - 220
Guyton-Morveau on manufactories prejudicial to health - - 290
Hæmatemesis, utility of purgatives in - - - - - - 109
Hairs found in the ovarium - 180
Hamilton, Dr, on purgative medicines - - - - 97, 454
Harrison's, Dr, letter on medical reform - - - - - 252
Head, and digestive organs, reaction of - - - - - 469
Health, board of, second report of 111
Health, public, care of - 290
Heart, affection of, subsequent to rheumatism - - - - 448
Hemorrhage, process employed by nature in suppressing - 224
———, secondary, means of preventing - - - - 176
Hemorrhoids, treatment of - 240
Hensler's, Prof. case of lepra tyria 32
Hernia, sphacelated, case of - 307
———, essay on - - 211
———, crural, anatomy of - 265
———, with unusual distribution of the obturator artery 203
Herpes, essay on - - 325
Hip-joint, amputation at - 222
Hooping-cough, use of alkali in 380
Hospital, general, at Vienna, account of - - - - 491
Humboldt's equinoctial botany 485
Hunter, Mr, on the external use of oil - - - - - - 185

Hunter,

INDEX.

Page

Hunter's, Dr W., opinions concerning the formation of the ovum 1
Hydatids, with ascites, case of 170
Hydrocephalus internus and worms, diagnosis between - - 52
————, connected with disease of the liver - 470
————, connection of, with scrofula - - - - - 409
Hysteria, use of purgatives in 110, 454
Iatraliptic medicine - - 189
Ichthyosis, systematic description of 67
Idiopathic fevers, distinguished from symptomatic - - - - 75
Incubus, remarkable case of 451
Induration, white, of organs 401
Infanticide, effects of, in depopulating Otaheite - - - - 289
Inflammation, theory of - 78
Inguinal hernia, treatise on - 244
Inoculated small-pox, preventive of the plague - - - - 182
Institutions for routiniers, mode of instruction in - - - 475
Intestines, uncommon conformation of - - - - - 397
Intermittent fevers cured by animal jelly - - - - - 479
Iron, carbonate of, effects, in cancer - - - - - 372
Jackson, Mr, on the effects of olive oil externally applied - 302
Jelly, animal, medical use of 479
——, in animal fluids, how estimated - - - - - 40
Jennerian society, report of - 254
Johnston's, Mr, supposed case of small-pox after vaccination 426
Jones, Dr, on the natural suppression of hemorrhage - - 224
Kellie's, Dr, case of sphacelated hernia - - - - - 307
————, case of chorea cured by purgatives - - - - 422
Kitson's, Mr, case of tic doloureux 319
Koutam-poulli, description of 172
Larrey's, M. surgery of the army in the East - - - - 213
Leeches, inconveniences from swallowing - - - - - 117
Leghorn, fever, epidemic, at - 83
Legislative interference in medical concerns deprecated - - 439
Lepra, systematic description of 63
——, induced in Egypt by the use of pork - - - - 219
Lepra, diagnosis between, and erythema mercuriale - - 33
Leucorrhœa cured by tincture of cantharides - - - 134
Lichen, systematic description of 58
Ligatures on arteries, effects of 230
———— on arteries, the best mode of - - - - - - 176
Linnæus, account of the life and writings of - - - - 91
Liverpool dispensary, annual report of - - - - - - 261
Local diseases, effects of, on general health - - - - 464
Lubbock's, Dr, theory of inflammation - - - - - 78
Lunatic asylum at Vienna, account of - - - - - - 493
Lunatics more frequently male than female - - - 379, 493
Lungs, uncommon conformation of - - - - - - 398
Lying-in hospital at Vienna, account of - - - - 495
M'Mullin, Dr, on erythema mercuriale - - - - - 25
Madras, letter from - - 503
Magnesia, phosphate of, found in bones - - - - - 262
Manufactories unwholesome, observations on - - - - 290
Marasmus infantilis, observations on - - - - - - 451
————, utility of purgatives in - - - - 104
Maton's, Dr, account of the life and writings of Linnæus - - 91
————, discovers the reaction of cinchona on astringents 480
Medical practitioners not obliged to attend the poor gratis - 475
———— routiniers, on the education of - - - - - 472
Men more subject to mental derangement than women 379, 493
Mental pathology, observations on 440
Merat, Dr, on cerebral tubercles 405
Mercury, excess of, very hurtful in India - - - - - 503
Mercurials hurtful in erythema mercuriale - - - - 33
Misletoe, use of, in epilepsy - 352
Moisture, bad effects of, prevented by oily frictions - - 199
Morning, bad time for cold bathing - - - - - 459

Mortification

Page

Mortification of the intestines 248
Mucus in animal fluids, how estimated - - - - - 40
Mursinna, Prof., cases of idiopathic tetanus - - - 430
Naevi materni, cured by pressure 471
Nephritis, gouty, or rheumatic 447
Noon, best time for cold bathing 459
Nosology, importance of - 73
Nourishment conveyed by oily frictions - - - - - 201
Nuisances, laws regarding - 297
Nurses, change of, useful in marasmus infantilis - - - - 452
Obturator artery, unusual distribution of - - - - - 203
Odier Prof. Manuel de Medécine practique - - - - 446
——— Account of the illness and death of Saussure - 393
Œdema of the ancles, produced by cold bathing - - - 461
Oil, on the external use of, in medicine - - - - - 185
Omentum, affection of - - 417
Ophthalmia, observations on - 233
——— Egyptian, M. Larrey on - - - - - 214
Opium, best remedy in tetanus 214
——— successful in idiopathic tetanus - - - - - 430
——— vinous tincture of, use of, in ophthalmia - - 234
Otaheite, remarkable depopulation of - - - - - 284
——— diseases prevalent at 503
——— syphilis unknown at 274
Ovarium, teeth and hair formed in 180
Ovum, structure and formation of 1
Palloni, Dr, on the Leghorn fever 83
Papulous diseases, systematic description of - - - - 58
Paralysis cured by Galvanism 426
Paralytic affections, symptomatic 467
Pathology mental, observations on 440
Pathological cabinet of Vienna Hospital - - - - - 494
Paton, Mr, cases of Guinea worm 150
Pearson, Dr G., observations on the vitality of the fœtus in protracted gestations - - 20
Pearson, D. R., on hooping cough 380
Pemphigus, diagnosis between, and erythema mercuriale - - 31
Pericardium fluid in, analysis of 42
Perspiration induced by exercise, useful in dyspepsia - - 5

Page

——— excessive, prevented by oily frictions - - - 193
Phosphat of magnesia formed in bones - - - - - 263
Phthisis pulmonalis cured by uva ursi - - - - - 346
Physicians, Royal College of, in London, advertisement from 487
Pityriasis, systematic description of 67
Plague, oily frictions in - - 201
——— prevented by small pox inoculation - - - - 183
——— does not attack the severely wounded - - - - 217
Plica Polonica, prize questions concerning - - - - 121
Poor, means of providing medical attendance for - - 474
Practice of Physic, Edinburgh 82
Practique, Manuel de Medécine 446
Pressure cures naevi materni 471
Prurigo, systematic description of 60
Pseudo-syphylitic affections, observations on - - - - 468
Psoriasis, systematic description of 65
Psorophthalmy, observations on 238
Pulteney, Dr, account of the life and writing of Linnaeus - 91
Purgatives, on the use of 371 454
———, success of, in chorea sancti viti - - - - 423
———, use of, in diseased spleen 412
Putrefaction, injurious effects of, on public health - - 293
Reeve, Dr, on the state of vaccination on the Continent - 126
Reform, medical, proceedings of, association for - 252, 489
———, observations on 206, 437
Reil, Prof., on medical education 472
Revolutions in medicine, observations on - - - - 206
Rheumatism, acute, fatal cases of 391
——— frequent at Otaheite 286
——— frequent in Switzerland - - - - - 448
Ring, crural, and abdominal, description of - - - - 341
Roberton, Mr, on the use of cantharides in gleet - - 134
Rosenmuller, Prof., account of Dr Gall's anatomical discoveries 320
Rousseau, Dr, on cutaneous absorption - - - - - 10
Routiniers, medical, on the education and necessity of - 473

Rowley,

Page
Rowley, Dr, refuted by Aculeus 240
Rubeola, systematic description of 68
——— diagnosis between, and erythema mercuriale - - 30
Saliva, analysis of - - 43
Salt water, effects of bathing in 459
Sarcocele, enormous, common in Egypt - - - - - 219
Saussure, M. de, illness and death of 393
Scaly diseases, systematic description of - - - - - 62
Scarlatina, systematic description of 68
——— diagnosis between, and erythema mercuriale - 31
——— utility of purgatives in 102
Scirrhus, character of - - 403
Scorpion, bite of, cured by oily frictions - - - - - 202
——— Indian remedy against the bite of - - - 304
Scrofula, connection of, with hydrocephalus - - - - 409
——— frequent at Otaheite 286 503
Scrofulous tumours, formed in the brain - - - - - 405
Sea air, effects of - - 462
Sea bathing, treatise on - 456
Sea water, effects of, taken internally - - - - - 461
Sedative effects of cold - 342
Seguin's theory of the medical use of gelatine - - - 479
Seminaries for routinier's, mode of instruction in - - - 475
Skin, diseases of, Dr Willan, on 56
——, syphilitic affection of - 133
——, dry state of, in dyspepsia, to be removed by exercise - 5
Small pox, supposed case of, after vaccination - - - 426
Soda carbonated, use of, in hooping cough - - - - - 380
Solanum dulcamara, good effects of, in Lepra - - - 65
Spasms occasioned by accumulation of faeces - - - 400
Sphacelated hernia, case of - 307
Spina bifida, analysis of, fluid in 41
Spleen, diseased case of - 409
Sprenger, Mr, cures of deafness by galvanism - - - 425
State not obliged to pay for medical assistance to the poor - 473
Stearoid tumour, analysis of - 14
Stock, Dr, on the medical effects of cold water - - 340
Page
———'s account of Dr Rousseau's experiments - - 10
Stoll's, Mr, case of Chorea S. Viti, cured by purgatives - 423
Stomach complaints, use of sulphurated hydrogen in - - 9
———, remarkable thickening of its coats - - - 417
———, action of gelatine upon 482
Strophulus, systematic description of - - - - - - 58
Sulphurated hydrogen, use of, in stomach complaints - - 9
Sulphuret of potass in stomach complaints - - - - - ib.
Surgery of the army of the East 213
Surgical observations - - 463
Sweating, a favourable symptom in idiopathic tetanus - - 434
Symptomatic fevers distinguished from idiopathic - - 75
Syphilis, till of late, unknown at Otaheite - - 274, 502
———, form of, in Egypt - 220
———, diseases resembling 468
Syphilitic affection of the skin 133
Teeth formed in the ovarium 180
Testicles, gradual disappearance of 218
Tetanus, M. Larrey on - 214
———, use of purgatives in 255
———, idiopathic, cured by opium - - - - - 430
Tic douloureux, case of - 319
Tongue, tumour of, cured by calomel and cicuta - - 318
Tonic effects of sea-bathing 457
Topography, medical, of Berlin 376
Toothach cured by slowly swallowing cold water - - 448
Trepanning successful in curing epilepsy - - - - 428
Trusses on the application of 249
Tubercles scrofulous formed in the brain - - - - - 405
Tuberculous degeneration, characters of - - - - 402
Tumour stearoid, analysis of - 14
Tympanites cured by entereotomy - - - - - 452
Typhus, utility of purgatives in 102
Universities, mode of instruction in - - - - - 475
Ulcers of the legs, effects of seabathing on - - - 461
Urethra, diseases of - - 471
Uterus, successful amputation of 419

INDEX.

Page

———, ossified with the fœtus 22
Uva ursi, effects of in pulmonary consumption - - - 346
Vacca Berlinghieri's theory of inflammation - - - - 79
Vaccine pock institution, report of - - - - - 117, 504
——— institution at Edinburgh, report of - - - - 257
Vaccination general at Geneva 449
———, state of, on the Continent - - - - - 126
———, irregularities in, at Madras - - - - - 504
——— erroneously supposed ineffectual - - - - 426
Vauquelin's analysis of palm wax 485
Vegetables, diseases of, prize questions concerning - - 121
Vena medinensis. *See* Guinea-worm.
Vienna, general hospital and medical school of - - - 491
———, effects of vaccination at, on deaths from small pox - 128
Viscus quercinus in epilepsy - 352
Voightel's cases of amputation of the uterus - - - - 421
Volta, Prof. on the use of galvanism in congenital deafness - 424

Page

Walter's, Prof. account of Dr Gall's cranioscopy - - - - 354
Wardrop's, Mr J. case of crural hernia - - - - 203
Ware's, Mr, surgical observations on the eye - - - - 233
Warm bath more useful than the cold in cutaneous disorders 461
Wax palm, account of - - 485
White's, Dr, description of the koutam-poulli - - - - 172
White indurations of organs 401
Wilkinson, Mr, on Pacchioni's experiments - - - - 381
Willan, Dr, on cutaneous diseases 56
Wilna, university of, described 499
——— prize questions from 118
Wilson, Dr A.P., on febrile diseases - - - - - 72
Wilson, Mr, on syphilis and other diseases at Otaheite - 274
Wine, acid, does not predispose to gravel - - - - - - 447
Women less subject to mental derangement than men - 493, 379
Wood's, Mr, W. observations on crural hernia - - - - 205
Worms and hydocephalus, diagnosis between - - - - 52
Yellow fever in Egypt - 218

ERRATA.

Mr G. Atkinson is the author of the Communication, No. VIII. of our last Number.

For *his*, page 372, line 13, read *this*.

Page 487, 8th line from the bottom, insert *the* before *London*.

Page 488, line 12, dele *legally*.

TO CORRESPONDENTS.

The communications from Mr Mudd, Mr J. Wardrope, Dr Millar, Mootoosawmy, Mr Hay, Dr Anderson, Aubert du Petit Thouars, Mr Cooke, and Dr Buchanan, and the Analysis of Dr Jeffrey's, and Dr Pemberton's recent publications arrived too late for insertion in the present Numbers. Communications may be addressed to the Editors of the Edinburgh Medical and Surgical Journal, to the care of Messrs Constable and Co. Edinburgh; John Murray, London, or Gilbert and Hodges, Dublin.

Lightning Source UK Ltd.
Milton Keynes UK
UKHW020244150119
335569UK00011B/1204/P